Successful Nursing Assistant Care

Diana L. Dugan, RN

SECOND EDITION

Hartman Publishing, Inc.   *hartman*online.com

CREDITS

Managing Editor
Susan Alvare

Proofreaders
Suzanne Wegner
Kristin Calderon

Illustrator
Thaddeus Castillo

Page Layout
Thaddeus Castillo

Cover and Interior Designer
Kirsten Browne

Photography
Art Clifton/Dick Ruddy/Pat Berrett

Sales/Marketing
Debbie Rinker
Ernest Culver
Caroyl Scott
Cheryl Garcia

Customer Service
Kim Williams
Juan Reynosa
Fran Desmond

SPECIAL THANKS

A heartfelt thank-you to our insightful
and wonderful reviewers:

Jill A. Walker, RN, BSN
Modesto, CA

Jill Holmes Long, MA, BSN, BS, RN
Hayesville, NC

Denice S. DeAntonio, RN, BSN, MEd
Pottstown, PA

Jenni Castle, RN, BSN, PHN
Modesto, CA

Jan Hunt, RNC
Decatur, IL

Peg Pearson, LPN
Glenside, PA

Anne Snyder, LPN
Ivyland, PA

Lyla Berry, Ed.D, MPM, RN
Beaverton, OR

NOTICE TO READERS

Though the guidelines and procedures contained in this text are based on consultations with healthcare professionals, they should not be considered absolute recommendations. The instructor and readers should follow employer, local, state, and federal guidelines concerning healthcare practices. These guidelines change, and it is the reader's responsibility to be aware of these changes and of the policies and procedures of her or his healthcare facility.

The publisher, author, editors, and reviewers cannot accept any responsibility for errors or omissions or for any consequences from application of the information in this book and make no warranty, expressed or implied, with respect to the contents of the book. The Publisher does not warrant or guarantee any of the products described herein or perform any analysis in connection with any of the product information contained herein.

GENDER USAGE

This textbook utilizes the pronouns "he," "his," "she," and "hers" interchangeably to denote healthcare team members and residents.

PERMISSIONS

Excerpt from "Falling into Life" by Leonard Kriegel. From *The American Scholar*, Volume 57, Number 3, Summer 1988. Copyright © 1988 by Leonard Kriegel. Reprinted with permission of Leonard Kriegel.

Excerpt on The Great Chicago Fire adapted from *To Be a Nurse* by Susan M. Sacharski. Copyright © 1990. Reprinted with permission of Susan M. Sacharski.

This book is dedicated to our dearest, loving children, Mark and Marissa. As you walk down that exciting path into the wonderful world of health care, keep following your dreams. We are so very proud of you. You inspire others to do their best.

"Blessed is he who has found his work." —Thomas Carlyle, 1795-1881

To my dearest John, my soulmate, for everything. "How do I love thee? Let me count the ways." * With deepest gratitude for your enduring love and devotion. My sincerest thanks for your help and support. For all that you do for me and for all of us, a heartfelt thank you. You have my never-ending love.

To Dad, for your wisdom, guidance, and love. To Paul, Paula, Matthew, and Leah for your love and support. To Thomas and Mary Alice, all of John's siblings and his entire family, especially George E. Barrett, for your love, support and encouragement. To our puppy, Cassandra, for your absolute love.

To all of our good friends for your help, support and love, especially Ruth Darling and Barbara J. Ramutkowski.

To Mark Hartman, publisher extraordinaire, for his vision, commitment, patience and encouragement. What a wondrous journey this has been for all of us since that very first e-mail! To Jennifer, for her efforts and strong support of Mark and the business, and to Elliott and Warren.

To Susan Alvare, the hardest-working and most dedicated editor on earth. As always, it was a joy working with you. My everlasting thanks for all of the things you have done for our books. To Mark Hedman, for his support of Susan and the company.

To the Hartman staff and their families: Thad Castillo, Debbie Rinker, Kim Williams, Suzanne Wegner, Ernest Culver, Cheryl Garcia, Juan Reynosa, Caroyl Scott, Fran Desmond, and Kristin Calderon, thank you for your daily hard work and efforts.

To our special book designer, the "other Mrs. D.," Kirsten Browne, thank you for your hard work and your inspiring creativity.

To our always-available reviewers, thank you for all of your efforts and work on behalf of this book.

To all of the instructors and students, thank you for your insights that helped craft this book. We listened carefully to you and have worked very hard to make this textbook everything you want it to be!

And finally, to Mom, for everything you have done for all of us. You always were the angel in our family, and now you have your wings!

With respect, admiration and sincere gratitude to all,

Diana

Diana L. Dugan

* from Elizabeth Barrett Browning, 1806-1861, Sonnets from the Portuguese, XLIII

Contents

8. Emergency Care, First Aid, and Disasters

9. Admission, Transfer, Discharge, and Physical Exams

10. Bedmaking and Unit Care

11. Positioning, Moving, and Lifting

12. Personal Care

13. Vital Signs

Procedures

Using this Textbook

Understanding how your book is organized and what its special features are will help you make the most of this resource!

look!

Carefully-chosen quotes begin each chapter and may be used for discussion. Additional information highlights how health care has changed over the years by detailing interesting events in medicine from the past.

We have assigned each chapter its own colored tab.
Each colored tab contains the chapter number.
The chapter title runs down the side of every page.

1. Explain HIPAA and related terms

Everything in this book, the student workbook, and the instructor's teaching material is organized around learning objectives. A learning objective is a very specific piece of knowledge or a very specific skill. After reading the text, if you can do what the learning objective says, you know you have mastered the material.

bloodborne pathogens

You'll find bold **key terms** at the beginning of each chapter and then again throughout the text. These terms are defined in the text and in the glossary at the back of this book.

Making an occupied bed

All care procedures are highlighted by the same black bar for easy recognition.

Guidelines:
Accurate Documentation

Guidelines are listed with colored bullet points for easy reference.

RESIDENTS' RIGHTS

Take your time when feeding resider
Feeding residents quickly is dangerous
the risk for choking and aspiration. Wl
helpi ⁀ take your time. L
̴ process. F

Residents' Rights boxes teach important information about abuse and neglect and how to recognize and prevent both. Ways to support and promote Residents' Rights are also included. Hot Tips and Trivia boxes show interesting and educational tidbits that you can use inside and outside of work.

CHAPTER REVIEW

Chapter-ending questions test your knowledge of the information found in the chapter. We have included the textbook's learning objective numbers to make it easier for you to go back and reread a section if you need to refresh your memory. When you see this notation after a question—(LO 3)—it refers to that particular learning objective number in the chapter on which you are working. If you have trouble answering a question, you can return to the text and reread the material.

See the Appendix at the end of the book for additional information.

1
The Nursing Assistant in Long-Term Care

Nurses' Aides: Helping Hands During WWII

One of the early times nurses' aides were used in America was during World War II. Various hospitals, along with the American Red Cross, trained nurses' aides in 1941 to help deal with a shortage of nurses due to the war. Employers in the United States expected nurses' aides to volunteer during this time. The country set a goal of training 100,000 nurses' aides to assist nurses with patient care. These aides worked each day without being paid. Imagine being hired today as a nursing assistant and being expected to do the job without pay!

"A professor can never better distinguish himself in his work than by encouraging a clever pupil, for the true discoverers are among them, as comets amongst the stars."

Carl Linnaeus, 1707-1778

"If one advances confidently in the direction of his dreams, and endeavors to live the life which he has imagined, he will meet with a success unexpected in common hours."

Henry David Thoreau, 1817-1862
from *Walden*

1. Define important words in this chapter

accountable: answerable for one's actions.

activities of daily living (ADLs): personal daily care tasks, including bathing, dressing, mouth care, hair care, toileting, and eating and drinking.

acute care: 24-hour skilled care for temporary illnesses or injuries; generally given in hospitals and ambulatory surgical centers.

adaptive devices: special equipment that helps a person who is ill or disabled perform ADLs; also called assistive devices.

adult daycare: care given to adults at a facility during daytime work hours.

assistive devices: special equipment that helps a person who is ill or disabled perform ADLs; also called adaptive devices.

assisted living: a setting for people who require some help with daily care, but who need less care than a long-term care facility offers.

care team: the group of people with different kinds of education and experience who provide resident care.

chain of command: the order of authority within a facility.

charge nurse (nurse-in-charge): a nurse responsible for a team of healthcare workers.

chronic: the term for an illness or condition that is long-term or long-lasting.

cite: to find a problem through a survey.

conscientious: guided by a sense of right and wrong; principled.

continuity of care: coordination of care for a resident over time, during which the care team is always exchanging information about the resident and working toward shared goals.

courteous: polite, kind, considerate.

delegation: transferring authority to a person for a specific task.

dementia: the loss of mental abilities, such as thinking, remembering, reasoning, and communicating.

diagnosis: the identification of a disease by its signs and symptoms and from the results of different tests.

empathetic: identifying with and understanding another's feelings.

first impression: a way of classifying or categorizing people at the first meeting.

functional nursing: method of care assigning specific tasks to each team member.

holistic: care that involves the whole person; this includes his or her physical, social, emotional, and spiritual needs.

home health care: care that takes place in a person's home.

hospice care: care for people who have six months or less to live.

inter-generational care: mixing children and the elderly in the same care setting.

Joint Commission: a not-for-profit organization that evaluates and accredits different types of healthcare facilities.

length of stay: the number of days a person stays in a healthcare facility.

liability: a legal term that means a person can be held responsible for harming someone else.

licensed practical nurse (LPN) or licensed vocational nurse (LVN): licensed nurse who has completed one to two years of education; LPN/LVN passes medications, gives treatments, and may supervise daily care of residents.

long-term care: 24-hour care provided usually in nursing homes for people with ongoing conditions.

nurse practitioner (CNP): a registered nurse with advanced education who is able to see patients and write prescriptions.

nursing assistant: an important member of the care team who performs assigned nursing tasks and gives personal care.

outpatient care: care usually given for less than 24 hours to people who have had treatments or surgery.

pet therapy: the practice of bringing pets into a facility or home to provide stimulation and companionship.

policy: a course of action to be followed.

primary nursing: method of care in which the registered nurse gives much of the daily care to residents.

procedure: a method, or way, of doing something.

professionalism: the act of behaving properly for a certain job.

registered nurse (RN): a licensed nurse who has completed two to four years of education; RNs assess residents, monitor progress, provide skilled nursing care, give treatments, and supervise the care given by nursing assistants and other members of the care team.

rehabilitation: a program of care given by a specialist to restore or improve function after an illness or injury.

resident: a person living in a long-term care facility.

resident-focused care: method of care in which the resident is the primary focus; team members are cross-trained in skills, allowing residents to see many of the same people performing their care.

sandwich generation: people responsible for the care of both their children and aging relatives.

skilled care: medically necessary care given by a skilled nurse or therapist.

subacute care: care given in a nursing home or a hospital; used for people who need a higher level of care and observation than some long-term care facilities can give.

team leader: a nurse in charge of a group of residents for one shift of duty.

team nursing: method of care in which a nurse acts as a leader of a group of people giving care.

trustworthy: deserving the trust of others.

2. Describe healthcare settings

Welcome to the rewarding world of caring for others! No work is more appreciated or valued. Your work will make an important difference in the lives of many people.

Nursing assistants have many job opportunities. Where you work will depend on you, your schedule, and the type of resident you prefer. More information on finding a job is in Chapter 28.

Each healthcare setting is unique; however, there are some similar tasks that will be performed in every setting. This textbook will focus on **long-term care** for elderly residents.

Long-term care (LTC) facilities provide 24-hour skilled care for people who are no longer eligible for hospital care but are unable to stay in their homes. **Skilled care** is medically necessary care given by a skilled nurse or therapist. This care is available 24 hours a day. It is ordered by a doctor, and involves a treatment plan.

Long-term care assists people with ongoing, chronic medical conditions, and is usually given for an extended period of time. **Chronic** means that the conditions last a long period of time, even a lifetime. Examples of chronic conditions include physical disabilities, heart disease, and recovery from stroke. Other terms for long-term care facilities are:

- nursing homes
- nursing facilities
- skilled nursing facilities
- extended care facilities

A long-term care facility is the resident's home. This is why we call people in these facilities "**residents**." It will be the resident's home until he or she returns home, moves to another place, or dies (Fig. 1-1). You must always remember that when you knock on the door and walk into a resident's room, it is the very same thing as knocking on the door of your neighbor's home. Always treat residents' rooms with respect.

Fig. 1-1. A long-term care facility is the resident's home. Treat their rooms and possessions with respect.

In **assisted living**, residents are generally more independent. Staff is available to provide whatever daily care the resident needs, such as bathing and dressing. Some assisted living facilities give help with medications. Residents in assisted living do not usually need skilled care.

Many assisted living centers have a stair-step method of handling residents' needs. The stair-step method means that a person is admitted to a facility when he is still fairly independent. As he requires more care, the level of placement within the facility changes. The advantage of this is that the resident is not moved from institution to institution.

Home health care is care that takes place in a person's home (Fig. 1-2). In some ways, working as a home health aide is similar to working as a nursing assistant. Almost all care in this textbook applies to home health aides. Most of the personal care and basic nursing procedures are the same. Home health aides may also clean the home, shop for groceries, do laundry, and cook. They will work more independently, although a supervisor monitors their work, and may have more contact with the family. The advantage of home health care is that clients do not have to leave home. They may have lived in their homes for many years, and staying at home is more comforting for most people.

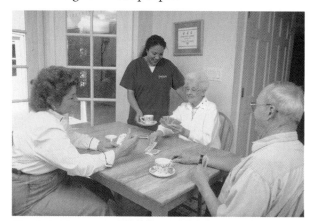

Fig. 1-2. Home care is performed in a person's home.

Adult daycare is given at a facility during daytime working hours. Generally, adult daycare cares for people who need some help, but are not seriously ill or disabled. In the past, aging family members were cared for mostly at home. Today, the **sandwich generation**—the generation caring for children and aging parents at the same time—is often unable to spend enough time at home. If no one can care for an elderly relative at home, or if a person needs a break from caregiving, adult daycare is a good option for busy families.

Some centers have merged adult and child daycare and offer **inter-generational care**. With this type of care, the young and the elderly are able to spend their days together (Fig. 1-3). Many elderly people live far away from close family or do not have family. This kind of care provides "grandparents" or "grandchildren" for those who have none or who live too far away from their own families.

Fig. 1-3. Inter-generational care provides an opportunity for the elderly and the young to spend time together.

Acute care is given in hospitals and ambulatory surgical centers (Fig. 1-4). It is for people who require care for illnesses or injuries. People are admitted for short stays for surgery or diseases. The length of time the person remains will vary depending upon the illness. Acute care is 24-hour skilled care for temporary, but serious, illnesses or injuries.

Fig. 1-4. Acute care is performed in hospitals.

Subacute care can be given in a nursing home or a hospital. It is used for people who need a higher level of care and observation than some long-term care facilities can give. The cost is usually less than a hospital but more than long-term care. Subacute care will be covered in depth in Chapter 26.

Outpatient care is usually given for less than 24 hours. It is for people who have had treatments or surgery and need short-term skilled care. They are sent home with instructions for further care. Families or friends may play a part in their successful recovery.

Rehabilitation is care given by a specialist. Physical, occupational, and speech therapists restore or improve function after an illness or injury. You will learn more about these specialists in Learning Objective 9 of this chapter. Information on rehabilitation is in Chapter 25.

Hospice care is for people who have six months or less to live. Hospice workers give physical and emotional care and comfort and they also support families during this process. Hospice care can take place in facilities or in homes.

HOT TIP

Pet Therapy

Another addition to adult daycare, inter-generational care, or nursing home care is pet therapy. **Pet therapy** provides different kinds of animals to brighten the days of older adults. The Delta Society, founded in 1977 by a physician and a veterinarian, is a national organization dedicated to the therapeutic bond between animals and humans. The group welcomes inquiries from owners interested in volunteering good-natured dogs for participation. You can contact the society by visiting their website, www. deltasociety.org. Many people love having animals nearby and become attached to them. Pet allergies or fear of pets must be taken into account when using pet therapy.

TRIVIA

Early Nursing Schools

The early nursing schools in the 1800s and early 1900s had very strict rules for their students. The classes at that time were made up of women, and they normally lived together in the same building. The schools usually had women who acted as housemothers for the students. Rigid curfews, rules restricting smoking, drinking and profanity, separation of the sexes, and specific dress codes were strictly enforced. Women were normally not allowed to date or marry, and those who broke the rules suffered severe punishment. The nursing students were expected to work long hours and, in addition to caring for patients, had to wash and wax floors and do chores that today are duties of other employees.

3. Explain Medicare and Medicaid

The Centers for Medicare & Medicaid Services (CMS), formerly the Health Care Finance Administration (HCFA), is a federal agency within the United States Department of Health and Human Services (Fig. 1-5). CMS runs two national healthcare programs, Medicare and Medicaid. They both help pay for health care and health insurance for millions of Americans. CMS has many other responsibilities as well.

Fig. 1-5. *The CMS website.*

Medicare is a health insurance program for people who are 65 years of age or older. Medicare also covers people younger than 65 who are disabled or ill and cannot work.

Medicare has two parts: Hospital Insurance (Part A), and Medical Insurance (Part B). Part A helps pay for care from a hospital, skilled nursing facility, home health agency, or hospice. Part B helps pay for physician services and other medical services and equipment. Medicare covers a percentage of healthcare costs. Medicare will only pay for care it determines to be medically necessary.

Medicaid is a medical assistance program for low-income people. It is funded by both the federal government and each state. Eligibility is determined by income and special circumstances. People must qualify for this program.

Medicare and Medicaid pay long-term care facilities a fixed amount for services. This is based on the resident's need upon admission.

4. Describe the residents for whom you will care

There are some general statements that can be made about residents in nursing homes. However, more important than understanding the entire population is understanding each individual for whom you will care. Make sure you know how to care for residents based on their specific needs, illnesses, and preferences.

According to the National Center for Health Statistics, almost 91 percent of long-term care residents in the U.S. are over age 65. Only nine percent are younger than 65. Almost 72 percent of residents are female. More than 85 percent are Caucasian (Fig. 1-6). This is a much larger percentage than the U.S. population as a whole. About one-third of residents come from a private residence; over 50 percent come from a hospital or other facility.

Fig. 1-6. Caucasian women make up a high percentage of nursing home residents.

The **length of stay** is the number of days a person stays in a healthcare facility. The length of stay of almost one-half of residents in long-term care is six months or longer. These residents need enough help with their activities of daily living to require 24-hour care. Often, they did not have caregivers available to give sufficient care for them to live in the community. The groups with the longest average stay are the developmentally disabled. They are often younger than 65. You will learn more about these groups in Chapter 5.

The other half of residents stay for less than six months. This group generally falls into two categories. The first category is residents admitted for terminal care. They will die in the facility. The second category is residents admitted for rehabilitation or temporary illness. They will recover and return to the community. As you can imagine, care of these residents may be very different.

Dementia is defined as the loss of mental abilities, such as thinking, remembering, reasoning, and communicating. Various studies place the number of nursing home residents with dementia between 50 and 90 percent. Dementia and other mental disorders are major causes of nursing home admissions. Many residents are admitted with other disorders as well. However, the disorders themselves are often not the main reason for admission. It is most often the lack of ability to care for oneself and the lack of a support system that leads people into a facility.

A support system is vital in allowing the elderly to live outside a facility. For every elderly person living in a long-term care facility, at least two with similar disorders and disabilities live in the community.

You may notice the lack of outside support given to your residents. It is one reason you will care for the "whole person" instead of only the illness or disease. Residents have many needs besides bathing, eating, drinking, and toileting. These needs will go unmet if staff do not work to meet them.

5. Describe the nursing assistant's role

Nursing assistants perform many tasks. Most of the tasks deal with helping care for residents. A **nursing assistant** (NA or CNA) does delegated or assigned nursing tasks. **Delegation** means transferring authority to a person for a specific task. Examples of nursing tasks include taking residents' temperature and blood pressure. A nursing assistant also assists residents with **activities of daily living (ADLs)**, which are personal daily care tasks, such as bathing, dressing, mouth care, toileting, and eating and drinking.

Common nursing assistant tasks include:

- Serving trays and feeding residents (Fig. 1-7)
- Helping residents dress and undress
- Bathing residents
- Shampooing hair
- Shaving residents
- Bedmaking
- Tidying residents' living areas
- Taking vital signs, including temperature, pulse, respiration, blood pressure and checking pain levels
- Helping residents with toileting needs
- Assisting with mouth care
- Giving back rubs
- Observing and reporting changes in residents' conditions
- Reporting residents' complaints to the nurse
- Helping residents move safely around the facility
- Caring for equipment

Fig. 1-7. Helping residents eat and drink will be an important part of your job.

Nursing assistants are generally not allowed to give medications. Other tasks that nursing assistants usually do not perform include inserting and removing tubes, giving tube feedings, and changing sterile dressings.

Nursing assistants can have many different titles. Examples include "nurse aide," "patient care attendant," "health care assistant," "patient care technician," and "personal care assistant." This book will use the term "nursing assistant (NA)."

6. Discuss professionalism and list examples of professional behavior

Understanding how to be professional is the first step to success in the healthcare field. Professional behavior is vital in the workplace. **Professionalism** has to do with behaving properly on the job. Everything about the way you present yourself to others in a healthcare setting will be closely observed. Dressing appropriately, speaking well, and being dependable and responsible are all part of professionalism. A healthcare facility is a place where professional behavior is expected. Follow these guidelines to behave professionally:

Guidelines
Professional Behavior

- Be neatly dressed and groomed. Keep your uniform and shoes clean.
- Do not discuss personal problems or personal situations with residents. At work, conversation focuses on the resident, not the caregiver.
- Be at work on time at your scheduled times. Call in a timely manner if you are sick or not reporting for duty as scheduled.
- Avoid unnecessary absences. When you are absent, your co-workers have more work to complete.
- Never leave your job early without permission. Report to the nurse in charge when leaving your unit for any reason.
- Do not report to work under the influence of drugs and/or alcohol.

- Keep a positive attitude.
- Do not gossip or speak badly about co-workers.
- Speak politely to all persons in the facility. Treat all visitors with courtesy and respect.
- Address residents, family members and visitors in the way they wish to be addressed. Never call someone names such as "honey" or "dear" or "sweetie."
- Do not curse or use inappropriate language.
- Keep all resident information confidential (private).
- Follow all facility procedures and policies.
- Report concerns or problems to your supervisor.
- Meet and maintain all educational requirements.
- Ask questions when you do not understand something.
- Be honest. Document and report carefully and truthfully (Fig. 1-8).
- Accept constructive criticism gracefully and learn from it. Constructive criticism is meant to help you improve your performance. An example is, "You need to document care more accurately."
- Do not accept tips or gifts from residents, their families, or other visitors.
- Be loyal to your facility. Be a positive role model.

Fig. 1-8. *Writing down what you observe is one of your most important duties.*

Behaving professionally will be an ongoing focus of this textbook. Pay attention to this in-

formation. Professionalism may earn you the respect of others and help you advance in your job.

7. List qualities that nursing assistants must have

The best nursing assistants have the qualities listed below. As you read through this list, ask yourself whether or not you have these qualities.

Patient and understanding. Working with ill or disabled people requires patience and understanding. People who are patient remain calm. They are able to put up with difficulties without complaining.

Honest and trustworthy. An honest person tells the truth and can be trusted. Co-workers will depend on honesty in planning care. Employers count on truthful records of care performed and observations. Residents count on nursing assistants to safeguard their belongings and to keep their confidential information private.

Conscientious. Nursing assistants must be conscientious. People who are conscientious are guided by a sense of right and wrong. They always try to do their best. They are always alert, observant, accurate, and responsible.

Enthusiastic. People who are enthusiastic have a positive attitude. They are encouraging. They show interest in others and their situations and problems (Fig. 1-9). Enthusiastic people have a positive influence on others.

Fig. 1-9. *Being enthusiastic, cheerful and positive is something that will be expected of you.*

Courteous and respectful. Nursing assistants must be kind, polite, and considerate. They should respect others' beliefs even if they are different from their own.

Empathetic. Empathetic people care about other people's problems. They can think about what it would be like to be ill and dependent on others for help.

Dependable and responsible. Nursing assistants must be at work on time and avoid too many absences. They should always follow policies and procedures. Nursing assistants must be able to be counted on to do their tasks properly.

Humble and open to growth. People who are humble are willing to admit when they have made a mistake. They can accept their limitations. They hold themselves **accountable** when they have made a mistake. This means that they can admit the mistake and apologize. They can ask others for help when they need it.

Tolerance. Nursing assistants must not judge others. They should keep their opinions to themselves and see people as individuals.

Lack of prejudice. Nursing assistants work with different people from many backgrounds. They must give each person quality care regardless of age, gender, sexual orientation, religion, race, ethnicity, or condition.

TRIVIA

NAs: In demand in 1945
Nursing assistants, it seems, have been in demand for many years. This list of "unfilled positions" in hospitals at that time appeared late in 1945:
- Registered Nurses 65,000
- Non-nursing personnel 90,000
- Nurses' Aides 90,000
- Untrained volunteers 45,000

8. Discuss proper grooming guidelines

Good **first impressions**, or ways of classifying people at the first meeting, can make a difference in getting a job, getting another date, or even getting good service in a store. Nursing assistants must pay attention to the way they present themselves to residents, their family members and friends, and to other staff members. Good grooming is essential to making a good first impression. Some important grooming guidelines are listed below:

Guidelines
Grooming
- Keep your uniform clean, neat, and pressed.
- Bathe or shower every day. Wear deodorant or anti-perspirant.
- Brush your teeth at least twice a day.
- Avoid using strongly-scented items, such as perfume, cologne, after-shave, body washes, body creams and lotions, hair spray, and fabric softeners.
- Keep your hair neatly tied back and away from your face (Fig. 1-10).
- Keep beards trimmed and neat-looking.
- Apply makeup lightly or use none at all.
- Keep nails short, filed, and clean. As older people have fragile skin, this is very important. Follow facility policy on whether nail polish is allowed.
- Do not wear false nails. False nails harbor bacteria no matter how well you wash your hands.
- Keep shoes and laces clean. Shoes should be in good condition. They should be comfortable. They should not look worn and old. Change or wash shoelaces when they become soiled.
- Wear as little jewelry as possible. Sharp edges on jewelry can scratch or tear fragile skin. Remove rings and bracelets while working. They collect bacteria and can cause infection. They may also cause problems with wearing gloves. Remove necklaces while working; necklaces may also hide bacteria. Wear small earrings that will not snag on things and that confused residents cannot pull on. The exceptions to this rule are a simple, waterproof watch and an identification badge. You will need a watch to take a resident's pulse and

respirations and record events. An identification badge identifies you to residents, visitors, and other staff members.

Fig. 1-10. *Keeping your hair neatly tied back and wearing a clean uniform are examples of professional behavior.*

HOT TIP

Kill the scent!
Residents may have allergies that are worsened by scents. Residents may also be very aware of scents because they do not feel well. Think about how you feel when you are sick. You must always try to meet the needs of residents in every way. That means respecting their individual problems and putting their comfort first. Avoid using heavily-scented items.

9. Define the roles of each member of the care team

The **care team** consists of many members who have had different training and experience to provide care for each resident (Fig. 1-11). The resident is the most important part—the center—of the care team. Members of the care team include the following:

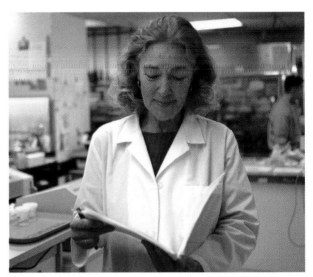

Fig. 1-11. *The care team is made up of many different types of professionals.*

Nurse: A nurse assesses residents, monitors progress, and gives treatments. Your immediate supervisor may be a registered nurse (RN), a licensed practical nurse (LPN), or a licensed vocational nurse (LVN). An explanation of the different types of nurses and their training follows.

Registered Nurse (RN): A person with a license by examination who has completed two to four years of education.

Nurse Practitioner or **Certified Nursing Practitioner (CNP)**: A person with advanced training who may see patients at offices and can write prescriptions. Usually the nurse has completed at least five years of education.

Licensed Practical or Licensed Vocational Nurse (LPN/LVN): A person with a license by examination who has completed one to two years of education.

Physician or Doctor [MD (medical doctor) or DO (doctor of osteopathy)]: A doctor diagnoses disease or disability and prescribes treatment. A **diagnosis** is the identification of a disease by its signs and symptoms and/or results from testing. Doctors have graduated from four-year medical schools after receiving a bachelor's degree. Many doctors also take specialized training programs after medical school.

Medical Social Worker (MSW): A medical social worker helps with social needs. For example, an MSW helps residents find compatible roommates. An MSW also helps with support services, such as counseling and financial assistance.

Physical Therapist (PT): A physical therapist gives therapy in the form of heat, cold, massage, ultrasound, electricity, and exercise to muscles, bones, and joints (Fig. 1-12). This is done to improve blood circulation, promote healing, ease pain, and help the resident regain mobility.

Fig. 1-13. *An occupational therapist will help residents learn to use adaptive devices, such as this special spoon and plate. (Photo courtesy of North Coast Medical, Inc. 800-821-9319.)*

Fig. 1-12. *A physical therapist helps exercise muscles, bones, and joints to improve strength or restore abilities.*

Occupational Therapist (OT): An occupational therapist works with people who need help with activities of daily living (ADLs). An OT evaluates a resident's ability to do these activities, and **assistive** or **adaptive devices** may be ordered to help. These devices help residents perform ADLs. An example is a special spoon that helps a person feed himself (Fig. 1-13).

Registered Dietitian (RDT): A registered dietitian or nutritionist assesses nutritional status and plans a care program. A dietitian creates diets for residents with special needs. These special diets can improve health and help manage illness.

Speech Language Pathologist (SLP): A speech language pathologist or speech therapist teaches exercises to help the resident improve or overcome speech problems. An SLP also evaluates a person's ability to swallow food and drink.

Activities Director: The activities director plans activities, such as bingo or special performances, to help residents socialize and stay physically and mentally active.

Nursing Assistant or Certified Nursing Assistant (NA/CNA): The nursing assistant does assigned tasks, such as taking a resident's temperature. NAs also give personal care, such as bathing residents, brushing their teeth, and assisting with toileting. Nursing assistants are one of the most important team members because they have the most direct contact with residents. If a resident's health changes from day to day, they will often be the first ones to notice this change. Nursing assistants must report any changes in residents' conditions to the nurse promptly. The federal government requires that nursing assistants have at least 75 hours of training. Some states require more than 75 hours of training. You will learn more about these requirements in Chapter 2.

Resident and Resident's Family: As stated earlier, the resident is the most important part of the care team. The care team revolves around the resident. Residents make choices about their care. They help plan their care. The resident's family and friends may help with these decisions. They play another important role, too. Family and friends may share vital information about the resident with the care team. This information includes the resident's health and medical record, personal preferences, rituals, and routines.

10. Discuss the facility chain of command

The **chain of command** describes the line of authority in the facility. For example, the nurse will usually be the nursing assistant's immediate supervisor. If a nursing assistant has a problem with another department, he or she will report this to the proper person. This is usually an immediate supervisor or the **charge nurse**, who is a nurse responsible for a team of healthcare workers. The nursing assistant would not go directly to the department to tell them of the problem. That would not be following the chain of command (Fig. 1-14).

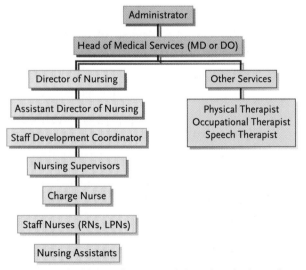

Fig. 1-14. *The chain of command describes the line of authority in a facility.*

The chain of command also helps to protect staff from **liability**. Liability is a legal term. It means a person can be held responsible for harming someone else. For example, a nursing assistant gives care to a resident and he is injured. If the care was assigned and was done according to policy and procedure, the nursing assistant may not be liable, or responsible, for hurting the resident. However, if a nursing assistant performs a task that is not assigned to her and it harms a resident, she could be held responsible. That is why it is important to follow instructions and the chain of command. Following the chain of command helps lessen the risk of liability. When handling any problem, speak with your supervisor first.

11. Explain "The Five Rights of Delegation"

When planning care, nurses have to decide which tasks to delegate to others. This includes nursing assistants. Everything you do in your job is delegated to you by a licensed healthcare professional. Licensed nurses are accountable for care, including all delegated tasks. The National Council of State Boards of Nursing has identified "The Five Rights of Delegation." This can be used as a mental checklist to help nurses in the decision-making process.

"The Five Rights of Delegation" are the "Right Task," "Right Circumstance," "Right Person," "Right Direction/Communication," and "Right Supervision/Evaluation." Before delegating tasks, nurses consider these questions:

- Is there a match between the resident's needs and the nursing assistant's skills, abilities, and experience?

- What is the level of resident stability?

- Is the nursing assistant the right person to do the job?

- Can the nurse give appropriate direction and communication?

- Is the nurse available to give the supervision, support and help that the nursing assistant needs?

There are questions you may want to ask yourself before accepting a task. Consider these questions:

- Do I have all the information I need to do this job? Are there questions I should ask?

- Do I believe that I can do this task? Do I have the necessary skills?

- Do I have the needed supplies, equipment and other support?

- Do I know who my supervisor is, and how to reach him/her?

- Have I told my supervisor of my special needs for help and support?

- Do we both understand who is doing what?

Never be afraid to ask for help. Always ask if you need more information or if you are unsure about something. If you feel that you do not have the skills for a task, talk to the nurse.

12. Describe four methods of nursing care

The nursing profession takes a holistic view of resident care. The word "holistic" comes from the Greek. It means "whole." **Holistic** means considering a whole system, such as a whole person, and not dividing the system up into parts. Holistic care is caring for the whole person. This includes his or her physical needs, as well as other needs, such as social contact, emotions, thought, and spirituality (Fig. 1-15). Meeting these needs helps improve residents' quality of life. You will learn more about these needs in Chapter 5.

Over the years, the nursing field has seen many changes. Many types of nursing care have been used at facilities. Four basic types of nursing care are outlined at right. Each facility chooses the type that provides the best care for their residents.

Fig. 1-15. Caring for residents holistically means considering their emotional needs as well.

Resident-Focused Care: This style of nursing care focuses on the resident, not on the staff. Care is carefully planned with each resident's needs and comfort in mind. Some members of the care team may be trained in many skills. This is called cross-training. For example, one caregiver is a nursing assistant who has been trained in drawing blood (phlebotomy). When a resident needs blood drawn, a familiar caregiver can do the procedure. This can reduce a resident's fear and anxiety. Cross-training allows residents to see many of the same faces regularly. Residents like seeing the same staff members. It makes the facility feel more like a home.

Team Nursing: In this method, a registered nurse has the role of the **team leader**. Assignments are made, care is given, and the team members report to the team leader throughout the day. The resident's care is managed efficiently and cooperatively. This is a true "team" approach to care.

Primary Nursing: In this method, a registered nurse gives much of the daily care to residents. This type of care allows for a closer relationship between the nurse and the residents. Consistency and continuity of care are positive results of this method. **Continuity of care** is coordination of care for a resident over time, during which the care team is always exchanging information about the resident and working toward shared goals.

Functional Nursing: In this method, staff provide care to large numbers of residents throughout the day. Each member is given one or more specific tasks to complete on a large number of residents living in a unit. For example, one nursing assistant makes all of the beds on the floor. Another completes all of the daily weights. One nurse passes medications, while another gives treatments. Some people find this method of care disorganized with less continuity of care. Staff may not have the time to really observe each resident, and changes in a resident's condition may be overlooked.

13. Explain policy and procedure manuals

All facilities have manuals outlining policies and procedures. A **policy** is a course of action to be taken every time a certain situation occurs. The policy manual has a complete list of every facility policy. For example, one very basic policy is that the chain of command must always be followed.

A **procedure** is a specific method, or way, of doing something. The procedure manual has information on the exact way to complete every procedure. For example, there will be a procedure on how to give a resident a bed bath.

Everyone needs a reminder on how to perform a task from time to time. The procedure manual serves as a guide if you want to review the steps in a procedure. Do not hesitate to look at the procedure manual. Nursing assistants who ask questions when they are unsure provide safer resident care. Acting confident when you are unsure of a procedure is dangerous. Always ask if you have questions.

The policy and procedure manuals are usually kept separate from each other. Know where these manuals are so that you may look at them when necessary.

14. Describe the long-term care survey process

Inspections are done to make sure long-term care facilities (and home health agencies) are following state and federal regulations. Inspections are done periodically by the state agency that licenses facilities. These inspections are called surveys. They may be done more often if a facility has been cited for problems. To **cite** means to find a problem through a survey. Inspections may be done less often if the facility has a good record. Inspection teams include a variety of trained healthcare professionals.

Surveyors study how well the staff cares for its residents. They focus on how residents' nutritional, physical, social, emotional, and spiritual needs are being met. They interview residents and families and observe the staff's interactions with residents and the care given. They review resident charts and observe meals. Surveys are one reason the "paperwork" part of a nursing assistant's job is so important.

If a facility is cited for not following a federal regulation, surveyors use special tags to note these problems. When surveyors are in your facility, try not to be nervous. Give the same great care you do every day. Answer any questions to the best of your ability. If you do not know the answer, be honest. Never guess. Tell the surveyor that you do not know the answer but will find out as quickly as possible. Then do just that.

The **Joint Commission**, formerly the Joint Commission on Accreditation of Healthcare Organizations (JCAHO), is an independent, not-for-profit organization whose standards focus on improving the quality and safety of care provided by healthcare facilities. The Joint Commission makes sure each facility is following the standards of care by inspecting and evaluating different types of healthcare facilities. The Joint Commission's surveys are not associated with state inspections.

Facilities join the Joint Commission on a voluntary basis; some do not participate in this process. In order to receive the Joint Commission's approval, facilities must pass evaluations at least every three years. A facility may be visited more often if problems are found.

CHAPTER REVIEW

1. Describe long-term care (LO 2).

2. Whom does Medicare insurance cover (LO 3)?

3. Who makes up the majority of nursing home residents—men or women (LO 4)?

4. List ten common nursing assistant tasks (LO 5).

5. What are three tasks that nursing assistants do not usually do (LO 5)?

6. List ten ways a nursing assistant can show professional behavior (LO 6).

7. List each of the ten qualities in Learning Objective 7. For each quality, write one example of a way that a nursing assistant can demonstrate that quality (LO 7).

8. Describe ten grooming guidelines for nursing assistants (LO 8).

9. Who is the most important part of the care team (LO 9)?

10. Choose four members of the care team and describe the roles they play (LO 9).

11. Define the chain of command (LO 10).

12. List the "Five Rights of Delegation" (LO 11).

13. Give a brief description of the four methods of nursing care (LO 12).

14. What is a policy? What is a procedure (LO 13)?

15. When surveyors visit a facility, what do they study and observe (LO 14)?

16. When a surveyor asks a nursing assistant a question she does not know the answer to, how should she respond (LO 14)?

2 Ethical and Legal Issues

The First Code of Ethics

An English physician named Thomas Percival wrote a code of ethics called "Percival's Medical Ethics" in 1803. Here is a sample from that first code of ethics: "A physician ought not to abandon a patient because the case is deemed incurable, for his attendance may continue to be highly useful to the patient, and comforting to the relatives around him . . ." In 1847, Percival's Medical Ethics was used to help develop the American Medical Association's first code of ethics. The American Medical Association Principles is still the code of ethics that physicians use today.

"It's a funny thing about life, if you refuse to accept anything but the best, you very often get it."

W. Somerset Maugham, 1874-1965

"Wherever there is a human being, I see God-given rights inherent in that being, whatever may be the sex or complexion."

William Lloyd Garrison, 1805-1879

1. Define important words in this chapter

abuse: purposely causing physical, mental, or emotional pain or injury to someone.

active neglect: purposely harming a person physically, mentally, or emotionally by failing to provide needed care.

advance directives: written documents or oral statements that allow people to decide what kind of medical care they wish to have if they are unable to make those decisions themselves.

assault: threatening to harm a person or leading a person to feel threatened that he or she will be touched without his or her permission.

battery: the actual touching of another person without the person's permission.

civil law: private law; law between individuals.

criminal law: public law; related to committing a crime against the community.

DNR (do-not-resuscitate): an order that tells medical professionals not to perform CPR.

domestic violence: abuse by spouses, intimate partners, or family members; can be physical, sexual, or emotional.

Durable Power of Attorney for Health Care: a signed, dated, and witnessed paper that appoints someone to make the medical decisions for a person in the event he becomes unable to do so.

ethics: the knowledge of what is right and wrong; standards of conduct.

etiquette: the code of proper behavior and courtesy in a certain setting.

false imprisonment: unlawfully restraining or confining someone against his or her will.

financial abuse: stealing, taking advantage of, or improperly using the money, property, or other assets of another.

HIPAA (Health Insurance Portability and Accountability Act): law passed to protect the privacy of health information and to facilitate the transferring of protected health information (PHI) for payment and research needs.

invasion of privacy: a violation of the right to be left alone and the right to control personal information.

involuntary seclusion: confinement or separation from others in a physical space; done without consent or against one's will.

laws: rules set by the government to help protect the public.

Living Will: a document that states the medical care a person wants, or does not want, in case he or she becomes unable to make those decisions.

malpractice: a negligent or improper act by a doctor or other medical professional that results in damage or injury to a person.

mandated reporters: people who are required to report suspected or observed abuse or neglect due to their regular contact with vulnerable populations, such as the elderly in nursing homes.

misappropriation: the act of taking what belongs to someone else and using it illegally for one's own gain.

NATCEP (Nurse Aide Training and Competency Evaluation Program): part of OBRA that sets minimum requirements for nursing assistants for training and testing.

negligence: actions, or a failure to act or give care, that results in injury to a person.

OBRA (Omnibus Budget Reconciliation Act): law originally passed in 1987; includes minimum standards for nursing assistant training, staffing requirements, resident assessment instructions, and information on rights for residents.

ombudsman: person assigned by law as the legal advocate for residents.

passive neglect: unintentionally harming a person physically, mentally, or emotionally by failing to provide needed care.

physical abuse: intentional or unintentional treatment that causes harm or injury to a person's body.

Protected Health Information (PHI): information that can be used to identify a person and relates to the patient's past, present, or future physical or mental condition, including any health care that patient has had, or payment for that health care.

psychological abuse: harming a person by threatening, scaring, insulting, humiliating, or treating him or her as a child; also includes verbal abuse.

Residents' Council: a group of residents who meet regularly to discuss issues related to the nursing home.

Residents' Rights: rights identified by OBRA for residents in long-term care facilities; purpose is to inform residents and others of their rights within these facilities and to provide an ethical code of conduct for healthcare workers.

scope of practice: the tasks that nursing assistants are permitted to perform as allowed by state or federal law.

sexual abuse: forcing a person to perform or participate in sexual acts against his or her will.

sexual harassment: any unwelcome sexual advance or behavior that creates an intimidating, hostile or offensive working environment.

substance abuse: the use of drugs, cigarettes, or alcohol in a way that harms oneself or others.

verbal abuse: oral or written words, pictures, or gestures that threaten or embarrass a person.

workplace violence: the abuse of staff by other staff members, residents, or visitors; includes both physical and verbal abuse.

2. Define the terms "law," "ethics," and "etiquette"

There are many legal and ethical terms that relate to resident care. **Ethics** are the knowledge of what is right and wrong; they help guide conduct. Ethics help us make decisions at home, in the workplace, or in the community. In healthcare, ethics guide the people giving care. For example, keeping a resident's information confidential is ethical behavior. It is also the law.

Laws are rules set by the government to help protect the public. In healthcare, laws protect those receiving care (Fig. 2-1). For example, there is a law against stealing a resident's belongings.

Fig. 2-1. Behaving ethically and following the law applies to all healthcare providers.

Laws can be civil or criminal. **Criminal laws** are written to protect society from people or organizations that try to do them harm. This type of law protects the public. It is also called "public law." **Civil law** refers to disputes between individuals. Problems with landlords, conflicts with neighbors, and divorce issues are examples of areas covered by civil law. Civil law is sometimes referred to as "private law."

Criminal law includes these offenses (crimes):

- A misdemeanor is any crime which is not a felony. It is not as serious an offense as a felony. Disturbing the peace is an example of a misdemeanor. Punishment may include community service time, a fine, and/or a short prison term.

- A felony is a more serious crime than a misdemeanor. Murder and bribery are examples of felonies. Punishment may include a longer prison term, such as life without parole, or even, a death sentence.

Etiquette is the code of proper behavior and courtesy in a certain setting. For example, asking "How may I help you?" when you answer the phone at your facility is proper telephone etiquette.

3. Discuss examples of ethical and professional behavior

A nursing assistant's ethics play an important part in his or her success as a care team member. Professional and ethical behavior is vital to the safety and well-being of the residents. Below are guidelines for behavior that nursing assistants must follow:

Guidelines
Legal and Ethical Behavior

- Keep all resident information confidential (private). This is one of the Residents' Rights covered later in this chapter. All team members must keep resident information confidential. You can only discuss residents with other members of the care team.

- Keep staff information confidential. Do not share private information about your coworkers at home or anywhere else.

- Be honest at all times. Communicate honestly and clearly with members of the care team. Be honest when documenting resident care. Be truthful when reporting the hours you have worked. Do not take items that do not belong to you.

- Be trustworthy. Trusting others is important in facilities. Residents must be able to trust staff members. Employers must be able to trust their employees. And employees need to trust their supervisors. For employers, trusting an employee means knowing that the employee will come to work each day on time. When an employee often fails to show up for work, the boss cannot trust or count on that employee. Employers also trust that employees will come to them if they have a problem. This is following the chain of command.

- Do not accept tips or gifts from residents or their family members or friends (Fig. 2-2).

- Report abuse or suspected abuse of residents. You will learn more about abuse in Learning Objective 7 of this chapter.

- Do not report to work under the influence of alcohol or drugs.

- Follow all facility policies, rules, and procedures. Document care you give accurately and promptly.

- Do your assigned tasks. If you make a mistake, report it promptly to the nurse. This can help minimize damage and prevent any further problems.

- Be positive and professional. Nursing assistants deal with a large number of people every day. Residents deserve people who will try to make their days as pleasant as possible. A person who is cheerful and encouraging is someone others like to be around.

- Be tactful. Tact is the ability to understand what is proper and appropriate when dealing with others. It is the ability to speak and act without offending others.

- Treat all residents with respect and be empathetic. Respect means allowing others to believe or act as they judge best. Empathy means being able to share in and understand the feelings and troubles of others. A caring person would be empathetic with a person who is ill. A caring person would also respect an ill person's actions or beliefs about the illness, despite her own feelings.

- Be patient. Nursing assistants have to deal with residents' troubles and pain without being frustrated. Activities of daily living (ADLs), such as eating, dressing, and toileting may take older people much longer and use up much of their energy, leaving them tired (Fig. 2-3). Residents should be allowed to do tasks at their own pace. The more patient you are, the better care you will provide.

Fig. 2-2. *Nursing assistants should not accept money or gifts because it is unprofessional and can lead to conflict.*

Fig. 2-3. *Older adults may need extra time with ADLs. Be patient and allow them to do tasks at their own pace.*

HOT TIP

Gifts and Tips

Accepting gifts or tips is not allowed in the health-care field. It is unprofessional and can lead to conflict. Nursing assistants and other staff receive payment from the facility for the work they do. If a resident, family member or visitor offers to tip you or tries to give you a gift, politely refuse. Explain that it would not be ethical for you to accept it and that it is against the facility's policies.

4. Describe a nursing assistant code of ethics

Many facilities have adopted a formal code of ethics. This helps their employees deal with issues of right and wrong. Codes of ethics differ, but all revolve around the idea that a resident is a valuable person who deserves ethical care. A sample code of ethics for nursing assistants is shown below:

1. I will strive to provide and maintain the highest quality of care for my residents. I will fully recognize and follow all of the Residents' Rights.

2. I will communicate well, serve on committees, and read all material as provided and required by my employer. I will attend educational in-services, and join organizations relevant to nursing assistant care.

3. I will show a positive attitude toward my residents, staff, family members, and other visitors.

4. I will always provide privacy for my residents. I will maintain confidentiality of resident, staff, and visitor information.

5. I will be trustworthy and honest in all dealings with residents, staff, and visitors.

6. I will strive to preserve resident safety. I will report mistakes I make, along with anything that I deem dangerous, to the right person(s).

7. I will have empathy for my residents, other staff, and all visitors, giving support and encouragement when needed.

8. I will respect all people, without regard to age, sex, ethnicity, religion, economic situation, sexual orientation, or diagnosis.

9. I will never abuse my residents in any way. I will always report any suspected abuse to my supervisor or the proper person immediately.

10. I will strive to have the utmost patience with all people at my facility.

HOT TIP

Never call yourself a nurse.

Nursing assistants must never identify themselves as nurses. Nurses have had more education and training than nursing assistants. Nurses have different responsibilities than nursing assistants do. Calling yourself a nurse could result in injury to yourself or others, a lawsuit, and/or being fired from your job. So never use the term "nurse" lightly; always identify yourself as a nursing assistant.

5. Explain the Omnibus Budget Reconciliation Act (OBRA)

The Omnibus Budget Reconciliation Act (OBRA) was passed in 1987. It has been updated many times since 1987. OBRA was written as a response to poor care and abuse in nursing homes. Reports of bad conditions in some nursing homes were common. Congress stepped in and set minimum standards of care. This included standardizing training of nursing assistants.

OBRA requires that the **Nurse Aide Training and Competency Evaluation Program (NATCEP)** sets minimum requirements for nursing assistants. Nursing assistants must complete at least 75 hours of training. However, programs may exceed these minimums. Many states require 80-150 program hours in theory and clinical skills. These skills include basic nursing skills, basic restorative skills, mental health and social service needs, personal care skills, Residents' Rights, and safety and emergency care.

Nursing assistants must also pass a competency evaluation (testing program) before they can be employed. The exam consists of both written and demonstrated nursing skills.

OBRA requires that nursing assistants attend regular in-service education (Fig. 2-4). OBRA also requires that states keep a current list of nursing assistants in a state registry. In addition, OBRA identifies standards that instructors must meet in order to train nursing assistants.

Fig. 2-4. *Completing in-service education successfully is an OBRA requirement for nursing assistants.*

OBRA also designates minimum staff requirements and specifies services that nursing homes must provide.

Another important part of OBRA is the resident assessment requirements. OBRA requires complete assessments on every resident. The assessment forms are the same for every facility. The MDS (Minimum Data Set) is a resident assessment system that was developed in 1990. It is revised periodically. The MDS is a detailed form with guidelines for assessing residents. You will learn more about the MDS in Chapter 3.

OBRA also identifies important rights for residents in nursing homes. You will learn about these rights in Learning Objective 6.

OBRA regulations are important to nursing assistant practice because they do these things:

1. Give recognition through certification and registration.

2. Help define the nursing assistant's **scope of practice**, which specifies the tasks that nursing assistants are permitted to perform as allowed by state or federal law.

3. Provide better uniformity of care.

4. Promote educational standards.

HOT TIP

What is the State Board of Nursing?
In your state, this agency might have a different name. However, the responsibilities will be similar. The State Board of Nursing is in charge of licensing of all nurses and testing or certification of nursing assistants. This agency may also handle issues and problems with nurses and nursing assistants.

HOT TIP

Reciprocity
When you have completed an approved nursing assistant course, you may be eligible for nursing assistant certification. When you move to another state, your certification may transfer to that state. This is called "reciprocity." Before moving to another state, contact the agency there that handles nursing assistant issues and find out if you qualify for reciprocity. If needed, gather important paperwork from your original state before you leave. Obtaining a new certificate in your new state is your responsibility and will be necessary before you can begin working.

6. Explain Residents' Rights

Residents' Rights specify how residents must be treated while living in a facility. They provide an ethical code of conduct for healthcare workers. You need to be familiar with these rights. Residents' Rights are very detailed. They include the following:

Quality of life: Residents have the right to the best quality of life possible. Residents must have dignity, be able to make choices in their care and be able to make decisions independently.

Services and activities to maintain a high level of wellness: Residents must receive the correct care. Facilities are required to develop a care plan that helps determine residents' daily activities. Residents' care must keep them as healthy as possible every day. Their health should not decline as a direct result of the facility's care.

The right to be fully informed about rights and services: Residents must be told about all services offered and the fee for each service. Residents must be given a copy of their legal rights, along with the facility's rules and regulations. These rights must be in a language that each resident can understand. Residents must be given the names and phone numbers of state agencies related to quality of care, such as the ombudsman. Survey results must be shared with residents if they request to see them. Residents have the right to be notified about any change of room or roommate. Residents have the right to communicate with someone who speaks their language. They have the right to assistance for any sensory impairment, such as hearing loss.

The right to participate in their own care: Residents have the right to receive proper care, be told of changes in their health, and make decisions regarding their care (Fig. 2-5). They have the right to change care providers at any time. Residents have the right to refuse medication and treatments and to not allow restraints to be used. They have the right to review their medical record.

Fig. 2-5. Residents have the right to be informed about their care and to make decisions about the kind of care they want.

The right to make independent choices: Residents have the right to make decisions about their daily lives, their doctors, and to take part in community activities. They have the right to decide what to wear and how to spend their time. They have the right to act within a Residents' Council.

A **Residents' Council** is a group of residents who meet regularly to discuss issues related to

the nursing home. This Council gives residents a voice in facility operations. Topics of discussion may include facility policies, decisions regarding activities, concerns, and problems. The Residents' Council offers residents a chance to provide suggestions on improving the quality of care. Council executives are elected by residents. Family members are invited to attend meetings with or on behalf of residents. Staff may participate in this process when invited by Council members.

The right to privacy and confidentiality: Residents have the right to speak privately with anyone, the right to privacy during care, and the right to confidentiality about every aspect of their lives. They have the right to send mail and receive mail that is unopened (Fig. 2-6). Their medical and personal information cannot be shared with anyone but the care team. You will learn more about confidentiality in Learning Objective 11 of this chapter.

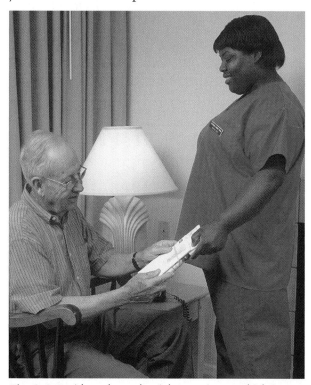

Fig. 2-6. Residents have the right to privacy, which includes being able to receive unopened mail.

The right to dignity, respect and freedom: Residents have the right to respectful treatment by caregivers. Residents cannot be abused in any way.

The right to security of possessions: Residents have the right to control their finances. They have the right not to be charged for any care covered by Medicaid or Medicare. Their personal possessions must be safe at all times. Residents have the right to file a complaint with the state agency for misappropriation of property. **Misappropriation** is taking what belongs to someone else and using it illegally for one's own gain.

Rights with transfers and discharges: Residents have the right to be informed of and to consent to any location changes. They can be moved from the facility if the resident's safety is at risk, if the resident's health has gotten better, if the move is needed to protect others at the facility, or if payment for care is not received by the facility. Residents also have the right to stay in a facility unless a transfer or discharge is needed.

The right to complain: Residents have the right to complain without any fear for their safety or care. They also have the right to a quick response to their concerns.

The right to visits: Residents have the right to visits from doctors, family members, friends, ombudsmen, legal representatives, or any other person (Fig. 2-7).

Fig. 2-7. *Residents have the right to receive visitors at any reasonable hour.*

Throughout this book you will see special boxes that will teach you how to promote Residents' Rights. Pay close attention to this informa-

tion. You must obey legal and ethical workplace guidelines.

7. Explain types of abuse and neglect

Abuse can occur in private homes or within any facility. **Abuse** is causing physical, mental, or emotional pain or injury to someone. There are many different types of abuse, including the following:

Physical abuse is intentional or unintentional treatment that causes harm to a person's body. Physical abuse includes hitting, kicking, cutting, burning, pushing or touching a resident in any way that causes pain or injury. It also includes rough handling of a person. Pushing a resident to move faster is one example of physical abuse. Hitting or pinching a resident is another example. Holding or restraining a resident is also considered abuse.

Psychological abuse is harming a person by threatening, scaring, insulting, humiliating, or treating him or her as a child. It also includes verbal abuse. **Verbal abuse** is oral or written words, pictures, or gestures that threaten or embarrass a person. Threatening to harm a resident if he tells another caregiver about a problem is one example of psychological abuse. Telling other residents about a private or embarrassing problem that a resident has is another example of psychological abuse.

Sexual abuse is forcing a person to perform or participate in sexual acts. Any kind of sexual behavior that causes a person to be fearful and feel threatened sexually is sexual abuse. For example, showing sexually explicit magazines to residents is sexual abuse. Rubbing against a resident inappropriately during personal care is also sexual abuse.

Financial abuse is stealing, taking advantage of, or improperly using the money, property, or other assets of another. For example, offering to give a resident "special" care if the resident pays the nursing assistant for it is financial abuse.

Stealing money from a resident is also financial abuse.

Assault happens when a person is threatened and feels fearful that he or she will be touched without his or her permission. Telling a resident that she will be slapped if she does not stop yelling is an example. Many lawsuits that include assault also include battery. **Battery** means a person is actually touched without his or her permission. An example is a nursing assistant hitting or pushing a resident. It is also physical abuse. Performing a procedure on a resident who has refused the procedure is also battery.

Domestic violence is abuse by spouses, intimate partners, or family members. It can be physical, sexual, or emotional. The victim can be a woman or man of any age or a child.

Workplace violence is the abuse of staff by other staff members, residents, or visitors. It includes both physical and verbal abuse. For example, one staff member hits another staff member during an argument. Another example is a resident who insults a nursing assistant's culture. Workplace violence also includes improper touching and discussion about sexual subjects.

False imprisonment is unlawfully restraining or confining someone against his or her will. Both the threat of being physically restrained and actually being physically restrained are false imprisonment. Not allowing a resident to leave the building is also false imprisonment.

Involuntary seclusion is confinement or separation from others into a separate physical space. It is done without consent or against one's will. For example, a resident is made to stay in her room with the door closed during the dinner hour.

Sexual harassment is any unwelcome sexual advance or behavior that creates an intimidating, hostile or offensive working environment. Requests for sexual favors, unwanted touching, and other acts of a sexual nature are examples of

sexual harassment. A supervisor telling a team member that if she has sex with him, she will get the work schedule she wants is one example of sexual harassment.

Substance abuse is the use of drugs, cigarettes, or alcohol in a way that harms oneself or others. Substances can be legal, or even prescribed, and still be abused. For example, alcohol and cigarettes are legal for adults, but are often abused. Over-the-counter medications can be addictive and harmful (Fig. 2-8). Even paint or glue may be abused. Information on the signs of substance abuse that must be reported is in Chapter 22.

Fig. 2-8. *Both prescription and non-prescription drugs can be abused.*

Neglect can be divided into two categories: active neglect and passive neglect. **Active neglect** is purposely harming a person physically, mentally, or emotionally by failing to provide needed care. Examples include deliberately leaving a bedridden resident alone for lengthy periods, ignoring a resident's call light, or willfully denying the resident food, medication, dentures, or eyeglasses. **Passive neglect** is unintentionally harming a person physically, mentally, or emotionally by failing to provide needed care. The caregiver may not know how to properly care for the resident, or may not understand the resident's needs. For example, a nursing assistant forgets to bring water to a resident who has a doctor's order to drink extra fluids.

ETHICAL AND LEGAL ISSUES

Negligence is actions, or a failure to act or give care, that results in injury to a person. For example, a nursing assistant forgets to lock the bed wheels before transferring a resident to a chair. The bed rolls backward and causes the resident to fall and injure herself. **Malpractice** occurs when a negligent or improper act by a doctor or other medical professional results in damage or injury to a person. Nursing assistants cannot be sued for malpractice; only licensed healthcare professionals can be sued for malpractice. However, nursing assistants can be named in other lawsuits because of the work they perform.

If you see or suspect that a resident is being abused in any way, you are legally required to report it. Report abuse immediately to your supervisor. Document any complaints of abuse reported to you and anything you witness yourself. If action is not taken, keep reporting up the chain of command. Do this until action is taken. If no appropriate action is taken at the facility, call the state abuse hotline. Usually this is an anonymous call. If no abuse hotline exists in your area, contact the proper state agency. Reporting abuse can be done in a way that protects you and does not identify you. These agencies are required to investigate reports of abuse.

If residents want to make a complaint of abuse themselves, you must assist in every possible way. This includes informing them of the process and their rights.

Never retaliate against a resident making a complaint of abuse. If you witness another team member retaliating against a resident who made a complaint, you must report it. Follow the chain of command. All care team members are responsible for residents' safety.

RESIDENTS' RIGHTS

They are all your residents.
All of the residents in your area or unit are your residents. Even though you may be assigned a certain number of residents, you must still respond to any resident in need. Never say, "He/she is not my resident."

8. Recognize signs and symptoms of abuse and neglect

Abuse can be suspected when staff observe certain signs and symptoms. All care team members must look for these signs and report them. Many of the signs of abuse are listed below.

Signs of physical abuse include:

- Unexplained broken bones
- Unexplained bruising
- Similar injuries that occur over and over, such as an injury shaped like a belt buckle
- Burns shaped in certain ways, like a cigarette burn or a burn caused by an iron
- Bite marks or scratches
- Unexplained weight loss, extremely dry and cracked skin, or signs of dehydration
- Missing hair
- Broken or missing teeth
- Blood in underwear
- Bruising in the genital area

Signs of psychological abuse include:

- Depression or withdrawal (Fig. 2-9)
- Mood swings
- Fear and anxiety, especially when a certain caregiver is present
- Lack of appetite
- Fear of being left alone

Fig. 2-9. *Withdrawal and depression are important signs to report.*

Signs of neglect include:

- Sores on the body
- Weight loss or signs of dehydration
- Frequent complaints of hunger or thirst
- Strong smell of urine
- Unclean body
- Dirty, matted, or unstyled hair
- Ragged or dirty fingernails
- Soiled clothes or bed linens
- Ripped or torn clothing
- Damaged or poorly-fitting hearing aids, glasses, or dentures
- Unanswered call lights

Other signs of abuse include:

- Missed doctor's appointments
- Changing doctors frequently
- Wearing makeup or sunglasses to hide injuries
- Family concern that abuse is occurring
- Person does not seem to be taking his medication
- Caregiver does not allow anyone to be alone with the resident

Remember that nursing assistants are legally required to report abuse or suspected abuse. Nursing assistants are considered "mandated reporters." **Mandated reporters** are people who are required to report suspected or observed abuse or neglect because they have regular contact with vulnerable populations, such as the elderly in nursing homes.

9. Describe the steps taken if a nursing assistant is suspected of abuse

After a report of nursing assistant abuse has been made, the NA is usually immediately suspended. The NATCEP (Nurse Aide Training and Competency Evaluation Program) is notified, as well as the facility administrator. A full, confidential investigation is done. The facility will protect the resident and the person who reported the abuse from retaliation. If the investigation does not prove the claim of abuse, the NA returns to work. If the investigation shows that there might be truth to the claim, specific actions are taken.

The NATCEP outlines steps that must be followed. These steps include investigation, notification, a hearing, decision of the hearing and the appeals process. If the findings show that abuse did occur, the nursing assistant is placed on the abuse registry, in addition to other possible legal penalties. The abuse registry is shared with other state abuse registries. Employers check this registry before hiring nursing assistants.

10. Discuss the ombudsman's role

The word "ombudsman" originally came from a Scandinavian word. In parts of Scandinavia, an ombudsman is a government official who investigates citizens' complaints. In nursing homes in the U.S., an **ombudsman** is the legal advocate for residents. The ombudsman visits the facility and listens to residents. He or she decides what course of action to take if there is a problem. An ombudsman can help settle disputes and resolve conflicts. He or she provides an ongoing presence in nursing homes to monitor care and conditions (Fig. 2-10).

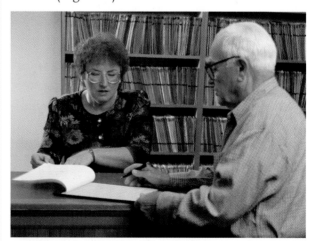

Fig. 2-10. An ombudsman is a legal advocate for residents who visits the facility and listens to residents. He or she also works with other agencies to resolve complaints.

An ombudsman typically performs these duties:

- Advocates for Residents' Rights and quality care
- Educates consumers and care providers
- Investigates and resolves complaints; works with investigators from the police, adult protective services, and health departments
- Appears in court and/or in legal hearings
- Gives information to the public

In some states, a group of specially-selected people may also investigate reports of abuse that occur in healthcare facilities.

There are also state agencies that can assist people with concerns about a facility. Know the name of your state's department that handles facility complaints. Some examples of departments that a resident or his family can contact are the State Department of Health and the State Department of Health and Human Services.

For more information about the ombudsman program, contact the department in your state that handles elder care or your legal aid society.

11. Explain HIPAA and related terms

One of the most important parts of a nursing assistant's job is to keep resident information confidential. Staff will learn residents' health information from the residents themselves, their families, or from their medical records. They may also learn personal information about a resident's finances or relationships. This information cannot be shared with anyone except other care team members.

The Health Insurance Portability and Accountability Act (HIPAA) was passed in 1996. It has been revised a few times since then. This law was written to protect the privacy of health information. It identifies certain **Protected Health Information (PHI)** that must remain confidential. It was also passed to facilitate the transferring of PHI for payment and research needs.

PHI is information that can be used to identify a person and relates to the patient's past, present, or future physical or mental condition; any health care that patient has had; or payment for that health care. PHI includes the patient's name, address, telephone number, medical record, social security number, e-mail address, and other information. This information must remain secure at all times in and out of the facility. All healthcare organizations must take special steps to protect health information. Only people who must have information for care or to process records can have access to this information (Fig. 2-11).

Fig. 2-11. HIPAA requires that special care be taken to keep medical records confidential. Only people who give care or process records should have access to this information.

HIPAA applies to all healthcare providers, including doctors, nurses, nursing assistants, and other care team members. Nursing assistants must never share any protected information with anyone who is not directly involved in the resident's care. For example, if a friend asks you about a resident's condition, the correct response is "I cannot share that information. It is confidential." Only people who have a legal reason to know about the resident, such as members of the care team, can share health information. Some ways that staff can keep information confidential are:

- Do not give health information on the telephone, unless you know you are speaking with an approved staff member.

- Do not give any personal information to any visitors, no matter who they are.

- Never share a medical record with anyone other than a staff member directly involved in the resident's care.

- Do not discuss residents in any public area, such as a restaurant, store, or waiting room (Fig. 2-12). Use private areas at the facility to give reports.

- Do not bring your family or friends to the facility to meet residents.

- Do not use cordless or cell phones to discuss resident information.

- Double-check fax numbers before faxing information. Use a cover sheet with a confidentiality statement.

- Return charts to their proper place after use. Hand charts directly to team members if transferring a resident to another unit or for a test.

- Turn off the computer when finished with your work.

- Do not include private information in e-mails.

- Give any documents you find with a resident's information to the nurse.

Fig. 2-12. *Do not discuss any information about residents in public places, such as grocery stores or restaurants. Only discuss residents' information with the care team.*

There can be serious penalties if you do not protect confidentiality and follow HIPAA guide-

lines. Team members may have to pay a fine and can even be sentenced to prison. All healthcare workers must follow HIPAA regulations.

Invasion of privacy is a legal term. It means violating a person's right to be left alone or exposing information about that person without his or her consent. This includes releasing private facts, such as a medical record or even a photograph, without the person's consent. For example, invasion of privacy could be charged if a caregiver released medical information about a resident to a newspaper.

Discussing a resident's care or personal affairs with anyone other than your supervisor or another member of the care team could be considered an invasion of privacy, which violates civil law.

12. Discuss The Patient Self-Determination Act (PSDA) and advance directives

The Patient Self-Determination Act (PSDA) is a federal law originally passed in 1990. This law encourages people to make decisions about advance directives. **Advance directives** are written documents or oral statements that allow people to decide what kind of medical care they wish to have if they are unable to make those decisions themselves. An advance directive can also designate someone else to make medical decisions for a person if that person is disabled. Rules on how to execute these documents vary from state to state.

Living Wills and a Durable Power of Attorney for Health Care are examples of advance directives. A **Living Will** states the medical care a person wants, or does not want, in case he or she becomes unable to make those decisions. For example, a person may specify that certain measures are to be taken or withheld if he is in a coma. It is called a "Living Will" because it takes effect while the person is still alive. It may also be called a "directive to physicians," "health care declaration," or "medical directive."

A **Durable Power of Attorney for Health Care** is a signed, dated, and witnessed paper that appoints someone to make the medical decisions for a person in the event he or she becomes unable to do so. This can include instructions about medical treatment the person wants to avoid. Because the term "power of attorney" indicates legal issues, people may think this means that someone can take control of a person's money, property, etc. This document, however, deals only with medical issues.

A **do-not-resuscitate (DNR)** order is another way to honor wishes about health care. A DNR order tells medical professionals not to perform CPR (cardiopulmonary resuscitation). CPR consists of the medical procedures used to restart a person's heart and breathing. You will learn more about CPR in Chapter 8. A DNR order means that providers will not attempt to give emergency CPR if breathing or the heartbeat stops. Generally these orders are used by people who are in the final stages of a terminal illness or who have a very serious condition.

Types of advance directives may be used together, or a person may elect to use one or none at all. Having an advance directive is not legally required. However, it is a good way to make sure a person's wishes regarding medical care are honored. An advance directive can be changed or canceled at any time, either in writing, or verbally, or both.

The PSDA requires that all facilities receiving Medicare and Medicaid money offer new residents information about their rights relating to advance directives. These rights include:

- The right to participate in and direct health-care decisions
- The right to accept or refuse treatment
- The right to prepare an advance directive
- Information on policies that govern these rights

The PSDA requires that facilities give new residents the facility's policies on handling advance directives. Each facility must ask residents what advance directives they have and obtain copies of these documents (Fig. 2-13). In addition, facilities must offer education to the staff about advance directives.

Fig. 2-13. *A sample form showing a person's wishes regarding advance directives. (Reprinted with permission of the Briggs Corporation, 800-247-2343.)*

HOT TIP

Wills and Living Wills
A Living Will is different from a will. A will is a legal document that details how a person wants his possessions to be disposed of after his death. If a resident tells you that he or she wants to prepare a will, notify the nurse. Many facilities have a rule that staff should not witness a will, even if a resident asks you to do so. Know your facility's policy about witnessing any legal documents.

CHAPTER REVIEW

1. What are ethics (LO 2)?

2. Give one example of a law that must be followed. (LO 2)

3. List five ways that a nursing assistant can behave ethically. Give an example of each that is not listed in the textbook (LO 3).

4. Describe five points of a typical nursing assistant code of ethics (LO 4).

5. Explain what OBRA covers (LO 5).

6. What is the minimum number of hours of training that a nursing assistant must complete (LO 5)?

7. What are ten different Residents' Rights (LO 6)?

8. Why do you think Residents' Rights are so important (LO 6)?

9. List eight different kinds of abuse and give one example of each (LO 7).

10. What are active neglect and passive neglect (LO 7)?

11. Give an example of negligence (LO 7).

12. What is a nursing assistant's responsibility if she sees or suspects abuse (LO 7)?

13. List 20 signs of abuse and/or neglect (LO 8).

14. What generally happens to a nursing assistant after a report of abuse has been made (LO 9)?

15. Describe some of the typical duties of an ombudsman (LO 10).

16. With whom can a nursing assistant share a resident's health information (LO 11)?

17. What does HIPAA protect (LO 11)?

18. List four examples of PHI (LO 11).

19. To which members of the care team does HIPAA apply (LO 11)?

20. What is an advance directive (LO 12)?

21. List four rights that apply to advance directives that the PSDA requires be given to new residents (LO 12).

3
Communication Skills

Hippocrates: The "Father of Medicine"

Hippocrates was a Greek physician who lived during the time period of about 400 B.C. Known as the "Father of Medicine," Hippocrates formed some of the earliest medical words in his writings. The Hippocratic Oath, a code of ethics, is named after him. Many new doctors continue to take this oath today.

In approximately 100 A.D. the early Romans developed the basis for the medical language of today. The Romans started keeping records of new words they developed from all of their experiences with wounded soldiers in the battlefield. The impressive record-keeping by the Romans, along with the prior work of Hippocrates, laid the groundwork for Greek and Latin to become the two primary languages of medicine.

"Old age, especially an honored old age, has so great authority, that this is of more value than all the pleasures of youth."

Marcus Tullius Cicero, 106-43 B.C.

"Never promise more than you can perform."

Maxim 45

1. Define important words in this chapter

active listening: a way of communicating that involves giving a person your full attention while he is speaking and encouraging him to give information and clarify ideas; includes nonverbal communication.

barrier: a block or an obstacle.

body language: all of the conscious or unconscious messages your body sends as you communicate, such as facial expressions, shrugging your shoulders, and wringing your hands.

care conference: a meeting to share and gather information about residents in order to develop a care plan.

care plan: a written plan for each resident created by the nurse; outlines the steps taken by the staff to help the resident reach his or her goals.

chart: written legal record of all care received within a facility.

charting: the act of noting care and observations; documenting.

code: when a group of specially-trained staff is called to provide advanced life support to a resident.

code status: whether a resident has a signed advance directive or not.

critical thinking: the process of reasoning and analyzing in order to solve problems; for the nursing assistant, critical thinking means making good observations and promptly reporting all potential problems.

culture: a set of learned beliefs, values, traditions, and behaviors shared by a social, ethnic, or age group.

edema: swelling in body tissues caused by excess fluid.

incident: an accident, problem, or unexpected event during the course of care.

incident report: a written report documenting the incident and the response to the incident.

Minimum Data Set (MDS): a detailed form with guidelines for assessing residents in nursing homes; also details what to do if resident problems are identified.

nonverbal communication: communication without words, such as gestures and facial expressions.

nursing process: an organized method used by nurses to determine residents' needs, plan the appropriate care to meet those needs, and evaluate how well the plan of care is working; five steps are assessment, diagnosis, planning, implementation, and evaluation.

prefix: a word part added to the beginning of a root to create a new meaning.

prioritize: to place things in order of importance.

objective information: factual information collected using the senses of sight, hearing, smell, and touch; also called signs.

root: the main part of the word that gives it meaning.

rounds: physical movement of staff from room to room to discuss each resident and the plans of care.

sentinel event: an unexpected occurrence involving death or serious physical or psychological injury.

subjective information: information collected from residents, their family members and friends; information may or may not be true but is what the person reported; also called symptoms.

suffix: a word part added to the end of a root or a prefix to create a new meaning.

verbal communication: communication involving the use of spoken or written words or sounds.

vital signs: measurements that monitor the function of the vital organs of the body.

2. Explain types of communication

Communication is the exchange of information with others. It is a process of sending and receiving messages. People communicate with signs and symbols, such as words, drawings, and pictures; they also communicate with behavior.

People have different roles during communication. A person can be the "sender" or the "receiver." The person who communicates first is the "sender," sending a message. The person who receives the message is called the "receiver." Receiver and sender switch roles as they communicate. The third step is giving feedback. The receiver repeats the message or responds to it to let the sender know the message was received and understood. All three steps must occur before the process is complete. During a conversa-

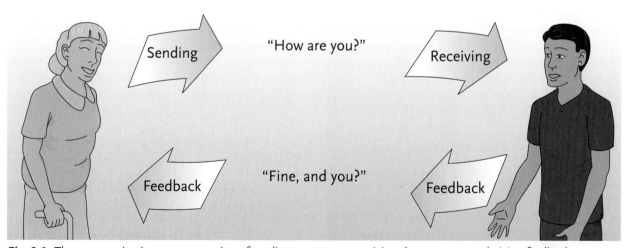

Fig. 3-1. The communication process consists of sending a message, receiving the message, and giving feedback.

tion, this process occurs over and over (Fig. 3-1).

Communicating verbally means using words. Speaking and writing are two ways of communicating verbally. Oral reports are an example of **verbal communication**. You will learn more about these reports in Learning Objective 18. Verbal communication also includes the way in which words are spoken or written. How the voice sounds when a person speaks says as much as the words he uses. For example, if a nursing assistant sounds irritated when saying, "Let me know if you need anything else," the resident may feel that the nursing assistant does not want to be bothered. The resident may not want to communicate a need because he fears it will make the nursing assistant angry. The words a person chooses send a message as well. Always use a pleasant tone of voice with residents, and carefully consider your choice of words before speaking.

When writing information, be clear and direct. Check to see if you are using the right words so that you will be understood. Also make sure to write clearly so that others can read your information correctly.

Nonverbal communication is communicating without using words. **Body language** is a form of nonverbal communication. Body language has to do with all of the conscious or unconscious messages your body sends as you communicate. It includes posture, body movements, facial expressions, and gestures (Fig. 3-2). Body language can add positive or negative messages during communication. For example, if you smile and tell a resident, "I'll be glad to help you find your glasses, Mrs. Martinez," that communicates that you are willing to help. However, if you roll your eyes while responding, it sends a message that you are annoyed by the request.

Touch is another important part of nonverbal communication. Some people are more comfortable with being touched than others. Some find it comforting, while others may be offended by

it. Nursing assistants have to touch residents during care. However, if a resident is more comfortable being touched less, limit touch as much as possible. Always ask permission before touching a resident.

Fig. 3-2. *Just as with speaking, body language sends messages. Which of these people seems more interested in their conversation—the person slouching in his chair or the person sitting up straight and smiling?*

Below are some examples of positive and negative nonverbal communication:

Positive Nonverbal Communication:

- smiling in a friendly manner
- leaning forward to listen
- with permission, putting your hand over a resident's hand while listening to her

Negative Nonverbal Communication:

- rolling your eyes or crossing your arms
- tapping your foot
- pointing at someone while speaking

As you read the examples of body language, think about how each would make you feel. If a resident seems offended by your behavior, think about what you might be communicating with your body. Make positive changes in your body language. It will improve the way you relate to other people.

To communicate properly, do the following:

- Use appropriate words. Make sure residents are able to understand what you say. Use proper words and terms with care team members.
- Be aware of your body language.

- Use an acceptable tone of voice. Communicate concern and caring.

- Wait for responses. Let pauses happen. Do not interrupt or try to finish the person's sentences.

- Practice active listening. **Active listening** involves giving residents your full attention while they are speaking. Maintain good eye contact. Use phrases that encourage them to keep speaking and to clarify their communication. Examples are "Yes," "Hmm," "I see," and "I understand." "Go on" is another example. Repeat the resident's message to show you have been listening closely. Active listening also includes nonverbal communication, such as nodding and smiling. Show residents you are really interested in what they have to say.

- Use facts when communicating. A fact is something that is definitely true. An opinion is something believed to be true, but is not proven to be true. For example, "Ms. Simpson weighs 155 pounds" is a fact. "I think Ms. Simpson looks thinner" is an opinion. It might be true, but cannot be backed up with evidence. If you give an opinion to the care team, make it clear that what you are saying is an opinion, not a fact. Both facts and opinions are valuable to the care team. However, using mostly facts will help you communicate more effectively.

3. Explain barriers to communication

Some residents will have trouble understanding or using verbal (spoken or written) communication. This is due to a barrier that prevents proper communication. A **barrier** is a block or an obstacle. For example, a resident who is hearing-impaired may not understand you when you are explaining a care procedure.

These are some barriers and ways to avoid them (Fig. 3-3):

Resident does not hear you, does not hear correctly, or does not understand. Stand directly facing the resident. Speak slowly. Make sure each word is spoken clearly. Do not shout, whisper or mumble. Speak in a low, pleasant voice. Use a professional tone of voice. If the resident wears a hearing aid, check to see that it is on and works properly.

Resident is difficult to understand. Be patient. Take the time to listen. Ask the resident to repeat or explain. State the message in your own words to make sure you have understood. If the resident becomes frustrated, take a break and try again in a few minutes or find someone else to listen with you.

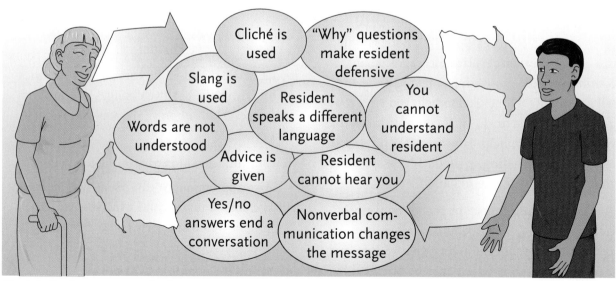

Fig. 3-3. Barriers to communication.

Message uses words receiver does not understand. Do not use medical terminology with residents or their families. Use simple, everyday words. Do not pretend to understand what a word means. Ask what a word means if you are not sure.

Do not use slang. Do not curse. Avoid slang; it can confuse the message. It may not be understood and is unprofessional. Never curse or use profanity even if the resident does.

Avoid clichés. Clichés are phrases that are used repeatedly and do not really mean anything. For example, "Everything will be okay" is a cliché. Instead of using a cliché, listen to what your resident is really saying. Respond with a meaningful and thoughtful message. For example, if a resident is afraid of having a bath, say "I understand that it seems scary to you. What can I do to make you feel more at ease?" Do not say, "Oh, it'll be over before you know it."

Asking "why" makes the resident defensive. Try not to ask "why" when a resident speaks. "Why" questions make people feel defensive. For example, a resident may say she does not want to participate in an activity. If you ask, "Why not?" you may get an angry response. Instead, ask, "Are you too tired to do this? Is there something else you want to do?" The resident may then be willing to discuss the issue.

Giving advice is inappropriate. Do not offer your opinion or give advice. Residents and family members should make decisions on their own or with help from doctors. Giving medical advice is not within the scope of your practice. It could be dangerous. People with more education and experience, such as doctors, can give medical advice.

Yes/no answers end a conversation. Ask open-ended questions that need more than a "yes" or "no" answer. Yes and no answers end conversation. For example, if you want to know what a resident likes to eat, do not ask "Do you like meatloaf?" Instead, try "What are some of your favorite foods?"

Resident speaks a different language. If a resident speaks a different language than you do, speak slowly and clearly. Keep your messages short and simple. Be alert for words the resident understands. Also be alert for signs that the resident is only pretending to understand you. You may need to use pictures and gestures to communicate. Ask the resident's family, friends, or other staff members who speak the resident's language for help. Be patient and calm.

Nonverbal communication changes the message. Be aware of your body language and gestures. Look for nonverbal messages from residents and clarify them. For example "Ms. Gold, you say you're doing well but you seem to be in pain. Is that true? Can I help in any way?"

4. List ways that cultures impact communication

The world is full of many different cultures. A **culture** is a set of learned beliefs, values and behaviors shared by a social, ethnic, or age group. Cultures communicate in many different ways.

The use of eye contact varies from culture to culture. One culture may believe a person should look another person in the eye when speaking. That culture may think it is a sign of honesty or respect. Another culture may find this rude or aggressive. People may view looking someone in the eye as disrespectful. Learn about your residents' behaviors and preferences. If a resident is sensitive to eye contact, try to limit it as much as possible.

As you learned earlier, touch is another important way to communicate. Touch practices differ from one culture to another (Fig. 3-4). Preferences regarding touch may also just be a part of a person's personality. You will need to touch residents during daily care. However, if a resident is uncomfortable with touch, respect this. Below are some examples of acceptable and unacceptable touch:

Fig. 3-4. How a person perceives touch may depend on his background.

Acceptable Touch

- Giving residents respectful personal care, such as bathing, dressing, feeding, and shaving

- Hugging, if the resident permits or asks for it

- Holding a resident's hand when she asks you to

Unacceptable Touch

- Sitting on a resident's lap or asking a resident to sit on your lap

- Kissing a resident

- Hugging a resident who pulls away from you

- Inappropriately touching or rubbing against a resident or staff member

Language barriers can be a problem in communication. A resident's first language may be different than yours. One way to deal with this is to use an interpreter. An interpreter is a person who speaks the resident's language and can translate words from another language to explain the message. A slight change in pronunciation can change the meaning of words.

An interpreter will make sure that residents can fully understand the information you are giving them. Picture cards and flash cards can also assist with communication.

You can also try to learn a few words or phrases in a resident's native language. An interpreter can help with that. A resident's family and friends may also be able to help. Hearing a few words in residents' native languages may be comforting to them. Do not speak with other staff in a different language in front of residents.

5. Identify the people you will communicate with in a facility

There are many people you will communicate with on a daily basis while in a facility. Some of these people are listed below.

Doctors, Nurses, Supervisors, Managers, and Other Staff Members

As you learned in Chapter 1, there are different care team members. Nursing assistants will communicate with the care team both verbally and nonverbally. Charting information and using the telephone and call systems are other ways you will communicate. You may use a computer and be involved in care planning. More information on each of these methods is listed later in the chapter. Be familiar with them, as they promote better communication with the care team.

Other Departments

Nursing assistants will communicate with other departments, such as the dietary department. This may happen in person or over the phone. A good relationship with other departments in a facility is very important. It helps deliver excellent, organized care. Be positive in your dealings with other departments. Keep communication open and friendly. If you experience a problem with another department, report it to the nurse.

Residents

The most important communication with residents happens each time you greet them. At that time, you will introduce yourself and identify the resident. You will explain the procedure you are going to be doing and encourage the resident's participation. You will do this for every resident each time you provide care. Facilities may use name bands or photos to help identify residents. Explaining care before you give it is an important part of communication. It's also part of Residents' Rights.

Families and Visitors

The care team should try to have a good, open relationship with residents' families and friends. One way to do this is to always respond immediately when a resident calls for help. This lets family and friends know that you are taking great care of their loved ones. Responding immediately to requests also helps prevent injury. Families are a rich source of information regarding residents' likes, dislikes, and histories (Fig. 3-5). Ask them about residents' preferences and experiences. You will learn more and be able to provide better care.

Fig. 3-5. *Take time to talk to residents' family members about residents' preferences, routines, and histories.*

The Community

Staff may receive calls from doctors' offices or clinics. Staff from these offices may visit the facility. Refer any questions to your supervisor. Keep all resident and staff information confidential, unless you have been instructed otherwise.

6. Understand basic medical terminology and abbreviations

In order to communicate well with care team members, you will need to learn medical language. You will use medical terms for specific conditions. For example, **edema** is swelling in body tissues caused by excess fluid.

Medical terms are made up of these word parts: roots, prefixes, and suffixes. A **root** is the main part of the word that gives it meaning. For example, the root "scope" means an instrument to look inside. The prefix "oto" means ear. An otoscope is an instrument used to examine the ear.

A **prefix** comes at the front of the word. It works with a word root to make a new term. For example, the prefix "brady" means slow. The root "cardia" means heart. "Bradycardia" means slow heart rate or pulse.

A **suffix** is found at the end of a word. A suffix by itself does not form a full word. When you add a prefix or a root, the suffix turns it into a working medical term. For example, the suffix "meter" means measuring instrument. The prefix "thermo" means heat. A thermometer is an instrument that measures body temperature. One of the most common suffixes is "-logy," which means the study of something. You will mostly see it when it refers to a medical specialty, such as cardiology. Cardiology is the study of the heart.

Very soon, you will be able to look at word parts and recognize them immediately. Your instructor has more examples of roots, prefixes, and suffixes for you to review.

When speaking with residents and their families, use simple, non-medical terms. When you speak with the care team, medical terms will help you give more complete information.

Abbreviations are another way to communicate more efficiently. For example, the abbreviation "p.r.n." means "when necessary." "Stat" means "immediately." "BP" or "B/P" means blood pressure. Learn the standard medical abbreviations your facility uses. Use them to report information concisely and accurately. You may need to know these abbreviations to read assignments, care plans, or medical charts. A brief list of abbreviations is below. A more comprehensive list is found at the end of this textbook, but it is not a complete list. Check with your facility to see if there are others you must know.

ADLs	activities of daily living
amb	ambulatory
b.i.d.	two times a day
BM	bowel movement
BP, B/P	blood pressure
$\bar{c}$	with
c/o	complains of
DNR	do not resuscitate
Dx, dx	diagnosis
h, hr	hour
H_2O	water
I&O	intake and output
inc	incontinent
isol	isolation
IV	intravenous (within vein)
meds	medications
min	minute
mL	milliliter
NKA	no known allergies
NPO	nothing by mouth
PPE	personal protective equipment
p.r.n., prn	when necessary
q2h, q3h, etc.	every 2 hours, every 3 hours, and so on
q.h., qh	every hour
$\bar{s}$	without
stat	immediately
T, temp	temperature
t.i.d., tid	three times a day
TPR	temperature, pulse, and respiration
v.s., VS	vital signs
w/c, W/C	wheelchair

7. Explain how to convert regular time to military time

Facilities may use the 24-hour clock, or military time, to document information (Fig. 3-6). Regular time uses numbers 1 to 12 to show each of the 24 hours in a day. In military time, the hours are numbered from 00 to 23. So, using this system, midnight is expressed as 00, 1 a.m. is 01, 1 p.m. is 13, and so on.

Fig. 3-6. *Divisions in the 24-hour clock.*

Both regular and military time list minutes and seconds the same way. The minutes and seconds do not change when converting from regular to military time. Regular time uses a.m. and p.m. to show what time of day it is. These are not used in military time, since specific numbers show each hour of the day.

To change the regular hours between 1:00 p.m. to 11:59 p.m. to military time, add 12 to the regular time. For example, to change 4:00 p.m. to military time, add 4 + 12. The time is expressed as 1600 hours. To change 1:42 p.m. to military time, add 1 + 12. The minutes do not change. The time is expressed as 1342 hours.

Midnight is the only time that differs. Midnight is often written as 0000. However, some places use 2400 to express midnight. This follows the rule of adding 12 to the regular time. Follow your facility's policy on this.

To change from military time to regular time, subtract 12 from the hours. Again, the minutes do not change. For example, to change 1600 hours to standard time, subtract 16 - 12. The time is expressed as 4:00 p.m. To change 2210 hours to standard time, subtract 22 - 12. The result is 10:10 p.m.

Examples of the way the numbers are written follow:

Regular to Military
3:00 p.m. = 1500 (fifteen-hundred hours)

Military to Regular
1115 = 11:15 a.m.

8. Describe a standard resident chart

The **chart**, or resident medical record, is the legal record of a resident's care. What is written in the chart is considered in court to be what actually happened. This chart is saved for as long as the law dictates it be kept. It is saved in case other care providers need to refer to the chart. A provider may need medical history or information about an advance directive. Lawyers or courts may also request to see a chart if there is a legal need. The information found in the medical chart includes:

- Admission forms
- Resident's history and results of physical examinations
- Care plans

- Doctor's orders
- Doctor's progress notes
- Nursing assessments
- Nurse's notes
- Notes from physical therapists, occupational therapists and other specialists
- Flow sheets
- Graphic record
- Intake and output record
- Consent forms
- Lab and test results
- Surgery reports
- Advance directives

Your responsibility with the resident's chart is to gather information and report it to the nurse. You will write down your observations and care. This is called **charting**. You may also use a computer to record this information. You will read more about documentation in Learning Objective 9.

Some facilities allow nursing assistants to chart in a medical record. Others will limit nursing assistants' charting to certain forms. Follow your facility's policies. Remember, all of the information you see or add to a chart is confidential.

RESIDENTS' RIGHTS

Confidentiality

The observations you gather about residents are private information. They cannot be shared with anyone except for the care team. You would not want anything private repeated about you or any of your loved ones. Remember that the resident is someone's mother, father, sister, brother, or friend. He or she feels the same way. However, confidentiality is not only about promoting respect and dignity. Keeping residents' information confidential is the law. You must obey it. See information on HIPAA in Chapter 2.

9. Explain guidelines for documentation

Nursing assistants chart, or document, all care that they give residents. They document their observations, too. It is very important to document accurately (Fig. 3-7). Documentation provides an up-to-date record of each resident's status and care. As you learned before, the medical chart is a legal document. Documentation is a legal record of all resident care. Documentation is also important for planning residents' care. General documentation guidelines are listed below.

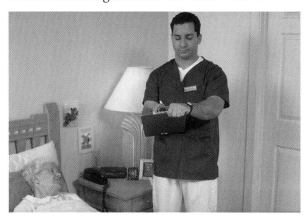

Fig. 3-7. *Documenting accurately provides important information about residents to the care team.*

Guidelines

Accurate Documentation

- Keep all information in the chart confidential.

- Document immediately after care is given. Record your notes carefully. Never record any care before it is done.

- Use black ink when documenting. Write neatly.

- Sign each note you make in the chart. Sign your name and title. Some states require you to list your full name; others require your first initial and last name. Write it the way your state requires. For example, Max Johnson, NA (or CNA) or M. Johnson, NA. Use the correct date and time.

- Use only facts, not opinions, when documenting. Write exactly what the person has said, or what you see, hear, smell, or touch. The words "seems," "appears to be," or "looks like" are not used in charting. For example, "The resident doesn't seem to like her family" is an opinion. "The resident yelled at her relatives and asked them to leave" is a fact.

- If you make a mistake, draw one line through it. Write the correct information. Put your initials and the date (Fig. 3-8). Do not erase what you have written. Do not use correction fluid.

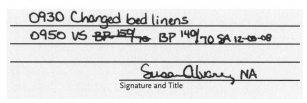

Fig. 3-8. *One example of how to correct a mistake.*

- Use only your facility's accepted abbreviations and terms. A sample list of abbreviations is at the back of this book.

- Use comparisons to describe size instead of words like "large," "medium," or "small." For example, "There is a spot of blood on her bandage the size of a dime."

All facilities will have policies and procedures for documenting. Follow them. Some facilities will require documentation on a "check-off" sheet. This is also called an ADL (activities of daily living) or flow sheet (Fig. 3-9). You will learn more about ADLs in Chapter 12.

HOT TIP

Little Letters, Big Meanings
Have you ever wondered what the following little abbreviations mean?
et al. (Latin "et alia"): means "and other things." Only "al" has a period at the end.
i.e. (Latin "id est"): means "that is." Both letters have a period.
e.g. (Latin "exempli gratia"): means "for example." Both letters have a period.

10. Describe the use of computers in documentation

Some care facilities require that computers be used to document information. Computers can easily store information that can be retrieved when it is needed. This is usually faster and more legible than writing by hand.

In some facilities, a computer is in every resident's room. Staff input information each time

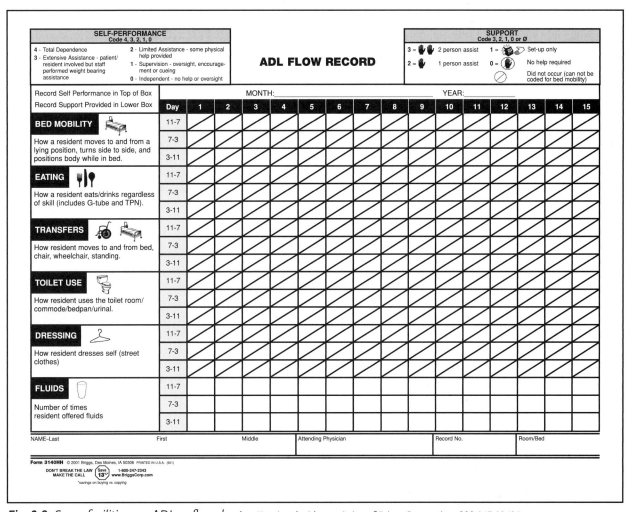

Fig. 3-9. *Some facilities use ADL or flow sheets. (Reprinted with permission of Briggs Corporation, 800-247-2343.)*

they enter and leave the room. This replaces time-consuming paper charting, although some paperwork still may need to be done.

Facilities will train staff on computer use. Nursing assistants must follow the rules for computerized charting. These are some general rules for computer use:

- Do not share your personal password or log-in ID with anyone.

- Do not access personal e-mail accounts at work.

- Do not view inappropriate websites from work.

- Log off the computer when you are done with charting or using the computer.

- HIPAA privacy guidelines apply to computer

use. Be careful about who can see private or protected health information (PHI) on the computer screen.

11. Explain the Minimum Data Set (MDS)

The **Minimum Data Set (MDS)** manual is an assessment tool developed by the federal government. It gives long-term care facilities a structured, standardized approach to care. The original edition was produced in 1990. The manual is revised periodically.

The MDS is a detailed form with guidelines for assessing residents. It also explains what to do if resident problems are identified. The manual provides examples and definitions for nurses to help them complete the assessments accurately (Fig. 3-10).

Numeric Identifier_____

MINIMUM DATA SET (MDS) – *VERSION 2.0*
FOR NURSING HOME RESIDENT ASSESSMENT AND CARE SCREENING
BASIC ASSESSMENT TRACKING FORM

SECTION AA. IDENTIFICATION INFORMATION

1. RESIDENT NAME ✱ — (Exactly as appears on Medicare Card)
a. (First)   b. (Middle Initial)   c. (Last)   d. (Jr./Sr.)

2. GENDER ✱ — 1. Male   2. Female

3. BIRTHDATE ✱ — (Complete all four digits)
Month – Day – Year

4. RACE/ETHNICITY ✱
1. American Indian/Alaskan Native   4. Hispanic
2. Asian/Pacific Islander   5. White, not of Hispanic origin
3. Black, not of Hispanic origin

5. SOCIAL SECURITY AND MEDICARE NUMBERS ✱ ✱
[C in 1st box if non Med. no.]
a. Social Security Number
b. Medicare number (or comparable railroad insurance number)

6. FACILITY PROVIDER NO. ✱
a. State No.   (Facility Medicaid Provider number)
(Facility Medicare Provider number)
b. Federal No.

7. MEDICAID NO. ["+" if pending, "N" if not a Medicaid recipient] ✱
(Resident Medicaid number)

8. REASONS FOR ASSESSMENT
Use 8a if NOT Medicare covered, leave 8b blank.
Use 8a & b if Medicare covered.

[Note–Other codes do not apply to this form]
a. Primary reason for assessment ☐
1. Admission assessment (required by day 14) - may be ➤
2. Annual assessment
3. Significant change in status assessment - may be ➤
4. Significant correction of prior full assessment - may be ➤
5. Quarterly review assessment
10. Significant correction of prior quarterly assessment
0. *NONE OF ABOVE*
b. Codes for assessments required for Medicare PPS or the State
1. *Medicare 5 day assessment*
2. *Medicare 30 day assessment*
3. *Medicare 60 day assessment*
4. *Medicare 90 day assessment*
5. *Medicare readmission/return assessment*
6. *Other state required assessment*
7. *Medicare 14 day assessment*
8. *Other Medicare required assessment*

9. Signatures of Persons who Completed a Portion of the Accompanying Assessment or Tracking Form

I certify that the accompanying information accurately reflects resident assessment or tracking information for this resident and that I collected or coordinated collection of this information on the dates specified. To the best of my knowledge, this information was collected in accordance with applicable Medicare and Medicaid requirements. I understand that this information is used as a basis for ensuring that residents receive appropriate and quality care, and as a basis for payment from federal funds. I further understand that payment of such federal funds and continued participation in the government-funded health care programs is conditioned on the accuracy and truthfulness of this information, and that I may be personally subject to or may subject my organization to substantial criminal, civil, and/or administrative penalties for submitting false information. I also certify that I am authorized to submit this information by this facility on its behalf.

Signature and Title	Sections	Date
a.		
b.		
c.		
d.		
e.		
f.		
g.		
h.		
i.		
j.		
k.		
l.		

GENERAL INSTRUCTIONS

Complete this information for submission with all full and quarterly assessments (Admission, Annual, Significant Change, State or Medicare required assessments, or Quarterly Reviews, etc.).

MDS RUG III CASE MIX GROUPS

RU = Rehabilitation Ultra High
RV = Rehabilitation Very High
RH = Rehabilitation High
RM = Rehabilitation Medium
RL = Rehabilitation Low
SE = Extensive Services
SS = Special Care
CC
CB } = Clinically Complex
CA

✱ = Key items for computerized resident tracking

▨ = When box blank, must enter number or letter

a. = When letter in box, check if condition applies

Code "–" if information unavailable or unknown

◆ = Quality Indicator/ Quality Measure

▬ = Related to the Top 26 RUG III Case Mix Classifications

☐ = Related to the Lower RUG III Case Mix Classifications

QM LEGEND: Chronic Care & Post-Acute
Percent of short stay residents who had moderate to severe pain
Percent of short stay residents with delirium
Percent of short stay residents with pressure sores
Percent of residents whose need for help with daily activities has increased
Percent of residents who have moderate to severe pain
Percent of residents who were physically restrained
Percent of high-risk residents who have pressure sores
Percent of low-risk residents who have pressure sores
Percent of residents with a urinary tract infection
Percent of residents who spent most of their time in bed or in a chair
Percent of residents who have become more depressed or anxious
Percent of low-risk residents who lose control of their bowels or bladder
Percent of residents who have/had a catheter inserted and left in their bladder
Percent of residents whose ability to move about in and around their room got worse

QI LEGEND
❶ Incidence new fractures
❷ Prevalence of falls
❸ Prevalence of behavioral symptoms affecting others
❹ Prevalence of symptoms of depression
❺ Prevalence of depression w/o antidepressants
❻ 9+ medications
❼ Incidence of cognitive impairment
❽ Prevalence of bladder or bowel incontinence
❾ Prevalence of occasional bladder or bowel incontinence w/o plan
❿ Prevalence of indwelling catheter
⓫ Prevalence of fecal impaction*
⓬ Prevalence of UTI
⓭ Prevalence of weight loss
⓮ Prevalence of tube feeding
⓯ Prevalence of dehydration*
⓰ Prevalence of bedfast residents
⓱ Incidence of decline in late loss ADLs
⓲ Incidence of decline in ROM
⓳ Prevalence of antipsychotic use in absence of psychotic conditions
⓴ Prevalence of antianxiety/hypnotic use
㉑ Prevalence of hypnotic use > 2x/wk
㉒ Prevalence of daily restraints
㉓ Prevalence of little or no activity
㉔ Prevalence of stage 1-4 pressure ulcers*

*SENTINEL HEALTH EVENT

TRIGGER LEGEND
1 - Delirium
2 - Cognitive Loss/Dementia
3 - Visual Function
4 - Communication
5A - ADL-Rehabilitation
5B - ADL-Maintenance
6 - Urinary Incontinence and Indwelling Catheter
7 - Psychosocial Well-Being
8 - Mood State
9 - Behavioral Symptoms
10A - Activities (Revise)
10B - Activities (Review)
11 - Falls
12 - Nutritional Status
13 - Feeding Tubes
14 - Dehydration/Fluid Maintenance
15 - Dental Care
16 - Pressure Ulcers
17 - Psychotropic Drug Use
17* - For this to trigger, O4a, b, or c must = 1-7
18 - Physical Restraints

For additional information on MDS required schedule and documentation to justify skilled care, see page 8.

Form 1728EHH © 1997 Briggs Corporation, Des Moines, IA 50306   (800) 247-2343   PRINTED IN U.S.A.
R104   Copyright limited to addition of trigger, coding, QI and QM recognition systems

MDS 2.0   September 2000

1 of 9

Fig. 3-10. A sample MDS form. (Reprinted with permission of the Briggs Corporation, 800-247-2343.)

Facilities must complete the MDS for each resident within 14 days of admission and again each year. In addition, the MDS for each resident must be reviewed every three months. A new MDS is done when there is any major change in a resident's condition.

The MDS helps the care team identify problems with a resident's health. Always report changes you notice to the nurse. The reporting you do on changes in your residents may "trigger" a needed assessment. Changes may be a sign of a problem or illness. By reporting them right away, a new MDS assessment can be done if needed.

12. Describe how to observe and report accurately

Nursing assistants spend more time with residents than any other care team member. Because of this, they may observe more changes in residents than other team members. Reporting these observations accurately and in a timely manner is very important. These observations are vital to the care plan.

A **care plan** is a written plan for each resident created by the nurse. It outlines the steps and tasks that the care team must perform to help the resident achieve his or her goals (Fig. 3-11). The care plan must be followed very carefully.

In order to plan care, nurses collect information from staff. Nursing assistants will report signs and symptoms that they observed. This information will be either objective or subjective.

Objective information is information based on what you see, hear, touch, or smell; it is collected

Fig. 3-11. *A sample resident care plan. (Reprinted with permission of Briggs Corporation, 800-247-2343.)*

using four of the five senses: sight, hearing, smell, and touch. It is also called "signs." **Subjective information** is information collected from something that residents or their families reported to you, and it may or may not be accurate. It is also called "symptoms." Subjective information is something you cannot or did not observe. This is information the "subject" is telling you, so it is an opinion. Objective information may confirm subjective information.

An example of objective information is "Mr. Hartman is rubbing his temples and holding his head." A subjective report might be, "Mr. Hartman says he has a headache." Both objective and subjective reports are valuable.

Your observations can alert staff to possible problems. To report accurately, observe accurately (Fig. 3-12). Use medical terminology when making and recording observations.

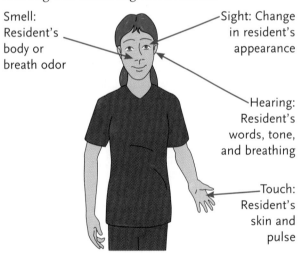

Smell: Resident's body or breath odor

Sight: Change in resident's appearance

Hearing: Resident's words, tone, and breathing

Touch: Resident's skin and pulse

Fig. 3-12. Reporting what you observe means using more than one sense.

To use the four senses listed above to gather information, do the following:

Sight: Look for changes in appearance, such as redness, swelling, rashes, discharge, changes in the eyes or ears or ability to move.

Hearing: Listen to what the resident tells you. Make sure he is making sense. Check to see if his breathing is normal. Note if he is coughing or gasping. Report if he is showing emotions, such as anger or sadness.

Smell: Check for odors coming from the resident's body or mouth. Odors can indicate an infection, a need for bathing, or poor mouth care.

Touch: Note if the skin seems hot or cool. Check to see if it is dry or moist.

Other ways for you to observe residents accurately include the following:

- Note any change in orientation. Does the resident know who he is, who you are, where he is, and what year it is?

- Check to see if the resident's vital signs are normal or abnormal. **Vital signs** are the measurements that monitor the function of the vital organs of the body. (Vital signs will be covered in depth in Chapter 13.)

- Report any change in ability. Has there been a change in the resident's ability to move any part of her body? Can the resident perform all of her regular daily activities that she could yesterday? Can the resident see, hear, smell, touch, and taste the same today?

- Report other important changes, such as changes in weight or overall appetite, changes in ability to go to the bathroom (urinating, bowel movement), and changes in mood.

Accurate documentation and prompt reporting are important to residents' well-being. How do you determine what to report immediately to the nurse and which signs and symptoms can wait until later? This involves critical thinking. Nursing assistants do not try to solve problems or make decisions about residents' health. This is the nurse's role. For the nursing assistant, **critical thinking** is making good observations and promptly reporting all potential problems.

Signs and symptoms that should be reported will be discussed in this book. In addition, anything that endangers residents should be reported immediately, including:

- Wheezing
- Difficulty breathing
- Chest pain and pressure
- Pain in calf of leg

- Blurred vision
- Slurred speech
- Vomiting
- Sudden limp
- Numbness or loss of feeling in one side of the body or one arm or leg
- Abdominal pain
- Change in vital signs
- Severe headache
- Resident fall

A resident's condition will need to be checked closely. Sometimes a nurse will ask you to report every change, no matter what the change is. If this is the case, you will report each change to the nurse as it happens.

13. Explain the nursing process

To communicate with other care team members, nurses use the **nursing process**. This is an organized method used by nurses to determine residents' needs, plan the appropriate care to meet those needs, and evaluate how well the plan of care is working. The process has five steps:

- assessment: getting information from many sources, such as medical history and a physical assessment, and reviewing it; the purpose is to identify actual or potential problems
- diagnosis: the identification of health problems after looking at all the resident's needs; completed to make a care plan
- planning: in agreement with the resident, goals are set and a care plan is created to meet the resident's needs
- implementation: putting the care plan into action; giving care
- evaluation: a careful examination to see if goals were met or progress was achieved; if progress is slow or if the problem worsened, the care plan must be changed

This process constantly changes as new information is collected. Good communication between all team members and the resident is vital. It helps ensure the success of this process. The nursing assistant's accurate observations and reports are an important part of helping to meet the resident's care needs.

14. Discuss the nursing assistant's role in care planning and at care conferences

Nursing assistants have an important role in care planning. Care plans are prepared from the observations of staff caring for the resident. At care planning meetings, do not be afraid to share your observations. If you are unsure about what information to share, talk to the nurse before the meeting to find out.

Care plans may be written at a special care conference. The **care conference** is a meeting to share and gather information (Fig. 3-13). This is done in order to develop care plans for residents. Care team members may attend. Each team member may share important information to be used to create or add to the care plan. Residents and their families and friends may also attend the care conference. Members of the community, such as ombudsmen, share helpful information, too. Care plans are usually kept at the nurse's station in a Kardex or by the resident's room. The Kardex is a type of card file that keeps resident information organized and easy to find. Information found in a Kardex includes the resident's diagnoses, special needs, and equipment used. It may include the resident's care plan.

Fig. 3-13. *A care conference is a meeting to share information and to develop a resident's care plan.*

Remember that HIPAA privacy guidelines apply to care plans and information in a Kardex. Do not share a resident's information with anyone not directly involved with the resident's care.

15. Describe incident reporting and recording

Incident reports are vital to the safety of the staff and residents. An **incident** is an accident, problem, or unexpected event during the course of care. It is something that is not part of the normal routine. An error in care, such as feeding the resident from the wrong meal tray, is an incident. A resident fall or injury is also an incident. Accusations by residents against staff and employee injuries are other types of incidents.

A **sentinel event** is an unexpected occurrence involving death or serious physical or psychological injury. Events are called "sentinel" because they signal the need for an immediate investigation and response. An example of this type of event is a resident falling out of bed and breaking a hip or a medication error that results in a resident's death.

An **incident**, or occurrence, **report** is a written report documenting the incident and the response to it. After the incident occurs, this report must be completed as soon as possible. This is so you do not forget important details. The information in an incident report is confidential. Give the report to the charge nurse (Fig. 3-14).

Always fill out an incident report if you are injured in any way, no matter how slightly, while on the job. This protects you and identifies that the injury occurred at work. Nurses may sign and add information to an incident report. The nurse will complete these reports for any accident or injury to residents or visitors. You may be asked to add information regarding residents or visitors.

Write exactly what you saw. State the time and the condition of the resident or visitor. Describe the reaction of the person to the incident. State the facts. Do not give your opinion.

HOT TIP

Incident Reports

Do not let anyone try to talk you out of filling out an incident report. It is important to have these reports on file. Complete it the same day the incident occurs, as soon as possible. You may want to keep a copy of the incident report for yourself. This will protect you should the report be lost by the facility.

16. Explain proper telephone etiquette

When you use the telephone during your shift, you are representing your facility to the community. You must follow rules for proper telephone etiquette. These include the following:

- When greeting a caller, cheerfully say, "Good morning," "Good afternoon," or "Good evening."
- Identify your facility: "Evergreen Facility."
- Identify yourself and your position: "Carol Scott, Nursing Assistant."
- Listen closely to the caller's request. Write down messages. Ask for correct spelling of names. In emergencies, take action immediately.
- Get a telephone number, if needed.
- Say "Thank you," and "Goodbye."

A few general rules for telephone use are:

- Do not give out any information about staff or residents over the phone. For example, if someone calls and asks, "Does Susie Hawkins work there?" you respond with, "Please hold and I will get my supervisor to help you." Most facilities have this policy due to the increase in domestic violence and other problems, like stalking. People may call and ask about a resident's condition. Creditors may call looking for people who owe them money. All resident and staff information is confidential. It must not be given out over the telephone. Refer this type of phone call to a supervisor.

Form 875/2 (if 2 part set) or
Form 875/3 (if 3 part set)

BRIGGS, Des Moines, IA 50306 (800) 247-2343

Printed in U.S.A.

INCIDENT REPORT

"An incident is any happening which is not consistent with the routine operation of the hospital or the routine care of a particular patient. It may be an accident or a situation which might result in an accident."

PERSON INVOLVED

(Last Name)   (First Name)   (Middle Initial)   Mr. ❑:   Mrs. ❑:   Child ❑:   Male ❑:   Female ❑:   Age _____

PATIENT ❑

Room No.   State Cause for Hospitalization

Patient's Condition Before Incident

Normal ❑:   Senile ❑:   Disoriented ❑:   Sedated ❑:   Other

Were Bed Rails Present?   Was Height of Bed Adjustable?

Yes ❑:   No ❑:   Up ❑:   Down ❑:   Ordered ❑:   Yes ❑:   No ❑:   Up ❑:   Down ❑:

EMPLOYEE ❑

Department   Job Title

VISITOR ❑

Home Address   Home Phone

OTHER ❑

Occupation   Reason for Presence at the Hospital

Exact Location of Incident   Date of Incident   Time of Incident   ❑ A.M.   ❑ P.M.

Property Involved ❑:   Equipment Involved ❑:   Describe

Description of Incident by Person Involved

_____

_____

Describe Exactly What Happened: Why It Happened: What Causes Were. If an injury, State Part of Body Injured. If Property or Equipment Damaged, Describe Damage.

_____

_____

_____

Name, Address & Phone No. of Witness(es)

Was It Necessary to Notify Physician?   Time of Notification   Time Responded

Yes ❑   No ❑   _____ a.m./p.m.   _____ a.m./p.m.

Was Person Involved Seen by a Physician?   Time Seen   Where

Yes ❑   No ❑   ❑ A.M.   ❑ P.M.

Physician's Name   T. _____ P. _____ R. _____ B.P. _____

Statement of Physician:

_____

_____

Date of Report   Title & Signature of Person Preparing Report

Additional Comments:

_____

Form 875 BRIGGS, Des Moines, IA 50306 (800) 247-2343
PRINTED IN U.S.A.

INCIDENT REPORT

Fig. 3-14. *A sample incident report. (Reprinted with permission of Briggs Corporation, 800-247-2343.)*

- You may place a caller on hold if you need to get someone to take the call. Ask the caller if she can hold first. Ask for help and training on this if you need it.

- You may have to transfer a call. If you do not know how to transfer, ask for training on this.

- Follow your facility's policy on personal phone calls.

- Follow your facility's policy on cell phone and pager use. These may not be allowed at work.

17. Describe the resident call system

Residents signal staff that they need them by using the facility call system. Other terms for this system are "signal light," or "call light." This system allows residents to call for help when needed. Think of this system as a resident's lifeline. A lifeline is something that connects another person to help when needed; it can literally save someone's life. Always respond to call lights promptly. Do not ignore call lights. Doing so can be considered abuse and/or neglect. Answer all call lights, even for people who are not your assigned residents. Always leave the call light within residents' reach before leaving their rooms (Fig. 3-15).

Fig. 3-15. *Keep call lights within residents' reach so they can call you when needed.*

18. Describe the nursing assistant's role in change-of-shift reports and "rounds"

There are two types of shift reports: start-of-shift report and end-of-shift report. Nursing assis-

tants usually are asked to be at the start-of-shift reports. Nurses are present for both types of reports. The care team gathers to discuss and plan residents' care for a shift. Shifts vary by facility; they are usually 8, 10, or 12 hours in length.

Guidelines
Shift Reports

For start-of-shift reports

- Arrive on time.

- Each staff member is given his or her assignment for the shift. This assignment lists residents for whom every staff member will be responsible during that shift. However, each resident is "your" resident. You must respond to any resident who needs your help. Listen for important information about all of the residents in your area.

- The staff listens to a nurse from the prior shift who reports on the care of each resident. Examples of information passed to the next shift are appetite problems, difficulties with urination, complaints of pain, or changes in the ability to move. Listen carefully to this information.

- The nurses give special instructions to the other staff members who will be providing resident care. Ask any questions you have about your residents. Special information shared during a report may include new admissions and transfers or discharges from the facility.

For end-of-shift reports

- Report to the nurses before the end-of-shift report. This gives nurses important information you gathered about residents during your shift. Examples are changes in pulse or temperature and skin changes that could signal the start of a pressure sore. Nurses will share this information with the staff for the next shift.

Some facilities use a method of reporting called "**rounds**." Staff members move from room-to-room and discuss each resident and the care plan. You may be involved in rounds at your facility. If you are, listen closely. Take notes (Fig. 3-16). Offer valuable information gathered about residents to staff. Sometimes, this method makes residents feel better cared for. Residents may be reassured by the fact that many people can help them when needed.

Fig. 3-16. *Take notes if you need to during rounds so that you can remember resident information.*

19. List the information found on an assignment sheet

An assignment sheet lists residents and has all of the tasks that you must do for them. Certain tasks are done daily. These daily tasks are called activities of daily living (ADLs). Range of motion (ROM) exercises may be listed on the sheet. These are exercises done to bring joints through a full range of movement. You will learn more about these in Chapter 25. A residents' **code status** tells the staff whether the resident has an advance directive or not. A "**code**" is when a group of specially-trained staff provide advanced life support during a medical emergency.

Assignment sheets contain the following information:

- names and room numbers of residents
- the medical diagnosis of each resident
- code status
- activity level
- range of motion (ROM) exercises
- bathing information
- diet orders

- fluid orders
- bowel and bladder information
- how often to measure vital signs
- treatments to be performed
- special tests and other procedures to be performed

HOT TIP
Show up!
Assignments are based on the number of residents and the number of staff members available on that shift. It is important to work every day you are scheduled. Missing a day can put residents in danger. It can also put staff at risk of injury due to having too many residents to care for. If you must be absent, call your facility early to tell them. This lets your supervisor start trying to replace you sooner.

20. Discuss how to organize your work and manage time

Following report, you will begin your day of caring for residents. Staff members will have duties to complete at certain times of the day. In order to complete your assignments each day, you must learn to organize your work. Here is an example of how you might organize a work day:

After you receive your assignment, make rounds on all of your residents. Check to see if any residents require immediate help or care. If residents have their call lights within reach and do not need immediate help, write down anything important on your assignment sheet. Write down any needed reminders on a notepad. For example, list special tests a resident needs. Ask the nurse if there are any special orders that may not have been added yet to the residents' care plan. When you feel you have all of the needed information, decide which resident you will care for first.

Each facility will have its own schedule of events and care. Duties that may begin the shift you will work include setting up residents for mealtime, bathing residents, and taking vital signs on all residents.

These are only a few of the starting duties you may have on a given day. Many things can happen to affect the work day. Adapt quickly to changing situations. A new admission, a staff member going home, or a resident transferring to a hospital are some things that may happen to change your day. Make sure each resident has the call light left in reach before you leave them to do anything else.

Here are some other basic tips for organization and time management:

Plan ahead. Take the time to list everything you have to do, including special tasks. Check to see if you have all the supplies needed for a procedure. This will get you focused.

Prioritize. Identify the most important things to get done. Do these first.

Make a schedule. Write out the hours of the day and fill in when you will do what. This will help you be realistic.

Combine activities. Can you visit with residents while providing care? Work more efficiently when you can.

Get help. It is not reasonable for you to try to do everything. Sometimes you will need help to ensure a resident's safety. Do not be afraid to ask for help. If you cannot complete an assignment for any reason, notify the nurse.

HOT TIP

Organizing Your Work
It is important to prioritize and organize your work every day. Do you use sticky notes to remind yourself to do things at home? Many nursing assistants use a similar method at work. A small notebook can make the difference between feeling organized and feeling overwhelmed.

CHAPTER REVIEW

1. What is the difference between verbal and nonverbal communication (LO 2)?

2. Write one example each of positive and negative nonverbal communication not listed in the textbook (LO 2).

3. Why should "yes" or "no" questions be avoided (LO 3)?

4. A resident tells a nursing assistant that he is scared of a medical test that is going to be performed. Instead of using a cliché, such as "Oh, everything will be fine," what could the nursing assistant say (LO 3)?

5. What does the word "culture" mean (LO 4)?

6. What can help overcome a language barrier with a resident (LO 4)?

7. What does a nursing assistant do each time he or she greets a resident (LO 5)?

8. Should nursing assistants use medical terms when speaking with residents (LO 6)?

9. Define "prefix," "root," and "suffix" (LO 6).

10. Convert 8:33 p.m. to military time (LO 7).

11. Convert 11:10 a.m. to military time (LO 7).

12. List eight items found on a resident's chart (LO 8).

13. With whom can a nursing assistant's observations about residents be shared (LO 8)?

14. When should care be documented (LO 9)?

15. Why is documentation so important (LO 9)?

16. Do HIPAA guidelines apply to computer use (LO 10)?

17. What is the MDS manual? How does a nursing assistant's reporting impact it (LO 11)?

18. List the four senses that are used in accurate observing and reporting (LO 12).

19. What does critical thinking mean for the nursing assistant (LO 12)?

For each of the following five statements, decide whether it is an objective sign or subjective symptom observation. Write "S" for subjective or "O" for objective (LO 12).

20. Resident says she has a sore throat. ____

21. Resident has dark red urine. ____

22. Resident states, "I have a hard time catching my breath." ____

23. Resident is running a fever. ____

24. Resident has blisters on her feet. ____

25. List the five steps in the nursing process (LO 13).

26. How does a nursing assistant contribute to care planning (LO 14)?

27. What is an incident (LO 15)?

28. When should an incident report be completed (LO 15)?

29. Give an example of a proper greeting when answering the phone (LO 16).

30. Why is a call light a resident's lifeline (LO 17)?

31. Describe the nursing assistant's role in rounds at a facility (LO 18).

32. List seven items found on an assignment sheet (LO 19).

33. Give an example of how to combine activities to manage time better (LO 20).

34. What does "prioritize" mean (LO 20)?

4

Communication Challenges

The Navajo Code Talkers

During World War II, the Japanese were able to break almost any American military code. So in 1942, a young Navajo man approached top-ranking U. S. military staff with an idea of how to use the Navajo language as a code. He believed the code would help communicate military messages securely. Many Native Americans, including some teenagers, became Marines and went to work as "Code Talkers." They used a form of the Navajo language to send top-secret messages during the war. In 1943, there were about 200 Navajo Code Talkers, and ultimately, around 400 Code Talkers went to the Pacific to serve in World War II. The code was never broken. The Navajo Code Talk remained classified information until 1968. The Navajo Code Talkers played a vital role in the victory of the United States in World War II. Some of the original Navajo Code Talkers were awarded Congressional Gold Medals in 2001.

"A wise old owl sat on an oak
The more he saw the less he spoke:
The less he spoke the more he heard;
Why aren't we like that wise old bird?"

Edward Hersey Richards, 1874-1957
from *Wise Old Owl*

"The important thing is to not stop questioning."

Albert Einstein, 1879-1955

1. Define important words in this chapter

airway: the natural passageway for air to enter into the lungs.

anxiety: uneasiness, often about a situation or condition.

artificial airway: any plastic, metal, or rubber device inserted into the respiratory tract for the purpose of maintaining ventilation.

coma: state of unconsciousness in which a person is unable to respond to any change in the environment, including pain.

combative: violent or hostile.

confusion: the inability to think clearly and logically.

defense mechanisms: unconscious behaviors used to release tension and/or help a person cope with stress.

depression: an illness that causes social withdrawal, lack of energy, and loss of interest in activities, as well as other symptoms.

disorientation: confusion about person, place, or time; may be permanent or temporary.

impairment: a loss of function or ability; can be a partial or complete loss.

masturbation: to touch or rub sexual organs in order to give oneself or another person sexual pleasure.

tracheostomy: an opening through the neck into the trachea that is surgically created.

2. Identify communication guidelines for visual impairment

Some residents you care for will be visually impaired. An **impairment** is a loss of function or ability, and it can be a partial or complete loss. Several diseases can cause visual impairment or blindness. Diabetes and glaucoma are two examples. You will learn more about these diseases in Chapters 22 and 23. A visual impairment is also something that can exist at birth. People of all ages can be visually impaired. It can affect one or both eyes.

Guidelines
Visual Impairment

- Announce yourself and greet the resident when you first enter the room. Do not touch him before you have identified yourself. Tell him why you are there.

- Look at the resident the entire time you are speaking with him.

- Make sure there is proper lighting in the room.

- Tell him about the care you are going to perform. Keep talking to him during care.

- Do not shout.

- Use the face of an imaginary clock to explain the position of objects (Fig 4-1). If you are taking the resident to a new area, orient him to the room. For example, "There is a table with four chairs around it at 3 o'clock. There is a sofa at 7 o'clock." Do not use words such as "see," "look," and "watch."

- Make sure the resident has his glasses on if he wears them. Check to see that they are clean, fit properly, and are in good condition (Fig. 4-2). If they are damaged or do not fit properly, report this to the nurse.

- Do not move personal items or furniture without the resident's permission. If he agrees, tell him the new location of the items.

- Put everything back where you found it.

- Read menus to the resident.

- Encourage the resident to use his other senses, such as smell, touch, and hearing.

- Announce when you are going to leave the resident's area.

- Do not play with or distract guide dogs if residents use them.

- There are many helpful items for people with visual impairments. Books on tape or CD, large-print books and newspapers, and large clocks are examples. Offer them when available.

- Be empathetic. Try to imagine what it feels like to not be able to see or see well.

Fig. 4-1. *The face of a clock can explain the position of objects.*

Fig. 4-2. *Glasses must be on the person and should be clean, fit properly and be in good condition.*

3. Identify communication guidelines for hearing impairment

Residents may have different kinds of hearing losses. Having a partial hearing loss in one ear is one example. Being completely unable to hear at all is another example. Hearing may also be temporarily impaired due to the noise level in the room.

Most hearing loss occurs gradually. The person will, over time, notice changes. The following list shows some symptoms of hearing loss. If you notice any of these, report them to the nurse.

- Trouble hearing high-pitched noises
- Trouble hearing soft consonants, such as "s" and "t"
- Trouble hearing what is said in a setting that has background noise
- Not understanding the meaning of words
- Being unable to hear people when they are not in the same room
- Favoring one ear over the other one
- Avoiding movies or special events due to not being able to understand the dialogue
- Resident complains of ringing in the ears
- Resident complains of pain in one or both ears

Guidelines

Hearing Impairment

- Get the resident's attention before speaking. Do not approach her from behind, as she may not hear you come in. Walk in front of her if possible.

- Stand or sit so that the resident can see your face. Make sure there is proper lighting in the room. The light should be on your face, rather than the resident's (Fig. 4-3).

- Look directly at the resident while speaking. A hearing-impaired resident may read lips.

- If the resident uses a hearing aid, make sure it is turned on (Fig. 4-4). More information on hearing aids is in Chapter 22.

- Be familiar with any hand gestures a hearing-impaired resident uses.

- Turn off TV or radios.

- Speak clearly in a low tone of voice. Do not shout. If the person favors one ear, speak to that side.

- Lower the pitch of your voice.

- Do not chew gum or cover your mouth with your hand while speaking.

- Do not exaggerate pronunciation of words.

- Use simple words and short sentences.

- Use pen and paper or picture cards when needed.

Fig. 4-3. *Speak face-to-face in good light.*

Fig. 4-4. *Make sure hearing aids are turned on.*

4. Explain defense mechanisms as methods of coping with stress

Communicating with residents under stress requires empathy and sensitivity. Words must be carefully chosen so that you do not increase the person's stress level. Residents who are stressed may use defense mechanisms. **Defense mechanisms** are unconscious behaviors used to release tension and/or help a person cope with stress.

They help to block uncomfortable or unpleasant feelings which may cause anxiety.

Defense mechanisms prevent the person from facing the real reason a situation has occurred. Overuse of these mechanisms keeps a person from understanding his or her emotional problems and actions.

Defense mechanisms include the following:

Denial: Blocking reality; rejecting the thought or feeling—A resident refuses to believe his diagnosis of cancer.

Displacement: Transferring a strong feeling to a less threatening object—A resident who is mad at her son yells at the nursing staff.

Projection: Seeing feelings in others that are actually one's own—A staff member says that a resident does not like her.

Rationalization: Making excuses to justify something—An elderly man fails a driving test and says the test was "unfair."

Repression: Blocking painful events or feelings from the mind—A woman cannot recall abuse she suffered as a child.

Regression: Going back to behavior from the past for comfort—A resident who is stressed starts to rock back and forth.

5. List communication guidelines for anxiety or fear

Anxiety is uneasiness, often about a situation or condition. Feeling anxious is not the same as feeling afraid. Anxiety is a vague emotional state. The unpleasant feelings are coming from the anticipation of something bad that could happen or a future danger. The danger is not happening at this time. With fear, one is dealing with the present. Fear is a reaction to an actual danger. The resident who is fearful is dealing with a threat of some kind.

There are physical symptoms of anxiety. They include nausea, shaking, sweating, chest pain

and chest palpitations. The goal of communicating with an anxious person is to reduce the anxiety and stress levels.

Guidelines
Anxiety or Fear

- Greet the resident when you first enter the room. Do not touch him before you have identified yourself. Use touch only if it does not upset the resident.

- Speak softly. Reduce the noise level.

- Speak slowly and calmly.

- Listen to the resident. Be patient. Ask gentle questions to try to identify what is causing the anxiety or fear.

- Be empathetic. Be calm and reassuring.

- Avoid demanding behavior.

- Reassure resident that he is safe.

More information on anxiety and related disorders is in Chapter 22.

6. Discuss communication guidelines for depression

Depression is a mental illness that causes withdrawal, lack of energy, and loss of interest in activities, as well as other symptoms. It can be managed or even cured. There are many different types and degrees of depression, and you will learn more about these in Chapter 22.

Residents who have recently moved into a facility may be depressed. They have had many changes and personal losses in their lives. Examples of losses include the loss of spouse, family, and friends. Other losses are the loss of health, independence, mobility, and the ability to care for oneself. A chemical imbalance may also cause depression.

Residents may have moved out of their home and into a facility full of strangers. Residents may not have family near, or close family may not choose to visit them. They will probably have to share a room with someone, possibly for the first time in their lives. One of these factors can be enough to make a person depressed. However, residents may have to deal with all of these problems at once. It is not surprising if they become depressed.

Depression is not something people can overcome by choosing to be well. It is an illness like any other illness. Your role is to be supportive and compassionate. Try to make each day as pleasant an experience as possible for residents.

Guidelines
Depression

- Be pleasant, respectful, and supportive.
- Use touch to help comfort the resident. Consider cultural differences before using touch.
- Sit down and listen carefully to the resident. Lean forward and keep good eye contact. This body language helps show you are interested (Fig. 4-5).
- Think before you speak. Try to empathize with the resident's feelings and situation.
- Use a normal tone of voice when speaking. Use simple, clear statements. Do not talk to adults as if they were children.
- Talk about feelings if the resident wishes.
- Encourage social interaction.

Maintain a posture that shows you are listening   Practice active listening

Maintain eye contact

Use a normal tone of voice

Fig. 4-5. *Practice good communication skills with depressed residents.*

Report a resident's depression to the nurse immediately. Signs of depression to report are in Chapter 22.

7. Identify communication guidelines for anger

Anger is a natural emotion. You may see residents, their families, and friends express it. Staff members may show anger, too. Anger can be due to many reasons. Disease, fear, pain, grief, loneliness, and loss of independence can all cause a resident to be angry. Even minor things, such as a change in the dinner menu, can trigger anger. Anger may also just be a part of someone's personality.

Some people express anger by yelling, throwing things, threatening, sarcasm, and pacing. Narrowed eyes, clenched fists, and raised fists are other signs of anger. Anger can also be expressed by withdrawing, being silent, or sulking. Anger can be difficult to handle. Always report angry behavior to the nurse at the first sign of it.

If a resident's anger makes it so that he or she requires more time from staff, a care conference may be scheduled. Care plans can be developed to reduce the behavior. Your input at a care conference is valuable. Offer ideas to help identify the cause of the anger and thoughts on how to stop it.

Guidelines
Angry Behavior

- Be pleasant and supportive. Let the resident know you are there for him and that you are available to help.
- Try to find out what caused the resident's anger. Listen closely as he speaks. Note the exact words the resident uses. Being silent may help him explain.
- Watch the resident's body language.
- Think before you speak. Empathize with the resident. Try to understand what he is feeling.
- Do not argue with the resident.
- Stay calm. Speak in a normal tone. Consider your responses carefully.

- Treat the resident with dignity and respect.
- Answer call lights promptly.
- If the resident's anger increases, get the nurse immediately. Stay at a safe distance if the resident becomes combative.
- Try to involve the resident in activities if he is willing. Examples are taking a walk or listening to music.

HOT TIP

Assertive vs. Aggressive Behavior

Assertiveness is a desired trait, both in and out of the workplace. Being assertive means being confident when dealing with other people. Expressing thoughts and feelings in a direct, honest, and respectful way shows assertive behavior. For example, a nursing assistant informs the charge nurse that she needs help moving a resident because it would be unsafe to handle it by herself.

Aggressiveness is different from assertiveness. Aggressiveness means expressing thoughts and feelings in a way that humiliates or overpowers another person. Aggressive behavior does not show respect for the needs or feelings of others.

Being assertive at work is important to help you provide the best care for residents. Do not be afraid to share your feelings, thoughts, and observations in a respectful way. Do not behave aggressively with residents or other staff. Aggressive behavior can result in injury to others, both physical and emotional.

8. Identify communication guidelines for combative behavior

When anger increases, a person may become combative. **Combative** means violent or hostile. Such behavior includes hitting, shoving, kicking, throwing things, and insulting others.

Combative behavior may be due to a disease affecting the brain. It may be due to a worsening of anger or frustration. Medication or changes in health may cause a resident to become combative. Combativeness may be linked to behaviors seen, expected, accepted or practiced in a person's childhood. In general, though, combative behavior is not a reaction to you. Try not to take it personally.

Even though it is probably not personal, a combative resident is a threat to you, other staff, residents, and visitors. Your responsibility is to keep everyone safe. If you see a resident becoming combative, call for the nurse right away. Combative behavior requires special techniques.

Guidelines
Combative Behavior

- Call for the nurse immediately or get someone to call her. Try not to leave the resident alone.
- Keep yourself and other people at a safe distance from the resident. If a resident tries to hit you, or does hit you, never hit back (Fig. 4-6).
- Stay calm. Do not appear threatening to the resident.
- Be reassuring.
- Try to find out what triggered the behavior.
- Do not respond to insults.
- Follow the direction of the nurses.
- Report facts you know.
- When anger passes, sit with the resident for awhile to provide comfort if instructed to do so.

Fig. 4-6. If a resident tries to hit you, step out of the way if you can. Never hit back even if a resident does strike you.

Never hit a resident.
Unfortunately, it is not uncommon to read or hear about physical abuse of the elderly by caregivers. These caregivers may be family, friends, or care team members. Often, physical abuse is due to stressful situations causing the caregiver to lash out quickly. You can never hit a resident, NO MATTER WHAT. Even if a resident strikes you first, you may not strike back.

9. Identify communication guidelines for inappropriate sexual behavior

Older adults, like all humans, are sexual beings. Residents have the right to choose how they express their sexuality. They have the right to make choices about sex. There is a variety of sexual behavior in all age groups. This is also true of residents.

However, sometimes residents will show inappropriate sexual behavior. This behavior does not seem normal or makes you or others uncomfortable. It includes sexual advances or comments. Inappropriate behavior also includes acts like residents removing clothing in public places, such as the dining room or hallway, or masturbating in public areas. **Masturbation** means to touch or rub sexual organs in order to give oneself or another person sexual pleasure.

This behavior can be due to illness, dementia, confusion, or medication (Fig. 4-7). Changes in the brain may make a person unable to tell the difference between proper and improper behavior. Use the following guidelines to help deal with inappropriate sexual behavior.

Guidelines
Inappropriate Sexual Behavior

- If you encounter an embarrassing situation, do not overreact. Be matter-of-fact. Remain calm and try to distract the person. If this does not work, gently direct the resident to a private area. Tell the nurse.

- Listen to the resident if he or she wants to talk.

Fig. 4-7. *Older adults are sexual beings and have the right to make choices about sex. However, illness, dementia, confusion, and medication may cause inappropriate sexual behavior, which is something that must be reported to the nurse.*

- Do not judge the behavior.

- Sometimes a confused resident will show inappropriate behavior that is really due to having a rash, or clothes that are too tight, too hot, or too scratchy. The resident might just need to go to the bathroom. Watch for these problems.

- Always report all inappropriate behavior to the nurse.

All human beings need love and affection. Aging can affect a person's ability to express sexual needs. It also may limit his or her access to partners. Residents have the right to engage in mutually-agreed-upon sexual relationships. Residents also have the right to masturbate. If you witness either of these situations, be sensitive. Provide privacy. Do not make fun of the situation.

See Chapter 5 for more information on sexual needs.

10. Identify communication guidelines for disorientation and confusion

Disorientation is confusion about person, place, or time. This condition may be permanent, due to an injury or disorder in the brain. It can also be temporary, due to dehydration, constipation, hypoxia (lack of oxygen to the brain) or medication. Orientation was first discussed as a way to observe residents accurately in Chapter 3. When a resident is oriented, it means he can identify who he is and who you are (person), the city, state, and facility he is in (place), and the correct year (time). A resident who is disoriented may not be able to express one or more of these things.

Confusion is the inability to think clearly and logically. A confused person has trouble focusing his attention and may feel disoriented. A confused resident may not remember to finish his meal or may not be able to locate his room. Confusion interferes with the ability to make decisions and may change a person's personality. When a resident is confused, he may not be able to identify his name, the date, other people or where he is. Confusion can be a temporary or permanent state.

Confusion is often due to a physical problem, such as a stroke. You will learn more about strokes, also called cerebrovascular accidents (CVA), in Chapter 22. Confusion also has these causes:

• low blood sugar

• head trauma or head injury

• dehydration

• nutritional problems

• fever

• sudden drop in body temperature

• lack of oxygen

• medications

• infections

• brain tumor

• illness

• loss of sleep

• seizures

• constipation

• not using hearing aids

Guidelines

Disorientation or Confusion

- Do not leave a confused resident alone.
- Stay calm. Provide a quiet environment.
- Speak in a lower tone of voice. Speak clearly and slowly.
- Introduce yourself each time you see the resident. Remind the resident of his or her location, name, and the date. A calendar can help with this (Fig. 4-8).
- Repeat directions if needed. Use short, simple sentences. Break tasks into steps.
- Be patient with the resident. Do not rush him or her.
- Listen to the resident closely. Observe how the resident is communicating. Watch his body language. Do not focus on the words alone.
- Tell the resident about plans for the day. Keep a routine.
- Encourage the use of glasses and hearing aids. Make sure they are clean and are not damaged.
- Tell the resident when you are leaving the area. Repeat if needed.
- Report observations to the nurse.

Fig. 4-8. Personal photos and a calendar can help remind a resident who he is, where he is, and what the date is.

11. Identify communication guidelines for the comatose resident

You may be assigned to care for a resident who is comatose. A **coma** is a state of unconsciousness. A person in a coma cannot respond to any change in the environment, including pain. It usually occurs due to an illness, such as meningitis, a condition, such as a drug overdose, or injury, such as a motor vehicle accident. A comatose resident deserves your respect in the same way that an alert resident does.

Guidelines

Comatose Resident

- Introduce yourself when entering the resident's room.

- Explain each procedure you will be performing. List the steps you will take.

- Do not hold personal discussions while caring for a comatose resident.

- Announce when you are going to leave the room.

RESIDENTS' RIGHTS

Unconscious Residents

Even when people are unconscious, they still may be able to hear what is going on around them. Unconscious people have been known to regain consciousness and relate many of the things they heard while they were unconscious. Limit your discussions to appropriate subjects. Speak respectfully, and explain what you are doing. Do not talk about anything personal while giving care. Speak to unconscious residents as you would to any resident.

12. Identify communication guidelines for functional barriers

Residents may have a functional problem that interferes with their ability to speak. Some causes of these problems are difficulty in breathing, physical problems with the mouth or lips, or an artificial airway.

When a resident has trouble breathing, never push him or her to speak. It can make breathing more difficult. Allow plenty of pauses between words and sentences.

Physical problems of the lips, mouth, and tongue make speech difficult. They include the following:

- lip, mouth or tongue sores of any kind

- dental problems of any kind, including missing teeth, mouth pain, and dental work

- poorly-fitting dentures (artificial teeth)

- birth defects like cleft palate

- paralysis of one side of the mouth due to stroke

An **airway** is the natural passageway for air to move into and out of the lungs. An **artificial airway** is any plastic, metal, or rubber device inserted into the respiratory tract for the purpose of maintaining ventilation. This is needed when the airway is obstructed from illness, injury, secretions, or inhaling fluid into the lungs. Some residents who are unconscious will need an artificial airway.

A **tracheostomy** is a common type of artificial airway seen in nursing homes. An opening is made surgically through the neck into the trachea (windpipe) for the air to reach the person's lungs. This may be done because a resident cannot breathe normally through the nose. This procedure is usually temporary, but it can be permanent. While the tracheostomy is in place, the resident may be unable to speak. More information on artificial airways is in Chapter 26.

Guidelines

Functional Barriers

- Give the resident plenty of time to speak. Be patient.

- Ask the resident to write down anything you do not understand.

- Do not tire the resident. Use a communication board or picture cards if the resident becomes tired. (You will learn more about these in Chapter 22.)

- Do not remove a resident's oxygen for any reason. Only nurses do this.

- Report mouth sores, poorly-fitting dentures, or complaints of mouth pain to the nurse.

- Use other methods of communication if the person cannot speak. Try writing notes, drawing pictures, and using communication boards (Fig. 4-9). Watch for hand and eye signals. For example, you can use one blink for "yes" and two blinks for "no."

Ⓖ Be reassuring and calm. Be empathetic to the resident's situation. It can be frightening and uncomfortable to have an artificial airway. Some residents may choke or gag. Imagine how it might feel to have a tube in your nose, mouth, or throat.

A	B	C	D	E	F	G	H	I	J	K	L	M
N	O	P	Q	R	S	T	U	V	W	X	Y	Z

1	2	3	4	5	6
7	8	9	10	11	12
13	14	15	16	17	18
19	20	21	22	23	24
25	26	27	28	29	30

CALL BELL	BED UP	BED DOWN	UP IN CHAIR
DOCTOR	NURSE	HUSBAND/SON	WIFE/DAUGHTER
ICE/WATER	MILK	BATHROOM	BEDPAN
RAZOR/SHAVE	GLASSES	MEDICINE	WATCH/TIME
WHEELCHAIR	BACK TO BED	TOO HOT	TOO COLD
CLERGY	HUNGRY	DRINK	TEA/COFFEE
URINAL	BRUSH TEETH	TISSUES	COMB/BRUSH
PEN/PAPER	TELEPHONE	RADIO/TV	MAGAZINE/NEWSPAPER

Fig. 4-9. A sample communication board.

CHAPTER REVIEW

1. What should the nursing assistant do first when dealing with a resident with a visual impairment (LO 2)?

2. How can a nursing assistant explain the position of objects in front of a visually-impaired resident (LO 2)?

3. When speaking with a hearing-impaired resident, whose face should the light be on, the nursing assistant's or the resident's (LO 3)?

4. Why do you think that a nursing assistant should not chew gum or cover her mouth while speaking with a hearing-impaired resident (LO 3)?

5. Look at the defense mechanisms listed in Learning Objective 4. Write one example of how a resident could display each defense mechanism listed (denial, displacement, projection, rationalization, repression, regression) (LO 4).

6. What is the difference between anxiety and fear (LO 5)?

7. List four losses that could cause residents to be depressed (LO 6).

8. Can a person who is depressed simply choose to be well (LO 6)?

9. List five possible causes of anger (LO 7).

10. If a resident hits a nursing assistant first, is it okay for the nursing assistant to strike back (LO 8)?

11. What can cause inappropriate sexual behavior (LO 9)?

12. What are reasons a resident might be doing what looks like inappropriate behavior, but actually is not (LO 9)?

13. Define "disorientation" and "confusion" (LO 10).

14. Are disorientation and confusion always permanent states (LO 10)?

15. Why should a nursing assistant explain procedures and introduce herself to an unconscious resident (LO 11)?

16. What are other possible methods of communication if a person cannot speak (LO 12)?

17. List three physical problems of the lips, mouth, and tongue that make speech difficult (LO 12).

18. What is an artificial airway (LO 12)?

5 Diversity and Human Needs and Development

The Black Death: The Plague That Didn't Discriminate

In the 14th century, the Black Death, also known as the bubonic plague, first reared its ugly head. The name "Black Death" came from the black areas on the skin commonly seen in plague patients. It is thought to have developed in the Far East. This plague moved across Asia and into North Africa, slipping into Europe by way of Italy. Italian merchants at the time traveled to Asia searching for beautiful wares to sell. When they set sail for home, they carried the specter of the Black Death with them to Italy without realizing it. The plague spread over Italy and then over England. An estimated 60 million people died of the plague from 1340 to 1350. The plague killed people from many cultures and ethnic groups. Disease strikes everyone from every age group. It truly does not discriminate.

"The great law of culture is: Let each become all that he was created capable of being."
Thomas Carlyle, 1795-1881

"Religion is a great force—the only real motive force in the world: but what you fellows don't understand is that you must get at a man through his own religion and not through yours."
George Bernard Shaw, 1856-1950

1. Define all important words in this chapter

ageism: stereotyping of, prejudice toward, and/or discrimination against the elderly.

agnostic: a person who claims that he does not know or cannot know if God exists.

atheist: a person who claims that there is no God.

Buddhism: a religion that follows the teachings of Buddha.

Christianity: a religion that follows the teachings of Jesus Christ.

cultural diversity: the variety of people living and working together in the world.

developmental disability: a chronic condition that restricts physical or mental abilities.

health: state of physical, mental, and social well-being.

Hinduism: a religion that believes in the unity of everything and that all are a part of God.

Islam: a religion that follows the prophet Muhammad and the Five Pillars of Islam.

Judaism: a religion that follows the teachings of God as given to Moses in laws and commandments.

mores: the accepted traditional customs of a particular social group.

need: something necessary or required.

psychosocial needs: needs which involve social interaction, emotions, intellect, and spirituality.

puberty: the period when a person develops secondary sex characteristics.

religion: a set of beliefs and practices followed by a group of people.

spirituality: of or relating to the concerns of the spirit, the sacred, or the soul.

stereotype: a biased generalization about a group that is usually based on opinions and distorted ideas.

wellness: successfully balancing things that happen in everyday life; includes five different types: physical, social, emotional, intellectual, and spiritual.

2. Explain health and wellness

The World Health Organization has defined the word **health** as "a state of complete physical, mental, and social well-being, and not merely the absence of disease or infirmity." This view of health looks at the whole person. It also takes the focus off disease and redirects it to healthy attitudes and lifestyles. In recent years, we have seen much information on health, wellness, and healthy living.

Wellness has to do with successfully balancing things that happen in our everyday lives. There are five types of wellness: physical, social, emotional, intellectual, and spiritual. Physical wellness includes things like being able to complete everyday tasks. Social wellness has to do with

relating to other people. Emotional wellness covers managing stress and expressing feelings. Intellectual wellness deals with growing and learning throughout the life span. Spiritual wellness includes religious beliefs, ethics, values, and mores. **Mores** are the accepted traditional customs of a particular social group.

3. Explain the importance of holistic care

You first learned about holistic care in Chapter 1. Care team members should view resident care in a holistic way. Holistic care involves considering the whole person, which includes his physical and psychosocial needs (Fig. 5-1). **Psychosocial needs** include social contact, emotions, thought, and spirituality. A simple example of holistic care is taking time to talk with residents while helping them bathe. You are meeting a physical need with the bath and meeting the psychosocial need for interaction with others at the same time. You will learn more about these needs in Learning Objective 4.

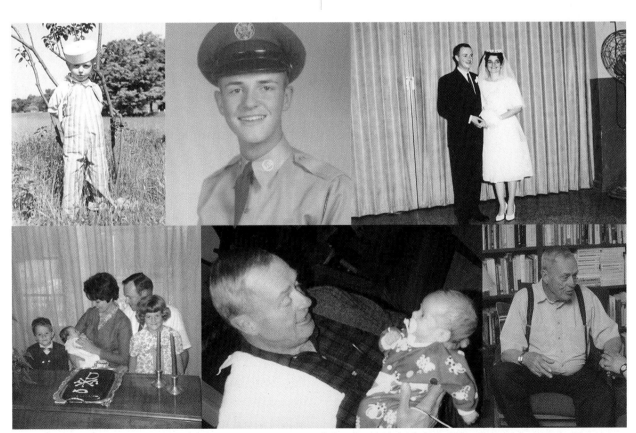

Fig. 5-1. Remember that residents are people, not just lists of illnesses and disabilities. They have many needs, like you. Many have had rich lives with wonderful experiences. Take time to care for your residents as whole people.

Health care is formed around the thought that harmony or balance in one's life promotes good health. If the balance is disturbed, illness can result. Holistic care supports the harmony, which can improve a resident's chances of living a better life.

4. Identify basic human needs and discuss Maslow's "Hierarchy of Needs"

All human beings have the same basic physical needs. A **need** is something necessary for a person in order to survive and grow. Physical needs include:

- Food and water

- Protection and shelter

- Activity

- Sleep and rest

- Safety

- Comfort, especially freedom from pain

Human beings also have psychosocial needs. Although they are not as easy to define as physical needs, psychosocial needs include:

- Love and affection

- Acceptance by others

- Security

- Self-reliance and independence in daily living

- Contact with others

- Success and self-esteem

One person who researched human behavior was Abraham Maslow. He developed a model to show how physical and psychosocial needs are arranged in order of importance. He believed that physical needs must be met before psychosocial needs can be met. His theory is called "Maslow's Hierarchy of Needs" (Fig. 5-2).

The needs at the bottom of the pyramid are physical needs. They are the ones that must be met to survive. For example, a person can live only a few days without water. Nursing as-

sistants can help residents meet these needs by encouraging them to eat and drink. NAs can provide a quiet place for residents to rest. They can also help residents with toileting whenever they need it.

Need for self-actualization: the need to learn, create, realize one's own potential

Need for self-esteem: achievement, belief in one's own worth and value

Need for love: feeling loved, accepted, belonging

Safety and security needs: shelter, clothing, protection from harm, and stability

Physical needs: oxygen, water, food, elimination, and rest

Fig. 5-2. *Maslow's Hierarchy of Needs*

The second level is safety and security needs. These include shelter, clothing, protection from harm, and stability. For example, moving a person from her home into a facility can cause anxiety. Because it is not yet a stable environment, new residents may find it hard to adapt. It may take time for them to feel comfortable in their new home. Nursing assistants can help residents by being compassionate and empathetic. They can listen to residents when they want to talk. NAs can reassure residents that they are being taken care of.

The third level is love, acceptance, and belonging. When residents move into a facility, they may be separated from their loved ones. Living in a new place with strangers can be very lonely. This is especially true if loved ones do not visit as often as before. Residents need to feel as if they belong in their new home. NAs can help by welcoming them and making them feel listened to and cared for. NAs can encourage residents to interact with other residents and staff.

The fourth level is the need for self-esteem. Residents may feel less of a sense of self-worth as they become dependent on others. They will need help with tasks they have performed alone all their lives. NAs can help by encouraging residents to be as independent as possible. You will learn more about doing this throughout this textbook. The more residents can care for themselves, the better they will feel about themselves. NAs should praise successes, no matter how small. This maintains dignity and self-esteem.

Self-actualization is the highest need a person can achieve, according to Maslow's theory. A person must reach his or her highest potential to be self-actualized. People rarely reach this level in every single part of their lives. Residents will each be at different stages in this process. Some residents will be content with the level they have reached in life. They may spend their days quietly watching television or reading. Other residents will still be striving to do more. This may mean that they help other residents read mail or write letters. They may help out at the facility gift shop or volunteer to oversee special activities.

RESIDENTS' RIGHTS

Ensure easy access to food and drink.
Refusing to help residents meet their basic needs, such as eating and drinking, is abuse. When food is delivered to residents' rooms, trays must be set up in a timely manner. Residents must have their trays prepared so they can eat as easily as possible. Not bothering to open a milk carton or to cut meat on a plate can prevent a resident from eating all of the food needed. This can be considered abuse or neglect.

5. Identify ways to accommodate cultural differences

As you learned in Chapter 3, "culture" refers to a set of learned beliefs, values and behaviors. The world is full of many different groups of people. Each group has its unique way of looking at the world. You will have the opportunity to take care of people from many cultures. Having an un-derstanding of cultures will help you give better care to your residents. Your own culture greatly influences you in many ways.

Cultural diversity has to do with the wide variety of people throughout the world. Each culture may have similar lifestyles, religions, traditions, customs, and behaviors. Culture and background often have an impact on how a person behaves while ill. Understanding other cultures will help you provide better care. Be sensitive to and respect people who are different from you. Respect and value each person as an individual. It is important to respond to new ideas with acceptance, not prejudice.

There are so many cultures that they cannot all be listed here. There are thousands of different groups in the United States alone. Some examples are Japanese-Americans, Native Americans, and Latinos. The U.S. also has people from many different regions. Each region has its own culture and traditions. For example, the rural U.S. is much different from the urban U.S. The culture of the Northeast is not the same as the culture of the South (Fig. 5-3).

Fig. 5-3. *There are many different cultures in the U.S.*

As you learned earlier, culture can affect ideas about touch or eye contact. It can affect the language people use and the need for an interpreter.

Culture also influences food choices. For example, some Korean people eat kimchi, which is a type of spicy cabbage. Some Mexican people eat queso fresco, which is a type of cheese. You will learn more about food choices in Chapter 14.

Culture also influences the way people seek health care or discuss health issues. Some people will be very comfortable with and open about discussing their health. Others will feel shy and be embarrassed by this. Nursing assistants must be sensitive to differences in how residents feel about their health.

A good nursing assistant is familiar with residents' cultures. People may be happy to talk about their backgrounds and educate others about where they are from. Ask residents, their families and friends about special customs or traditions. When nursing assistants are sensitive to cultural differences, residents benefit.

Do not make fun of or disrespect any culture, behavior or belief. When people accept and do not judge others' beliefs or way of life, they can create lasting relationships. Residents will feel comfortable with you and will look forward to seeing you each day.

RESIDENTS' RIGHTS

Rights with Language

Residents have the right to communicate with someone who speaks their language. They must understand all forms before signing them. They also must understand all care before it is performed. Sometimes a change in pronunciation will change the meaning of what is said. Tell the nurse if you feel you need an interpreter to make sure your meaning is clear.

6. Discuss the role of the family in health care

Families play an important part in most people's lives. The concept of "family" is always changing. Often the support people give each other defines the family more than the particular people involved. Many different kinds of families exist (Fig. 5-4). They include:

Fig. 5-4. *Families come in all shapes and sizes.*

- Nuclear families (a father and a mother and one or more children)

- Single-parent families (one parent and one or more children)

- Unmarried couples of the same sex or opposite sex, with or without children

- Extended families (parents, children, grand-parents, aunts, uncles, cousins, other relatives, and even friends)
- Blended families (divorced or widowed parents who have remarried and have children from previous relationships and/or the current marriage)

Treat all kinds of families with respect. Do not judge families, even if they are different from your own idea of what a family is. No family is a "right" or "wrong" kind of family. The only time the staff should be involved is when there are concerns about a resident's safety around one or more family members.

Families have an important role in residents' health care. They may provide some of their loved one's care. Friends may also help with their care. They help in many other ways, such as:

- Helping make care decisions
- Relating routines and preferences to care team members
- Connecting residents to what is going on outside of the facility
- Reading mail
- Helping to prepare menus
- Taking residents on walks
- Going with residents to activities or outside functions
- Bathing or helping with other personal care
- Washing special clothing at home
- Shopping for special items, gifts or cards
- Helping to prepare cards, letters and gifts

When families visit, do all you can to help residents prepare. Assist them to dress, apply makeup, buy gifts, or anything else they ask. Help them find a private place for the visit if needed. Pay attention to the needs of the resident and family during the visit. Report questions from the family promptly to the nurse.

7. Explain how to meet emotional needs of residents and their families

Nursing assistants may be of great help to residents and their families and friends since NAs are the primary caregivers. They play a large role in the comfort and well-being of residents.

Nursing assistants may be the people residents or their family members turn to when they feel fear, anger, or stress. They may go to NAs during an emotional crisis. For example, if a resident's friend dies, he may come to you needing comfort. If a resident dies, his family may seek you out for comfort or to talk.

When residents come to you with problems or needs, listen closely to what they say. Do not interrupt. Sometimes being quiet while someone talks is enough. Offer support and encouragement. Show that you care. Do not respond with cliches, such as "You will be fine." You do not know that for a fact. You can ask questions, such as "How can I help?"

Respond to worry or fear with a meaningful message. Answer any questions asked, if it is within your scope of practice. If any questions have to do with medical issues or advice, report them to the nurse.

Residents sometimes feel that nursing assistants are a part of their family. However, it is important for NAs to maintain professional boundaries. Understanding the limits of professional relationships with residents means behaving in an ethical and responsible way. Residents who are ill and lonely may feel that they need more from staff than what is appropriate. Staff who are overworked, have poor relationships at home, or who are prone to substance abuse may be at risk for inappropriate relationships with residents. It is important to be aware of these factors. If you are unsure about how to maintain a proper emotional distance from residents, always ask a supervisor for help.

NAs should be available for family members or friends of residents, too. Spend as much time with them as possible. Families often seek out nursing assistants because they see them more than other staff. Take time to listen to them when they want to talk (Fig. 5-5). Be reassuring. Families may ask questions regarding residents' ADLs. They may want to know when a resident is bathed or when meals are offered. Answer these types of questions. However, when families ask questions regarding a resident's diagnosis, treatments and therapies, refer them to the nurse.

Fig. 5-5. *Sometimes listening to a resident's family member is the best way to provide emotional support.*

NAs can provide comfort and compassion to residents' families and friends just by being there. When families get sad or upset for any reason, stay with them and seek other help as needed.

8. Explain ways to help residents with their spiritual needs

People have different spiritual needs. Nursing assistants can help residents meet these needs. Residents may feel strongly about their spiritual beliefs. This can help them cope with problems they face. Remember that spirituality is a sensitive area.

Residents may have varying beliefs in God from very strong to no belief. Residents may consider themselves spiritual, but may not believe in God or a higher power. The important thing for nursing assistants to remember is to respect all residents' beliefs, whatever they are. Do not make

judgments about residents' spiritual beliefs or try to push your own beliefs on residents.

It may help if you know a little about some of the different **religions** and religious practices. It is important to know that even if a resident belongs to a religious group, he may not believe or practice everything that religion teaches. There is a variety of faiths and non-faiths. Within each of these, there are many different beliefs. Your job is to accommodate religious practices and requests when possible. Common types of religions, listed alphabetically, follow:

Buddhism: Buddhism evolved from Siddhartha Gautama, who reached enlightenment and took the title of "Buddha." Buddhists believe that morality, meditation and wisdom are the path to enlightenment. They believe in reincarnation, and that people must travel through birth, life, and death. After these travels, a person can reach Nirvana. Nirvana is the state of peace and happiness and freedom from worry and pain. It is the highest spiritual plane one person can attain. There are many Buddhist texts. The Tipitaka or Pali Canon is the standard scripture collection. The Dalai Lama is considered to be the highest spiritual leader.

Christianity: Christians believe that Jesus Christ was the son of God and that he died so that their sins would be forgiven. Christians believe in heaven and that those who repent their sins before God will be able to go to heaven. Christians may be Catholic or Protestant. There are many subgroups, such as Baptists, Episcopalians, Evangelicals, Lutherans, Methodists, Mormons, and Presbyterians. Christians may attend church regularly once a week or many times a week. They may be baptized and take communion as a symbol of Christ's sacrifice. The Christian Bible is the sacred text and is divided into two parts: the Old Testament and the New Testament. Religious leaders may be called priests, preachers, pastors, ministers, or deacons.

Hinduism: Hindus believe in the unity of everything, called "Brahman." The purpose of life is to realize that all are part of God. People move through birth, life, death and rebirth. How a person moves toward enlightenment is determined by karma. Karma is the result of actions in past lives, and actions in this life can determine one's destiny in future lives. Good thoughts and deeds can cause one to be reborn at a higher level, but bad thoughts and deeds may cause a person to be born at a lower level. The Vedas are the primary texts of Hinduism. Holy men are called Sadhus.

Islam: Muslims are followers of the prophet Muhammad [Mohammed]. Muslims worship God; the Arabic term for God is "Allah." The Five Pillars of Islam include reciting the profession of faith, ritual prayer five times daily at certain times of the day, fasting during the month called "Ramadan," charitable donations to the poor and needy, and pilgrimage to Mecca. Mecca is the Muslim holy city. Muslims worship at mosques and follow specific religious practices related to food and drink. For example, Muslims usually do not eat pork or drink alcohol. The sacred text of Islam is the Qur'an [Koran]. The Qur'an is believed to be the literal word of God as revealed to Muhammad. There is a variety of Islamic religious leaders.

Judaism: Judaism is the religion of the Jewish people. It is divided into Reform, Conservative, and Orthodox movements. Jewish people believe there is one God. They believe God is merciful and that they should follow God's laws. Jewish people believe that God gave them laws and commandments through Moses in the form of the Torah. Jewish services are held on Friday evenings and sometimes on Saturdays in synagogues or temples. The Sabbath day, called "Shabbat," is a special day of rest. Jewish people may not do certain things on the Sabbath. This lasts from Friday sundown to Saturday sundown. Religious leaders are called rabbis.

Spirituality refers to concerns of the spirit, the sacred or the soul. Some consider themselves to be spiritual, but not religious. Others believe that their spiritual self is the same as their religious self. Spirituality centers around thoughts of a spiritual aspect of life and nature beyond worldly things. It may be associated with inner peace and well-being. It may refer to a person's beliefs about the overall meaning or purpose of life.

Many Native American tribes follow spiritual traditions. Their belief systems often include the idea that everything has a spirit, such as people, animals, oceans, trees, etc. The importance of community and a love of the environment can play an important part for Native Americans. Traditions generally include special ceremonies and rituals.

As mentioned earlier, some people may not believe in God or a higher power at all. They may identify themselves as "**agnostic**." Agnostics claim that they do not know or cannot know if God exists. They do not deny that God might exist, but they feel there is no true knowledge of God's existence.

Atheists are people who claim that there is no God. This is different from what agnostics believe. Atheists actively deny the existence of God. For many atheists, this belief is as strongly held as any religious belief.

Here are some ways you can help residents meet their spiritual needs:

- Honor dietary restrictions. Dietary restrictions are rules about what and when followers can eat. For example, Muslims may not eat shellfish. Catholics may not eat meat on Fridays during Lent. Orthodox and Conservative Jewish people may eat only kosher foods and may not eat pork. Do not judge any dietary restrictions. Report fasting requests to the nurse.

- Report requests to see clergy to the nurse promptly. Give privacy for clergy visits (Fig. 5-6).

- Help residents to the chapel when asked.

- Respect all religious items. Handle religious items carefully. When asked, help residents apply religious articles of clothing.

- Allow time and privacy for prayer. If you are asked to do so, read religious materials aloud.

- Residents have the right to attend religious services if they choose to do so. Make sure residents who want to go to these services are ready on time and are helped to the proper site.

- Report to the nurse or social worker if a resident needs help finding spiritual resources.

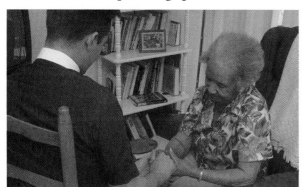

Fig. 5-6. *Be welcoming and give privacy when residents receive a visit from a spiritual leader.*

Residents' spiritual or religious beliefs or non-beliefs may be different from yours. Do not try to change someone's religion or tell a resident that his belief or religion is wrong. Do not express judgments or say anything negative about a religious group. Never insist that a resident join in a religious activity or interfere with a religious practice.

Spiritual needs are different for each person. Respect residents' religions or beliefs. Listen carefully when they want to talk about them. When you respect and provide support for each resident's spiritual concerns, you are helping to meet their needs.

9. Identify ways to accommodate sexual needs

Humans are sexual beings, and they continue to have sexual needs throughout their lives. Sexuality is not just about having sex. Sex and sexuality have been defined in this way: sex is something a person does, while sexuality is something a person is. Sexual orientation is a person's preference for one gender or the other. Sexual orientation or identity plays a big part in human sexuality.

Terms defining sexual identity include:

- Heterosexual: A person whose preference is for persons of the opposite sex; also known as "straight."

- Homosexual: A person whose preference is for persons of the same sex. The terms "gay" and "lesbian" are usually preferred.

- Gay: 1. A person whose preference is for persons of the same sex. 2. A man whose sexual orientation is to men.

- Lesbian: A woman whose sexual orientation is to women.

- Bisexual: A person whose orientation is for persons of both sexes.

- Transsexual: 1. One who wishes to be accepted by society as a member of the opposite sex. 2. One who has undergone a sex change operation.

A common myth is that elderly people no longer have sexual needs or desires. That is not true. Sexual urges do not end due to age or admission to a nursing home. Many things can affect residents' sexual needs. Illness and disability can affect sexual desires, needs, and abilities. However, do not assume you know what impact a disability has had on sexuality. A disability may limit the ability to meet sexual needs, but not lessen sexual desire. Many people in wheelchairs can have sexual and intimate relationships.

Living environments may also affect sexuality. In nursing homes, a lack of privacy and no available partner are often reasons for a lack of sexual expression. Be sensitive to privacy needs.

Sexuality is a very important part of every human being. And in every age group, there is a variety of sexual expression and behavior. Do not judge any sexual behavior you see (Fig. 5-7). An attitude that any expression of sexuality by the elderly is either "disgusting" or "cute" is inappropriate. It deprives residents of their right to dignity and respect.

Fig. 5-7. *Elderly people continue to have sexual needs and desires. Do not judge any sexual behavior you see.*

Here are ways you can help residents with their sexual needs:

- Always knock and wait for permission to enter before going into residents' rooms. Honor "Do Not Disturb" signs if your facility uses them.

- If you encounter any sexual situation between consenting adults, provide privacy and leave the room. Do not discuss what you saw with other staff members. Consenting adults are allowed to have sexual relationships. Residents may also masturbate, which means to rub or touch sexual organs to give oneself pleasure.

- Do not judge sexual choices or residents' sexual orientation. Do not judge the sexual orientation of residents' family members or friends.

- If you ever see a resident being sexually abused, remove the resident from the situation. Make sure he or she is taken to a safe place, then report this to the nurse immediately. Never delay in reporting sexual abuse.

If a sexual situation is disturbing or inappropriate, ask a nurse for help. Tips on dealing with sexually-inappropriate behavior are in Chapter 4. More information on sexual needs of the elderly is in Chapter 17.

10. Describe the stages of human growth and development

Human growth and development is an ongoing and complex process. Growth refers to the physical changes that can be measured. Development means the emotional, social and physical changes that occur. Each person's growth and development will differ. One child may walk at nine months old, while another will not walk until over a year old.

Many things affect growth and development. These include the parent's involvement, the child's surroundings, nutrition, exercise, medical care and overall lifestyle.

There are different types of development. Cognitive development focuses on how children think and learn. Language development focuses on gaining language skills. Moral development deals with forming a sense of right and wrong. Motor development is gaining an ability to do things like grasp things, use scissors, and draw. Physical development deals with the changes that happen to the body during growth. Sexual development has to do with the reproductive changes that occur when people reach puberty. Social development is the process of learning to relate to other people.

Infants (Birth to 12 months)

Babies grow quickly during the first year. Infants tend to triple birth weight in the first year of life. Physical development in infancy moves from the head down (Fig. 5-8). For example, infants gain control over the neck muscles before the muscles in their shoulders. Infants learn to grasp, lift their heads, and crawl. They may be able to pick things up towards the end of the first year. Infants are totally dependent on others for care. Lots of touch is important as a communication tool during this time. Touch helps babies grow and thrive.

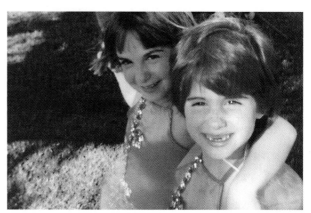

Fig. 5-8. *An infant's physical development moves from the head down.*

Toddler (Ages 1 to 3)

Toddlers grow fast between the ages of one and three. Most toddlers can move about quickly, and run and jump. During the toddler years, speech improves. Toddlers gain coordination of their limbs and learn to control their bladders and bowels (Fig. 5-9). It is important to protect toddlers as they explore their world, for they can take risks. They do not understand what kinds of things can harm them. Parents begin to teach them language, the difference between right and wrong, and accepted behavior.

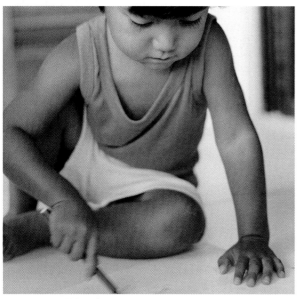

Fig. 5-9. *Toddlers learn to speak and gain coordination of their limbs.*

Pre-School (Ages 3 to 6)

Pre-school aged children become more independent and have social relationships. They play better with other children, and they can play in groups (Fig. 5-10). Their language ability improves. Pre-schoolers learn to care for themselves. They become more physically coordinated, and their sense of imagination develops. Playing dress-up in parents' clothing is common.

Fig. 5-10. *Children in pre-school years develop social relationships.*

School-Age (Ages 6 to 12)

School-age children's development centers on cognitive and social development. Entering school is a big adjustment for children and their families. Children learn to get along with each other. They begin to develop a conscience, morals, and self-esteem. During this time, boys develop more muscle, but girls may be larger than boys. The period between nine and twelve is called "pre-adolescence." Hormonal changes occur. There is a growing interest in the opposite sex. Girls may reach puberty in the later years of this stage. **Puberty** is when a person develops secondary sex characteristics. In females, secondary sex characteristics include growth of body hair and development of breasts and hips. In males, they include growth of body hair, growth of the testes and the penis, broadening of the shoulders, and a lowered voice.

Adolescence (Ages 12 to 18)

During adolescence, genders become sexually mature. Boys tend to reach puberty. If girls did not reach puberty during the prior stage, it will start here. Adolescents may have a hard time adapting to changes caused by puberty (Fig. 5-11). This group becomes more independent. They must make important decisions, mostly by themselves, each day. Moral values that the child has learned play a part in these decisions. Adolescents can sometimes become stubborn and difficult for their parents to handle. They may have mood swings. They are concerned with acceptance from others.

Fig. 5-11. Adolescence is a time of adapting to change.

Young Adulthood (Ages 18 to 40)

Growth has usually been completed by this time. However, boys can continue to grow up to the age of 25. During this stage, people make decisions on whether to continue their education or join the work force. They may meet a life partner. Many couples marry (Fig. 5-12). Some people decide to have children during this time.

Fig. 5-12. Young adulthood often involves finding long-term mates.

Middle Adulthood (Ages 40 to 65)

During middle adulthood, people usually become more comfortable and stable. Their chil-

dren may have left home to go to college or to live on their own. This can be a very happy time for people (Fig. 5-13). They may find there is more time and money to spend on themselves. Couples may take trips and spend more time together. A person may decide to start on a second career.

Fig. 5-13. Middle adulthood can offer more free time to take trips and pursue hobbies.

Some people may find themselves in a "mid-life crisis" during this stage. This is a period of unrest due to a desire for change and fulfillment of unmet goals. It has to do with the reality of getting older. A mid-life crisis can occur in both men and women. People can change the way they dress, act or behave during this time.

Late Adulthood (65 years and older)

People in late adulthood can see many changes. They may retire from jobs. Couples may travel more and see children, friends and family. Medical care may be needed for problems that develop during this time. Mobility can become limited due to these health problems. People may have to cope with a loved one's illness or death. Staying connected to others is vital to staying healthy and mentally alert (Fig. 5-14). Hobbies and volunteering can help the person stay connected. It is important to encourage people in this stage to stay as active and involved as possible.

Fig. 5-14. *In late adulthood, staying connected with others is important to help stay healthy and active.*

Figure 5-15 outlines the developmental tasks that are required throughout all of the stages of life.

11. Discuss stereotypes of the elderly

It is common for people to have false beliefs about the elderly. A **stereotype** is a biased generalization about a group. These generalizations are usually based on opinions and distorted ideas and often come from television or the movies. These unfair ideas create prejudices against the elderly. Stereotyping of, prejudice toward, and/or discrimination against the elderly is called **ageism**.

Some common stereotypes of the elderly are:

* They cannot remember things.
* They are totally dependent on others.
* They do not have an active sex life.
* They do not like to leave home.
* They are grumpy or grouchy.
* They cannot manage their money.
* They have no friends.
* They have no interests.

Infant (Birth to 12 months)	Toddler (Ages 1 to 3)	Pre-School (Ages 3 to 6)	School-Age (Ages 6 to 12)
• Rapid physical growth • Physical development moves from the head down • Learns to grasp and lift head • Begins to crawl and climb • Picks up objects • Smiles, cries, coos, babbles, and laughs	• Learns to walk, run and jump • Speech improves • Gains coordination of limbs • Learns to control bladder and bowels	• Becomes more independent • Has social relationships • Language ability improves • Learns to care for self • Becomes more physically coordinated	• Learns to get along with other children • Begins to develop a conscience, morals, and self-esteem • During "pre-adolescence" hormonal changes occur • Growing interest in the opposite sex • Girls may reach puberty in the later years of this stage—body hair grows and breasts and hips develop

Adolescence (Ages 12 to 18)	Young Adulthood (Ages 18 to 40)	Middle Adulthood (Ages 40 to 65)	Late Adulthood (65 years and older)
• Boys reach puberty—body hair grows; the testes and the penis grow; shoulders broaden; and voice lowers • Girls reach puberty if they haven't before • Has a difficult time adapting to changes caused by puberty • Becomes more independent • Makes important decisions • Can become stubborn • May have mood swings • Concerned with acceptance from others	• Growth has usually been completed • Makes decisions about education or careers • May select a mate • May marry • May have children	• Becomes more comfortable and stable • Some changes of aging appear • Children may have left home • May travel	• Retires from jobs • May travel more • Changes of aging more apparent • May require medical care for problems • Mobility can become limited • May have to cope with a loved one's and friends' illnesses or death

Fig. 5-15. *The stages of growth and development.*

These ideas are not true of most elderly people. Research has shown that most older people are active and have many interests (Fig. 5-16). They exercise, continue to learn, work, manage their finances, and have intimate relationships. They are relatively independent.

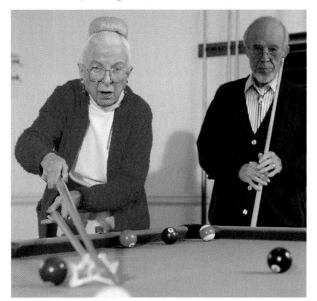

Fig. 5-16. *Most older people lead active lives.*

Aging is a normal process. There are many emotional and physical changes that occur as people age. These normal changes of aging do not mean that people will always become ill or dependent. You must be able to tell the difference between what is true and what is not true about the aging process. This will help you better care for your residents.

12. Discuss developmental disabilities

Developmental disabilities are present at birth or emerge during childhood. A **developmental disability** is a chronic condition; it will exist throughout a person's life. Developmental disabilities restrict physical or mental ability. These disabilities prevent a child from developing at a "normal" rate. These disabilities include cerebral palsy, autism, visual or hearing impairment, and the most common disability, mental retardation.

Developmental disabilities cause problems with language, mobility, and learning. They also cause difficulty with self-care and the things people do every day. For example, a person may struggle with eating, bathing, walking, or speaking. A brief description of some developmental disabilities follows.

Cerebral Palsy (CP): Cerebral palsy is a developmental disability that affects movement and balance. It can also cause mental disabilities. A person with cerebral palsy suffered brain damage while in the uterus or during birth. The part of the brain that was damaged controls muscle tone. People with CP may lack control of their head and have trouble using their arms and hands. They can have poor balance or posture. They may be stiff or limp. CP can cause problems with speech and intelligence.

CP generally does not worsen as the person gets older. Cerebral palsy includes four types: ataxic, athetoid, spastic and mixed. Most people with CP have spastic cerebral palsy. This means they might move awkwardly and have stiff muscles.

Signs and symptoms of CP can be different for each person. Some people have very mild symptoms. Others are much more severe. Some people with CP also have other disorders, such as mental retardation, hearing or visual impairment or a seizure disorder.

Autism: Autism is a group of developmental disabilities called "ASDs" or "Autism Spectrum Disorders." Autism starts prior to age three and continues through the person's lifetime. It is seen more often in boys. People with autism disorders have trouble with speech, language, and communication. They may have problems relating to other people socially. Autistic people may do specific actions over and over again, such as rocking back and forth.

Mental Retardation: The most common developmental disability is mental retardation. It causes below-average mental functioning. People have difficulty in learning and problems with social skills. People with mental retardation develop at a below-average rate.

There are different degrees of mental retardation. It is not a disease or mental illness. One method used to identify this disability is the testing of intelligence (IQ). People who are mentally retarded need some support in their day-to-day lives. They may need help with ADLs, such as bathing, eating, moving and positioning. People who are mentally retarded can work and live independently, depending upon the severity of the disability (Fig. 5-17).

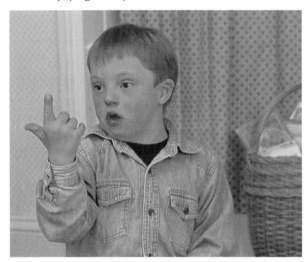

Fig. 5-17. *People who are mentally retarded have the same emotional and physical needs as others do.*

There are other terms used for mental retardation that some people find more preferable. Examples include developmental disability, developmental delay, intellectual disability and learning disability. Respect each person's wishes on how to refer to this disability.

Guidelines
Developmental Disabilities

- Treat adult residents as adults, regardless of their behavior.

- Praise and encourage them often, especially for positive behavior.

- Help teach ADLs by dividing tasks into small steps.

- Repeat words to make sure they understand.

- Talk to the resident, even if he or she cannot speak.

- Help residents with cerebral palsy move slowly. They may take longer to adjust their body position.

- Promote independence. Assist with activities and motor functions that are difficult.

- Encourage social interaction.

- Always be patient.

Other developmental disabilities are visual or hearing impairments. You learned about these impairments in Chapter 4. A person with a visual or hearing impairment may need a little or a lot of outside support throughout their lives. Having one of these impairments may affect a person's ability to drive, work and communicate. See Chapters 4 and 22 for guidelines for these impairments.

CHAPTER REVIEW

1. What do the terms "health" and "wellness" mean (LO 2)?

2. Define "holistic care" and describe what it involves (LO 3).

3. What are psychosocial needs (LO 3)?

4. The needs listed at the bottom of Maslow's "Hierarchy of Needs" are physical needs. What needs are physical needs (LO 4)?

5. List one example of how a nursing assistant can help with the following needs: physical needs, safety and security needs, need for love, need for self-esteem (LO 4).

6. What is cultural diversity (LO 5)?

7. List three things that culture affects (LO 5).

8. List five ways families and friends help with a resident's care (LO 6).

9. Name three ways nursing assistants can respond to the emotional needs of residents and their families (LO 7).

10. Describe five ways nursing assistants can help residents meet their spiritual needs (LO 8).

11. If a nursing assistant encounters a sexual

situation between two consenting residents, what should she do (LO 9)?

12. What should a nursing assistant do if she sees a resident being sexually abused (LO 9)?

13. Name one thing that occurs in each stage of human development (LO 10).

14. What is a stereotype (LO 11)?

15. Why should stereotyping be avoided (LO 11)?

16. List three facts about developmental disabilities (LO 12).

17. Why do you think it is important for nursing assistants to treat developmentally disabled residents as adults, regardless of their behavior (LO 12)?

6
Infection Control

Semmelweis and Childbed Fever: It was handwashing, plain and simple!

Ignaz Semmelweis (1818-1865) was a Hungarian doctor who practiced and taught medicine in Vienna, Austria during the mid-1800s. He noted that the death rate on a certain maternity ward was higher than on a similar ward at the same facility. The only difference he could find was that doctors and medical students came to the ward where the death rate was higher right after dissecting corpses in the autopsy rooms. The second ward, where the midwives worked, had a much lower death rate. The midwives did not go into the autopsy rooms.

Semmelweis asked the doctors and the medical students to first wash their hands and then soak them in a special solution before and after examining the maternity patients. After this process was initiated, the death rate from childbed fever dropped dramatically. Semmelweis eventually wrote a book on his discovery.

"Cleanliness is a great virtue ..."
Charles B. Fairbanks 1827-1859

"The sick are the greatest danger to the healthy; it is not from the strongest that harm comes to the strong, but from the weakest."
Friedrich Wilhelm Nietzsche, 1844-1900

1. Define important words in this chapter

antimicrobial: an agent that destroys or resists pathogens.

autoclave: machine creating steam or a type of gas that kills all microorganisms.

barrier: block or obstacle; object(s) worn by healthcare providers to prevent the transmission of infectious diseases.

biohazard container: hard, leakproof containers into which sharp objects and items contaminated with infectious material are placed.

bloodborne pathogens: microorganisms found in human blood that can cause infection and disease in humans.

Bloodborne Pathogen Standard: federal law requiring that healthcare facilities protect employees from bloodborne health hazards.

body fluids: tears, saliva, sputum (mucus coughed up), urine, feces, semen, vaginal secretions, and pus or other wound drainage.

carrier: person who carries a pathogen without signs or symptoms of an illness or disease and who can spread the disease.

catheter: tube inserted through the skin or into a body opening; used to add or drain fluid.

C. difficile (C. diff, clostridium difficile): a bacterial illness that can cause diarrhea and colitis; spread by spores in feces that are difficult to kill.

The Centers for Disease Control and Prevention (CDC): federal government agency responsible for improving the overall health and safety of the people of the United States.

clean: a condition in which an object has not been contaminated with pathogens.

clean technique: process of removing pathogens; also called medical asepsis.

communicable disease: disease transmitted when a pathogen is spread from one person to another.

contagious disease: a communicable disease that is spread easily from person to person.

contaminated: soiled, unclean; having disease-causing organisms or infectious material on it.

cross-infection: acquiring an infection from someone else; also called cross-contamination.

dehydration: a condition that occurs when a person does not have enough fluid in the body.

direct contact: way to transmit pathogens through touching the infected person or his or her secretions.

direct spread: method of transmission of disease from one person to another.

dirty: a condition in which an object has been contaminated with pathogens.

disinfection: a measure used to decrease the spread of pathogens and disease by destroying pathogens.

drainage: flow of fluids from a wound or cavity.

exposure control plan: plan that identifies the step-by-step method of what to do if exposed to infectious material; also includes specific work practices that must be followed.

exposure incident: situation that occurs when a person is exposed to infectious blood or material.

fomite: an object that is contaminated with a pathogen and can now spread the pathogen to another person.

hand hygiene: handwashing with either plain or antiseptic soap and water and using alcohol-based hand rubs.

healthcare-associated infection (HAI): an infection associated with various healthcare settings, such as long-term care facilities, hospitals, ambulatory settings and home care.

hepatitis: inflammation of the liver caused by infection.

immunity: resistance to infection by a specific pathogen.

incubation period: the period of time between the time the pathogen enters the body and the time it causes an infection.

indirect contact: a way to transmit pathogens by touching something contaminated by the infected person.

indirect spread: method of transmission of disease from an object, insect, or animal to a person.

infection: the state resulting from pathogens invading and growing within the human body.

infection control: set of methods used to control and prevent the spread of disease.

infectious disease: any disease caused by growth of a pathogen.

isolate: to keep something separate, or by itself.

localized infection: infection limited to a specific part of the body; has local symptoms.

malnutrition: a serious condition in which a person is not getting proper nutrition.

medical asepsis: process of removing pathogens; also called clean technique.

microbe: a tiny living thing visible only by microscope; also called a microorganism.

microorganism (MO): a tiny living thing not visible to the eye without a microscope; also called a microbe.

MRSA (methicillin-resistant *Staphylococcus aureus*) infection: an infection caused by bacteria that are resistant to many antibiotics; can develop when people do not take all of the medication prescribed to them.

mucous membranes: the membranes that line body cavities that open to the outside of the body, such as the linings of the mouth, nose, eyes, rectum, and genitals.

multidrug-resistant organisms (MDROs): microorganisms, mostly bacteria, that are resistant to one or more antimicrobial agents.

non-communicable disease: a disease not capable of being spread from one person to another.

non-intact skin: skin that is broken by abrasions, cuts, rashes, acne, pimples, lesions, surgical incisions or boils.

normal flora: the microorganisms that normally live in and on the body and do not cause harm in a healthy person.

nosocomial infection: an infection acquired in a hospital.

Occupational Safety and Health Administration (OSHA): a federal government agency that makes rules to protect workers from hazards on the job.

pathogen: the microorganisms that cause disease.

perineal care: care of the genitals and anal area by cleansing.

PPE (personal protective equipment): a barrier between a person and disease; includes gloves, gowns, masks, goggles, and face shields.

reinfection: being infected a second time with an infection.

resistance: the body's ability to prevent infection and disease.

sanitation: ways communities maintain clean, hygienic conditions that help prevent disease, such as the disposal of sewage and solid waste.

Standard Precautions: a method of infection control in which all blood, body fluids, non-intact skin (like abrasions, pimples, or open sores), and mucous membranes (lining of mouth, nose, eyes, rectum, or genitals) are treated as if they were infected with a disease.

sterilization: a measure used to decrease the spread of pathogens and disease by destroying all microorganisms, including pathogens.

surgical asepsis: method that makes an area or an object completely free of microorganisms; also called sterile technique.

systemic infection: an infection that occurs when pathogens enter the bloodstream and move throughout the body; causes general symptoms, such as chills and fever.

transmission: transfer of a disease.

vaccine: a substance prepared from weakened or killed microbes that is used to give immunity to disease.

VRE (vancomycin-resistant *enterococcus*): a mutant strain of the bacterium *enterococcus*; a resistance caused by a person not taking all of a powerful antibiotic Vancomycin.

2. Define "infection control" and discuss types of infections

Communities strive to maintain clean conditions in order to help prevent the spread of disease. This is known as **sanitation**. In facilities, infection control is used to help prevent the spread of disease. **Infection control** is the set of methods used to control and prevent the spread of disease. It is the responsibility of all members of the care team. Know your facility's policies on infection control and follow them. They help protect you, residents, visitors, and other staff members from disease.

A **microorganism** (**MO**) is a tiny living thing visible only by a microscope. It is also called a **microbe**. Microorganisms are always present in the environment (Fig. 6-1). **Infections** are caused by **pathogens**, which are harmful microorganisms. For infections to develop, pathogens must invade and grow within the human body.

Fig. 6-1. *Microorganisms are always present in the environment. They are on almost everything we touch.*

There are two main types of infections, localized and systemic. A **localized infection** is limited to a specific part of the body. It has local symptoms, which are near the site of infection. For example, if the eye becomes infected, the area around it might be red, swollen, painful, and warm to the touch. A **systemic infection** occurs when pathogens enter the bloodstream and move throughout the body. It causes general symptoms, such as fever, chills, or mental confusion. AIDS (Acquired Immune Deficiency Syndrome) is an example of a systemic infection. You will learn more about AIDS later in this chapter and in Chapter 24.

A special type of infection that can be localized or systemic is a **healthcare-associated infection** (**HAI**), an infection associated with various healthcare settings, including long-term care facilities, hospitals, ambulatory settings and home care. A second type of infection that can be localized or systemic is a nosocomial infection. A **nosocomial infection** is an infection acquired in a hospital. For example, a resident gets a urinary tract infection (UTI) from a urinary catheter after entering a facility. A **catheter** is a tube inserted through the skin or into a body opening that is used to add or drain fluid. HAIs and nosocomial infections can be mild or life-threatening. There are signs and symptoms of infections that you need to know to be able to report them to the nurse. It is important to report these signs promptly. Not reporting immediately can put residents at risk for even greater infections. For example, you forget to report a resident's symptoms before leaving the facility. By the time you return the next day, the infection has traveled into the bloodstream and has become systemic. Always report the following signs and symptoms right away.

Signs and symptoms of a localized infection include the following:

- Redness
- Swelling
- Pain

- Heat
- **Drainage** (fluid from a wound or cavity)

Signs and symptoms of a systemic infection include the following:

- Fever
- Chills
- Headache
- Change in other vital signs
- Nausea, vomiting, and diarrhea
- Mental confusion

An **infectious disease** is a disease caused by a pathogen. The pathogen will cause an infection if conditions are right. Pathogens grow best in warm, dark, and moist places where food is present, and in hosts who have low resistance. **Resistance** is the body's ability to prevent infection and disease. There are two types of infectious diseases: communicable and non-communicable.

A **communicable disease** occurs when a pathogen is spread from one person to another. A **contagious disease** is a communicable disease that is spread easily from person to person. A **non-communicable disease** is a disease not capable of being spread from one person to another. For example, a person who has emphysema, a disease of the lungs, is not contagious to others.

By using proper infection control methods, you can prevent all people in your care, as well as other staff members and visitors, from acquiring an infection from someone else. This is called **cross-infection**, or cross-contamination. Infection control methods will also help protect residents from being infected a second time, called **reinfection**.

3. Discuss terms related to infection control

Infection control is about breaking the chain of infection, which is discussed in the next learning objective. **Transmission**, or transfer, of disease can be blocked by using good infection control. This is done by using a method called **clean technique** or **medical asepsis**. It is the process of removing pathogens. Medical asepsis is used in all healthcare facilities. Before asepsis is explained in more detail, some terms must be understood.

In health care, an object can be called "**clean**" if it has not been **contaminated** with pathogens. An object that is "**dirty**" has been contaminated with pathogens.

Measures like disinfection and sterilization decrease the spread of pathogens that could cause disease. **Disinfection** means that only pathogens are destroyed. **Sterilization** means all microorganisms are destroyed, including pathogens. Spores are special hard-shelled microorganisms. They are not killed by disinfection; they are killed by sterilization. An **autoclave** is usually used to sterilize equipment. This machine creates steam or a type of gas that kills all microorganisms.

The goal of medical asepsis is to prevent the spread of pathogens by keeping a facility as clean as possible. This does not mean that the facility is free from microorganisms. The only way to make an area or object completely free of microorganisms is to use **surgical asepsis**. Another term for surgical asepsis is sterile technique. Surgical asepsis makes an object or area sterile. This means it is completely free of all microorganisms. There may be times when you will assist a nurse with a procedure that requires sterile technique. You will have special training to help with this type of procedure. Chapter 18 has more information on the sterile field, sterile gloves, and sterile dressings. These are all measures used in surgical asepsis.

Facilities will have separate areas for clean and dirty items, such as equipment, linen and supplies. They are normally called the "clean" and the "dirty" or "contaminated" utility rooms. Before entering a clean utility room, wash your hands. This helps keep the equipment in this room clean.

The contaminated or dirty utility room is separate from the clean utility room. It is used to store equipment that is not needed by the resident. Supplies in this room are not "clean," such as trash bags. A sink is usually in this room. Wash your hands before leaving this room so that you do not transfer pathogens to other areas in the facility. After washing your hands, do not touch anything in the dirty utility room. If you do, you must wash your hands again.

Know the location of the clean and dirty utility rooms and what is stored in each. You will learn more about handling linen and equipment in Learning Objective 9 of this chapter.

4. Describe the chain of infection

The chain of infection describes how disease is transmitted from one being to another (Fig. 6-2). There are six links in the chain of infection:

- Link 1: Causative agent
- Link 2: Reservoir
- Link 3: Portal of exit
- Link 4: Mode of transmission
- Link 5: Portal of entry
- Link 6: Susceptible host

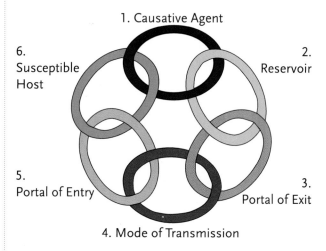

Fig. 6-2. *The chain of infection.*

If one of the links in the chain of infection is broken, the infection can be prevented.

Chain Link 1: Causative agent

The causative agent is a pathogen or microorganism that causes disease. As you learned, microorganisms are small living bodies that cannot be seen without a microscope. They are everywhere—on skin, in food, in the air, and in water. Causative agents include bacteria, viruses, fungi, and parasites.

Normal flora are the microorganisms that normally live in and on the body without causing harm to a healthy person. When they enter a different part of the body, they may cause an infection.

There is a waiting period between the time the pathogen enters the body and the time it causes an infection. This period is called an **incubation period**. Some examples of incubation periods are as follows:

- Chickenpox: 10-21 days

- Influenza (flu): 1-3 days

- Measles: 10-21 days

Infection Control Example for Link 1: Vaccines.

Vaccines, substances prepared from weakened or killed microbes, can give **immunity** to a disease without causing the symptoms of the particular disease. The immunity may not last forever.

Chain Link 2: Reservoir

A reservoir is where the pathogen lives and grows. A reservoir can be a human, animal, plant, soil, or substance. Microorganisms grow best in warm, dark, and moist places where food is present. Some microorganisms need oxygen to survive, while others do not. The blood and the lungs are examples of reservoirs.

There are two main ways of spreading an infection from a reservoir: direct and indirect. **Direct spread** occurs when a person gets a disease directly from another person (reservoir). The human reservoir may be a person with an active disease or a person carrying the disease (a carrier). A human carrier "carries" the disease, but does not show any signs or symptoms at the time he or she spreads the disease. This "carrier" may or may not get the disease later.

Indirect spread occurs when a person gets a disease from an object, insect, or animal (reservoir). Objects are also called "fomites." A **fomite** is an object that is contaminated with a pathogen and can now spread the pathogen to another person. Fomites may be things like infected food, water, food utensils, bedpans, or bed linens.

Infection Control Example for Link 2: Keeping surfaces clean and dry.

Chain Link 3: Portal of exit

There can be different exit routes, or portals of exit, from a reservoir. The portal of exit is any opening on an infected person allowing pathogens to leave. These include the nose, mouth, eyes, or a cut in the skin (Fig. 6-3).

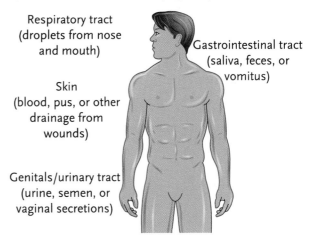

Respiratory tract (droplets from nose and mouth)

Gastrointestinal tract (saliva, feces, or vomitus)

Skin (blood, pus, or other drainage from wounds)

Genitals/urinary tract (urine, semen, or vaginal secretions)

Fig. 6-3. Portals of exit.

Infection Control Example for Link 3: Covering the mouth when sneezing.

Chain Link 4: Mode of transmission

The mode of transmission describes how the pathogen travels. The actual transmission of an infectious disease occurs in different ways. The main routes of transmission are contact, droplet, and airborne transmission.

Contact transmission occurs through contact with the person's blood or body fluids that are contaminated by the pathogen. **Body fluids** include tears, saliva, sputum (mucus coughed up), urine, feces, semen, vaginal secretions, and pus or other wound drainage. **Direct contact** happens by touching the infected person or his or her secretions. **Indirect contact** results from touching something contaminated by the infected person, such as a needle, instrument, or dressing.

Droplet transmission occurs when the pathogen travels short distances after being expelled. Droplets normally do not travel more than three feet, but they may travel further. Droplets can be created when the infected person coughs, sneezes, or talks. Laughing, suctioning, singing, and spitting may also transmit droplets. A susceptible host (Link 6) inhales contaminated droplets and gets an infection.

In airborne transmission, the pathogen is transmitted through the air after being expelled. The pathogen is carried a distance, usually more than three feet, by moisture in the air. A pathogen can also be carried by dust. A susceptible host (Link 6) may inhale contaminated moisture or dust, which causes an infection.

Infection Control Example for Link 4: Handwashing.

Chain Link 5: Portal of entry

Pathogens enter the human host through different portals of entry. The portal of entry is any body opening on an uninfected person that allows pathogens to enter. This includes the nose, mouth, eyes, and other mucous membranes, cuts in the skin, and cracked skin (Fig. 6-4). **Mucous membranes** are the membranes that line body cavities that open to the outside of the body. These include the linings of the mouth, nose, eyes, rectum, and genitals.

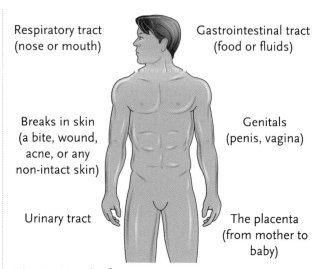

Fig. 6-4. *Portals of entry.*

When a pathogen invades the body, it causes an infection. Many areas of the body are protected from invading pathogens. A sort of body "armor" works with the immune system to help protect the body from harmful bacteria (Fig. 6-5). The box on the next page describes how the body keeps itself healthy.

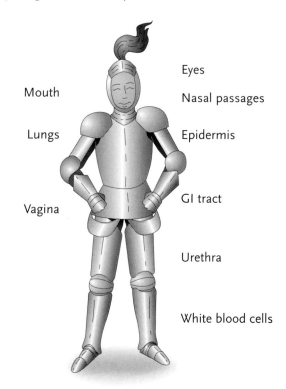

Fig. 6-5. *The body's natural "armor."*

The Human Body's Defensive Armor

Nasal passages: Mucous membranes have cilia, tiny hairs in the nose that trap microorganisms.

Epidermis: As long as skin stays unbroken and undamaged, microorganisms cannot get inside.

Lungs: Cilia move microbes, mucus, and debris up and out of the airways.

Mouth: Saliva has a protein called lactoferrin that blocks the growth of pathogens.

Eyes: The eyes have tears that protect them by cleaning out microorganisms.

GI (gastrointestinal) tract: The GI tract has "good" microorganisms, called "normal flora," that prevent the growth of "bad" microorganisms, or pathogens.

Vagina: The vagina has a low pH of about 3.5 to 4.5, which blocks the growth of pathogens.

Urethra: Urine rinses out pathogens from the urinary tract.

Blood cells: White blood cells defend the body from microorganisms and play a role in the secretion of antibodies.

Infection Control Example for Link 5: Wearing gloves.

Chain Link 6: Susceptible Host

A susceptible host is an uninfected person who could get sick. A person becomes a susceptible host when his or her resistance to disease decreases. Some reasons for lowered resistance include age, existing illnesses, fatigue, and stress. The elderly have weaker immune systems and a lower resistance to pathogens. When a pathogen invades the body, it will start reproducing itself. As pathogens grow, they damage healthy tissue.

Infection Control Example for Link 6: Staying healthy and protecting the elderly and ill from pathogens.

TRIVIA

The Amazing Discovery of Edward Jenner

In 18th-century England, smallpox was a very common, horribly disfiguring disease. A doctor at that time, Edward Jenner (1749-1823), noticed that people who were exposed to cowpox, such as the milkmaids who milked cows, would develop a small sore and then never get smallpox. He then developed a vaccine from the cowpox sores to give immunity to smallpox. After he injected the matter from the sore into a boy, James Phipps, he tested the vaccine by trying to give James the disease more than once. Each time, Jenner found that little James was immune to the disease.

5. Explain why the elderly are at a higher risk for infection

Residents are at great risk for acquiring infections while living in a facility. As people get older, multiple changes of aging tend to make the elderly more susceptible to infections (Fig. 6-6). Immune systems become weaker, which puts them at a higher risk for infection. Elderly people are hospitalized more often, which increases their chances of getting nosocomial and other infections. When the elderly get sick, recovery may take longer. Also, the infections themselves may be more dangerous. A simple cold can turn into a life-threatening illness, such as pneumonia.

Fig. 6-6. *The elderly are at higher risk for infection due to weaker immune systems, limited mobility, thinner skin, slow wound healing and many other reasons.*

As people age, their skin becomes thinner, which makes it easy to tear. When fragile skin tears, pathogens can enter the body. Limited mobility is another risk factor. Both thinner skin and limited mobility increase the risk of pressure sores and skin infections.

Bones become more brittle and can break more easily. Broken bones increase the risk of infection. Decreased circulation and slow wound healing also contribute to infections in the elderly.

Elderly people may require catheters for urinary elimination. Catheters, and other types of tubing, such as feeding tubes, can greatly increase the risk of infections.

Older adults are at risk for dehydration and **malnutrition**. A person who is malnourished is not getting the proper nutrition. **Dehydration** occurs when a person does not have enough fluid in the body. Both dehydration and malnutrition are serious problems. They may be caused by a lack of thirst and appetite, certain illnesses, or medications. When cells do not get proper nutrients and fluids, the chance of infection greatly increases.

One method of reducing infection is to keep residents as healthy as possible by promoting good health habits and using proper infection control methods. This is required of all staff members. You will learn more methods on how to keep residents infection-free in Chapter 24.

6. Describe The Centers for Disease Control and Prevention (CDC) and explain Standard Precautions

The Centers for Disease Control and Prevention (CDC) is a federal government agency that issues guidelines to protect and improve health. It promotes public health and safety through education and tries to control and prevent disease. In 1996, the CDC created new guidelines to protect people in health care from contracting infectious diseases. In 2007, the CDC released some changes to this system.

There are two levels of precautions in the infection control system recommended by the CDC. They are Standard Precautions and Transmission-Based, or Isolation Precautions. To **isolate** means to keep something separate, or by itself.

Standard Precautions must be used with every resident in your care. **Standard Precautions** means treating blood, body fluids, non-intact skin, and mucous membranes as if they were infected. Body fluids include tears, saliva, sputum (fluid coughed up from the lungs), vomit, urine, feces, pus or other fluid from a wound, vaginal secretions, and semen. It does not include sweat. Standard Precautions are always followed because you cannot tell by looking at residents or their charts if they have a contagious disease (Fig. 6-7). The guidelines for Standard Precautions are listed below.

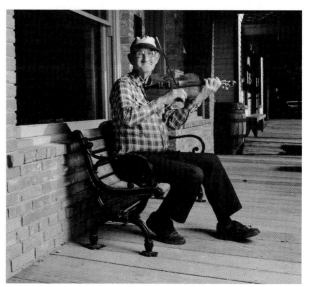

Fig. 6-7. Standard Precautions must be practiced on every person in your care, no matter how healthy or unhealthy he seems. You cannot tell by looking at a person whether he has an infectious disease or not.

Guidelines
Standard Precautions

- Wash your hands before putting on gloves. Wash them immediately after removing gloves. Do not touch clean objects with contaminated gloves. Follow the handwashing guidelines listed in the next Learning Objective.

- Immediately wash all skin surfaces that have been contaminated with blood and body fluids.

- Wear gloves if you may come into contact with blood, body fluids, secretions and excretions, broken or open skin, human tissue, or mucous membranes (linings of the eyes, nose, mouth, vagina, penis, or rectum). See Learning Objective 8 for more information.

- Wear a gown if you may come into contact with blood, body fluids, secretions or excretions, or when splashing or spraying blood or body fluids is likely. See Learning Objective 8 for more information.

- Wear a mask, protective goggles, and/or face shield if you may come into contact with blood, body fluids, secretions or excretions, or when splashing or spraying blood or body fluids is likely. See Learning Objective 8 for more information.

- Bag all disposable contaminated supplies. Dispose of them according to your facility's policy. Special containers are used for disposal. Place non-disposable contaminated supplies, such as linens and reusable equipment, into the proper container.

- Wear gloves and use caution when handling razor blades and other sharps. Be careful not to cut yourself or nick or cut residents when using razor blades. Place sharps carefully in a biohazard container. **Biohazard containers** are hard, leakproof containers. They are clearly labeled and warn of the danger of the contents inside (Fig. 6-8).

- Never attempt to cap needles or sharps. You might stick yourself. Dispose of them in an approved container.

- Clean all surfaces that may be contaminated with infectious waste. Examples of these areas are overbed tables, beds, wheelchairs, and shower chairs.

- Remember that Standard Precautions must be practiced on every single person in your care. Standard Precautions help reduce the risk of getting disease from those in your care. It also helps prevent residents' infections from being passed to other residents.

Fig. 6-8. *One type of biohazardous waste container.*

In addition to Standard Precautions, here are general guidelines for controlling infection in a facility:

- Clean a cut or break in your skin immediately with a facility-approved disinfecting product.

- Cover your mouth and nose when coughing or sneezing. Immediately wash your hands afterward.

- Keep yourself as healthy as possible.

- Never use one resident's personal items for another resident. Keep all personal items separate.

- Never transfer personal items or any kind of equipment from one room to another. An exception is something like your stethoscope. You must disinfect the part of your stethoscope that touches a resident after each use.

- Hold all equipment or personal care items you carry away from your uniform while walking.

- Completely clean objects before using them if they have dropped to the floor.

- Clean all equipment used by residents after use. Follow the facility's guidelines for disinfection.

- Clean all common areas (areas used by more than one resident) after use.

- Remove food or soiled eating utensils in residents' rooms after food trays have been picked up.

- Change water cups often.

- Clean resident toothbrushes and shaving equipment often.

- Never place contaminated items like bedpans or any other dirty items on the overbed table. You will learn more about resident's unit equipment in Chapter 10.

- When cleaning anything, move from the cleanest to the dirtiest area.

Respiratory/Cough Etiquette

Guidelines for all persons entering facilities who show any signs of respiratory illnesses have been developed as a new part of Standard Precautions. The guidelines consist of covering the nose and mouth when coughing or sneezing, using tissues for respiratory secretions, and promptly disposing of the tissues in a hands-free waste container. People who are coughing must wear special masks, and turn their head away from others. When coughing, they must keep a distance of more than three feet from others.

7. Define "hand hygiene" and identify when to wash hands

In your work you will use your hands constantly. Microorganisms are on everything you touch. People have developed serious illnesses due to the lack of handwashing by staff. Washing your hands is the single most important thing you can do to prevent the spread of disease (Fig. 6-9).

Fig. 6-9. *All people in health care must wash their hands often. Washing your hands is the most important thing you can do to prevent the spread of disease.*

Hand hygiene is defined by the CDC as any method that removes or destroys microorganisms on hands. This includes using plain or an-

tiseptic soap and water and using alcohol-based hand rubs. Alcohol-based hand rubs (hand sanitizers) include gels, rinses, and foams which do not require the use of water. Alcohol-based hand rubs are not a substitute for frequent and proper handwashing. When hands are visibly soiled, wash them with plain or antimicrobial soap and water. An **antimicrobial** agent destroys or resists pathogens. Once hands are clean, alcohol-based products can be used in addition to handwashing.

Keep your nails short and clean. Do not wear artificial nails or extenders because they harbor more bacteria, even if you wash your hands often. Rings and other jewelry collect bacteria and can cause infection. Keep them at home if possible.

Use unscented lotions to keep your hands soft and intact. It is dangerous for you to work with cracked, broken skin. Use lotions at home, as well, to reduce the risk of broken skin.

You must wash your hands at these times:

- When you first arrive at work
- When you enter a resident's room
- When you leave a resident's room
- Before and after feeding residents
- Before you put on gloves and after you remove gloves or if gloves rip or tear
- After contact with blood or any body fluids
- After handling contaminated items
- After touching garbage
- Before entering a "clean" supply room
- Before getting clean linen
- Before and after touching meal trays and/or handling food
- After cleaning spills or picking up anything from the floor
- Before and after drinking and eating
- After smoking
- After handling your hair or touching areas on your body, such as your nose, mouth, eyes, and face

- Before and after applying makeup
- Before and after inserting contact lenses
- After using the bathroom
- After coughing, sneezing, or blowing your nose
- Before leaving the facility
- When you get home from work before touching anything or anyone

Washing hands

Equipment: soap, paper towels

1. Identify yourself by name. Identify the resident. Greet the resident by name.

2. Turn on water at the sink.

3. Angle your arms downward, with your fingertips pointing down into the sink. Your hands should be lower than your elbows. Wet your hands and wrists thoroughly (Fig. 6-10).

Fig. 6-10.

4. Apply skin cleanser or soap to your hands.

5. Lather all surfaces of your hands, wrists, and fingers. Use friction for at least 20 seconds (Fig. 6-11).

Fig. 6-11.

6. Clean your nails by rubbing your fingertips in the palm of your other hand.

7. Rinse all surfaces of wrists, hands, and fingers. Keep your hands lower than your elbows and your fingertips down.

8. Use a clean, dry paper towel to dry all surfaces of your hands, wrists, and fingers.

9. Use clean, dry paper towel or your knee to turn off the faucet. Do not contaminate your hands by touching the inside of the sink or the faucet at any time (Fig. 6-12).

Fig. 6-12.

10. Dispose of used paper towels in wastebasket immediately after shutting off faucet.

RESIDENTS' RIGHTS

Wash hands before resident care.
As you move between residents' rooms, always wash your hands. Taking care of residents means you will get many microorganisms on your hands. Wash your hands before giving care. It will help prevent the spread of disease.

8. Discuss the use of personal protective equipment (PPE) in facilities

Personal protective equipment (**PPE**) is a **barrier** (a block or obstacle) between a person and disease. PPE is what you wear to prevent the transmission of disease. You will need to know how to apply and use PPE correctly.

PPE includes gloves, gowns, masks, goggles, and face shields. Gloves protect hands, and gowns protect the skin and clothing. Masks protect the mouth and nose. Goggles protect the eyes, and face shields protect the entire face—the eyes, nose and mouth.

Your employers will provide you with the proper PPE to wear. The type of PPE you wear depends on what kind of exposure you may encounter. For example, a chance of coming into contact with spraying or splashing blood or body fluids is one type of exposure that requires gown, gloves, and mask and goggles, or face shield. PPE selection also depends on the type of Transmission-Based Precautions that are ordered for a resident. You will learn more about these Precautions in Learning Objective 11. PPE use is determined by the type of task you will perform. Hand hygiene is always the final step after removing and disposing of PPE.

Gloves

There are two types of gloves: non-sterile and sterile. Non-sterile gloves are used for basic care in a facility. These come in different sizes and may be made of nitrile, vinyl, or latex. Some people are allergic to latex. If you are, let the nurse know so that alternative gloves can be provided. Gloves should fit your hands comfortably. They should not be too loose or too snug.

When wearing gloves, always work from clean to dirty. This means you should touch clean surfaces or areas before touching contaminated ones.

Always wear gloves when:

- You may come into contact with blood or any body fluids, open wounds, or mucous membranes

- Performing or helping with mouth care

- Performing or helping with **perineal care** (care of the genital and anal area)

- Performing care on a resident who has **non-intact skin**—broken by abrasions, cuts, rashes, acne, pimples, lesions, surgical incisions, or boils

- You have any open sores or cuts on your hands

- Shaving a resident

- Disposing of soiled bed linens, gowns, dressings, and pads

- You will have direct contact with residents who require Contact Precautions (a type of Transmission-Based Precaution; see Learning Objective 11)

- When touching surfaces or equipment or handling equipment that is either visibly contaminated or may be contaminated

If you do have sores or cuts on your hands, cover them first with gauze, then put on gloves. Disposable gloves cannot be washed or re-used. Wear them only once and then discard them.

Change gloves right before contact with mucous membranes or broken skin. Change gloves immediately if they become wet, worn, soiled, or torn. Do not contaminate skin or clothing when removing gloves. Wash your hands before putting on new gloves. Do not touch anything with contaminated gloves that anyone else may touch without wearing gloves.

For example, if you are carrying a used bedpan, do not touch the doorknob or open the door with gloved hands. The doorknob would be contaminated if you did. Change gloves if your hands will move from a body site that is contaminated to a body site that is not contaminated. Before touching any surface, remove your gloves, wash your hands, and put on new gloves if needed.

Putting on gloves

Equipment: clean gloves in the correct size

1. Wash your hands.

2. If you are right-handed, slide one glove on your left hand (reverse if left-handed).

3. Using your gloved hand, slide the other hand into the second glove.

4. Interlace fingers to smooth out folds and create a comfortable fit.

5. Check for tears, holes, cracks, or discolored spots in the gloves. Replace the glove if needed.

6. Adjust gloves until they are pulled up over the wrist and fit correctly. If wearing a gown, pull the cuff of the gloves over the sleeve of the gown (Fig. 6-13).

Fig. 6-13.

Remove gloves immediately after use and before caring for another resident. Wash your hands. Never touch your face or adjust PPE with clean or dirty gloves.

Taking off gloves

1. Touch only the outside of one glove. Pull the first glove off by pulling down from the cuff toward the fingers (Fig. 6-14).

Fig. 6-14.

2. As this first glove comes off, it should be turned inside-out.

3. With the fingertips of your gloved hand, hold the glove you just removed.

4. With your ungloved hand, reach two fingers inside the remaining glove. Be careful not to touch any part of the outside of the glove (Fig. 6-15).

Fig. 6-15.

5. Pull down, turning this glove inside-out and over the first glove as you remove it.

6. You should now be holding one glove from its clean inner side. The other glove should be inside it.

7. Drop both gloves into the proper container.

8. Wash your hands.

Gowns

Gowns protect the skin and the clothing from contamination. Wear a gown if you may come into contact with blood, body fluids, secretions or excretions, tissue, or when splashing or spraying blood or body fluids is likely. Wear a gown if your clothing will have direct contact with the resident or any contaminated equipment or surfaces near the resident or that may have come into contact with the resident. Wear a gown when handling any equipment that is visibly soiled or may have had contact with blood or body fluids.

Gowns should fully cover your torso. They should fit comfortably over your body, and have long sleeves that fit snugly at the wrist. If a gown does not fit you properly, report it to your supervisor. If one gown is too small to safely and completely cover your torso, you may need to wear two gowns. One ties in the front and one ties in the back.

Gowns are usually made of a fluid-resistant material. However, they may still become wet or soiled. If this happens, remove the gown. Check your clothing and put on a new gown. Gowns must be changed immediately if they become wet or soiled. Gowns are used once and disposed of properly. Remove gown promptly after care. Do not contaminate skin or clothing when removing gowns. After gown removal, avoid touching any surface in the room with your uniform or your skin before exiting the room.

Putting on a gown

Equipment: clean gown in correct size

1. Wash your hands.

2. Remove watch and place it on a clean paper towel. If wearing long sleeves, push or roll them up.

3. Open the gown. Hold it out in front of you and allow it to open (Fig. 6-16). Do not shake gown or touch it to the floor. Slip your arms into the sleeves and pull the gown on.

Fig. 6-16.

4. Cover torso from the neck down to and covering the knees. Cover the arms to the end of the wrists and wrap gown completely around the back. Securely fasten at the neck and the waist. Tie the neck ties into a bow so they can be easily untied later, or seal the tapes closed if gown has tapes.

5. Reach behind you. Pull the gown until it completely covers your clothing. Tie the back ties (Fig. 6-17).

6. Use gowns only once and then remove and discard. Do not contaminate skin or clothing when removing gowns. Untie neck strings, then waist strings of gown. Peel gown away

from body. Hold gown away from body and roll inside-out into a bundle. Discard gown in proper container.

7. Put on gloves after putting on a gown.

Fig. 6-17.

Masks and Goggles

Masks should be worn when caring for residents who cough or sneeze or have respiratory illnesses. Masks can prevent inhalation of microorganisms through the nose or mouth. Masks protect the nose and mouth and mucous membranes from contamination during resident care or activities. Wear a mask along with protective goggles if you anticipate that during resident care or activities, you may come into contact with blood or body fluids.

Goggles are worn with a mask and are used whenever it is likely that blood or body fluids may be splashed or sprayed into your eye area or your eyes. Eyeglasses alone do not provide enough protection. Goggles should fit snugly over and around your eyes or eyeglasses.

Masks should fully cover your nose and mouth and prevent fluid penetration. Masks should fit snugly over the nose and mouth. Masks are worn once and disposed of. Masks that become wet or soiled must be changed immediately. Remove masks after a procedure. Change masks between resident care. Never wear a mask in the hall between resident rooms.

When removing a mask and/or goggles, remove your gloves first and then wash your hands. Be careful to not touch the mask or goggles to your clothing or your skin. The pieces used to secure the mask or goggles to the head are clean and can be touched with your ungloved hands. The mask and goggles themselves are considered contaminated. Do not contaminate skin or clothing when removing masks or goggles. Wash hands every time after removing a mask and/or goggles.

Putting on a mask and goggles

Equipment: mask, goggles

1. Wash your hands.

2. Pick up the mask by the top strings or the elastic strap. Do not touch the mask where it touches your face.

3. Adjust the mask over your nose and mouth. Tie top strings, then bottom strings. Never wear a mask hanging from only the bottom strings (Fig. 6-18).

Fig. 6-18.

4. Pinch the metal strip at the top of the mask (if part of the mask) tightly around your nose so that it feels snug. Fit mask snugly around face and below the chin.

5. Put on the goggles. Position them over the eyes. Secure them to the head using the headband or earpieces.

6. Put on your gloves after putting on mask and goggles.

Some respiratory diseases, such as tuberculosis (TB), require special PPE to be worn. More information on TB is in Chapter 20. This equipment helps keep staff safe from this disease. Special masks must be worn because a standard mask does not protect the caregiver from TB. These masks, called respirators, have a filter that protects the face and lungs. An N95 respirator mask is one type of special mask. The caregiver must be fitted for this mask. Each time the person puts the respirator on, a "user-seal check," formerly called a "fit-check," must be done to minimize the leaking of any air from around the respirator. You will be taught how to perform a user-seal check.

Face Shields

Face shields may be worn when contact with blood or body fluids may occur. Face shields are used whenever it is likely that blood or body fluids may be splashed or sprayed into your eye area or your eyes. Face shields can be used instead of wearing goggles and may offer more protection from sprays and splashes than goggles can provide. Face shields may be worn with a mask. Follow facility policy with face shields. The face shield should cover your forehead, go below the chin, and wrap around the side of the head. Secure it on your head using the headband.

When removing a face shield, remove your gloves first and wash your hands. Be careful to not touch the shield to your clothing or your skin. The pieces used to secure the shield to the head are clean and can be touched with your ungloved hands. The face shield itself is considered contaminated. Do not contaminate skin or clothing when removing face shields. Wash hands every time after removing a face shield.

You are responsible for knowing where the PPE is kept in your facility. If you have questions on what PPE is needed, ask the nurse. When applying PPE, you must follow a specific order. Removing PPE requires a specific order, too. The order depends on what PPE you are wearing and whether special precautions have been ordered (Fig. 6-19).

Fig. 6-19. Using PPE is an important way to reduce the spread of infection.

Applying and removing the full set of PPE

Equipment: gown, mask or respirator, goggles or face shield, gloves

Applying:

1. Wash your hands.

2. Put on gown.

3. Apply mask or respirator.

4. Apply goggles or face shield.

5. Apply gloves last.

Removing:

1. Remove gloves first. Discard gloves in proper container.

2. Wash your hands.

3. Remove face shield or goggles if used.

4. Remove gown next. Discard in proper container.

5. Remove mask or respirator. Discard in proper container.

6. Wash your hands.

9. List guidelines for handling linen and equipment

Facilities handle storage and disposal of linen and equipment by following guidelines set by the CDC. As you have learned, facilities have separate areas for clean and dirty items, called the "clean" and the "dirty" or "contaminated" utility rooms. Linen and equipment will be placed in separate containers to be cleaned or discarded.

There will be disposal containers for:

• Linen disposal

• Trash disposal

• Equipment disposal

• Special disposal of infectious waste

Guidelines
Handling Linen and Equipment

⊕ Wear gloves when handling, transporting and processing soiled linens.

⊕ When removing linen, handle it carefully. Check linen to make sure no items are left inside, especially sharps, as you remove it from the bed. Fold or roll linen so that the dirtiest area is inside.

⊕ Hold and carry dirty linen away from your uniform (Fig. 6-20).

⊕ Do not shake dirty linen or clothes.

⊕ Place or dispose of linen, trash, used equipment, and infectious waste in the proper containers. All sharps must be safely placed in puncture-proof biohazard containers.

⊕ Do not touch the inside of any disposal container.

⊕ Do not use "re-usable" equipment again until it has been properly cleaned and reprocessed. Dispose of all single-use equipment properly.

⊕ Wear gloves when cleaning and disinfecting surfaces. Clean and disinfect beds, bedrails and all bedside equipment. Clean all frequently-touched surfaces, such as doorknobs.

Fig. 6-20. *Hold dirty linen away from your uniform.*

10. Explain how to handle spills

Spills happen when blood, body fluids, or other fluids get on any person, object, or area in a facility. Spills pose a serious risk of infection and in addition, put residents at risk for falls. Clean spills using proper equipment and procedures, and follow these guidelines:

- Apply gloves immediately. You may need to use special heavy-duty gloves, depending on the spill.

- Wipe up spill immediately. Clean from the outside "cleanest" to the inside "dirtiest" to keep from spreading the spill. Follow facility policy.

- A cleaning solution of one part bleach to ten parts water can be used to finish cleaning the area. You may have ready-to-use spray bottles available at your facility. These bottles will be clearly labeled. Make sure the date on the bottle is current.

- Be careful if any glass or other sharp objects are in the spill. Get help when picking up and disposing of sharps and other objects. Never pick up glass, even with gloved hands. If you do accidentally cut yourself, follow exposure incident guidelines listed below.

- For large spills, call for the nurse and she will follow your facility's policy for large-spill clean-up. Dispose of gloves and cleaning equipment and supplies according to facility policy.

- If you spill a substance on your body, immediately wash that area using the proper cleaning agent. Follow exposure incident guidelines (see Learning Objective 13).

- Wash your hands after cleaning spills.

Some facilities have special "spill areas" that have equipment to handle spills. Colored cones are placed to identify the area where the spill occurred. Pads that come in different sizes are placed over the spill. Then the proper department is notified to clean the area.

11. Discuss Transmission-Based Precautions

In 1996, the CDC set forth a second level of precautions beyond Standard Precautions. These guidelines were for persons who are infected or may be infected with diseases. They are known as Transmission-Based or Isolation Precautions.

The three categories of Transmission-Based Precautions are Airborne Precautions, Droplet Precautions, and Contact Precautions. The type used depends on what type of disease the person has or may have and how it spreads. They may also be used in combination for diseases that have multiple routes of transmission.

Airborne Precautions

Airborne Precautions prevent the spread of pathogens that travel through the air for a distance after being expelled (Fig. 6-21). The pathogens remain floating for some time. They are carried by moisture and are also carried by dust. An example of an airborne disease is tuberculosis (TB). TB is a disease that is transferred through droplets in the air that can travel a long distance. TB can be fatal if not treated. More information on TB is found in Chapter 20. For Airborne Precautions:

- Follow all Standard Precautions.

- Residents will be placed in a room called an airborne infection isolation room (AIIR), formerly known as a negative pressure isolation room. These rooms have a controlled flow of air. All the air inside the room will be exhausted directly to the outside, or all air will first be re-circulated through a special HEPA filter before being returned to circulation. Keep windows to these rooms closed; keep doors closed when not going in or out of the room. Do not open or close the door quickly when entering the room.

- Wear a special mask during resident care. All people entering the room must wear a special mask, such as an N95 respirator mask, prior to entering the AIIR. A standard mask is not safe to use because the TB bacterium is small enough to penetrate a regular mask.

- Follow facility policy on where to remove masks.

- Residents will wear masks if they must leave the room.

Fig. 6-21. *Airborne diseases stay suspended in the air.*

Droplet Precautions

Droplet Precautions are used for diseases that are spread by droplets in the air. Droplets normally do not travel further than three feet, but they may travel further. Talking, singing, sneezing, laughing, or coughing can spread droplets (Fig. 6-22). An example of a droplet disease is the mumps. For Droplet Precautions:

- Follow all Standard Precautions.

- Apply a mask before entering the room. Wear the mask during resident care.

- Facilities should limit transport of residents outside of the room to medical necessities. Residents must wear masks if they must

leave the room and observe Respiratory/Cough Etiquette (see earlier box).

- Cover your nose and mouth with a tissue if you sneeze or cough and place tissues in a hands-free disposal. Ask others to do the same. Wash your hands promptly if you sneeze or cough on them.

- Visits from uninfected people will be restricted.

- Pull the privacy curtain between beds of any residents placed in the same room.

Fig. 6-22. *Droplet Precautions are followed when the disease-causing microorganism does not remain in the air.*

Contact Precautions

Contact Precautions are used when a resident may spread an infection by direct contact with another person or object. The infection can be spread when a nursing assistant touches a contaminated area on a resident's body or his contaminated blood or body fluids (Fig. 6-23). It may also be spread by touching contaminated personal items, linen, equipment, or supplies. Conjunctivitis (pink eye) and *Clostridium difficile* (*C. diff*) are examples of a contact disease. You will learn more about *C. diff* later in the chapter. For Contact Precautions:

- Follow all Standard Precautions.

- Wear proper PPE. Put on gloves before entering a resident's room. Change gloves if they are contaminated with infected material. Remove gloves before leaving the room.

- While still in the room, wash hands with an antimicrobial soap after removing gloves. Do not touch any surface with your hands before exiting.

- Put on a gown before entering a resident's room. Remove gown before leaving the room. Dispose of gown properly. Wash hands after removing gown before leaving. Do not touch any surface in the room with your uniform or your skin before exiting.

- Do not share residents' equipment with other residents. Any equipment that must be used by more than one resident will be disinfected before being used again.

- Residents will most likely be placed in a private room. If they are not, keep the privacy curtain closed between beds.

Fig. 6-23. *Contact Precautions are followed when the person is at risk of transmitting a microorganism by touching an infected object or person.*

When Transmission-Based Precautions are ordered, they are always used in addition to Standard Precautions.

12. Describe care of the resident in an isolation unit

Residents who require Transmission-Based Precautions are referred to as being in "isolation." A sign should be on the door indicating "isolation" or alerting people to see the nurse before entering the room.

Residents in isolation units experience big changes. They cannot move about freely because they are separated from everyone else. Empathize with them. Think about how you would feel if you were in isolation. Spend as much time with the resident as possible. This can help reduce loneliness and gives them a connection to the outside world. Listen to the resident and encourage him or her to talk about feelings and concerns. Reassure the resident that it is the disease, not the person, that is being isolated.

Explain why these special steps are being taken. In addition, follow these guidelines:

Guidelines
Residents in Isolation

- Clean and disinfect all equipment properly. Follow facility policy on equipment that belongs to staff and does not stay in the room, such as a stethoscope. Some facilities do not allow staff to take their own items into the room. If so, there will be a stethoscope that stays in the isolation room at all times. Disinfect the stethoscope each time before using.

- Dispose of trash in proper containers.

- Place disposable food trays, eating utensils, cups and dishes in the proper containers, which may be separate from regular disposal areas or containers.

- Dispose of waste containing blood or body fluids and sharps in biohazard containers.

- Double-bag used linen or equipment. This means putting it in one bag, and then putting the first bag in a second, clean trash bag and closing it. For more information on double-bagging, see Learning Objective 13.

- Disinfect all furniture and surfaces (doorknobs, sinks, other bathroom surfaces) regularly.

- If the resident is allowed visitors, assist them with putting on gowns and masks as needed.

- Before you leave the room, make sure the TV, telephone, and radio are all in working order.

- Encourage reading material that can be disposed of, such as magazines and newspapers. Make sure the resident has access to eyeglasses, if needed.

- Always place the call light within the resident's reach when leaving the isolation room.

You may assist in setting up an isolation unit. Before doing anything in the isolation area, wash your hands and put on gloves. Follow the nurse's instructions on what to do in the room. Adjust the bed to the proper height. Put away clean towels and other supplies. Leave clean pajamas or gown in an easy-to-reach spot. Check to make sure the following are in working order:

- The bed controls, including the call light
- Lights in the room
- The television and radio controls
- Telephone
- Closet and dressers/cabinets
- Windows and latches

Re-stock bathroom supplies. Refill the soap dispenser and paper towel dispenser. Check to make sure garbage cans have been emptied. If anything is damaged or not working properly, tell the nurse immediately.

If asked to set up an isolation cart outside of the resident's room, make sure the cart is stocked with all PPE needed. This includes gloves in various sizes, gowns, masks, goggles, and face shields. Gather extra plastic bags and laundry bags, too. Some facilities use an anteroom just outside of the isolation room. This anteroom may have a sink. Follow facility policy when using the anteroom. Special steps may need to be taken in that room.

Information on collecting specimens from a resident in isolation will be discussed in Chapter 15.

RESIDENTS' RIGHTS

Residents in Isolation

Residents' rights must be protected when they are in isolation. Their dignity, privacy and confidentiality must be maintained at all times. Residents can participate in their care as much as possible. They have the right to choose what care they receive and to file complaints. They have the right to visits from family, friends, or clergy. Visitors must receive training on the safe and proper use of PPE before entering the isolation room.

13. Explain OSHA's Bloodborne Pathogen Standard

Bloodborne pathogens are microorganisms found in human blood. They can cause infection and disease in humans. They may also be found in body fluids, draining wounds, and mucous membranes. These pathogens are transmitted by infected blood entering the bloodstream, or if infected semen or vaginal secretions contact mucous membranes. Sharing infected drug needles is another way to spread bloodborne diseases. Infected pregnant women may transmit bloodborne disease to their babies. In health care, contact with infectious blood or body fluids is the most common way to get a bloodborne disease. Infections can be spread by having accidental contact with contaminated blood or body fluids, skin, needles or other sharp objects, or contaminated supplies or equipment.

The Occupational Safety and Health Administration (OSHA) is a federal government agency that is responsible for the safety of workers in the U.S. OSHA makes rules to protect workers from hazards on the job. OSHA conducts workplace inspections to check on worker safety and updates safety standards that are needed at work. OSHA also provides training for employers and employees on workplace safety (Fig. 6-24). The employer is responsible for meeting all safety standards and providing a workplace that is free of hazards. Employees are responsible for doing their job in a way that meets OSHA's safety standards.

Fig. 6-24. *The OSHA website.*

OSHA sets standards for equipment use and special techniques to use when working in facilities. One of these standards is the **Bloodborne Pathogen Standard**. This law was passed in

1991. It requires that healthcare facilities protect employees from bloodborne health hazards.

By law, employers must follow these rules to reduce the risk of acquiring infectious diseases. The Standard also guides employers and employees through the steps to follow if exposed to infectious material. Types of waste that are considered infectious are blood, body fluids, and human tissue. Significant exposures include:

- Exposure by injection; a needle stick

- Mucous membrane contact

- Cut from an object containing a potentially infectious body fluid (includes human bites)

- Non-intact skin (OSHA includes acne in this category)

Guidelines employers must follow include:

- Employers must give in-service training on the risks from bloodborne pathogens and updates on any new safety standards.

- Employers must have an exposure control plan should an employee accidentally become exposed to any infectious waste. The **exposure control plan** identifies the step-by-step method of what to do if exposed to infectious material. It also includes specific work practices that must be followed. All employees must be trained on it and know where to find it.

- Employers must give all employees, visitors, and residents proper PPE to wear when needed.

- Employers must place biohazard containers in each resident's room and in other areas in the facility to dispose of equipment and supplies contaminated with infectious waste.

- If bags are used without hard containers for any type of waste, use the right bag for the right type of infectious waste disposal. The bag must be sealed tightly before leaving the resident's room. Double-bagging is generally only done when there is a high risk of leakage through one bag. Bags must be safely taken to the proper area for biohazard infectious waste.

- Employers are required to provide a free hepatitis B vaccine to all employees after hire.

When an employee is exposed to infectious blood or material, it is called an **exposure incident**. After an exposure incident, specific steps must be taken:

- Immediately follow facility policy regarding a spill, splash, or cut. (More information on skin and eye splashes is in Chapter 7.)

- Report an exposure incident immediately to your supervisor.

- Fill out an exposure report form. Keep a copy for yourself. Exposure reports help you get the follow-up care you need after an exposure. They also help employers find ways to prevent future exposures.

- Go to your employer's health service department to get any needed tests.

In 2001, OSHA revised the Bloodborne Pathogens Standard. The revisions address the need for employers to select safer needle devices and to involve employees in choosing these devices. They also require employers to keep a log of injuries from contaminated sharps.

14. Discuss two important bloodborne diseases

Two major bloodborne diseases in the U.S. are acquired immune deficiency syndrome (AIDS) and hepatitis.

AIDS is a disease caused by the human immunodeficiency virus (HIV). Over time, HIV damages the immune system so that the body cannot fight infections. These types of infections are called "opportunistic infections." In addition to these infections, tumors and central nervous system symptoms may appear. This stage of the disease is known as AIDS. People with AIDS lose all ability to fight infection. They can die from illnesses that a healthy immune system could fight.

HIV is transmitted by blood, infected needles, and from mother to fetus. It is also a sexually-transmitted disease. You will learn more about HIV and AIDS in Chapter 24.

Hepatitis is an inflammation of the liver caused by infection. Liver function can be permanently damaged by hepatitis. Several different viruses can cause hepatitis, including hepatitis A, B, C, D, and E. The most common are hepatitis A, B, and C. Hepatitis B and C are blood-borne diseases that can cause death. Many more people have hepatitis B (HBV) than HIV. The risk of getting hepatitis is greater than the risk of acquiring HIV.

Hepatitis A (HAV) is spread by an oral/fecal route. Transmission occurs when a person puts an object into his mouth that has been contaminated with another person's feces who has HAV. Symptoms are jaundice (yellow skin or eyes), fatigue, abdominal pain, nausea, diarrhea and fever. There is a vaccine available for Hepatitis A.

Hepatitis B (HBV) is a bloodborne form of hepatitis. The infection is usually spread by blood and body fluids. HBV can cause few symptoms or become a severe infection. Some of the symptoms are fatigue, nausea, vomiting, diarrhea, jaundice, lack of appetite, joint pain and abdominal pain. Hepatitis B can lead to serious problems with the liver, such as cirrhosis (liver damage) or liver cancer. In some cases, HBV can be fatal.

HBV is spread through sexual contact, sharing infected needles, from a mother to her baby during delivery, improperly sterilized needles used for tattoos, and grooming supplies, such as razors and toothbrushes. It is also spread by exposures at work from accidental contact with a used infected needle or other sharp instrument, or from splashing blood.

HBV poses a serious threat to healthcare workers. It is important to use proper PPE to help prevent HBV. Also handle needles and other sharps carefully. Dispose of them properly in a biohazard container. Do not share a resident's razor, toothbrush, or other grooming supplies with other residents.

Equally important is to get the vaccine for hepatitis B when it is offered. Employers must offer a free vaccine to protect you from hepatitis B. Talk to your supervisor about getting this vaccine.

Hepatitis C (HCV) is transmitted by blood or body fluids. Many people have no symptoms of Hepatitis C. If symptoms do occur, they include fatigue, nausea, jaundice, dark urine, lack of appetite, and abdominal pain. Hepatitis C can be fatal if it leads to serious illness, such as liver cancer or cirrhosis. A liver transplant may be required. There is no vaccine for hepatitis C.

Hepatitis D (HDV) is transmitted by blood or body fluids. Hepatitis D can be caught at the same time as hepatitis B (HBV). HBV must be present for the person to get hepatitis D. The symptoms are fatigue, nausea, vomiting, jaundice, dark, tea-colored urine, lack of appetite, joint pain, and abdominal pain. Many people with hepatitis D develop cirrhosis of the liver.

Hepatitis E (HEV) is spread by an oral/fecal route or by contaminated food or water. People generally get this virus while traveling in developing countries. Hepatitis E is normally an acute, not a chronic, illness. The symptoms are fatigue, nausea, vomiting, jaundice, dark, tea-colored urine, lack of appetite, and abdominal pain.

RESIDENTS' RIGHTS

Know the facts.

Do not be afraid of a resident who has HIV or AIDS. Simple touches, handshakes or hugs cannot spread the HIV virus (Fig. 6-25). It is important to provide emotional support. Do not ignore or avoid residents with HIV or AIDS.

Fig. 6-25. *Hugs cannot spread HIV or AIDS.*

15. Discuss MRSA, VRE, and *C. Difficile*

Multidrug-resistant organisms (**MDROs**) are microorganisms, mostly bacteria, that are resistant to one or more antimicrobial agents. As you learned earlier, an antimicrobial agent destroys or resists pathogens. There has been an increase in MDROs in healthcare facilities and it is a serious problem. Two common types of MDROs are MRSA and VRE.

MRSA stands for methicillin-resistant *Staphylococcus aureus*. *Staphylococcus aureus* is a common type of bacteria that can cause illness. Methicillin is a powerful antibiotic drug. **MRSA infection** is an antibiotic-resistant infection often acquired in healthcare facilities.

MRSA is mostly spread by direct physical contact with infected people. If a person has MRSA on her skin, especially her hands, and touches someone else, she may spread MRSA. Indirect contact by touching equipment or supplies contaminated by a person with MRSA can also spread MRSA.

Common MRSA infection sites include the respiratory tract, surgical wounds, perineum, rectum, and the skin. Symptoms of MRSA infection include drainage, fever, chills, and redness. The single most important way to control MRSA is through proper hand hygiene. Always follow Standard Precautions, along with Transmission-Based Precautions as ordered.

VRE is vancomycin-resistant *enterococcus*. *Enterococcus* is a bacterium that lives in the digestive and genital tracts. It does not cause problems in healthy people. Vancomycin is a powerful antibiotic used to prevent or kill bacterial infections. It is often the antibiotic of last resort. Its use is generally limited to bacteria that are resistant to other antibiotics. Vancomycin-resistant *enterococcus* is a mutant strain of *enterococcus*. It originally developed in people who were exposed to the antibiotic. VRE is very dangerous because it cannot be controlled with antibiotics. It causes life-threatening infections in those with weak immune systems—the very young, the very old, and the very ill. VRE is spread through direct and indirect contact.

Symptoms of VRE infection include fever, fatigue, chills, and drainage. Once it establishes itself, it is very hard to get rid of. Preventing VRE is much easier. Proper hand hygiene can help prevent the spread of VRE. Always follow Standard Precautions, along with Transmission-Based Precautions as ordered.

Residents with MRSA may be placed in contact or droplet isolation depending upon the site of the infection. Residents with VRE may be placed in contact isolation.

As with VRE and MRSA, tuberculosis can become resistant to available treatments. This is called multidrug-resistant tuberculosis (MDR-TB). Risk of MDR-TB increases when people do not complete their prescribed course of medications. See Chapter 20 for more information.

Current CDC guidelines state that residents with MRSA or VRE should remain as active as possible. They may be allowed to eat with others and participate in activities as long as any open sores or wounds are completely covered. All bodily fluids, such as urine, must be contained. Residents with MRSA or VRE must practice good hygiene. They should wash their hands often or have staff assist them if they are not able to do this on their own. Some residents with MRSA or VRE will be restricted to their rooms.

In addition, all staff members should:

- Wash their hands with soap and water after any physical contact with residents with MRSA or VRE.

- After handwashing, discard paper towels immediately in a hands-free disposal.

- Wear disposable gloves when any contact with blood or body fluids may occur.

- Wash linen whenever soiled.

- Clean the resident's room with the proper disinfectant whenever body fluids soil surfaces.

- Alert other caregivers and visitors to take proper precautions prior to any contact with residents with MRSA or VRE.

- Attend all in-service programs on infection control methods used with MRSA and VRE residents.

Clostridium difficile is commonly known as "**C. diff**" or "**C. difficile**." It is a spore-forming bacterium which can be part of the normal intestinal flora. When the normal intestinal flora is altered, *C. difficile* can flourish in the intestinal tract. It produces a toxin that causes a watery diarrhea. Enemas, nasogastric tube insertion, and GI tract surgery increase a person's risk of developing the disease. The elderly are at a higher risk of getting *C. difficile*. The overuse of antibiotics may alter the normal intestinal flora and increase the risk of developing C. *difficile* diarrhea. *C. difficile* can also cause colitis, a more serious intestinal condition. It can also cause sepsis, a bloodstream infection, which can be fatal. More information about sepsis can be found in Chapter 26.

C. difficile is spread by spores in feces that are difficult to kill. These spores can be carried on the hands of people who have direct contact with infected residents or with environmental surfaces (floors, bedpans, toilets, etc.) contaminated with *C. difficile*. Touching an object contaminated with *C. difficile* can transmit *C. difficile*. Alcohol-based hand sanitizers are not considered effective on *C. difficile*. Soap and water must be used each time hand hygiene is performed.

Symptoms of *C. difficile* include frequent, foul-smelling, watery stools. Other symptoms include fever, diarrhea that contains blood and mucus, nausea, lack of appetite and abdominal cramps. Proper handwashing and handling of contaminated wastes can help prevent the spread of the disease. Additional Transmission-Based Precautions are used with residents who have *C. difficile*. Cleaning surfaces with the appropriate disinfectant containing bleach can also

help. Limiting the use of antibiotics helps lower the risk of developing *C. difficile* diarrhea. All caregivers and visitors must be advised to take proper precautions before any contact with a resident who has *C. difficile*.

There is a quick test that can diagnose *C. difficile*. If you note any of the symptoms, promptly report them to the nurse. The risk of serious illness, along with transmission, increases if the infection is not identified and cared for promptly.

CHAPTER REVIEW

1. What does "infection control" mean (LO 2)?

2. How does infection occur (LO 2)?

3. Describe the difference between localized and systemic infections (LO 2).

4. Define communicable disease and non-communicable disease (LO 2).

5. Describe the difference between "clean" and "dirty" in health care (LO 3).

6. What is the difference between sterilization and disinfection (LO 3)?

7. What is surgical asepsis (LO 3)?

8. Describe the six links in the chain of infection and list an infection control practice for each link (LO 4).

9. What are mucous membranes (LO 4)?

10. List four reasons the elderly are at a higher risk for infection (LO 5).

11. Under Standard Precautions, what does the term "body fluids" include (LO 6)?

12. On whom should Standard Precautions be practiced (LO 6)?

13. When do Standard Precautions require gloves to be worn (LO 6)?

14. What is hand hygiene (LO 7)?

15. Why should nursing assistants avoid using false nails (LO 7)?

16. List ten situations that require handwashing (LO 7).

17. When should gloves be worn (LO 8)?

18. When should gowns be worn (LO 8)?

19. When should a mask and goggles be worn (LO 8)?

20. In what order should PPE be applied and removed (LO 8)?

21. How should soiled linen be carried (LO 9)?

22. When can re-usable equipment be used again (LO 9)?

23. Is it okay to pick up glass with gloved hands (LO 10)?

24. List and describe three categories of Transmission-Based Precautions (LO 11).

25. List six guidelines to use for residents in isolation (LO 12).

26. How are bloodborne diseases transmitted (LO 13)?

27. List five guidelines employers must follow to meet The Bloodborne Pathogen Standard (LO 13).

28. What is hepatitis (LO 14)?

29. What does HIV do to the immune system (LO 14)?

30. How is Hepatitis B (HBV) spread (LO 14)?

31. What is one of the best ways to prevent the spread of MRSA and VRE (LO 15)?

32. What are two ways that can help prevent *C. difficile* (LO 15)?

7
Safety and Body Mechanics

The Great Chicago Fire and Daisy the Cow

Legend has it that a cow named Daisy kicked over a lantern and started the Great Chicago Fire of October 8, 1871. That fire killed more than 300 people and left 100,000 more homeless, including patients at Deaconess Hospital of Chicago (later Passavant Memorial Hospital), who were forced to flee for their lives as the fires burned out of control.

Two weeks after the fire, Reverend Passavant arrived in Chicago to survey the damage and assist the homeless and destitute. He observed that "ruin reigns supreme." In fact, the remains of the hospital were sold for the pathetic sum of $8.50.

If the story of Daisy the Cow is true, then the fire that devastated the nation's fourth-largest city in 1871 didn't have to happen. It could have been prevented with a little care and caution.

(Adapted from "To Be a Nurse" by Susan M. Sacharski, © 1990.)

"The biggest problem in the world could have been solved when it was small."
Witter Bynner, 1881-1968,
The Way of Life According to Laotzu

"When you see a rattlesnake poised to strike, you do not wait until he has struck before you crush him."
Franklin Delano Roosevelt, 1882-1945

1. Define important words in this chapter

aspiration: inhaling food or drink into the lungs.

atrophy: weakening or wasting of muscles.

body mechanics: the way the parts of the body work together when you move.

chemical restraint: medications used to control a person's behavior.

combustion: the process of burning.

cyanosis: blue or pale skin and/or mucous membranes due to decreased oxygen in the blood.

disorientation: confusion about person, place and time.

dysphagia: difficulty in swallowing.

flammable: easily ignited and capable of burning quickly.

hoarding: collecting and putting things away in a guarded way.

Material Safety Data Sheet (MSDS): sheets that provide information on the safe use, hazards, and emergency steps to take when using chemicals.

PASS: acronym for use of a fire extinguisher; stands for Pull-Aim-Squeeze-Sweep.

postural support: device that maintains good posture or body alignment; also considered a restraint.

protective device: another word for a physical restraint or postural support.

RACE: acronym for steps taken during a fire; stands for Remove-Activate-Contain-Extinguish.

restraint: a physical or chemical way to restrict voluntary movement or behavior.

restraint alternatives: measures used instead of physical or chemical restraints.

restraint-free care: an environment in which restraints are not kept or used for any reason.

scalds: burns caused by very hot liquids.

slip knot: a special quick-release knot used to tie restraints.

suffocation: death from a lack of air or oxygen.

synthetic: artificial or man-made.

2. List common accidents in facilities and ways to prevent them

There are many accidents that can occur in a long-term care facility. Always be on your guard to try to keep residents, other staff, visitors, and yourself safe. Being proactive is the goal. Being proactive means trying to *prevent* an accident from occurring. It is much better than being reactive. Reacting or responding to an accident means that it has already taken place. You can change policy, but you cannot change that an accident happened after it has occurred. Prevention is the key to safety.

Maintaining safety is also a way to protect your residents' rights. Residents have the right to be safe and secure.

Some common resident accidents include:

- Falls
- Failing to identify residents before performing procedures or serving food
- Burns and scalds
- Poisoning
- Choking
- Cuts

Fall Prevention

Most of the accidents in a facility are related to falls. Many things increase the risk of falls. Unsafe environments, loss of abilities, diseases, and medications raise the risk for falls. Conditions that put a person at risk for falls include problems with walking, muscle weakness, poor vision, and **disorientation**, which is confusion about person, place and time. Follow these guidelines to help prevent falls:

Guidelines
Preventing Falls

- Identify residents who may be at risk and guard against falls. Report residents who seem unsteady to the nurse.

- Know which medications cause unsteadiness or problems moving about. Be especially watchful of residents taking those medications.

- Respond to call lights promptly. Never wait to respond.

- Wipe up spills immediately.

- Remove clutter from walkways. Pick up anything that has fallen on the floor right away.

- Get help when moving a resident. Never assume you can handle it alone. When in doubt, ask for help.

- Lock bed wheels before giving care (Fig. 7-1). Lock bed wheels before moving a resident into or out of bed.

- Lock wheelchair wheels before helping residents into or out of them (Fig. 7-2).

- If side rails are ordered, check to make sure they are raised before leaving the room. Return beds to their lowest position when you are done with care.

- Residents should wear clothing that fits properly. For example, it should not be too long. Residents must be wearing non-skid shoes at all times when out of bed. Make sure shoelaces are tied. Report if you think a resident needs safer shoes.

- Use non-skid mats or rugs to prevent slipping. Always report any rugs that move. Use non-skid mats in the bath or shower each time residents bathe. If allowed, stay with residents while they are showering or in the tub.

- Report loose hand rails in halls or rooms immediately. Report cracks or holes in floors, tile, walls, furniture, bathrooms, ceilings or stairwells.

- Report damage in outdoor furniture or benches, walkways, or ramps in outdoor common areas.

- Use brightly-colored tape to mark uneven areas on stairs or the floor.

- Keep frequently-used items close to the bedside or chair and in easy reach in the room, especially call lights.

- Keep walkers and canes close by residents. Allow residents to sit for short periods before getting up to prevent lightheadedness.

- Do not move furniture without an order from the nurse. Tell the resident before moving furniture.

- Offer trips to the bathroom often. Respond to residents' requests promptly.

- Keep night light on in room if approved by facility and resident. Keep halls and other areas well-lit. Report any problems with lighting.

- Make sure resident has eyeglasses within reach.

- If a resident begins to fall, do not try to stop it or to catch him. Use your body to slide him to the floor safely (Fig. 7-3). You or the resident may be injured if you try to stop the fall.

Fig. 7-1. *Always lock the bed wheels before helping a resident into or out of bed and before giving care.*

Fig. 7-2. *Always lock wheelchairs before a resident transfers into or out of them.*

Fig. 7-3. *If a resident starts to fall, do not try to stop the fall. Bring the resident's body close to you to break the fall. Bend your knees and support the resident as you gently lower her to the floor.*

HOT TIP

Safety with Wheelchairs

Lock wheelchairs before moving residents into or out of them. Push wheelchairs slowly and carefully. This helps to ensure safety, as well as making residents feel more secure.

Resident Identification

Residents must always be identified before providing care or serving food. Not doing so can result in serious problems, illnesses, and even death. There is never an excuse for not checking identification. Do it each time you see a resident before providing care or serving food.

Most people are used to seeing armbands as a form of ID on patients in hospitals (Fig. 7-4). However, residents in a facility may not wear name bracelets or armbands. Sometimes photos are placed above the bed or outside the door to identify residents.

Fig. 7-4. Identify all residents before giving care. This is an armband, which may or may not be used at your facility to identify residents. The abbreviation "NKA" means "no known allergies."

For disoriented or confused residents, some facilities use special bands that have alarms on them. The alarm will sound when a resident tries to leave the facility. Check alarms often to make sure they are working.

Regardless of which method the facility uses, identify each resident before giving care and serving food. Check the resident's identification and call the resident by name. Check diet cards against the resident's identification. Do this every time you see a resident.

Burn/Scald Prevention

99 - 105°F

Burns and scalds are a common concern in facilities. **Scalds** are burns caused by very hot liquids, such as coffee or tea. It does not take long for a serious burn to occur. When the temperature of a liquid reaches 140°F, it can take five seconds or less to cause a burn.

Burns are extremely painful. They can require surgery. They can cause a resident's condition to deteriorate quickly, depending on the person's physical state prior to the burn. Elderly people and people who have a loss of sensation due to paralysis are at the greatest risk for burns.

In addition, burns are costly because they require a lot of care. Follow these guidelines to help prevent burns:

Preventing Burns and Scalds

- Check water temperature before giving a resident a bath or shower. Temperature should not be over 110°F. Do not allow a resident to get into a bath or shower without checking first.

- Check for proper temperature of warm water applications, such as warm packs. A resident's skin is fragile. Warm or cold water applications may only be applied for 20 minutes at a time. (See Chapter 18 for more information.)

- Use low settings on hair dryers.

- Spills can cause burns. Residents may spill drinks on themselves if they are unsteady. Drinking hot liquids can also cause burns. Make sure the drink has cooled before encouraging the resident to drink.

- Serve residents drinks only when they are seated.

- Tell residents when you are about to pour or set down hot liquids.

- Use lids on hot liquids if possible. Keep hot drinks away from edges of tables.

- Pour hot liquids away from residents.

- If plate warmers are used to keep food warm, check the plates carefully. They may be hot. Warn residents if they are hot.

- Make sure anything that was left in the sun, such as a wheelchair, has cooled off completely before letting a resident sit in it. Residents themselves should not be left out in the sun too long. Use sunscreen and hats when residents are going outside.

- Tell residents about smoking precautions. Smoking may be allowed in specific areas. Serious burns, and even fires, can occur if a resident falls asleep with a cigarette, pipe, or cigar burning.

Poison Prevention

There are many poisonous items in a facility that should not be eaten. Cleaning products, glue, soaps, perfumes, and paints are some examples. These items might be of interest to or be consumed by a confused person. Medication can also be poisonous if taken in the wrong amount and/or by the wrong person. Follow these guidelines to help prevent poisoning:

Guidelines
Preventing Poisoning

- Keep fresh flowers or plants away from disoriented residents. Store or lock away items like nail polish remover, soaps, perfumes, or hair products. Lock up cleaning products and paints. Do not leave cleaning products in residents' rooms. All of these items may also be eaten by a disoriented person. The number of the Poison Control Center should be posted by all telephones.

- Check dates of foods to ensure that they are fresh.

- Check bedside table drawers for food that was hoarded and has spoiled. Residents who are confused or have dementia may hoard items; **hoarding** is collecting and putting things away in a guarded way.

- Residents can be overcome by fumes when using chemical products. Make sure there is proper ventilation. Always report to the nurse any situation that you believe to be risky.

Choking Prevention

Residents must be watched closely during meals for signs of choking. Residents who are weak or who have dysphagia are at a high risk for choking. **Dysphagia** means difficulty in swallowing. Residents who have swallowing problems may have special diets consisting of thickened liquids. Thickened liquids are easier to swallow.

Swallowing problems cause a high risk for choking on food or drink. Inhaling food or drink into the lungs is called **aspiration**, which can cause pneumonia or death. You will learn more about dysphagia, thickened liquids, and aspiration in Chapter 14. Follow these guidelines to help prevent choking:

Guidelines
Preventing Choking

- Residents should be sitting up straight while eating (Fig. 7-5). This is true whether the resident is in bed or in a chair.

- Assist with feeding slowly. Never rush a resident during a meal.

- Cut food into small pieces.

- If you believe a resident would be helped by softer foods or thickened liquids, report this to the nurse.

- Make sure dentures are in place and fit properly.

- Know any swallowing precautions residents have.

Fig. 7-5. *Residents must be sitting up straight when eating, whether in a bed or a chair.*

Cuts and Other Injuries

Cuts, tears, and scrapes can happen quickly. Follow these guidelines to help prevent injuries:

Guidelines

Preventing Cuts, Scrapes, and Other Injuries

- Do not leave any sharp objects out. Put away residents' supplies, such as razors, after use.

- When approaching doors, move slowly. If there is a window in the door, look on the other side before opening.

- When moving residents in wheelchairs or stretchers, protect their arms and legs. Hands and feet can be hit or bumped into walls or doors. Fingers may be caught in a wheelchair. Make sure arms and legs are inside of the chair or stretcher (gurney).

- Push wheelchairs forward; do not pull them behind you. When entering elevators, turn the chair around so that residents are facing forward. Watch for doors closing before arms and legs are inside.

Other general safety guidelines include:

- Do not run in a facility. Pay attention to your environment. Look for wet areas or things that you might trip over. Place a sign, such as "Wet Floor," near spills, and then wipe up spilled liquids right away. Remove clutter from walkways.

- Do not stick your hand into a bed or anywhere else without looking first. Be on the lookout for sharp objects or needles.

- Ask for help any time you feel you need it when lifting or assisting residents. Follow facility guidelines on lifting. Use proper equipment provided for lifting.

- Know which residents are combative and watch them closely. Learn the triggers of this behavior. If a resident tries to hit you, protect yourself with your arm or step out of the way. Do not hit back.

- Follow facility policy if a skin splash occurs. Immediately rinse your skin with large amounts of water.

- Follow facility policy if an eye splash occurs.

If no eye wash station is available, immediately rinse with large amounts of water at a sink. If an eye wash station is available, follow directions listed there. If you need to use an emergency eye wash, flip the cup lid open. Open your eyelid with your thumb and index finger. Press cup against eye and squeeze bottle repeatedly. Notify the nurse as soon as possible and get checked by a doctor.

- Report all injuries immediately.

3. Explain the Material Safety Data Sheet (MSDS)

The Occupational Safety and Health Administration (OSHA - see Chapter 6) is responsible for the safety of employees at work. OSHA requires that all dangerous chemicals have a **Material Safety Data Sheet** (**MSDS**) (Fig. 7-6). These sheets are placed where all staff can access them.

The important information the MSDS provides includes:

- The chemical ingredients of the product
- The dangers of the product
- The protective items to wear when using the chemical
- The correct method of using and cleaning up a chemical
- The emergency response actions to be taken when a chemical is splashed, sprayed, or ingested by a person
- The safe handling procedures for the product

Some facilities use a toll-free number to access MSDS information. Your employer will have an MSDS for every chemical used. Easy access to these sheets must be provided. You must know where they are located and how to read them. If you do not know how to read them, ask for help. Some facilities will have an annual MSDS class. Attend this class when it is offered.

Material Safety Data Sheet
May be used to comply with OSHA's Hazard
Communication Standard, 29 CFR 1910 1200. Standard
must be consulted for specific requirements.

U.S. Department of Labor
Occupational Safety and Health Administration
(Non-Mandatory Form)
Form Approved
OMB No. 1218-0072

IDENTITY *(as Used on Label and List)*

*Note: Blank spaces are not permitted. If any item is not
applicable or no information is available, the space
must be marked to indicate that.*

Section I

Manufacturer's name	Emergency Telephone Number
Address *(Number, Street, City, State and ZIP Code)*	Telephone Number for Information
	Date Prepared
	Signature of Preparer *(optional)*

Section II—Hazardous Ingredients/Identity Information

Hazardous Components (Specific Chemical Identity, Common Name(s))	OSHA PEL	ACGIH TLV	Other Limits Recommended	% (optional)

Section III—Physical/Chemical Characteristics

Boiling Point		Specific Gravity (H$_2$0 = 1)	
Vapor Pressure (mm Hg)		Melting Point	
Vapor Density (AIR = 1)		Evaporation Rate (Butyl Acetate = 1)	

Solubility in Water

Appearance and Odor

Section IV—Fire and Explosion Hazard Data

Flash Point (Method Used)	Flammable Limits	LEL	UEL

Extinguishing Media

Special Fire Fighting Procedures

Unusual Fire and Explosion Hazards

OSHA 174 Sept. 1985

***Fig. 7-6.** A Material Safety Data Sheet.*

4. Describe safety guidelines for sharps and biohazard containers

As you learned in Chapter 6, sharps and biohazard containers are the containers that hold sharp objects and infectious waste. Follow these safety guidelines when using these containers:

Guidelines
Safe Use of Sharps and Biohazard Containers

Ⓑ Always wear gloves before touching a sharps container.

Ⓑ When dropping an object into the biohazard container, keep your hands above the opening at the top (Fig. 7-7).

Ⓑ When touching a sharps container, touch the bottom of the container only. If you need to carry the container, carry it by the bottom. Be sure it is closed.

Ⓑ Replace the sharps container when it is ¾ full (or follow your facility policy). Ask the nurse about your facility's guidelines for replacing these containers.

Ⓑ Wash your hands after putting anything into the sharps container.

Ⓑ Use the biohazard container for anything contaminated with infectious waste (blood, body fluids, or human tissue), except for anything sharp.

Ⓑ Always wear gloves when disposing of infectious waste.

Ⓑ Wash your hands after putting anything into the biohazard container.

Fig. 7-7. Wear gloves and keep your fingers above the opening of a sharps container.

5. Explain the principles of body mechanics and apply them to daily activities

Back and body strains and injuries are important problems that nursing assistants face. They are common risks of working in a facility. Preventing injury by using proper techniques is very important. Every time you move, lift, or transfer a resident you will need to use good body mechanics.

Body mechanics is the way the parts of the body work together when you move. Good body mechanics help save energy and prevent injury and muscle strain. When muscles are used correctly to push, pull and lift objects or people, it reduces the risk of injury. Basic principles of body mechanics will help keep you and your residents safe.

Alignment: Alignment is based on the word "line." When you stand up straight, a vertical line could be drawn right through the center of your body and your center of gravity (Fig. 7-8). When the line is straight, the body is in alignment. Whether standing, sitting, or lying down, try to have your body in alignment. This means that the two sides of the body are mirror images of each other, with body parts lined up naturally and properly supported. Maintain correct body alignment when lifting or carrying an object by keeping it close to your body. Point your feet and body in the direction you are moving. Do not twist at the waist.

Fig. 7-8. Proper body alignment is important when standing or when sitting.

Base of Support: The base of support is the foundation that supports an object. Something that has a wide base of support is more stable than something with a narrow base of support. The feet are the body's base of support. Standing with your legs shoulder-width apart gives a greater base of support. You will be more stable than someone standing with his feet together.

Center of Gravity: The center of gravity in your body is the point where the most weight is concentrated (Fig. 7-9). The location of this point will depend on the position of the body. When you stand, your weight is centered in your pelvis. A low center of gravity gives a more stable base of support. Bending your knees when lifting an object lowers your pelvis. It lowers your center of gravity. This gives you more stability and makes you less likely to fall. It also makes you less likely to strain your muscles. If you are moving or transferring a resident, the center of gravity includes the resident. When you are transferring a resident, the resident needs to be as close to your body as possible.

Fig. 7-9. Holding things close to you moves weight toward your center of gravity. In this illustration, who is more likely to strain his back muscles?

Consider some activities that require moving or lifting something:

- Lifting a resident
- Picking up a resident's bag of laundry
- Carrying a new resident's luggage
- Taking heavy trash bags to the appropriate site
- Cleaning a floor
- Moving a resident's bed into another room

Each task could cause serious injury if done without using proper body mechanics. Even a simple task, such as picking up something light from the floor, could cause injury to your back. By applying the principles of body mechanics to daily activities, you can avoid injury and use less energy. Here are ways to use proper body mechanics:

- Raise beds to a safe working level before making them. This is usually waist high.
- Stand close to the object.
- Stand with a wide base of support.
- Push, slide, or pull objects rather than lifting them.
- Use the largest muscles of your upper arms and upper thighs to lift.
- Bend at your knees (squat) instead of at your waist (Fig. 7-10).
- Avoid twisting or choppy movements; keep movements smooth. Face the object or person you are moving. Pivot your feet instead of twisting at the waist.
- Do not try to lift with just one hand. Use both arms and hands to lift, pull, push, or carry objects.
- Hold objects close to your body when you are lifting or carrying them (Fig. 7-11).
- Avoid bending and reaching.
- Get help from co-workers when lifting or helping residents.
- Talk to residents before moving them. Let them know what will be happening so that they can help if possible. Agree on a signal, such as counting to three. Lift or move on three so that everyone moves together.

Fig. 7-10. In this illustration, which person is lifting correctly?

Fig. 7-11. *Keeping objects close while carrying them decreases stress on the back.*

Back injuries are a common problem in facilities. These injuries can be serious. Using good body mechanics is important in preventing injury.

HOT TIP

Bend your knees for ease.

When preparing to move or position a resident in bed, always bend your knees. You should be able to feel the bed with your knees before you begin the procedure. If you do not bend your knees properly, you can seriously injure your back.

6. Define two types of restraints and discuss problems associated with restraints

A **restraint** is a physical or chemical way to restrict voluntary movement or behavior. Common physical restraints are the vest restraint, belt restraint, wrist/ankle restraint, and mitt restraint. Physical restraints are also known as **postural supports** or **protective devices,** which are devices that maintain good posture or body alignment. Side rails and special chairs, such as geriatric chairs, are also considered physical restraints (Fig. 7-12 and 7-13).

Fig. 7-12. *Side rails are considered restraints because they restrict movement.*

Fig. 7-13. *When the tray table is attached, a geriatric chair, or geri-chair, is considered a restraint.*

Chemical restraints are medications used to control a person's behavior. Overuse of chemical restraints was once a common problem. In the past, residents were routinely restrained for different reasons. They were restrained to prevent falls and to keep a confused person from wandering. Residents were also commonly restrained to keep them from hurting themselves or others and to keep them from pulling out tubing. Restraint usage was often abused by caregivers. This abuse led to new laws restricting their use. Today, the use of both physical and chemical restraints in facilities has greatly decreased.

Restraints can never be used without a doctor's order. It is against the law to apply restraints for staff convenience or to discipline residents. Residents who are restrained must be continually monitored. This is important. Residents have been severely injured and have died due to improper restraint use and lack of monitoring. You will learn more about what to do if a resident is restrained in Learning Objective 9.

There are many complications of restraint use. Some of the negative effects of restraint use are:

- Bruises and cuts

- Pressure sores

- Pneumonia

- Reduced blood circulation

- Risk of suffocation (**suffocation** is death from a lack of air or oxygen)

- Stress on the heart
- Incontinence
- Constipation
- Muscle **atrophy** (weakening or wasting of muscles)
- Loss of bone mass
- Poor appetite and malnutrition
- Depression
- Sleep disorders
- Loss of dignity
- Loss of independence
- Stress and anxiety
- Increased agitation
- Loss of self-esteem
- Severe injury
- Death

7. Define the terms "restraint free" and "restraint alternatives" and list examples of restraint alternatives

Facilities are moving away from restraint use altogether. State and federal agencies encourage them to take steps to create restraint-free environments. **Restraint-free care** means that restraints are not kept or used for any reason. Creative ideas that help avoid the need for restraints are being used instead. These creative ideas are called **restraint alternatives**.

Studies have shown that restraints are not truly needed. People tend to respond better to the use of creative ways to reduce tension, pulling at tubes, wandering, and boredom. If you have ideas on ways to avoid using restraints, tell the nurse. You may be able to come up with successful restraint alternatives. Examples of restraint alternatives are outlined below:

- Answer call lights immediately. Make sure call lights are within reach.
- Improve lighting to prevent falls and other accidents.

- Use postural devices to support and protect the residents' bodies.
- Take the resident on a walk. Add more exercise into the care plan.
- Let confused residents wander in designated safe areas.
- Give frequent help with toileting. Make sure residents are clean and dry and comfortable.
- Encourage independence with all tasks. Provide meaningful activities.
- Encourage participation in social activities. Escort the resident to social activities when needed.
- Get the resident involved with hobbies.
- Create activities for those who wander at night.
- Offer reading materials, such as a newspaper. Read to the resident if needed.
- Offer backrubs.
- Increase visits and social interaction.
- Increase the number of familiar caregivers. Use more volunteers when possible.
- Get the family involved. Family members may decrease tension just by being with residents.
- Offer snacks or drinks.
- Redirect the resident's interest.
- Decrease the noise level.
- Use soothing music. Music has been shown to have a calming effect on some people.
- Report complaints of pain to the nurse immediately.

Bed or body alarms are other examples of restraint alternatives. They can be used in place of side rails. They can also be used with wheelchairs or chairs. They help prevent falls by alerting staff when residents attempt to leave the bed or chair. Alarms can also be used for confused residents who wander. If a resident is ordered to have a body alarm (bed or chair), make sure it is on the resident and turned on.

In addition to alarms, there are several types of pads, wheelchair inserts, and special chairs that may be used instead of restraints (Fig. 7-14). They are listed below:

- Saddle cushion
- Wedge cushion
- Self-releasing belt
- Lap pillow
- Lap tray
- Foam body support
- Safety sensors
- Wheelchair positioner cushion

Fig. 7-14. *a) A Posey Torso Support, b) A Posey Deluxe Wedge Cushion, c) A lap-top cushion.* (Photos courtesy of North Coast Medical, Inc., www.ncmedical.com, 800-821-9319.)

Some people use music to relax. Residents may also respond to music in a positive way. Their tastes will vary. Some may prefer classical or reggae, while others may like country, rhythm and blues, jazz, or rock and roll. When new residents are admitted, ask them the type of music they prefer. It may help guide the staff in choosing soothing music. Music may be just the right "medicine."

8. Describe beginning and ending steps in care procedures

For most care procedures, the beginning and ending steps are repeated each time. Understanding why each step is important will help you remember to perform each step every time care is provided.

Beginning Steps

Identify yourself by name. Identify the resident. Greet the resident by name. A resident's room is his home. Residents have a right to privacy. Before any procedure, knock and wait for permission to enter the resident's room. Upon entering his room, identify yourself. Residents have the right to know who is providing their care. Greeting residents shows courtesy and respect. It also establishes correct identification. This prevents care from being performed on the wrong person.

Wash your hands. Handwashing provides for infection control. Nothing fights infection in facilities like consistent, proper hand washing. Handwashing may need to be done more than once during a procedure. Practice Standard Precautions on every resident.

Explain procedure to resident. Speak clearly, slowly, and directly. Maintain face-to-face contact whenever possible. Encourage resident to assist if possible. Residents have a right to know exactly what care you will provide. It promotes understanding, cooperation, and independence. Residents are able to do more for themselves if they know what needs to happen.

Provide for the resident's privacy with a curtain, screen, or door. Doing this maintains residents' right to privacy and dignity. Providing for privacy in a facility is not simply a courtesy; it is a legal right.

Practice good body mechanics. Adjust the bed to a safe level, usually waist high. Lock the bed wheels. Locking the bed wheels is an important safety measure. It ensures that the bed will not move as you are performing care. Raising the bed helps you to remember to use good body mechanics. This prevents injury to you and to residents. Remember that side rails are considered restraints. Side rails should only be used when specifically ordered.

Ending Steps

Make resident comfortable. Make sure sheets are wrinkle-free and lie flat under the resident's body. This helps prevent pressure sores. Replace bedding and pillows. Check that the resident's body is in proper alignment. This promotes comfort and health after you leave the room.

Return bed to low position if raised. Ensure resident's safety. Remove privacy measures. Lowering the bed provides for residents' safety. Side rails are only raised when specifically ordered by the doctor. Remove extra privacy measures added during the procedure. This includes anything you may have draped over and around residents, as well as privacy screens.

Leave call light within resident's reach. A call light allows residents to communicate with staff as necessary (Fig. 7-15). Remember that the decision not to respond to a call light is considered neglect.

Fig. 7-15. *Always leave the call light within the resident's reach.*

Wash your hands. Handwashing is the most important thing you can do to prevent the spread of infection.

Be courteous and respectful at all times. Say "thank you" before you leave. It is the polite and proper thing to do. Ask residents if they need anything else (Fig. 7-16). Let them know that you are leaving. This promotes respect.

Fig. 7-16. *After performing care, ask residents if they need anything else. Let them know you are leaving.*

Report any changes in the resident to the nurse. Document procedure using facility guidelines. You will often be the person who spends the most time with a resident, so you are in the best position to note any changes in a resident's condition. Every time you provide care, observe the resident's physical and mental capabilities, as well as the body's condition. For example, a change in a resident's ability to dress himself may signal a greater problem. After you have finished giving care, document the care using facility guidelines. Do not record care before it is given. If you do not document the care you gave, legally it did not happen.

In addition to the beginning and ending steps listed above, remember to follow infection control guidelines. Even if a procedure in this book does not tell you to wear gloves, masks, or other PPE, there are times when it is appropriate. For example, the procedure for giving a back rub will not include gloves. Gloves are usually not required for a back rub. However, if the resident has open sores, gloves are necessary. Wearing gloves or other PPE when they are not required can be considered abuse. However, not wearing gloves when a risk of contact with body fluids exists is dangerous.

Another important step to remember in every procedure is to use proper body mechanics. The procedures will describe the correct way to perform the task. Remembering the basic rules of body mechanics during each step is up to you. These rules help prevent injury to you and to your residents.

9. Identify what must be done if a restraint is ordered

OBRA sets specific rules for restraint use. Restraints are used only after everything else has been ruled out and only with a doctor's order. Restraints cannot be used for staff convenience or discipline. Do not use a restraint unless the nurse has told you to do so and you have been trained to use it. When restraints have been ordered, follow these guidelines:

Guidelines
Restraints

- Know your state's laws and facility rules regarding applying restraints. Make sure there is a written doctor's order for a restraint before applying one.

- Follow manufacturer's instructions when applying restraints.

- Use the correct size and style of restraint. Ask the nurse for help if needed.

- Always use a slip knot. A **slip knot** is a quick-release knot used to tie restraints so that they can be removed quickly when needed.

- Never tie the restraint to side rails. Only tie the restraint to the movable part of a bed frame.

- Check to make sure the restraint is not too tight. You should be able to place your hand in a flat position between the resident and the restraint. This helps to ensure that the device fits properly and is comfortable.

- Apply vest or belt style restraint over clothing. Be careful not to catch the resident's breasts or skin in the restraint. The criss-cross in a vest restraint must be placed on the front of the body.

- Place the call light within the resident's reach. Residents with mitt restraints will not be able to press regular call lights. They will either need a special "easy touch" call light or they must be checked every five minutes. An "easy touch" call light is a soft, vinyl, air-filled bulb that when slightly depressed will activate the call light system.

- Document the following when restraints are used:
  - Type of restraint and time applied
  - Each time of removal
  - Care given when released
  - Any circulation, skin, or other problems

When a resident is restrained, he must be monitored constantly. Check the resident at least every 15 minutes (every five minutes for a mitt restraint). Look at the skin around the restraint to check for blue-tinged, gray or pale skin (**cyanosis**), which could mean lack of oxygen in the blood. With dark-skinned residents, the skin color may darken or appear purple. Check for redness or swelling of the body part.

At least every two hours, remove the restraints for at least 15 minutes. Provide personal care. Offer help with toileting. Take the resident to the bathroom or change the incontinent brief. Make sure the resident is clean and dry. Offer fluids. Reposition the resident. Help the resident walk if he or she is able. Give the resident anything else he or she needs.

Applying a physical tie restraint safely

Equipment: correct size and type of restraint

1. Identify yourself by name. Identify the resident. Greet the resident by name.

2. Wash your hands.

3. Explain procedure to the resident. Speak clearly, slowly, and directly. Maintain face-to-face contact whenever possible. Encourage resident to assist if possible.

4. Provide for the resident's privacy with a curtain, screen, or door.

5. Apply the restraint carefully. Follow manufacturer's directions and facility policy. For each type of restraint, make sure that it is not too tight.

   CHEST or BELT-STYLE RESTRAINTS: Make sure you do not catch breasts or skin in the restraints. Double-check before actually tying together or attaching buckle.

   VEST: The criss-cross in the vest restraint must be placed on the front of the body.

   MITT: Place a rolled-up washcloth or commercial hand roll in the mitt restraint. This helps the hand stay in proper alignment and helps prevent contractures (permanent and painful shortening of a muscle).

   WRIST/ANKLE: Make sure the restraint will not slide off the wrist or ankle.

6. Use slip knot to tie the restraint. Make sure it is not too tight. If restraint is used on a resident who is in bed, tie it to the movable part of the bed frame. Do not tie it to the side rail.

7. Make resident comfortable.

8. Leave call light within resident's reach.

9. Wash your hands.

10. Be courteous and respectful at all times.

11. Report any changes in the resident to the nurse. Document procedure using facility guidelines.

    Check resident every 15 minutes. (Residents with mitt restraints must be checked every five minutes because they are unable to use the call light.)

    Release the restraint(s) every two hours for at least 15 minutes and provide all care, such as giving fluids, toileting, walking (if ambulatory), or range of motion exercises.

10. List safety guidelines for oxygen use

Oxygen is used by residents who have breathing problems. Oxygen use is prescribed by a doctor. Nursing assistants do not turn off or adjust oxygen levels. This is the nurse's responsibility. You will learn more about oxygen in Chapter 20.

Working with oxygen requires special safety precautions because oxygen is a dangerous fire hazard. Oxygen makes other things burn; however, oxygen itself does not burn. It merely supports combustion. **Combustion** means the process of burning. There are strict safety rules that must be followed when working around oxygen.

Guidelines
Safety with Oxygen

- Post "No Smoking" and "Oxygen in Use" signs. These should be posted on each door and over the resident's bed. **Do not** allow smoking anywhere around oxygen equipment. If you find smoking materials in a resident's room or on a resident, report to the nurse immediately.

- Remove fire hazards from the room. This includes electrical equipment, such as electric razors, hair dryers, or radios. Tell the nurse if residents do not want fire hazards removed.

- Remove flammable liquids from the area. **Flammable** means easily ignited and capable of burning quickly. Examples of flammable liquids are alcohol and nail polish remover. Read the label on liquids if you are unsure. If it says "flammable," remove them from the area.

- Do not allow candles, lighters, or matches around oxygen.

- Residents using oxygen must not use wool or nylon or any other synthetic clothing or bedcovers. **Synthetic** means artificial or man-made fabric. Staff must not wear wool clothing or sweaters near a resident with oxygen.

- Check the nasal area and behind the ears often and report signs of irritation from the tubing from the nasal cannula or face mask (Fig. 7-17).

- Learn how to turn oxygen off in case of a fire if your facility allows this. Never adjust oxygen levels.

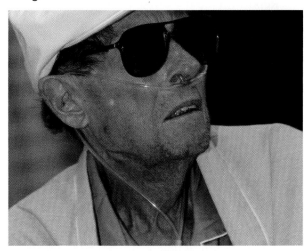

Fig. 7-17. *A resident with a nasal cannula.*

HOT TIP

Watch for flammables!

Do you know anyone who smokes while polishing her nails or using nail polish remover? If so, advise them to stop this practice. Nail polish and nail polish remover are flammable and are dangerous when around sparks or flames. Lighting a cigarette or smoking a cigarette near flammable liquids can cause the product to explode. This can cause injury or possibly a fire.

11. Identify safety guidelines for intravenous (IV) lines

"IV" is an abbreviation for "intravenous," which means into a vein. A resident with an IV is receiving medication, nutrition, or fluids through a vein (Fig. 7-18). When caring for residents who have IVs, follow these guidelines:

Fig. 7-18. *A resident with an IV.*

Guidelines

IVs

Always wear gloves if you have to touch the IV area.

- Do not do any of the following when caring for a resident with an IV:

  - Take blood pressure on an arm with an IV.

  - Get the IV site wet.

  - Pull on or catch the tubing in anything during positioning, such as clothing.

  - Leave the tubing kinked.

  - Lower the IV bag below the IV site.

  - Touch the clamp.

  - Disconnect IV from pump or turn off alarm.

- Report to the nurse if any of the following occurs:

  - The needle or catheter has fallen out or moves out of the vein. If an IV catheter comes out of the vein, it can cause an infiltration; an infiltration is the administration of fluids into surrounding tissue.

- The armboard or handboard (device taped to the arm or hand, used to help keep the IV catheter inside the vein) becomes loose.

- The tubing is disconnected.

- Blood appears in the tubing.

- The IV fluid in the bag or container is gone or almost gone.

- The IV fluid is not dripping, is leaking, or the bag breaks.

- The IV pump is beeping.

- The area around the IV is wet, bleeding, swollen, red, or warm to the touch.

- The resident complains of pain, has difficulty breathing, or has a fever. Pain and fever may indicate phlebitis, which is inflammation of a vein.

- The resident pulls out or attempts to pull out the IV.

RESIDENTS' RIGHTS

Oxygen and IVs

Residents who use oxygen or have IVs have the continued right to freedom of movement. They must be kept safe from the hazards of oxygen use and from the risks of having an IV.

12. Discuss fire safety and explain the "RACE" and "PASS" acronyms

There are many causes of fire. For a fire to occur, it must have these three things:

1. Heat: makes the flame

2. Fuel: the object that burns

3. Oxygen: gas that will keep the fire burning

There are many potential causes of a fire in facilities, including:

- Smoking

- Frayed or damaged electrical cords

- Electrical equipment in need of repair

- Space heaters

- Overloaded electrical plugs

- Oxygen use

- Careless cooking

- Flammable liquids or rags with oils on them

- Stacks of newspapers or other clutter

Ways to prevent fires from occurring include:

- Stay with a resident who is smoking at all times.

- Check ashtrays for lit cigarettes or matches. Put out burning cigarettes.

- Make sure cigarettes or other smoking materials have not fallen on an area where a fire may start.

- If emptying an ashtray, make sure there are no hot ashes, matches, or cigarette butts in the ashtray.

- Report immediately if electrical equipment or cords are damaged or frayed. Check to see that cords are not too short. Do not use cords that have electrical tape around them. Report this to the nurse promptly.

When a fire occurs, make sure you know the location of alarms. Also, two acronyms will help you remember what to do. The first is the **RACE** acronym, which outlines what to do in case of a fire:

Remove residents from danger.

Activate alarm (or call 911).

Contain the fire by closing all doors and windows, if possible.

Extinguish the fire, or fire department will extinguish. Evacuate if instructed to do so.

There will be many fire extinguishers at every facility (Fig. 7-19). Learn where they are located. In order to understand how to use an extinguisher, follow the **PASS** acronym:

Pull the pin.

Aim at the base of the fire when spraying.

Squeeze the handle.

Sweep back and forth at the base of the fire.

Fig. 7-19. *Know the location of your facility's fire extinguishers and how to use them.*

All facilities have fire safety plans. Learn your facility's plan. It will help you know what to do in the event of a fire. Here are general procedures to follow in case of a fire:

- Call for immediate help.
- Know the location of the fire evacuation plan.
- Remain calm. Do not panic.
- Remove all persons in the immediate area of the fire (see RACE acronym).
- If a door is closed, always check it for heat before opening it.
- Stay low in a room when trying to escape a fire.
- Use wet towels to block doorways to prevent smoke from entering a room.
- Use a covering over the face to reduce smoke inhalation.
- If clothing is on fire, remember to stop, drop, and roll to put out fire.
- Never get into an elevator during a fire.

In case of fire, nursing assistants may be asked to turn off all oxygen and electrical equipment in the area if possible. Follow your facility's policies.

13. List general safety steps to protect yourself and residents in a facility

Living or working in a facility may sometimes put a person at risk of crime. Many people go in and out of a facility during the day. Delivery people, visitors, clergy, temporary workers, and others may enter facilities regularly. Unfortunately, not everyone is honest and trustworthy. It is best to watch for any suspicious behavior. If you notice any suspicious behavior, report it immediately. In addition, follow these safety guidelines:

- Keep valuable personal items at home.
- Ask the nurse to lock up residents' valuable items.
- If any visitor or staff member makes you uneasy, do not leave a resident alone with the person.
- Follow guidelines for the number of visitors allowed at one time in a resident room.
- Do not share your personal information with anyone. Do not share residents' or other staff members' information with anyone.

CHAPTER REVIEW

1. List each of the six common resident accidents in facilities and list two ways to prevent each one (LO 2).

2. In what position should a resident be placed for eating (LO 2)?

3. What is the important information the MSDS provides about chemicals (LO 3)?

4. What should be disposed of in a biohazard container (LO 4)?

5. Define "body mechanics" (LO 5).

6. Should objects be held close to the body or far away from the body when lifting or carrying them (LO 5)?

7. How should legs be positioned when standing to give a better base of support (LO 5)?

8. When lifting, is it better to bend at the waist or at the knees (LO 5)?

9. Define "restraint" (LO 6).

10. Why was restraint usage restricted (LO 6)?

11. List 12 complications of restraint use (LO 6).

12. List ten examples of restraint alternatives (LO 7).

13. What does a "restraint-free" environment mean (LO 7)?

14. List each beginning and ending step in care procedures and briefly explain why they are important (LO 8).

15. When can a restraint be applied (LO 9)?

16. How can a nursing assistant check to make sure that a restraint is not too tight (LO 9)?

17. Should restraints be tied to side rails (LO 9)?

18. When a resident is restrained, how often should he be checked (LO 9)?

19. List four guidelines for working safely around oxygen (LO 10).

20. List six signs to report to a nurse about an IV (LO 11).

21. What three things need to happen for a fire to occur (LO 12)?

22. Identify what the acronyms "RACE" and "PASS" stand for (LO 12).

23. If a door is closed and a fire has started, what should the nursing assistant do first (LO 12)?

24. List two general safety steps to protect residents in a facility (LO 13).

8

Emergency Care, First Aid, and Disasters

Emergency Transfer of Victims During the 1500s

Compare the rescue of a traveler in ancient times to the care our emergency squads give today. "The misfortune befell me in the manner which follows: wishing to pass across the water and trying to make my hackney enter a boat, I struck [the horse] . . . with a riding crop [and] the animal gave me such a kick that she broke entirely the two bones of my left leg . . . . I was quickly carried into the boat to cross to the other side in order to have me treated. But its shaking almost made me die, because the ends of the broken bones rubbed against the flesh, and those who were carrying me could not give it fit posture. From the boat, I was carried into a house of the village with greater pain than I had endured in the boat . . . . Finally, however, they placed me on a bed to regain my breath a little . . . while my dressing was being made . . ."

**Ambroise Paré, 1510-1590,
from *Ten Books of Surgery***

"It is by presence of mind in untried emergencies that the native metal of a man is tested."
James Russell Lowell, 1819-1891

" . . . the truly noble and resolved spirit raises itself, and becomes more conspicuous in times of disaster and ill fortune."
Plutarch, A.D. 46-120

1. Define important words in this chapter

abdominal thrusts: the method of attempting to remove an object from the airway of someone who is choking.

cardiac arrest: the medical term for the stopping of the heartbeat.

code team: group of people chosen for a particular shift that respond to resident emergencies.

conscious: the state of being mentally alert and having awareness of surroundings, sensations, and thoughts.

CPR (cardiopulmonary resuscitation): refers to medical procedures used when a person's heart or lungs have stopped working.

diabetic ketoacidosis: a life-threatening complication of diabetes that can result from undiagnosed diabetes, not enough insulin, eating too much, not getting enough exercise, and stress; also known as ketoacidosis or hyperglycemia.

dyspnea: difficulty breathing.

emesis: the medical term for vomit or vomitus.

epistaxis: the medical term for a nosebleed.

expressive aphasia: inability to express needs to others through speech or written words.

fainting: loss of consciousness; also called syncope.

first aid: care given by the first people to respond to an emergency.

hemiparesis: weakness on one side of the body.

hemiplegia: paralysis of one side of the body.

hyperglycemia: a life-threatening complication of diabetes that can result from undiagnosed diabetes, not enough insulin, eating too much, not getting enough exercise, and stress; also known as diabetic ketoacidosis (DKA) or ketoacidosis.

hypoglycemia: a life-threatening complication of diabetes that can result from either too much insulin or too little food; also known as insulin reaction and insulin shock.

insulin reaction: a life-threatening complication of diabetes that can result from either too much insulin or too little food; also known as hypoglycemia or insulin shock.

myocardial infarction: a condition in which blood flow to the heart is completely blocked and muscle cells die; also called a heart attack.

obstructed airway: a condition in which a person has something blocking the tube through which air enters the lungs.

receptive aphasia: inability to understand what others are communicating through speech or written words.

respiratory arrest: the medical term for the stopping of breathing.

shock: a condition in which there is decreased blood flow to organs and tissues.

syncope: loss of consciousness; also called fainting.

2. Demonstrate how to respond to medical emergencies

Medical emergencies can happen when you least expect them (Fig. 8-1). Choking, diabetic emergencies, falls, poisoning, heart attacks, strokes, and gunshot wounds are all medical emergencies. The most serious medical emergencies involve one or more of the following:

- the person is unconscious
- the person is not breathing
- the person has no pulse
- the person is bleeding severely

Fig. 8-1. Medical emergencies can happen at any time. Being calm and prepared is the best way to respond to emergencies.

Two Types of PPE for Emergencies

There are many potential diseases that people can come into contact with when they respond to an emergency. Make sure you have proper protection in the event of an emergency. Always keep this PPE with you:

- two sets of gloves
- a special face mask or other oral/nasal barrier device

A face mask is a small mask that can protect you if you must give rescue breaths to help a victim breathe (Fig. 8-2). Keep two sets of gloves in your vehicle, purse or bag, or your pocket. Look at the gloves periodically to make sure they are not damaged or torn. Two sets of gloves are a good idea in case one glove tears or if you have to replace your gloves with clean gloves.

Fig. 8-2. One type of face mask.

In an emergency, try to remain calm. Act quickly and communicate clearly. Take your gloves/face mask kit with you. Look around to make sure the area is safe. Make sure you are safe before providing necessary care. Once you have your gloves on, follow these steps:

- Assess the situation. Notice the time. Try to find out what has happened.

- Assess the victim. Ask the injured or ill person what has happened. If the person cannot respond, he may be unconscious. Being **conscious** means being mentally alert and having awareness of surroundings, sensations, and thoughts. Determine whether the person is conscious. Tap the person and ask if he is all right. Speak loudly. Use the person's name if you know it. If there is no response, assume that the person is unconscious. This is an emergency. Call for help right away, or send someone else to call.

When calling 911 or activating Emergency Medical Services (EMS), know the procedure for dialing an outside line. Be prepared to let the operator know the phone number and address of the emergency, directions, and the location of the building. Report the victim's condition, including any medical background you know. Give your name and position and the details of any first aid being given. Do not hang up the phone until the dispatcher hangs up or tells you to hang up. If another person calls 911, have her return after making the call so that you know the call was placed.

If a person is conscious and able to speak, then he is breathing and has a pulse. Talk with the person about what happened and check him for injury. Look for these things:

- severe bleeding
- changes in consciousness
- irregular breathing
- unusual color or feel to the skin
- swollen places on the body
- medical alert tags
- any complaints of pain

If any of these exist, you may need professional medical help. Always get help before doing anything else. If the injured or ill person is conscious, he may be frightened. Listen to the person. Tell him what is being done to help him. Be calm and confident. Reassure him that he is being taken care of.

After the emergency, while still on duty, document the emergency in your notes. You may need to complete an incident report. Try to remember as many details as you can. Remember, only report the facts. If you think a resident suffered a heart attack, write only the signs and symptoms you observed. Record the actions you took. Knowing what information you will have to document will help you remember the important facts. For example, it is especially important to remember the time a person became unconscious.

"Flying Ambulances"

Napoleon invaded Italy in 1796. During that invasion, Dominique Jean Larrey (1766-1842) developed "flying ambulances." These were horse-drawn vehicles that were able to quickly remove the wounded from the front lines for treatment. During the American Civil War, around 1863, "ambulance trains" similar to the legendary wagon trains of western lore appeared.

3. Describe basic CPR and demonstrate knowledge of first aid procedures

Emergency situations can happen to anyone. When a person is involved in a serious accident, such as drowning or choking, respiratory arrest can occur. **Respiratory arrest** means that breathing stops. If the person is not helped quickly, cardiac arrest may soon follow. **Cardiac arrest** is when the heart stops. When respiratory arrest or cardiac arrest occurs, **cardiopulmonary resuscitation (CPR)** is necessary. CPR refers to medical procedures used when the heart or lungs have stopped working and is used until medical help arrives.

Quick action is necessary. The first few minutes of any emergency can determine the victim's ability to survive the accident. CPR must be started immediately to help prevent or minimize brain damage. Brain damage can occur within four to six minutes after the heart stops beating and breathing stops.

Only properly trained people should perform CPR. In an emergency situation, never do anything that is beyond your ability or training. Performing CPR incorrectly can further injure a person. Give basic first aid until the emergency medical team arrives. **First aid** is the care given by the first people to respond to an emergency.

This textbook is not a CPR course. If your employer does not arrange for you to be trained in CPR, the American Heart Association and the American Red Cross, among others, offer courses in CPR. Keep your CPR certification current. A separate first aid course, to stay up-to-date on life-saving methods, is also available.

Some facilities do not allow nursing assistants to begin CPR without the direction of a nurse even if they have been trained. This is due, in part, to residents' advance directives. Some residents have made the decision that they do not want CPR. Know your facility's policies on whether you can initiate CPR if you have been trained.

Here is a brief CPR review. This review is for procedures used by trained healthcare providers (HCP). It follows the American Heart Association guidelines. This procedure is intended for use on adults, not children:

1. Before starting CPR, make sure the person is not asleep. Check to see if the person is responsive. Gently shake the person and shout, "Are you okay?"

2. If there is no response, call 911 immediately or send someone to call 911. Stay calm.

3. Kneel at the person's side near his head to start CPR. An easy way to remember the CPR steps is "ABCD." "A" stands for airway. "B" stands for breathing. "C" stands for circulation. "D" stands for defibrillation.

4. **AIRWAY**. Open the airway. Tilt the head back slightly. Lift the chin with one hand while pushing down on the forehead with the other hand (head tilt-chin lift method) (Fig. 8-3). This method is used if a neck injury is not suspected.

Fig. 8-3. The head tilt-chin lift method.

5. Hold the airway open and check for adequate breathing:

   • Look for the chest to rise and fall.

   • Listen for sounds of breathing. Put your ear near the person's nose and mouth.

   • Feel for the person's breath on your cheek.

6. **BREATHING**. If adequate breathing is not present, you will have to breathe for the person. Give two rescue breaths. To give rescue breaths:

   • Use a barrier device, such as a special face mask, to give rescue breaths.

   • Pinch the nose to keep air from escaping. Cover the person's mouth completely with your mouth.

   • Blow into the person's mouth slowly. Watch for the chest to rise. Blow two full breaths, about one second each. Take a "regular" (not a deep) breath (Fig. 8-4). Turn your head to the side to listen for air. If the chest does not rise when you give a rescue breath, reopen the airway. Use the head tilt-chin lift method. Try to give rescue breaths again.

Fig. 8-4. Give two rescue breaths while covering the person's mouth and pinching the nose to keep air from escaping.

7. **CIRCULATION**. After giving rescue breaths, look for signs of response. The person may start moving, breathing normally, or coughing. If you do not see a response, check the carotid pulse in the neck for not longer than 10 seconds (a CPR trainer will teach you how to locate the carotid pulse). If pulse is not felt within 10 seconds, give 30 chest compressions. Do this only if you have been trained to do so. Be sure the person

EMERGENCY CARE, FIRST AID, AND DISASTERS

is lying flat on a hard surface. To give chest compressions:

- Place your hands in the center of the person's chest between the nipples. Place one hand on top of the other. Interlace your fingers to help maintain hand position.

- Place knees shoulder-width apart and as close to the person as possible. Bring your body up and forward. Your shoulders should be directly above your hands. Lock your elbows and shoulders.

- Keeping one hand on top of the other one, press the heel of the hand that is underneath into the chest. Do not allow hands to lose contact with the chest during compressions.

- Maintaining position of both hands, use the heel of one hand to give 30 chest compressions (Fig. 8-5). Push hard and fast. Allow for complete recoil of chest between compressions. After about a minute of CPR, check for signs of response. If you see signs of response, stop compressions. Continue to provide rescue breathing as necessary (one breath every five seconds).

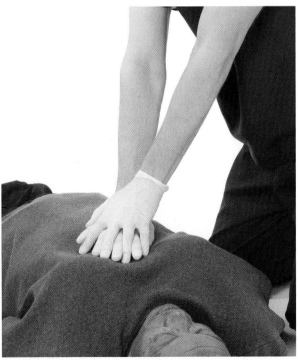

Fig. 8-5. *To give chest compressions, elbows and shoulders must be locked and fingers should be interlaced.*

8. **DEFIBRILLATION**. For a sudden cardiac arrest (SCA), a defibrillator (a device that gives an electrical shock), or AED (Automated External Defibrillator) may be available to help a victim. When the heart suddenly stops, this device gives the heart an electrical shock to bring back a normal heartbeat. The AED can restart the heart and transport oxygen throughout the body.

AEDs may be used at your facility. They are also located in airports, on many airplanes, and in some stores and offices. A clear, computerized voice inside the AED takes the user through each step. It is important to listen closely to the voice prompts when using the AED.

Your CPR trainer will give you specific guidelines on when to use the AED first and when to use CPR first with sudden cardiac arrest (SCA). In certain situations, CPR and defibrillation have been found to work together to improve survival rates of cardiac arrest victims.

People must be properly trained to give CPR and use the AED. Caregivers must be careful when using the AED around oxygen. Fires can occur due to sparks. AEDs must be properly maintained for best performance. Follow manufacturer's instructions to make sure the AED is in working order. Doing regular checks can prevent problems with AEDs during use.

When medical help arrives, follow their directions. Assist them as necessary.

PPE SCC

Performing first aid is something for which many people are not prepared. If you have to perform first aid, remember this acronym: PPE SCC.

- **PPE**: Grab and apply Personal Protective Equipment!

- **S**afety first! Are you safe?

- **C**all for help or point to person and say: "You, call 911 now!"

- **C**are for victims.

Choking

Residents who have difficulty chewing or swallowing, are confused, or have poor vision may be at risk of choking. When something is blocking the tube through which air enters the lungs, the person has an **obstructed airway**. When people are choking, they usually put their hands to their throats and cough (Fig. 8-6). As long as the person can speak, cough, or breathe, do nothing. Encourage her to cough as forcefully as possible to get the object out. Ask someone to get a nurse. Stay with the person until she stops choking or can no longer speak, cough, or breathe.

Fig. 8-6. A common sign of choking is when a person puts her hands to her throat and coughs.

If a person can no longer speak, cough, or breathe, or turns blue, call for help immediately. Time is of extreme importance. **Abdominal thrusts** are a method of attempting to remove an object from the airway of someone who is choking. These thrusts work to remove the blockage upward, out of the throat.

The procedure for giving abdominal thrusts is described below. Follow your facility's procedure for clearing an obstructed airway. For obese people or women in the later stages of pregnancy, training on chest thrusts will be provided. Keep any first aid certifications current, as practices do change.

Make sure the person needs help before giving abdominal thrusts. The person must show signs of a severely obstructed airway. These include poor air exchange, an increase in trouble breathing, silent coughing, blue-tinged skin (cyanosis), or inability to breathe or speak. You must ask the person, "Are you choking?"

If the person nods her head "Yes," she has a severe airway obstruction and needs immediate help. Give abdominal thrusts. Do this only if your facility allows you to perform this procedure. Do not practice this procedure on a live person. This risks injury to the ribs or internal organs.

Abdominal thrusts for the conscious person

1. Stand behind the person. Bring your arms under her arms. Wrap your arms around the person's waist.

2. Make a fist with one hand. Place the flat, thumb side of the fist against the person's abdomen, above the navel but below the breastbone.

3. Grasp the fist with your other hand. Pull both hands toward you and up (inward and upward), quickly and forcefully (Fig. 8-7).

Fig. 8-7. Pull both hands toward you and up (inward and upward), quickly and forcefully.

4. Repeat until the object is pushed out or the person loses consciousness.

If the person becomes unconscious while choking, stop what you are doing. Help her to the floor gently. Lie her on her back with her face up. Activate Emergency Medical Services (EMS) and begin CPR. Make sure help is on its way. The person may have a completely blocked airway and needs professional medical help immediately. Stay with the victim until help arrives.

Shock

Shock occurs when organs and tissues in the body do not receive an adequate blood supply. Bleeding, heart attack, severe infection, and falling blood pressure can lead to shock. Shock can become worse when the person is frightened or in severe pain.

Shock is a dangerous, life-threatening situation. Signs of shock include pale or cyanotic (bluish) skin, staring, increased pulse and respiration rates, decreased blood pressure, and extreme thirst. Always call for help if you suspect a person is in shock. To prevent or treat shock, do the following:

Shock

1. Notify the nurse immediately. Victims of shock should always receive medical care as soon as possible.

2. Control bleeding. The next procedure will explain how to do this.

3. Have the person lie down on her back. If the person is bleeding from the mouth or vomiting, place her on her side (unless you suspect that the neck, back, or spinal cord is injured).

4. Check pulse and respirations if possible (Chapter 13). Begin CPR if breathing or pulse is absent.

5. Keep the person as calm and comfortable as possible. Loosen clothing or ties around the neck and any belts or waist strings.

6. Maintain normal body temperature. If the weather is cold, place a blanket around the person. If the weather is hot, provide shade.

7. Elevate the feet unless the person has a head, neck or abdominal injury, breathing difficulties, or a fractured bone or back (Fig. 8-8). Never elevate a body part if a broken bone exists or if it causes pain.

Fig. 8-8. Elevate the feet, unless the person has head, neck, or abdominal injuries, breathing problems, or fractures.

8. Do not give the person anything to eat or drink.

Bleeding

Severe bleeding can cause death quickly and must be controlled. Follow these steps to control bleeding:

Bleeding

1. Notify the nurse immediately.

2. Put on gloves. Always take time to do this. If the resident is able, he can hold his bare hand over the wound until you can put on gloves.

3. Hold a thick sterile pad, a clean pad, or a clean cloth, handkerchief, or towel against the wound.

4. Press down hard directly on the bleeding wound until help arrives (Fig. 8-9). Do not decrease pressure. Put additional pads over the first pad if blood seeps through. Do not remove the first pad.

Fig. 8-9. *Press down hard directly on the bleeding wound; do not decrease pressure.*

5. If you can, raise the wound above the level of the heart to slow down the bleeding. If the wound is on an arm, leg, hand, or foot, and there are no broken bones, prop up the limb on towels, blankets, coats, or other absorbent material.

6. When bleeding is under control, secure the dressing to keep it in place. Check the person for symptoms of shock (pale skin, increased pulse and respiration rates, decreased blood pressure, and extreme thirst). Stay with the person until help arrives.

7. Remove gloves and wash hands thoroughly when finished.

Burns

You learned about preventing burns and scalds in Chapter 7. Care of a burn depends on its depth, size, and location. There are three types of burns: first degree, second degree, and third degree burns. You will learn more about burns in Chapter 18.

If a resident is burned, call or have someone call for the nurse immediately.

Burns

To treat a minor burn:

1. Notify the nurse immediately.

2. Use cool, clean water to decrease the skin temperature and prevent further injury (Fig. 8-10). Do not use ice as ice may cause further skin damage. Dampen a clean cloth and place it over the burn.

Fig. 8-10. *Use cool, clean water, not ice, on burned skin.*

3. Once the pain has eased, you may cover the area with dry, sterile gauze.

4. Never use any kind of ointment, salve, or grease on a burn.

For more serious burns:

1. Remove the person from the source of the burn. If clothing has caught fire, smother it with a blanket or towel to put out flames. Protect yourself from the source of the burn.

2. Notify the nurse immediately.

3. Check for breathing, pulse, and severe bleeding.

4. Do not apply water. It may cause infection.

5. Remove as much of the person's clothing around the burned area as possible. Do not try to pull away clothing that sticks to the burn. Cover the burn with thick, dry, sterile gauze if available, or a clean cloth. A dry, insulated cool pack may be used over the dressing (Fig. 8-11). Again, never use any kind of ointment, salve, or grease on a burn.

Fig. 8-11. *A dry, insulated cool pack may be used over the dressing.*

EMERGENCY CARE, FIRST AID, AND DISASTERS

6. Ask the person to lie down. Elevate the affected part if this does not cause greater pain.

7. If the burn covers a larger area, wrap the person or the limb in a dry, clean sheet. Take care not to rub the skin or break any blisters.

8. Wait for emergency medical help.

Fainting (Syncope)

Fainting, or **syncope**, occurs as a result of decreased blood flow to the brain, causing a loss of consciousness. Fainting may be the result of hunger, fear, pain, fatigue, standing for a long time, poor ventilation, pregnancy, or overheating. Signs and symptoms of fainting include dizziness, perspiration, pale skin, weak pulse, shallow respirations, and blackness in the visual field. If someone appears likely to faint, follow these steps:

Fainting

1. Notify or have someone notify the nurse immediately.

2. Have the person lie down or sit down before fainting occurs.

3. If the person is in a sitting position, have her bend forward and place her head between her knees (Fig. 8-12). If the person is lying flat on her back, elevate the legs.

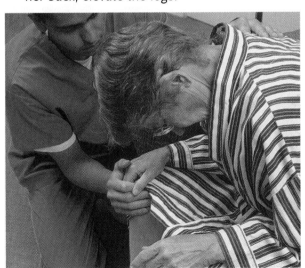

Fig. 8-12. Have the person bend forward and place her head between her knees if she is sitting.

4. Loosen any tight clothing.

5. Have the person stay in position for at least five minutes after symptoms disappear.

6. Help the person get up slowly. Continue to observe her for symptoms of fainting. Assist her to sit down if needed. Stay with her until she feels better. If you need help but cannot leave the person, use the call light.

If a person does faint, lower her to the floor or other flat surface. Position her on her back. If she has no head, neck, back or spinal injuries, elevate her legs 8 to 12 inches. If unsure about injuries, leave her flat on her back. Check to make sure the person is breathing. She should recover quickly, but keep her lying down for several minutes. Report the incident to the nurse immediately. Fainting may be a sign of a more serious medical condition.

Poisoning

As you learned in Chapter 7, facilities contain many harmful substances that should not be swallowed. Always have the Poison Control Center phone number available. Suspect poisoning when a resident suddenly collapses, vomits, and has heavy, difficult breathing. If you suspect poisoning, take the following steps:

Poisoning

1. Notify the nurse immediately.

2. Put on gloves. Look for a container that will help you determine what the resident has taken or eaten. With your gloves on, open mouth and look inside to check the mouth for chemical burns. Do not place your fingers inside the mouth. Note the breath odor.

3. The nurse may have you call the local or state Poison Control Center. Follow their instructions.

Nosebleed

A nosebleed can occur suddenly when the air is dry, when injury has occurred, or due to some medications. The medical term for a nosebleed is **epistaxis**. If a resident has a nosebleed, take the following steps:

Nosebleed

1. Notify the nurse immediately.

2. Elevate the head of the bed. Tell the resident to remain in a sitting position. Offer tissues or a clean cloth to catch the blood. Do not touch blood or bloody clothes, tissues or cloths without gloves.

3. Put on gloves. Apply firm pressure over the bridge of the nose. Squeeze the bridge of the nose with your thumb and forefinger (Fig. 8-13). You can have the resident do this until you are able to put on gloves.

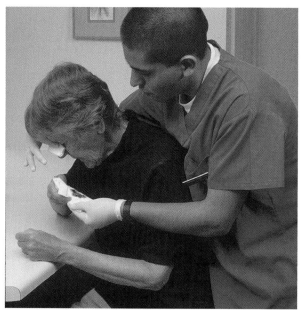

Fig. 8-13. With gloves on, squeeze the bridge of the nose with your thumb and forefinger.

4. Apply pressure until the bleeding stops.

5. Use a cool cloth or ice wrapped in a cloth on the back of the neck, the forehead, or the upper lip to slow the flow of blood. Never apply ice directly to skin.

6. Keep person still and calm until help arrives.

Vomiting

Vomiting, or **emesis**, is the act of ejecting stomach contents through the mouth. It can be a sign

of a serious illness or injury. Because you may not know when a resident is going to vomit, you may not have time to explain what you will do and assemble supplies ahead of time. Talk to the resident soothingly as you help him clean up. Tell him what you are doing to help him. If a resident has vomited, take the following steps:

Vomiting

1. Notify the nurse immediately.

2. Put on gloves.

3. Place an emesis basin under the chin. If an emesis basin is not nearby, use the wash basin. Remove it when vomiting has stopped.

4. Provide comfort to the resident. Wipe his face and mouth (Fig. 8-14). Position him comfortably, and offer a drink of water or a sip to swish in the mouth and spit. Provide oral care (see Chapter 12). It helps get rid of the taste of vomit in the mouth.

Fig. 8-14. Be calm and comforting when helping a resident who has vomited.

5. Remove soiled linens or clothes and replace with fresh linens or clothes.

6. If resident's intake and output (I&O) is being monitored (see Chapter 14), measure and note amount of vomitus. Find out if a specimen of the emesis should be sent to a laboratory.

7. Flush vomit down the toilet and wash and store the basin.

8. Put the soiled linen in proper containers.

9. Remove gloves.

10. Wash your hands again.

11. Document time, amount, color, odor and consistency of vomitus. Look for blood in vomitus or blood-tinged vomitus. Show the nurse the emesis before discarding if required or if blood is noted.

Myocardial Infarction or Heart Attack

When blood flow to an area of the heart is completely blocked, oxygen and nutrients fail to reach its cells. Waste products are not removed and the muscle cells die. This is called a **myocardial infarction** (MI), or heart attack. The area of dead tissue may be large or small. This depends on the artery involved. See Chapter 19 for more information.

A myocardial infarction is an emergency that can result in serious heart damage or death. The following are signs and symptoms of MI:

- sudden, severe pain in the chest, usually on the left side or in the center, behind the breastbone

- pain or discomfort in other areas of the body, such as one or both arms, the back, neck, jaw, or stomach

- indigestion or heartburn

- nausea and vomiting

- **dyspnea**, or difficulty breathing

- dizziness

- pale, gray, or cyanotic skin color or mucous membranes, indicating lack of oxygen

- perspiration

- cold and clammy skin

- weak and irregular pulse rate

- low blood pressure

- anxiety and a sense of doom

- denial of a heart problem

The pain of a heart attack is commonly described as a crushing, pressing, squeezing, stabbing, piercing pain, or, "like someone is sitting on my chest." The pain may go down the inside of the left arm. A person may also feel it in the neck and/or in the jaw. The pain usually does not go away.

Women often experience different symptoms than men. Often women do not have chest pain or discomfort. Women are more likely than men to experience shortness of breath, nausea/vomiting, indigestion, and extreme fatigue. Many women report back or jaw pain or a hot or burning sensation in the back, shoulders, arms or jaw.

You must take immediate action if a resident experiences any of these symptoms. Follow these steps:

Myocardial infarction

1. Call or have someone call the nurse.

2. Place the resident in a comfortable position. Encourage him to rest. Reassure him that you will not leave him alone.

3. Loosen clothing around the resident's neck (Fig. 8-15).

Fig. 8-15. Loosen the clothing around the person's neck if you suspect he is having an MI.

4. Do not give the resident liquids or food.

5. Monitor the resident's breathing and pulse. If the resident stops breathing or has no pulse, perform rescue breathing or CPR if you are trained to do so and your facility allows it.

6. Stay with the resident until help has arrived.

Insulin Reaction and Diabetic Ketoacidosis

Insulin reaction and diabetic ketoacidosis are complications of diabetes that can be life-threatening. **Insulin reaction**, or **hypoglycemia**, can result from either too much insulin or too little food. It occurs when insulin is given and the person skips a meal or does not eat all the food required. Even when a regular amount of food is eaten, additional physical activity may cause the body to rapidly absorb the food. This causes too much insulin in the body. Vomiting and diarrhea may also lead to insulin reaction in people with diabetes.

The first signs of insulin reaction include feeling weak or different, nervousness, dizziness, and perspiration (see list below for further signs). These signal that the resident needs food. The food should be in a form that can be rapidly absorbed. A lump of sugar, a hard candy, or a glass of orange or grape juice should be consumed right away. A diabetic may have other quick sources of sugar handy, such as glucose tablets. Call the nurse if the resident has shown signs of insulin reaction. Signs and symptoms of insulin reaction include:

- hunger
- weakness
- rapid pulse
- headache
- low blood pressure
- cold, clammy skin
- confusion
- trembling
- blurred vision
- numbness of the lips and tongue
- unconsciousness

Having too little insulin in the body causes **diabetic ketoacidosis** (DKA), also known as ketoacidosis or **hyperglycemia**. It can result from undiagnosed diabetes, not enough insulin, eating too much, not getting enough exercise, or physical and emotional stress. If left untreated, DKA can lead to diabetic coma.

The signs of diabetic ketoacidosis include increased thirst or urination, abdominal pain, deep or difficult breathing, and breath that smells sweet or fruity (see list below for further signs). Call the nurse immediately if you suspect your resident is experiencing DKA. Other signs and symptoms include the following:

- hunger
- weakness
- rapid, weak pulse
- headache
- low blood pressure
- dry skin
- flushed cheeks
- drowsiness
- nausea and vomiting
- unconsciousness

See Chapter 23 for more information on diabetes and related care.

Seizures

Seizures are involuntary, often violent, contractions of muscles. They can involve a small area or the entire body. Seizures are caused by an abnormality in the brain. They can occur in young children who have a high fever. Older children and adults who have a serious illness, fever, or head injury may also have seizures.

The main goal of a caregiver during a seizure is to make sure the resident is safe. During a seizure, a person may shake severely and thrust arms and legs uncontrollably. He may clench his jaw, drool, and be unable to swallow. Most seizures last a short amount of time. Take the following emergency measures if a resident has a seizure:

Seizures

1. Note the time.

2. Lower the person to the floor. Cradle and

protect his head. Loosen clothing to help with breathing. Attempt to turn his head to one side to lower the risk of choking. This may not be possible during a violent seizure.

3. Have someone call the nurse immediately. Do not leave the person unless you must do so to get medical help.

4. Move furniture away to prevent injury. If a pillow is nearby, place it under his head.

5. Do not try to stop the seizure or restrain the person.

6. Do not force anything between the person's teeth. Do not place your hands in his mouth for any reason. You could be bitten.

7. Do not give liquids or food.

8. When the seizure is over, note the time. Gently turn the person to his left side if you do not suspect a head, neck or spinal injury. This reduces the risk of choking on vomit or saliva. If the person begins to choke get help immediately. Check for adequate breathing and pulse. If breathing and pulse are absent post-seizure, call 911 and begin CPR if trained and allowed to do so. Do not begin CPR during a seizure.

9. Report the length of the seizure and your observations to the nurse.

Types of General Seizures

Absence or Petit Mal: Absence, or petit mal, seizures are brief episodes of staring in which the levels of awareness and responsiveness are limited. People who have them do not usually realize when they have had one. There is no warning before this type of seizure, and being completely alert afterward is common.

Myoclonic: Myoclonic seizures are brief jerks of a muscle or a group of muscles. They usually do not last more than a few seconds.

Atonic: With atonic seizures (also called "drop attacks" or "drop seizures"), the muscles suddenly lose strength, which can cause drooping of the eyelids and nodding of the head. The person may drop things and fall to the ground. The person usually remains conscious while having this seizure. The seizure usually lasts less than 15 seconds.

Tonic: In tonic seizures, muscle tone is greatly increased temporarily, and the body, arms, or legs can suddenly stiffen. The person usually remains conscious. Tonic seizures most often occur during sleep. They usually last less than 20 seconds.

Clonic: Clonic seizures consist of rhythmic jerking of the arms and legs. This can occur on one or both sides of the body. The length of time this seizure lasts varies.

Tonic-Clonic: During a tonic-clonic seizure (formerly known as a "grand mal" seizure), all the muscles stiffen. The person may groan and lose consciousness, falling to the floor. He may bite his tongue or cheek and may turn blue. The arms and legs may make rhythmic jerking and bending movements. The person may lose control of his bladder and/or bowels. These seizures usually last one to three minutes. After the jerking stops, consciousness returns slowly. The person may be confused, tired, or agitated.

CVA or Stroke

The medical term for a stroke is cerebrovascular accident (CVA). A CVA, or stroke, occurs when the blood supply to a portion of the brain is cut off (Fig. 8-16). A clot, a ruptured blood vessel, or pressure from a tumor compressing a vessel may cause a stroke.

Fig. 8-16. *A CVA, or stroke, occurs when the blood supply to the brain is suddenly cut off.*

Symptoms that a stroke is beginning include dizziness, ringing in the ears, blurred vision, headache, nausea, vomiting, slurring of words, and loss of memory. These signs and symptoms should be reported immediately.

A transient ischemic attack, or TIA, is a warning sign of a CVA. It is the result of a temporary lack of oxygen in the brain. Symptoms may last up to 24 hours. They include tingling, weakness, or some loss of movement in an arm or leg. These symptoms should not be ignored. Report them to the nurse immediately. More information on CVAs can be found in Chapter 22. Signs that a TIA or stroke is occurring include the following:

- dizziness
- confusion
- loss of consciousness
- seizures
- shaking or trembling
- redness in the face
- facial droop, inability to smile
- drooping of one eyelid or eye
- sudden loss of sight in one eye
- pupil of one eye is larger
- blurred vision
- trouble with hearing or ringing in the ears
- intense headache that will not go away
- nausea and vomiting
- loss of bowel and bladder control
- numbness or tingling on one side of the body
- paralysis on one side of the body, called **hemiplegia**
- weakness on one side of the body, called **hemiparesis**
- inability to express needs to others through speech or written words, called **expressive aphasia**
- inability to understand what others are communicating through speech or written words, called **receptive aphasia**
- use of strange words
- noisy breathing
- elevated blood pressure
- slow pulse rate

4. Explain the nursing assistant's role on a code team

Facilities often use codes to inform staff of emergencies without alarming residents and visitors. For example, "Code Red" usually means fire, and "Code Blue" usually means cardiac arrest. Know the codes for your facility.

When staff are given their assignments at the beginning of shifts, some facilities also assign positions on the "code team." The **code team** is the team chosen for that shift to respond in case of a resident emergency. Staff on the code team may be asked to get a special cart or other emergency equipment, such as a suction machine, CPR equipment, oxygen, or other items. Although nursing assistants will not do many of the code team procedures, they may be asked to do chest compressions during CPR. If your facility uses code teams, note whether or not you are on this team at the start of your shift.

Should a code be called during your shift, respond from wherever you are in the facility. Respond calmly. Do not panic when you hear a code announced. If you are caring for a resident, get another staff member to take over. After the resident is secured, respond to the code.

Annual classes to update proper responses to codes may be held in your facility.

RESIDENTS' RIGHTS

Responding to Codes
When a resident goes into cardiac or respiratory arrest, it can be difficult for staff, other residents, and visitors. When a code occurs, the staff's main concern is the victim's survival. Sometimes, staff do not consider the impact of a code on other people in a facility.
Be aware of the people who are near the emergency. Staff not involved in responding to the code can move these people away from the area until the problem has been resolved. In some facilities a "Code Watcher" team is established to respond to a code and deal only with the emotional concerns of residents, staff, and visitors. This team is made up of nursing staff, social workers, trained volunteers, unit clerks, and administrative staff.

When a code occurs, do not leave a roommate in his room or close to where the code is occurring. Unconscious residents may also be aware of everything that is happening. Reassure unconscious residents, too, during emergency situations.

5. Describe guidelines for responding to disasters

A disaster can occur during your shift at a facility. Disasters can include fire, flood, earthquake, hurricane, tornado, or severe weather. Many facilities also now consider acts of terrorism as disasters.

Nursing assistants are expected to respond calmly and skillfully to disasters. You need to be responsible and efficient.

Facilities will have an area-specific disaster plan available for employees to learn. Know where the plan is located and what to do in the event of disasters. There will be general guidelines, as well as specific guidelines for the area in which you work. For example, NAs working where hurricanes occur, such as Florida, need to know guidelines for hurricanes, as well as other disasters.

During an emergency, a nurse or the administrator will give directions. Listen carefully to all directions. Know what your responsibilities are, and follow instructions. Know the locations of all exits and stairways. Know where the fire alarms and extinguishers are located. Emphasize that everyone should keep calm in an emergency.

Being educated and prepared for emergencies helps decrease panic and ensure the appropriate response in a timely fashion. This helps to protect you and your residents.

Classes on disasters and disaster drills are held at facilities so that staff can prepare for disasters ahead of time. Take advantage of these sessions. Pay close attention to the instructions.

HOT TIP

Evacuation Carries

If an evacuation is required, be familiar with different types of evacuation carries. An evacuation carry is a method of removing an immobile resident safely from a dangerous situation. Make sure you attend emergency care and disaster plan in-services at your facility. Practice evacuation carries during disaster drills. Contact your local fire department for information and/or training.

CHAPTER REVIEW

1. List two types of PPE you should always have with you in case of an emergency (LO 2).

2. List the two steps to follow in an emergency after making sure the area is safe and putting on gloves (LO 2).

3. When checking a person for injury, what should a nursing assistant look for (LO 2)?

4. What is the difference between a respiratory and cardiac arrest (LO 3)?

5. How soon can brain damage occur after the heart stops beating and breathing stops (LO 3)?

6. Why should only properly trained people perform CPR (LO 3)?

7. What do the ABCDs of CPR stand for (LO 3)?

8. When a person is choking, but can speak, cough, and breathe, what should the nursing assistant do (LO 3)?

9. In what position should a person be placed if he is in shock (LO 3)?

10. List a reason why gloves should always be applied before helping a resident who is bleeding (LO 3).

11. If blood seeps through the first pad over a wound, should the first pad be removed before applying a second pad (LO 3)?

12. What should never be applied to a burn (LO 3)?

13. Why should water not be applied to serious burns (LO 3)?

14. If a person feels faint and is sitting down, what should the nursing assistant do (LO 3)?

15. When should a nursing assistant suspect a resident has been poisoned (LO 3)?

16. After putting on gloves, what should a nursing assistant do for a resident who has a nosebleed (LO 3)?

17. What is a medical term for vomit (LO 3)?

18. Explain why a nursing assistant should give oral care to a resident who has vomited (LO 3).

19. List ten general signs or symptoms of a myocardial infarction (MI) (LO 3).

20. What symptoms are women more likely to experience than men if they are having an MI (LO 3)?

21. What causes insulin reaction (LO 3)?

22. What causes diabetic ketoacidosis (LO 3)?

23. What are three things a nursing assistant should never do when a resident is having a seizure (LO 3)?

24. What is a transient ischemic attack (TIA) (LO 3)?

25. List eight signs that a stroke is beginning (LO 3).

26. What does the term "Code Blue" usually stand for during an emergency (LO 4)?

27. List five types of disasters. Give one example of a disaster that occurred in your area within the last two years (LO 5).

9
Admission, Transfer, Discharge, and Physical Exams

"A Walk Through a Ward of the Eighteenth Century" by Grace Goldin

The old ward of St. John's Hospital, Bruges, housed patients continuously from the 12th century, when its first section was built, until the 20th . . . . A division was customary in medieval times. . . forming two wards side by side with separate entrances; or two wards built one above the other to separate the sexes . . . . The . . . hospital of the 18th century was a dangerous place, mortality there was higher than among patients nursed at home, and therefore it catered only to wretches with no alternative; but among these, many got better. The bonneted beldame at the rear of the center aisle, being shown out the door with a pat on the shoulder, is very likely being discharged "cured."

Excerpt from "A Walk Through a Ward of the Eighteenth Century" by Grace Goldin. From *Journal of the History of Medicine and Allied Sciences*, Volume XXII, Number 2, 1967. Reprinted with permission of Oxford University Press.

"Where we love is home, Home that our feet may leave, but not our hearts."

Oliver Wendell Holmes, 1809-1894

"The best thing we can do is to make wherever we're in look as much like home as we can."

Christopher Fry, 1907-2005

1. Define important words in this chapter

abdominal girth: a measurement of the circumference around the abdomen at the umbilicus (navel).

admission: the initial entry of a resident into a facility or a unit.

admission pack: personal care items supplied upon a resident's admission.

baseline: initial value that can be compared to future measurements.

bedridden: confined to bed.

contracture: the permanent and often painful shortening of a muscle, usually due to a lack of activity.

discharge: a doctor's order that releases a resident to leave a facility to go home or to another facility.

dorsal recumbent: position with the person flat on her back with knees flexed and slightly separated; feet are flat on bed.

kilogram: 1000 grams; 1 kilogram = 2.2 pounds.

knee-chest: position with the person lying on his abdomen with knees pulled up towards the abdomen and with legs separated; arms are pulled up and flexed; the head is turned to one side.

lithotomy: position with the person on her back with her hips at the edge of the exam table; legs are flexed and feet are in padded stirrups.

metric: system of weights and measures based upon the meter.

pound: measurement of weight equal to 16 ounces.

transfer: an order that moves a resident from one unit to another within the same facility.

2. List factors for families in choosing a facility

Choosing the right facility for a loved one can be a challenging, emotional, and difficult process. To help guide their choice, family and friends may look at information from federal agencies, such as the Centers for Medicare & Medicaid Services (CMS). They may ask for recommendations from friends. Families may review facilities' results from past state surveys or inspections. They may check to see if the facility has been accredited by The Joint Commission.

Early in the process, families usually visit each facility they are considering (Fig. 9-1). In some cases, a single visit is enough to decide if a facility is right or not. For example, if a strong smell of urine is present, they may not return again to see if it was an isolated incident. Some factors families consider before placing a loved one in a facility include:

- Do the staff seem courteous and friendly?

- Do most of the staff speak the resident's native language? Is an interpreter available?

- Are there enough staff members on duty at the facility? What is the ratio of nurses and nursing assistants to residents? How is the facility staffed on evenings and weekends?

- Is there a strong smell of urine or other foul odors in the facility?

- What is the food like at the facility? Is attention paid to individual food preferences? Is a dietician available for meetings?

- Are the residents up and dressed early in the morning?

- Do the staff interact with the residents positively?

- Do residents look groomed, taken care of, and happy?

- How are residents' complaints resolved?

- Is the facility licensed?

- Have the state survey and other inspection results been satisfactory?

- Does the facility explain Residents' Rights?

- Does the facility provide assistance with activities of daily living (ADLs)? If so, how is it provided, and what are the fees?

- Are physical, occupational, and speech therapists available?

- Do volunteers work with residents? If so, are their interactions positive?

- How involved can the family be in creating the resident's care plan?

- Does the facility provide the level of care the resident needs? What about future needs?

- Is the environment safe, functional, and homelike?

- Is there an activities department? What kinds of activities are offered?

- What are the steps to take if a resident wants to move out of the facility?

- What policies does the facility have on advance directives and end-of-life decisions?

Fig. 9-1. *Before choosing a facility for a loved one, families may tour the facility. They may observe the environment, how the residents look and what types of activities are offered.*

These are only some of the things families watch for when choosing a facility for a loved one.

3. Explain the nursing assistant's role in the emotional adjustment of a new resident

Moving into a facility requires a big adjustment. New residents may have been independent for a long time. They may be moving from a family member's home. Either way, there is a huge emotional adjustment to be made.

Think about some of the life-altering changes residents have had to make. The move into a facility may have been sudden due to health reasons. They may have had to leave their homes and get rid of their personal belongings (Fig. 9-2). They may have had to give away beloved pets. There may have been a loss of family and friends. Due to all of these things, new residents may be experiencing fear, loss, anger, and uncertainty, along with a decline in health and independence.

Fig. 9-2. Understand and be empathetic to the fact that many residents had to leave familiar places. They may have had to give away personal items and beloved pets.

Nursing assistants should empathize with new residents. Think about how you would feel if you had to give up many of your things to move into an unfamiliar place full of strangers. Understanding some of what residents are going through will help you provide compassionate care. Your residents will need it during those early days and weeks in their new home.

Nursing assistants are the team members most involved with residents on a daily basis. You will have an important role in helping new residents feel comfortable in the facility. Other guidelines to help new residents adjust follow:

Guidelines

Helping New Residents Adjust

- Have a positive attitude. New residents, like most people, want to be near others who are nice and pleasant. Residents want to feel comfortable around staff who provide their care. Residents should not feel as though they are a burden to staff.

- Be tactful. Think before you speak.

- Communicate clearly. Giving a simple reminder about meal times helps the resident feel more connected.

- Show respect for residents' belongings. New residents may be frightened of their new surroundings. They may feel very protective of their personal items. Treat items carefully. Show that you are trustworthy.

- Be responsible. If you make a mistake with care, report it to the nurse immediately. People respect and trust you more when you admit mistakes.

- Be honest. Do not make promises you cannot keep. If you tell residents you are coming by to visit, they will look for you. If you forget, apologize and reschedule the visit as soon as possible.

- Listen to residents if they want to talk. New residents may want to express their feelings about what they are going through (Fig. 9-3). They may want to share some of their stories and backgrounds. Make time to listen.

- Pay attention to residents' wishes. For example, if a resident wants to be alone instead of joining others for an activity, let him do that. You can say, "Maybe next time," and leave him alone. Residents have the right to make choices about what to do and how to spend their time. If they choose to be alone, honor this decision.

- Respect residents' privacy. The right to privacy is a legal right, and it is always important. It can be especially important when residents are first admitted. Take care to make sure residents have as much privacy as possible.

- Be patient and kind. A new resident might have a good day followed by a not-so-good day. Allow residents to adapt at their own pace. Everyone is different. The process of adjusting may take some time. Dealing with multiple losses initiates the grieving process.

Fig. 9-3. *A new resident may have just lost someone very close to him. Be supportive. Listen to him if he wants to talk.*

HOT TIP

The Welcome Committee

To assist new residents with the transition into a facility, a "Welcome Committee" can be helpful. Team members from each department can be chosen to greet the new resident. Each department can make or buy a card for the resident. The special cards can be brought to the resident's new room one-by-one or as a group. This idea can be expanded to include other niceties, such as having flowers waiting for a resident in her new room. Small ways of showing care and warmth can help new residents feel better about the transition to a facility.

4. Describe the nursing assistant's role in the admission process

Admission is often the first time you meet new residents. Staff will be told the approximate time that the new resident will arrive. When the resident arrives, give him a good first impression of the staff and the facility. Welcome him in a friendly manner. Introduce yourself to the resident and all family members. Answer any questions residents and their family members have. Ask questions to get information on the resident's personal preferences, history, rituals,

and routines. Family members are great sources of information about the resident; take time to ask them questions.

The facility will have specific procedures for admitting new residents. Follow these general guidelines to help make the experience pleasant and successful:

Guidelines
Admission

- Wash your hands. Then gather any necessary equipment to bring to the resident's room. This equipment may include:

  - An **admission pack** or kit contains personal care items for the resident. The pack usually has a wash basin, bedpan, urinal (for male residents), toothpaste, soap, and a water pitcher and cup. Other items may be in the pack, such as a specimen cup and transport bag, special lotions or soaps.

  - A stethoscope and a sphygmomanometer (used to measure blood pressure; you will learn about this in Chapter 13) (Fig. 9-4).

  - A thermometer

  - A facility gown or pajamas, depending upon the resident

- Prepare the resident's room before the resident arrives to help make him feel welcome. Know the condition of the resident. Know if he or she is bed-bound or is able to walk.

- Prepare the bed according to the nurse's instructions. Open the curtains or blinds.

- If a roommate is in the room, notify him or her of the new resident's arrival.

- When the resident arrives, introduce yourself. State your position. Call the person by his formal name until he tells you what he wants to be called.

- Do not rush the process or the resident. He should not feel as if he is an inconvenience. Make sure that he feels welcome and wanted.

Ⓑ Introduce the new resident to his roommate and other residents in the rooms on either side and across the hall. This helps the resident feel more comfortable. It may also help the family feel better.

Ⓑ Explain day-to-day life in the facility. Offer to take him and his family on a facility tour. Show them the dining room, chapel, and all other important areas, such as the activity room. If available, show them activity schedules. Point out information about menus. During the tour, introduce residents to all staff and residents you see (Fig. 9-5).

Ⓑ Show the resident how to work the new bed controls.

Ⓑ Make sure the call light is close to the bed. Show the resident how to work the call light and explain its use.

Ⓑ Explain how to work the television and phone.

Ⓑ Handle all of the resident's personal items with care and respect. These are the items he has chosen to bring with him to the facility. Treat them carefully. Assist the resident to unpack everything. Ask him where he wants the items and how he would like the room set up (Fig. 9-6).

Fig. 9-4. a) A stethoscope and b) one type of sphygmomanometer.

Fig. 9-5. Take new residents on a tour of the facility and introduce them to all residents and staff you see.

Fig. 9-6. Handle a resident's personal items carefully. Set up the room according to her preference.

Admitting a resident

Equipment: may include admission paperwork (checklist and inventory form), gloves, and vital signs equipment

1. Identify yourself by name. Identify the resident. Greet the resident by name.

2. Wash your hands.

3. Explain procedure to the resident. Speak clearly, slowly, and directly. Maintain face-to-face contact whenever possible. Encourage resident to assist if possible.

4. Provide for the resident's privacy with a curtain, screen, or door. Ask the family to step outside until the initial admission process is complete. Show them where they may wait and let them know how long they will have to wait. Tell them where they can get refreshments.

5. If part of facility procedure, do these things:

   Take the resident's height, weight, and vital signs. (Height and weight procedures follow; vitals signs are in Chapter 13.) Most facilities require baseline height, weight, and vital sign measurements. **Baseline** signs are initial values that can be compared to future measurements. Document on admission form and elsewhere per facility policy.

   Obtain a urine specimen if required (see Chapter 16).

Complete the paperwork. Take an inventory of all of the personal items. Help the resident put personal items away. Label each item if it is facility policy. If the resident has valuables, ask the nurse for instructions.

Fill the water pitcher with fresh water unless the nurse has instructed you not to.

6. When the initial portion of the admission is complete, locate the family and let them know they may return to the resident's room.

7. Show the resident the room and bathroom. Explain how to work the bed controls and the call light. Point out the lights, telephone, and television and how to work them. Give the resident any information on menus, dining times, and activity schedules.

8. Introduce the resident to his roommate, if there is one. Introduce other residents and staff.

9. Make resident comfortable. Remove privacy measures.

10. Leave call light within resident's reach.

11. Wash your hands.

12. Be courteous and respectful at all times. Let the resident know when you are leaving. Ask if he needs anything else.

13. Document procedure using facility guidelines.

Residents' weight and height will be checked when they are admitted. Nursing assistants also check weight as part of regular care. Height is usually not checked as often as weight. Report weight loss or gain, no matter how small, promptly to the nurse. Changes in a resident's weight can be a sign of illness.

Weight will be measured using **pounds** or kilograms. **Kilograms** are units of **metric** measurement. Bedridden residents will need to be weighed, too. Being **bedridden** means that residents are unable to get out of bed.

A paper towel may need to be placed on the scale before the resident's weight is obtained. This

is done to prevent the transfer of bacteria or fungus to or from the bare feet. Follow your facility's policy on whether or not to place a paper towel on the scale first.

Measuring and recording weight of an ambulatory resident

Equipment: standing/upright scale, pen and paper to record your findings

1. Identify yourself by name. Identify the resident. Greet the resident by name.

2. Wash your hands.

3. Explain procedure to the resident. Speak clearly, slowly, and directly. Maintain face-to-face contact whenever possible. Encourage resident to assist if possible.

4. Provide for the resident's privacy with a curtain, screen, or door.

5. Start with the scale balanced at zero. If you do not know how to balance the scale, ask the nurse.

6. Help the resident remove shoes and step onto the center of the scale. The resident should be facing the scale. Once on the scale, his arms must hang free.

7. Weigh the resident. This is done by balancing the scale by making the balance bar level. Move the small and large weight indicators until the bar balances. Read the two numbers shown (on the small and large weight indicators) when the bar is balanced. Add these two numbers together. This is the resident's weight (Fig. 9-7).

Fig. 9-7. Move the small and large weight indicators until the bar balances.

8. Help the resident off the scale before recording weight.

9. Record the resident's weight.

10. Remove privacy measures.

11. Leave call light within resident's reach.

12. Wash your hands.

13. Be courteous and respectful at all times.

14. Report any changes in the resident to the nurse. Document procedure using facility guidelines.

When residents are not able to get out of wheelchairs easily, they are weighed using a special wheelchair scale. With this scale, wheelchairs are rolled directly onto the scale (Fig. 9-8). With some wheelchair scales, you will need to subtract the weight of the wheelchair from the resident's weight. If the weight of the wheelchair is not listed on the chair, weigh the empty wheelchair first. Then subtract the wheelchair's weight from the total. Some scales automatically adjust for the wheelchair's weight."

Fig. 9-8. *A type of wheelchair scale.*

When residents cannot get out of bed, they are weighed on special bed scales (Fig. 9-9). Before using a bed scale, know how it works and how to use it properly and safely. Follow your facility's procedure and any manufacturer's instructions. This is a general procedure for weighing someone on a bed scale.

Fig. 9-9. *A type of bed scale.* (Photo courtesy of Detecto, www. detecto.com, 800-641-2008)

Measuring and recording weight of a bedridden resident

Equipment: scale, pen and paper to record your findings

Have another co-worker assist.

1. Identify yourself by name. Identify the resident. Greet the resident by name.

2. Wash your hands.

3. Explain procedure to the resident. Speak clearly, slowly, and directly. Maintain face-to-face contact whenever possible. Encourage resident to assist if possible.

4. Provide for the resident's privacy with a curtain, screen, or door.

5. Practice good body mechanics. Adjust the bed to a safe level, usually waist high. Lock the bed wheels.

6. Start with the scale balanced at zero. If you do not know how to balance the scale, ask the nurse.

7. Examine the sling, straps, chains, and/or pad for any damage. Do not use the scale if you find damage.

8. Turn linen down so that it is off the resident.

9. Turn resident to one side away from you (Chapter 11) or if flat pad scale is used, slide resident onto pad using a helper. If sling is used, remove from the scale and place underneath the resident without wrinkling.

10. With a sling, turn the resident back to the supine (back) position and straighten sling.

11. Attach the sling to the scale or if using a flat pad scale, position resident securely on the pad.

12. Check the straps or other connectors, and raise the sling or the pad until the resident is clear of the bed. With some scales, you can keep the resident directly over the bed while weighing him. With others, you have to move the scale away from the bed. Either way, secure the resident before moving the scale.

13. For digital scales, turn them on and note reading. With other scales, move the weights until you get a reading. Note the weight.

14. Lower the resident back down on the bed. If using a sling, turn resident to both sides to remove the sling. If using a pad scale, carefully slide the resident back onto the bed.

15. Record the resident's weight.

16. Make resident comfortable. Replace bed linens.

17. Return bed to low position if raised. Ensure resident's safety. Remove privacy measures.

18. Leave call light within resident's reach.

19. Wash your hands.

20. Be courteous and respectful at all times.

21. Report any changes in the resident to the nurse. Document procedure using facility guidelines.

For measuring height, the rod measures in inches and fractions of inches. Record the total number of inches. If you have to change inches into feet, remember that there are 12 inches in a foot, and 60 inches equal five feet.

Measuring and recording height of an ambulatory resident

Equipment: standing/upright scale, pen and paper to record your findings

1. Identify yourself by name. Identify the resident. Greet the resident by name.

2. Wash your hands.

3. Explain procedure to the resident. Speak clearly, slowly, and directly. Maintain face-to-face contact whenever possible. Encourage resident to assist if possible.

4. Provide for the resident's privacy with a curtain, screen, or door.

5. Help the resident to step onto scale, facing away from the scale.

6. Ask the resident to stand straight. Help as needed.

7. Pull up measuring rod from back of scale. Gently lower measuring rod until it rests flat on the resident's head (Fig. 9-10).

Fig. 9-10. To determine height, gently lower measuring rod until it rests flat on resident's head.

8. Determine resident's height.

9. Help the resident off scale before recording height. Make sure measuring rod does not hit resident in the head while trying to help resident off the scale.

10. Record height.

11. Remove privacy measures.

12. Leave call light within resident's reach.

13. Wash your hands.

14. Be courteous and respectful at all times.

15. Report any changes in the resident to the nurse. Document procedure using facility guidelines.

Measuring and recording height of a bedridden resident

Equipment: measuring tape (Fig. 9-11), pencil, pen and paper to record your findings

Fig. 9-11. *A tape measure.*

1. Identify yourself by name. Identify the resident. Greet the resident by name.

2. Wash your hands.

3. Explain procedure to the resident. Speak clearly, slowly, and directly. Maintain face-to-face contact whenever possible. Encourage resident to assist if possible.

4. Provide for the resident's privacy with a curtain, screen, or door.

5. Practice good body mechanics. Adjust the bed to a safe level, usually waist high. Lock the bed wheels.

6. Turn linen down so it is off the resident.

7. Position resident lying straight in the supine (back) position.

8. Using a pencil, make a small mark on the bottom sheet at the top of the resident's head.

9. Make another pencil mark at the bottom of the resident's feet (Fig. 9-12).

Fig. 9-12. *Make marks on the sheet at the resident's head and feet.*

10. Using the tape measure, measure the area between the pencil marks. This is the resident's height.

11. Record the resident's height.

12. Make resident comfortable. Replace bed linen.

13. Return bed to low position if raised. Ensure resident's safety. Remove privacy measures.

14. Leave call light within resident's reach.

15. Wash your hands.

16. Be courteous and respectful at all times.

17. Report any changes in the resident to the nurse. Document procedure using facility guidelines.

Some residents cannot lie straight due to contractures. A **contracture** is the permanent and often painful shortening of a muscle. Some facilities require a tape measure be used to follow the curves of the spine and legs. The number of inches is totaled and recorded. This is the least accurate way of measuring height.

Another method used on residents with contractures is called the demi-span. Using this method, you measure the distance from the middle of the top of the chest, called the "sternal notch," to the tip of the middle finger. Ideally, the left arm is used. The arm is held up straight out from the shoulder. Once this measurement is obtained, a calculation is done for females and males. The final height is recorded in centimeters. You will receive special training if you are required to use this procedure.

Some residents require abdominal girth to be measured. **Abdominal girth** is a measurement of the circumference around the abdomen at the umbilicus (navel). These are taken and noted on an admission checklist form.

Measuring abdominal girth

Equipment: measuring tape, pen and paper to record your findings

1. Identify yourself by name. Identify the resident. Greet the resident by name.

2. Wash your hands.

3. Explain procedure to the resident. Speak clearly, slowly, and directly. Maintain face-to-face contact whenever possible. Encourage resident to assist if possible.

4. Provide for the resident's privacy with a curtain, screen, or door.

5. Practice good body mechanics. Adjust the bed to a safe level, usually waist high. Lock the bed wheels.

6. Position resident lying straight in the supine (back) position.

7. Turn linen down and raise gown or top enough to expose only the abdomen. Keep all areas covered that do not need to be exposed. Promote resident's right to dignity and privacy.

8. Gently wrap measuring tape around the resident's abdomen at the level of the navel.

9. Read the number where the ends of the tape meet (Fig. 9-13).

Fig. 9-13. *After wrapping the measuring tape around the resident's abdomen, read the number where the ends of the tape meet.*

10. Carefully remove the tape measure. Record abdominal girth measurement.

11. Make resident comfortable. Replace clothing and bed linen.

12. Return bed to low position if raised. Ensure resident's safety. Remove privacy measures.

13. Leave call light within resident's reach.

14. Wash your hands.

15. Be courteous and respectful at all times.

16. Report any changes in the resident to the nurse. Document procedure using facility guidelines.

5. Explain the nursing assistant's role during an in-house transfer of a resident

Residents may be transferred to another room within a facility. Residents may need to be transferred to a different unit that offers more intensive care. Whatever the reason for the **transfer**, it may be a difficult time for the resident. Change is always hard, but this is especially true if the resident has an illness or his condition has worsened. Nursing assistants should try to make the transfer as smooth as possible for residents.

Notifying residents as soon as possible of the transfer can help lessen the stress. Explain all the details you know, including where, when and why the transfer is happening. Refer any questions to the nurse. Residents have the right to be notified of any room or roommate change.

Nursing assistants are usually responsible for packing all of the resident's belongings. Packing up all of the items may take some time. Pack personal items carefully so that nothing breaks, is damaged, or is lost.

The resident may be transferred in a bed, in a stretcher, or in a wheelchair. Find out the method of transfer from the nurse so that you can plan the move.

When you arrive at the new unit, introduce the resident to everyone. If you unpack the resident's belongings, do it carefully. Try to re-create the way the belongings were set up in the former room. It is a good idea to check on the resident later in the day to make sure he is settled. After that, it is nice to stop in sometimes to say hello. This helps the resident feel that staff members care about him.

When you leave the resident's room, report to the nurse in charge of that resident. At that point, you will have formally transferred responsibility to the new unit.

Transferring a resident

Equipment: may include a wheelchair or stretcher, cart for belongings, all of the resident's personal care items

1. Identify yourself by name. Identify the resident. Greet the resident by name.

2. Wash your hands.

3. Explain procedure to the resident. Speak clearly, slowly, and directly. Maintain face-to-face contact whenever possible. Encourage resident to assist if possible.

4. Provide for the resident's privacy with a curtain, screen, or door.

5. Collect the items to be moved onto the cart, and ask another staff member to help take them to the new location.

6. Lock wheelchair or stretcher wheels. Help the resident into the wheelchair or onto the stretcher. Take him or her to the new area.

7. Introduce the resident to the new residents and staff.

8. Lock wheelchair or stretcher wheels. Transfer the resident to the new bed, if needed.

9. Unpack all belongings. Help the resident to put personal items away.

10. Make resident comfortable. Remove privacy measures.

11. Leave call light within resident's reach.

12. Wash your hands.

13. Be courteous and respectful at all times.

14. Report any changes in the resident to the nurse. Document procedure using facility guidelines.

6. Explain the nursing assistant's role in the discharge of a resident

A **discharge** is official after the doctor writes the discharge order that releases the resident to leave the facility to go home or to another facility. The nurse will then complete instructions for the resident to follow after discharge. These instructions may include future doctor appointments, medications, ambulation instructions, and special dietary requirements (Fig. 9-14). They may also contain special exercises for the resident to do and community resources for the resident.

Fig. 9-14. *After a resident is discharged, she may continue to receive physical therapy and have other medical appointments.*

Your responsibility is to collect the resident's belongings and to pack them carefully. You may be asked to check each item against the inventory list done at admission. This helps make sure everything is included.

A resident who is going home may be happy, although he may be unsure if he is ready for this important change. Be positive and reassuring. If he has additional questions, inform the nurse.

Know the resident's condition and whether or not he will need a wheelchair or stretcher for discharge. When it is time to move him to the car, you are responsible for him until he is safely in the car. Stay with the resident until he and his belongings are in the car. Residents have the right to a safe and secure discharge. Your responsibility does not end until the car doors are closed.

Discharging a resident

Equipment: may include a wheelchair or stretcher, cart for belongings, the discharge paperwork, including the inventory list done on admission, all of the resident's personal care items

1. Identify yourself by name. Identify the resident. Greet the resident by name.

2. Wash your hands.

3. Explain procedure to the resident. Speak clearly, slowly, and directly. Maintain face-to-face contact whenever possible. Encourage resident to assist if possible.

4. Provide for the resident's privacy with a curtain, screen, or door.

5. Compare the inventory list to the items being packed. Ask the resident to sign if all items are there.

6. Carefully put the items to be taken onto the cart, and ask another staff member to help transport items to the pick-up area.

7. Help the resident dress in clothing of his choice. Make sure the nurse has removed all dressings, IVs and tubes that need to be removed prior to discharge.

8. Lock wheelchair or stretcher wheels. Help him safely into the wheelchair or onto the stretcher (Chapter 11).

9. Help the resident to say his goodbyes to other residents and the staff.

10. Take him to the pick-up area. Lock wheelchair or stretcher wheels. Help the resident into the vehicle. Transfer personal items into the vehicle.

11. Say goodbye to the resident. You are responsible for the resident until he or she is safely in the car and the door is closed.

12. Wash your hands.

13. Document procedure using facility guidelines.

Leaving a facility AMA

Sometimes a resident decides to leave a facility without the approval of the doctor. This is called leaving AMA or "against medical advice." When this occurs, a process must be followed to protect the facility and staff.

If you see signs that a resident might be leaving the facility, notify the charge nurse. Signs that a resident wants to leave include appearing anxious and nervous. The resident may mention leaving or start gathering her belongings.

When residents want to leave AMA, they are usually asked to sign a form that says he or she has been informed of and understands the risks of leaving the facility.

7. Describe the nursing assistant's role during physical exams

Some residents need a physical exam when arriving at a facility. Others need a physical exam after they have been there for a while. Know your role during a physical exam so the process runs smoothly. Doctors or nurses will do part or all of the exam. Nursing assistants may be asked to help.

You can help residents with their emotional needs by being there for them. Exams can make people anxious. They may fear what the examiner will do or what he or she will find. Exams can cause discomfort and embarrassment. Help residents by listening to them, talking to them, or even holding their hands.

Nursing assistants are often responsible for gathering equipment for the nurse or doctor. Some of the equipment you will collect includes:

- sphygmomanometer (for blood pressure)
- stethoscope
- alcohol wipes
- flashlight
- thermometer
- tongue depressor
- eye chart for vision screening
- tuning fork (tests hearing with vibrations)
- reflex hammer (taps body parts to test reflexes)
- otoscope (lighted instrument that examines the outer ear and eardrum)
- ophthalmoscope (lighted instrument that examines the eye)
- specimen containers
- lubricant
- Hemoccult™ card (tests for blood in stool)

- vaginal speculum for females (opens the vagina so that it and the cervix can be examined)
- gloves
- drape

During the exam, the nursing assistant will place the resident in the correct position and stay with the resident as needed. The NA may help drape the resident for privacy and comfort. Expose only the body part being examined.

Some positions are embarrassing and uncomfortable. You can help by explaining why the position is needed. Explain how long the resident can expect to stay in the position.

Common positions used during physical exams include the following:

- The **dorsal recumbent** position. This position is used to examine the breasts, chest, abdomen, and perineal area. A person in this position is flat on her back. The knees are flexed and feet flat on the bed. The drape is put over the resident, covering her body. Her head remains uncovered (Fig. 9-15).

- The **lithotomy** position. This position is used to examine the vagina. The resident lies on her back and her hips are brought to the edge of the exam table. Her legs are flexed and her feet are in padded stirrups. The drape is put over the resident, covering her body. Her head remains uncovered. The drape is also brought down to cover the perineal area (Fig. 9-16).

- The **knee-chest** position. This position is used to examine the rectum or, sometimes, the vagina. A resident in the knee-chest position is lying on his or her abdomen. The knees are pulled towards the abdomen and legs are separated. Arms are pulled up and flexed. The head is turned to one side. In the knee-chest position, the resident will be wearing a gown and possibly socks. The drape should be applied in a diamond shape to cover the back, buttocks and thighs (Fig. 9-17).

Fig. 9-15. The dorsal recumbent position.

Fig. 9-16. The lithotomy position.

Fig. 9-17. The knee-chest position.

More information on different body positions is in Chapter 11.

In addition to helping with equipment, positioning and draping, the nursing assistant should:

- Wash your hands before and after the exam.
- Provide other privacy measures throughout the exam, such as closing the privacy screen or curtain and closing the door. Let the resident know that he or she will not be exposed more than necessary during the exam.
- Provide enough light for the doctor or nurse.
- Ask the resident to urinate before the exam. Collect any urine needed for a specimen at this time. Gather and label specimens as needed.
- Listen to the resident throughout the exam. Try to help him or her remain calm.
- Follow any of the doctor's or nurse's instructions.
- Make sure the resident does not fall.

- Put instruments in the proper place for the doctor or nurse. Hand instruments to the doctor or nurse as needed.
- Follow Standard Precautions.

After the exam, help the resident clean up and get dressed. Help the resident safely back to his or her room and secure the resident. Dispose of any trash and disposable equipment in the exam area. Bring all reusable equipment to the proper cleaning room. Clean and store reusable equipment according to facility policy. Label and bring any specimens to the proper place so that they can go to the lab.

RESIDENTS' RIGHTS

Residents' Rights During Exams

Residents have the right to know why exams are being done and who is doing them. Residents have the right to choose examiners and to have family members present during the exam.

RESIDENTS' RIGHTS

Knock first, then listen.

At some point in your life, you may have had a healthcare provider knock on the door to an examination room and not wait to hear you say "come in." If so, you may have felt uncomfortable. When a resident is in an examination room, not waiting to hear him say "come in" may expose him not only to you, but also to people walking through the hallway. Respect your residents' rights to privacy and dignity. Knock and wait to hear "come in" before you enter an examination room.

CHAPTER REVIEW

1. Name ten factors families may consider when choosing a facility (LO 2).

2. Why is moving into a facility a big emotional adjustment for new residents (LO 3)?

3. Name seven ways nursing assistants can help new residents adjust to a facility (LO 3).

4. Why is it a good idea for nursing assistants to ask family members questions about residents upon admission (LO 4)?

5. Why do you think it is important to introduce new residents to all other staff and residents in the area during admission (LO 4)?

6. What should the scale be balanced at before measuring a resident's weight (LO 4)?

7. Why might a transfer be difficult for a resident (LO 5)?

8. During discharge of a resident, when does a nursing assistant's responsibility for the resident end (LO 6)?

9. List and describe three common positions used during physical exams (LO 7).

10. How can a nursing assistant provide privacy for a resident during an exam (LO 7)?

11. List ten examples of equipment nursing assistants may collect for physical exams (LO 7).

10 Bedmaking and Unit Care

1. Define important words in this chapter

anxiety: uneasiness or fear, often about a situation or condition.

biorhythms: natural rhythms or cycles related to bodily functions.

circadian rhythm: the 24-hour day-night cycle.

closed bed: bed completely made with the bedspread and blankets in place.

depressant: a substance that causes calmness and drowsiness.

disposable: designed to be thrown away after one use.

draw sheet: an extra sheet placed on top of the bottom sheet; used for moving residents.

incontinence: the inability to control the bladder or bowels, which leads to an involuntary loss of urine or feces.

insomnia: the inability to fall asleep or remain asleep.

occupied bed: a bed made while the resident is in the bed.

open bed: bed made with linen folded down to the foot of the bed.

parasomnias: sleep disorders.

sleep: natural period of rest for the mind and body during which energy is restored.

stimulant: a drug that increases or quickens actions of the body.

surgical bed: bed made so that a person can easily move onto it from a stretcher.

unoccupied bed: a bed made while no resident is in the bed.

2. Discuss the importance of sleep

Sleep is a natural period of rest for the mind and body during which energy is restored. Sleep and rest are two basic needs, as described in Chapter 5. The human body cannot survive long without sleep. Sleep is needed to replace old cells with new ones and provide new energy to organs.

Sleep is vital to proper physical and mental development. Dreams help the brain sort out all of the things that it has been dealing with during the day. Deep sleep helps the body to renew.

The study of the rhythms of the body is called biorhythmology. **Biorhythms** are the natural rhythms or cycles related to body functions that occur due to daily, monthly or yearly changes. Light and darkness, gravity, and temperature changes are examples of changes that can affect living organisms.

The most famous biorhythm is the circadian rhythm. The **circadian rhythm** is the 24-hour day-night cycle. It usually appears in infants when they are about three weeks old. The circadian rhythm can affect the body in many ways. In addition to sleep patterns, other changes in the body can occur during the 24-hour cycle. These include variations in blood pressure and body temperature.

HOT TIP

Sleep cycles in your genes?

Have you ever wondered why two children in the same family have different sleep cycles? During non-school times, one child wakes up early in the morning and falls asleep at 10:00 p.m., while the other wakes up after noon and stays up well past midnight. The early riser is often called a "lark," and the person who stays up late is called an "owl." These are common terms given to people who have different body clocks, or circadian rhythms. Some believe that this is due to genetics—that sleep cycles are in our genes.

3. Describe types of sleep disorders

The inability to fall asleep or to remain asleep is called **insomnia**. A person may have difficulty falling asleep, may not stay asleep through the night, or may wake up too early in the morning. There are many different causes of insomnia. Some of the reasons that people develop sleep disorders, or **parasomnias**, are illness, anxi-

ety, fear, stress, medications, trouble breathing, noise, hunger or thirst. Some common sleep disorders are described in the box below:

Parasomnias

Somnambulism is sleepwalking. With this sleep disorder, the person performs activities that people normally perform while awake. In most cases, the episodes do not result in injury.

Sleeptalking is talking during sleep. This usually occurs without the person being aware of what he is saying, or even that he was talking. Episodes are usually brief and do not occur often.

Bruxism is grinding and clenching the teeth. It can cause headaches, jaw problems and pain, neck aches, and can loosen teeth.

REM sleep behavior disorder is talking, often along with violent movements, during REM (dreaming) sleep. The person may be acting out his dreams. This disorder is more common among elderly people who have illnesses affecting the nervous system, such as Parkinson's or Alzheimer's disease. (See Chapter 22.)

4. Identify factors affecting sleep

Many elderly people, especially those living away from their homes, have sleep problems (Fig. 10-1). Many factors can affect residents' sleep. The more you pay attention to these factors and try to improve conditions, the better residents will sleep.

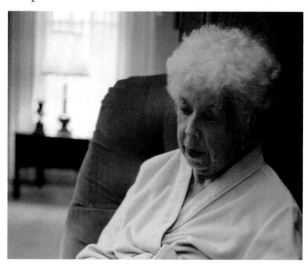

Fig. 10-1. *Living away from home can interfere with quality sleep.*

Factors affecting residents' sleep include:

Environment: Residents may have been used to sleeping with a mate or alone when they lived at home. Adjusting to a new place and a roommate is very difficult. Even if married residents are in the same room at a facility, sleep can be difficult because they are no longer in their home. Ways to help with environmental issues include:

- Listen to residents if they wish to talk. Be compassionate and reassuring.

- Have enough pillows and blankets.

- Make sure mattresses fit properly and are not damaged or lumpy. If a mattress does not fit properly, report it to the nurse or proper department.

Noise level and/or lighting can affect a resident's ability to sleep. Keeping the room dark is very important to some residents. Other residents prefer to sleep with a light or a night-light on. Ways to help address noise level and/or lighting include:

- Keep the noise level low. Closing doors at night may help.

- Keep your voice low.

- Do not bang equipment or meal trays.

- Use blinds or shades to help darken a room for sleep. Keep light controls within residents' reach.

Problems with odors and inadequate ventilation can cause a person to have difficulty sleeping. Residents may be **incontinent** (unable to control the bladder or bowels, which leads to an involuntary loss of urine or feces) which can cause odors. Vomit and wound drainage can cause odors. Certain diseases cause odors as well. Body odors can be offensive, too. Ways to help with odors and ventilation include:

- Change incontinent briefs often.

- Keep equipment and supplies clean.

- Give personal care often to help avoid breath and body odors.

- Change soiled bed linens and clothing as soon as possible.

- Open a window to help eliminate odors.

- Housekeeping may have a spray deodorizer available for persistent odors.

Temperature problems can affect sleep. Some people will want the room to be cooler; others like a warmer temperature in which to sleep. Ways to help with temperature include:

- Help find a comfortable temperature for residents.

- Report to the nurse if the temperature is a problem.

- Layer clothing and bed covers for warmth.

Anxiety: **Anxiety** is uneasiness or fear, often about a situation or condition. The resident may be anxious about sleeping alone in a private room. He may have anxiety about sleeping in a new environment with a roommate. He may be worried about illness and a decline in independence. If the resident has lost a mate and/or friends and family, he may be sad. Ways to help with anxiety include:

- Sit with residents and listen if they want to talk.

- Use touch and soothing words.

- Offer to give a back rub.

Illness: Some illnesses or diseases cause chronic or occasional pain and discomfort. For example, arthritis can cause chronic pain in different areas of the body. Arthritis is a disease that refers to inflammation, or swelling, of the joints. It causes stiffness, pain, and decreased mobility. Ways to help with illness, pain, and discomfort include:

- Make sure residents are clean and comfortable before bed.

- Observe and report signs of pain promptly to the nurse. The nurse may give the resident medication or you may be asked to help by giving a back rub or a bath. Signs of pain and measures to reduce pain are found in Chapter 13.

Aging changes: Sleep patterns are different for elderly people than for younger people. They may sleep a similar number of hours, but those hours may be spread out over the 24-hour day. The elderly may take frequent naps during the day, which affects sleep at night. They take longer to fall asleep. Elderly people may get up more often during the night to go the bathroom and have a hard time falling asleep again. Hormonal changes can cause difficulty sleeping. A lack of regular, moderate exercise affects sleep as well. Ways to help with aging changes include:

- Assist residents to the bathroom just before bedtime.

- Honor fluid restrictions in the evening if they are ordered.

- Use music or reading to help the resident fall asleep.

- Provide naps as needed throughout the day.

- Encourage residents to exercise if it is in their care plan. Exercise often helps people sleep longer and more soundly.

- Encourage residents to wear day wear instead of night clothes during the day.

Dietary habits: Drinking or eating products with caffeine, such as soda or chocolate, can prevent sleep (Fig. 10-2). Eating heavy meals before bedtime can cause restlessness or discomfort. Sugar can cause a person to be excited and anxious. This can make it harder to fall asleep or can cause wakefulness during the night. Ways to help with dietary habits include:

Fig. 10-2. Caffeinated drinks, such as coffee or some teas, can prevent sleep.

- Limit caffeine intake.

- Avoid serving heavy meals.

- Serve meals earlier in the evening, not late at night.

Medications, alcohol, and cigarettes: Some medications cause wakefulness and interfere with sleep. For example, antihistamines can either cause the person to become very sleepy or to be unable to fall asleep. Antihistamines are medications used to treat allergic reactions or allergies. Alcoholic drinks, including beer and wine, are depressants and can cause problems with sleep (Fig. 10-3). A **depressant** is a substance that causes calmness and drowsiness. Smoking can also cause problems with sleeping. Nicotine, which is found in cigarettes, is a stimulant. A **stimulant** is a drug that increases or quickens actions of the body. Ways to help with medications, alcohol, and cigarettes include:

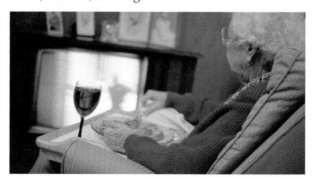

Fig. 10-3. Wine and other alcoholic beverages can prevent a person from sleeping well.

- The nurse or doctor will assess the resident's medications if a change in the sleep cycle occurs.

- Report if residents are not taking medications ordered for sleep.

- Report any evidence of unusual sleepiness or sudden inability to fall asleep.

- Discourage smoking and drinking alcohol before bedtime.

Not sleeping well can cause many problems, such as decreased mental function, reduced reaction time, decreased immune system function, and irritability. It is important to observe and report residents' complaints of lack of sleep.

A care conference may be planned to correct a resident's sleeping problems. Family members may participate. Offer any suggestions you have to help improve a resident's ability to sleep.

5. Describe a standard resident unit and equipment

Residents' units are their living spaces. They contain their beds, other furniture and personal items. These units must be kept clean and neat, while also honoring residents' personal choices. As you learned earlier, this room is the resident's home. You must always knock and wait for permission before entering.

Residents' belongings are very important to them. Treat their personal items with respect. Once personal items are in place within a room or unit, do not move them without the resident's permission. If a safety hazard exists, inform the nurse, and let him or her handle the situation.

Each unit may have slightly different equipment, because residents may bring furniture or other belongings from home. Personal items that bring the resident happiness should be encouraged. Resident rooms should be personal and home-like.

Standard unit equipment includes the following:

- Bed
- Bedside stand and possibly a dresser
- Overbed table
- Chair
- Bath basin
- Emesis basin
- Bedpan
- Urinal for males
- Water pitcher and cup
- Privacy screen or curtain
- Call light

The bedside stand is used for storing equipment like emesis basins, bath basins, urinals, and bedpans. Facility policy may require these items

to be placed in plastic bags to promote infection control. Soap, toothbrushes, toothpaste, combs and brushes, and other items may also be placed in the bedside stand but have to be kept separate from basins, urinals, and bedpans. Personal articles are usually in the top drawer. Basins are generally placed in the top shelf, and bedpans and urinals are in the lower shelf in the section underneath. A telephone and/or a radio, along with other personal items, may be placed on the top of the stand.

The overbed table may be used for residents' meals or personal care. It is a clean area and must be kept clean and free of clutter. Bedpans, urinals and soiled linen should not be placed on overbed tables because these tables are used for food (Fig. 10-4). Right before mealtime, clear these tables so that the meal tray may slide smoothly onto it. A water pitcher and cup are routinely kept on the overbed table.

Fig. 10-4. *Overbed tables are often used for residents' meals; they must be kept clean. Do not place bedpans, urinals, or soiled linens on overbed tables.*

RESIDENTS' RIGHTS

Making fun is not funny!
Making fun of any resident's personal items is inappropriate and cruel. Treat residents' belongings with respect.

6. Explain how to clean a resident unit and equipment

General care of the unit must be done whenever needed throughout the day. You should clean up spills promptly. Bedpans and urinals must be emptied and cleaned after securing residents.

Bed linens should be straightened before leaving the resident's room.

You will be taught how to use many different types of equipment. Make sure that you use and care for equipment properly. This prevents infection and injury.

There are many types of equipment that will be used one time and then thrown away. This is called "**disposable**" equipment. Some types of disposable equipment are cups, tissues, gloves, paper gowns, masks, disposable razors, and pads. Disposable equipment prevents the spread of microorganisms. Dispose of this equipment in the proper container. Wear gloves when using or disposing of some types of equipment, such as razors and pads.

Some equipment, such as urinals and bedpans, is cleaned after each use. You must wear gloves when handling this equipment. Follow facility policy on how to clean and disinfect these items.

Many facilities designate a person to clean equipment at the end of each shift. Equipment is cleaned using the proper disinfectant and heavy-duty gloves. The equipment is then placed in the proper area for clean items. If you are responsible for cleaning these items and notice damage to equipment, report it promptly to the nurse.

If equipment is to be re-used, it may need to be sterilized in the autoclave. Follow facility policy for this type of equipment. Do not use a piece of equipment on another resident if it has not been properly sterilized.

Guidelines
Resident's Unit

- Keep residents' units neat and clean. Clean the overbed table after use. Use a paper towel or cloth and facility-approved cleaning fluid. When cleaning, move the damp paper towel or cloth away from you so as to not wipe dirt or dust onto your uniform (Fig. 10-5). Place the table within the resident's reach before leaving.

- Keep the call light within the resident's reach. Make sure it is within reach before you leave the room. Report to the nurse immediately if the call light is not working.

- Straighten bed linens and remove crumbs from the bed after meals and before leaving.

- Re-stock all resident supplies daily, including facial tissues, bathroom tissue, paper towels, soap, or any other needed item. If this is not your responsibility, write out a supply order for the appropriate department to fill.

- If the bathroom needs cleaning, notify the housekeeping department. If the toilet, sink, or tub/shower are not working, report this promptly to the nurse or proper department.

- Check equipment daily to make sure it is working properly and not damaged in any way. Cords may be frayed or cracked; TVs or radios may not work. Report this immediately to the nurse or appropriate department.

- Refill water pitchers regularly unless resident has a fluid restriction. Promptly report to a nurse if a resident is not drinking fluids.

- Remove anything that might cause odors or safety hazards, like trash, clutter or spills. Dispose of any disposable supplies and trash. Clean up spills promptly. Empty trash often, following facility policy. Replace any equipment that is stained or has an odor.

- Report signs of insects or pests immediately.

- Leave residents' belongings where you find them. Do not throw away residents' personal items.

Fig. 10-5. *When cleaning an overbed table, move the cloth away from you so as to not wipe dirt or dust onto your uniform.*

After providing care, leave the unit neat and tidy. Put away equipment after properly cleaning and disinfecting it. Make sure the call light is within the resident's reach.

If you notice other equipment that is damaged, such as wheelchairs, IV poles, canes, crutches, or walkers, promptly report it. If you wait, a resident may become injured when using broken equipment.

Nursing assistants may be responsible for more thorough unit cleaning. When a resident is transferred, discharged, or dies, the unit will have to be completely cleaned and disinfected. Carefully follow facility policy when cleaning units. General guidelines for doing this type of thorough unit cleaning are listed below:

Guidelines

Unit Cleaning After Transfer, Discharge, or Death

- Wash your hands before doing unit cleaning.

- Wear gloves and the proper PPE as required by your facility.

- Remove and dispose of equipment and supplies carefully. These may include oxygen tubing, suction canisters, tissue boxes, water pitchers, and cups. Also remove towels, washcloths, and equipment that will be sent for cleaning. If you find any of the resident's personal items, take them to the new unit, or inform the nurse so that they can be sent to the resident or the family.

- Raise the bed to a safe working level, and remove soiled linen. Roll dirty linens away from you, watching for personal items. Wash all surfaces of the bed, including both sides of the mattress, with the facility-approved disinfectant. Allow to dry completely. Remove gloves, wash your hands, and then make a neat, wrinkle-free bed. See Learning Objective 7 for more information on bedmaking guidelines and the procedures for making a bed.

- Make sure the area is well-ventilated when using strong cleaning solutions. Clean all other unit items and equipment following facility policy. This may include items such as the telephone, TV and bed controls, bedside stand, overbed table, chairs, bathrooms, windows and window sills, and door handles.

- Write repair orders for any damaged or broken furniture.

- Remove all PPE and wash your hands.

- Place new equipment and supplies in the room for a new resident.

HOT TIP

Central Supply (CS) or Supply, Processing and Distribution (SPD)

The CS or SPD department is responsible for ordering, processing and delivering equipment to units and other departments in a facility. Residents usually bring items from home; however, they may need additional items that CS can obtain. If you are responsible for ordering new supplies, you will be trained in the proper procedure. Some facilities also train NAs on how to bill items for residents.

7. Discuss types of beds and demonstrate proper bedmaking

The resident's bed is a place in which he or she will spend a great deal of time. Neat, well-made beds help residents sleep better each night. In addition, careful bedmaking prevents infection. A clean, neat, dry bed helps prevent skin breakdown and odors and promotes good health and overall comfort. Skin breakdown and pressure sores are serious problems in long-term care facilities and are covered in detail in Chapter 18.

Many facilities have electric beds for residents. Electric beds have the ability to raise the head and the knee area (Fig. 10-6). Some electric beds have a safety lock that helps prevent the resident or visitor from accidentally moving the bed up or down.

BEDMAKING AND UNIT CARE

Fig. 10-6. *One type of electric bed.* (Photo courtesy of Invacare Continuing Care Group, 1-800-347-5440, www.invacare-ccg.com.)

The controls on electric beds vary. Generally, a person controls the electric bed by pressing buttons on a control panel. There will be a button to move the entire bed, one for the head of the bed, and another for the bottom of the bed (Fig. 10-7). There may also be controls for the bed to move into special doctor-ordered positions. These controls should only be used by the nurses. Residents and families will be taught to use the bed control on admission.

Fig. 10-7. *Controls for an electric bed.* (Photo courtesy of Invacare Continuing Care Group, 1-800-347-5440, www.invacare-ccg.com.)

Beds can be equipped with a variety of functions. Some beds have built-in weight scales. With these beds, bedridden residents do not have to be transferred to a scale to be weighed.

Some beds have special mattresses for residents who are at risk for pressure sores or who

have pressure sores. The mattresses are called alternating pressure mattresses. They are able to alternate the pressure inside the mattress so that one area of the body does not rest on a spot for too long. This type of mattress helps prevent pressure sores.

There are special beds for residents who weigh more than the average person. These beds are called bariatric beds. They are usually ordered for residents who weigh from 350 to 600 pounds. Special step stools help larger residents move from the bed to the floor. These stools are wider, longer and closer to the floor.

Some electric beds are able to be lowered very close to the floor, such as six or seven inches off of the floor. This makes it easier for residents to get out of bed and prevents unnecessary lifting by staff. This can also help reduce the risk of falling out of bed.

Beds should remain locked in their lowest positions whenever residents are in the beds. Special floor cushions, mats, or pads may be placed on the floor by the bed to protect residents if they should fall. If ordered by the doctor, special pads can also be placed inside the bed on both sides to prevent falls. These pads may be used with side rails.

Guidelines
Bedmaking

- Bed linens must be changed when they are wet, soiled or when they are too wrinkled for comfort. Residents can develop pressure sores when left in wet, wrinkled, or soiled linens. Make sure to remove and change disposable pads whenever they become soiled or wet (Fig. 10-8).

- Before getting clean linen, wash your hands. Always use proper infection control procedures. Wear gloves when removing soiled linens.

- Gather linen in order of placement on the bed. This means first pick up mattress pad, then all sheets, blankets, bedspreads, and pillowcases.

- Carry clean linen away from your uniform. If it touches your uniform, the linen becomes contaminated (Fig. 10-9).

- Bring linen into one resident's room at a time. Put it down after flipping the stack of linen so that the first item to be placed on the bed (mattress pad) is now on the top of the stack.

- Never pick up linen from one room and transfer it to another room.

- Place clean linen on a facility-approved spot, such as a chair, overbed table, or bedside stand. Do not place clean linen on the floor or on a contaminated area.

- Look at linens closely for any personal items, such as dentures, hearing aids and batteries, glasses, rings, watches, and money, before removing them.

- Roll dirty linen away from you as you remove it from the bed. Rolling puts the dirtiest surface of the linen inward, which lessens contamination.

- Do not shake linen because it may spread air-borne contaminants.

- Place used linen into proper container. Do not place used linen on the floor or on any piece of furniture in the room.

- Use proper body mechanics when making beds. Bend your knees, use a good stance, and raise the bed height to a safe working level.

- To save energy, make one side of the bed first. Then go to the other side of the bed to complete bedmaking.

- Keep beds wrinkle-free and free of all crumbs. Remove lumps of any kind in the bed, such as from pads, etc. If a lumpy mattress cannot be smoothed out, inform the nurse. Lumps, crumbs, and wrinkles increase the risk of pressure sores.

- Wash your hands after handling linen.

Fig. 10-8. *One type of absorbent pad.*

Fig. 10-9. *Carry clean linen away from your uniform.*

RESIDENTS' RIGHTS

Give prompt, compassionate care.
Some residents will unintentionally soil or wet the bed. Change the sheets, along with all clothing and pads, immediately when this happens. Do so with compassion and respect. Act professionally. Do not draw attention to the resident or tell other residents what happened. Clean the resident and make him feel comfortable again. When residents are left in soiled beds, it may be considered physical and emotional abuse, as well as neglect.

There are four basic types of beds: closed, open, occupied, and surgical (also called postoperative, post-op, recovery, gurney, or stretcher bed). A **closed bed** is usually made for a resident who will be out of bed all day. It is a bed completely made with the bedspread, blankets and pillows in place. A closed bed is turned into an **open bed** by folding the linen down to the foot of the bed. This makes it easier for a resident to get into the bed in the afternoon for a nap or at bedtime. You will also open a bed when a new resident has been assigned to that room.

Making a closed bed

Equipment: mattress pad (if used), fitted or flat bottom sheet, waterproof bed protector if needed, blanket(s), cotton **draw sheet***, flat top sheet, bedspread (if used), pillowcases, gloves*

1. Wash your hands.

2. Gather linen. Transport linen correctly.

3. If resident is in the room, identify yourself by name. Identify the resident. Greet the resident by name.

4. Explain procedure to the resident. Speak clearly, slowly, and directly. Maintain face-to-face contact whenever possible.

5. Using facility-approved barrier, place clean linen on clean surface within reach (e.g. bedside stand, overbed table, or chair).

6. Adjust bed to safe working level, usually waist high. Put bed in flattest position.

7. Apply gloves.

8. Loosen soiled linen and roll soiled linen (soiled side inside) from head to foot of bed. Avoid contact with your skin or clothes. Place it in a hamper or linen bag. Do not place on overbed table, chair, or floor.

9. Remove and dispose of gloves properly. Wash your hands.

10. Remake the bed. Place the mattress pad (if used) on the bed, attaching elastic at corners as necessary.

11. Place bottom sheet on bed without shaking linen. If using a flat sheet with seams, this sheet must be placed with the crease in the center of the mattress. The seams on both ends must be placed down. If using a fitted bottom sheet, place right-side up and tightly pull over all four corners of the bed.

12. Make hospital, or mitered, corners to keep bottom sheet wrinkle-free (Fig. 10-10).

Fig. 10-10. Hospital corners help keep the sheet smooth under the resident.

13. Put on waterproof bed protector and then the draw sheet, if used. Place them in the center of the bed on the bottom sheet. Smooth, and tightly tuck the bottom sheet and draw sheet together under sides of bed. Move from the head of the bed to the foot of the bed.

14. Place the top sheet over the bed and center it. The seam must be up.

15. Place blanket over the bed and center it.

16. Place the bedspread over the bed and center it.

17. Tuck top sheet, blanket, and bedspread under the foot of the bed and make hospital corners.

18. Fold down the top sheet to make a cuff of about six inches over the blanket and bedspread.

19. Take a pillow, and with one hand, grasp the clean pillowcase at the closed end. Turn it inside out over your arm. Next, using the hand that has the pillowcase over it, grasp the center of the end of the pillow. Pull the pillowcase over it with your free hand (Fig. 10-11). Do the same for any other pillows. Place them at the head of the bed with open end away from the door. Make sure zippers or tags are on the inside.

Fig. 10-11.

20. Return bed to low position if raised.

21. Dispose of soiled linen in proper container.

22. Leave call light within resident's reach.

23. Wash your hands.

24. Document procedure using facility guidelines.

HOT TIP

Seams and the Skin
Residents' skin may be very fragile. Seams rubbing against an elderly person's skin can cause the skin to tear or crack. Remember to follow these rules for placing linens properly on beds:
BOTTOM SHEET: Seam DOWN = Bottom-DOWN
TOP SHEET: Seam UP = Top-UP

Making an open bed

Equipment: mattress pad (if used), fitted or flat bottom sheet, waterproof bed protector if needed, blanket(s), cotton draw sheet, flat top sheet, bedspread (if used), pillowcases, gloves

1. Wash your hands.

2. Make a closed bed, as described in previous procedure.

3. Stand at the head of the bed. Grasp the top sheet, blanket, and bedspread and fold them down to the foot of the bed. Then bring them back up the bed to form a large cuff.

4. Bring the cuff on the top linens to a point where it is one hands-width above the linen underneath. This way, when the resident gets into bed, he will not pull all the linen out at the foot of the bed.

5. Make sure all linen is wrinkle-free.

6. Wash your hands.

7. Document procedure using facility guidelines.

An **occupied bed** is a bed made while the resident is in the bed. A resident may have a doctor's order to stay in bed at all times. These orders are called "absolute bedrest (ABR)," "strict bedrest," or "complete bedrest (CBR)." This type of bed may be completed more safely working with a co-worker. Remember to lock the bed wheels, and bend your knees while making the bed. Raise the height of the bed to a safe working level.

An **unoccupied bed** is a bed made while no resident is in the bed. If the resident can be safely moved out of bed, making the bed will be easier.

Making an occupied bed gives you an opportunity to observe a resident's skin for signs of breakdown. Bed-bound residents are at great risk for pressure sores.

RESIDENTS' RIGHTS

Side Rails
The use of side rails has become uncommon because they are considered restraints and can put residents at risk for injury. If side rail use is ordered by a doctor, they must be raised and lowered for resident care. Only one side rail should be lowered on the working side of the bed when one person is giving care. If care is being given by two caregivers, both side rails may be lowered as long as both caregivers stay at the bedside. They must be raised when care is completed before all caregivers leave the resident's bedside.

Making an occupied bed

Equipment: mattress pad (if used), fitted or flat bottom sheet, waterproof bed protector if needed, blanket(s), cotton draw sheet, flat top sheet, bedspread (if used), bath blanket, pillowcases, gloves

1. Wash your hands.

2. Gather linen. Transport linen correctly.

3. Identify yourself by name. Identify the resident. Greet the resident by name.

4. Explain procedure to the resident. Speak clearly, slowly, and directly. Maintain face-to-face contact whenever possible. Encourage resident to assist if possible.

5. Using facility-approved barrier, place clean linen on clean surface within reach (e.g. bedside stand, overbed table, or chair).

6. Provide for the resident's privacy with a curtain, screen, or door.

7. Put on gloves.

8. Avoid trauma or pain to the resident throughout the procedure.

9. Loosen top linen from the end of the bed on the working side.

10. Unfold the bath blanket over the top sheet and remove the top sheet. Keep resident covered at all times with the bath blanket.

11. Practice good body mechanics. Adjust bed to safe working level, usually waist high. Lower head of bed. Lock bed wheels.

12. You will make the bed one side at a time. Raise side rail (if bed has them) on far side of bed. After raising side rail, go to the other side of the bed. Lower side rail on the working side. Help resident to turn onto his side slowly, moving away from you toward raised side rail (see Procedure: Turning a Resident in Chapter 11) (Fig. 10-12).

13. Loosen bottom soiled linen on working side.

14. Roll bottom soiled linen toward resident and center of bed, soiled side inside. Tuck it snugly against resident's back.

Fig. 10-12.

15. Place the mattress pad (if used) on the bed attaching elastic at corners on working side.

16. Place clean bottom linen or fitted bottom sheet with the center crease in the center. If flat sheet is used, tuck in at top and on working side. Make hospital corners to keep bottom sheet wrinkle-free. If fitted sheet is used, tightly pull two fitted corners on working side.

17. Smooth the bottom sheet out toward the resident. Be sure there are no wrinkles in the mattress pad. Roll the extra material toward the resident. Tuck it under the resident's body (Fig. 10-13).

Fig. 10-13.

18. If using a waterproof bed protector, unfold it and center it on the bed. Smooth it out toward the resident.

19. If using a draw sheet, place it on the bed. Tuck in on your side, smooth, and tuck as you did with the other bedding.

20. Raise side rail nearest you. Go to the other side of the bed. Lower side rail on the working side. Help resident roll or turn onto clean bottom sheet (Fig. 10-14). Explain that he will be moving over a roll of linen.

Fig. 10-14.

21. Loosen soiled linen. Look for personal items. Roll linen from head to foot of bed, avoiding contact with your skin or clothes. Do not shake soiled linen. Place it in a hamper or linen bag. Do not place on overbed table, chair, or floor.

22. Pull the clean linen through as quickly as possible. Start with the mattress pad and wrap around corners. Pull and tuck in clean bottom linen, just like the other side. Pull and tuck in waterproof bed protector and draw sheet, if used. Make hospital corners with bottom sheet. Finish with bottom sheet free of wrinkles.

23. Place resident on his back. Keep resident covered and comfortable, with a pillow under his head.

24. Unfold the top sheet. Place it over the resident and center it. Ask the resident to hold the top sheet and slip the bath blanket out from underneath (Fig. 10-15). Put in the hamper/bag.

Fig. 10-15.

25. Place the blanket over the top sheet and center it. Place the bedspread over the blanket and center it. Tuck the top sheet, blanket and bedspread under the foot of the bed and make hospital corners on each side. Loosen the top linens over the resident's feet.

26. At the top of the bed, fold down the top sheet to make a cuff of about six inches over the blanket and bedspread.

27. Gently hold and lift resident's head and remove pillow. Do not hold it near your face. Remove the soiled pillowcase by turning it inside out. Place it in the hamper/bag.

28. With one hand, grasp the clean pillowcase at the closed end. Turn it inside out over your arm. Next, using the hand that has the pillowcase over it, grasp the center of the end of the pillow. Pull the pillowcase over it with your free hand. Do the same for any other pillows. Place them gently under resident's head with open end away from the door. Make sure zippers or tags are on the inside.

29. Make sure bed is wrinkle-free. Make resident comfortable.

30. Return bed to low position if raised. Ensure resident's safety. Return side rails to ordered position. Remove privacy measures.

31. Leave call light within resident's reach.

32. Dispose of soiled linen in proper container.

33. Remove and dispose of gloves properly.

34. Wash your hands.

35. Be courteous and respectful at all times.

36. Report any changes in the resident to the nurse. Document procedure using facility guidelines.

A **surgical bed** is made so that it can easily accept residents who must return to bed on stretchers or gurneys. Residents on stretchers are usually returning from treatment or hospital visits. Use caution when transferring residents from stretchers to beds. The bed and stretcher wheels must be locked, and the bed and stretcher must be close together during the transfer.

Discuss the preparation for the arrival of a resident on a stretcher with the nurse. When preparing the room, you may need to set up equipment in the room. Check with the nurse for instructions on gathering any extra equipment/supplies.

Making a surgical bed

Equipment: clean linen (see Procedure: Making a closed bed), gloves

1. Wash your hands.

2. Gather linen. Transport linen correctly.

3. Using facility-approved barrier, place clean linen on clean surface within reach (e.g. bedside stand, overbed table, or chair).

4. Adjust bed to safe working level, usually waist high. Lock bed wheels.

5. Apply gloves.

6. Remove all soiled linen, rolling it (soiled side inside) from head to foot of bed. Avoid contact with your skin or clothes. Place it in a hamper or linen bag.

7. Remove and dispose of gloves properly.

8. Wash your hands.

9. Make a closed bed. Do not tuck top linens under the mattress.

10. Fold top linens down from the head of the bed and up from the foot of the bed (Fig. 10-16).

Fig. 10-16.

11. Form a triangle with the linen. Fanfold the linen triangle into pleated layers and position opposite the stretcher side of the bed (Fig. 10-17). Fanfolding means folding several times into pleats. After fanfolding, form a tiny tip with the end of the linen triangle. The tip can be grasped quickly and pulled over the returning resident. This step quickly provides much-needed warmth to the resident.

Fig. 10-17.

12. Put on clean pillowcases. Place the clean pillows on a clean surface off the bed, such as on the bedside stand or chair.

13. Leave bed in its highest position. Leave both side rails down.

14. Move all furniture to make room for the stretcher.

15. Do not place call light on bed. That is placed after the resident returns to bed.

16. Dispose of soiled linen in the proper container.

17. Wash your hands.

18. Document procedure using facility guidelines.

CHAPTER REVIEW

1. List three functions that sleep performs (LO 2).

2. List six reasons that residents can develop parasomnias (LO 3).

3. List five factors that can affect a resident's ability to sleep. For each item listed, describe one thing that can be done to help promote better sleep (LO 4).

4. What is usually stored in the bedside stand (LO 5)?

5. What is the overbed table used for? Can a bedpan be placed on it (LO 5)?

6. Where should the call light always be placed (LO 6)?

7. Define disposable equipment (LO 6).

8. List three ways that careful bedmaking and clean, neat, and dry beds help residents (LO 7).

9. Why is it important that linen always be changed when it is wet, damp, wrinkled, or soiled (LO 7)?

10. Why should nursing assistants carry clean linen away from their uniforms (LO 7)?

11. Why should linen never be shaken (LO 7)?

12. Describe the difference between a closed bed and an open bed (LO 7).

13. While making an occupied bed, what should be observed by a nursing assistant (LO 7)?

14. When is a surgical bed made (LO 7)?

11
Positioning, Moving, and Lifting

A View from the Past: "Falling into Life"

"Having lost the use of my legs during the polio epidemic that swept across the eastern United States during the summer of 1944, I was soon immersed in a process of rehabilitation that was . . . as much spiritual as physical. That was a full decade before the discovery of the Salk vaccine ended polio's reign as the disease most dreaded by America's parents and their children. Treatment of the disease had been standardized by 1944: following the initial onslaught of the virus, patients were kept in isolation for a period of ten days to two weeks. Following that, orthodox medical opinion was content to subject patients to as much heat as they could stand. Stiff paralyzed limbs were swathed in heated, coarse woolen towels known as 'hot packs.' As soon as the hot packs had baked enough pain and stiffness out of a patient's body so that he could be moved on and off a stretcher, the treatment was ended, and the patient faced a series of daily immersions in a heated pool. I would ultimately spend two full years at the appropriately named New York State Reconstruction Home . . . . We would learn during our days in the New York State Reconstruction Home to confront the world that was . . . . My future had arrived."

Leonard Kriegel

"Take her up tenderly/Lift her with care..."

Thomas Hood, 1798-1845

1. Define important words in this chapter

ambulation: walking.

body alignment: body positioning that promotes proper body functioning; posture.

dangling: position with the resident sitting up with the feet over the side of the bed to regain balance, equalize blood flow in the body, and return blood flow to the head; helps prevent dizziness and lightheadedness that can cause fainting.

draw sheet: turning sheet that is placed under residents who are unable to assist with turning, lifting, or moving up in bed.

ergonomics: the science of designing equipment and setting up areas to make them safer and to suit the worker's abilities.

Fowler's: position with the person lying on his or her back with the head of bed elevated about 45 to 60 degrees.

gait belt: a belt made of canvas or other heavy material used to help residents walk; also called a transfer belt.

lateral: position with person on his or her side.

logrolling: moving a person as a unit, without disturbing the alignment of the body.

mechanical lift: special equipment used to lift and move or lift and weigh a person.

MSDs: acronym that stands for work-related musculoskeletal disorders.

positioning: helping people into positions that will be comfortable and healthy for them.

prone: position with person lying on his or her stomach.

shearing: rubbing or friction resulting from the skin moving one way and the bone underneath it remaining fixed or moving in the opposite direction.

Sims': position with person lying on his or her left side with one leg drawn up.

supine: position with person lying flat on his or her back.

transfer: moving a resident from one place to another.

transfer belt: a belt made of canvas or other heavy material used to assist residents who are weak, unsteady, or uncoordinated; also called a gait belt.

2. Explain body alignment and review the principles of body mechanics

The positioning of the body plays an important part in the proper functioning of the body. **Body alignment** is also known as posture. Good body alignment helps the body achieve balance without causing muscle or joint strain. In addition, good body alignment allows the body to function at its highest level. The lungs are able to expand and contract, blood circulation is more efficient, digestion is easier, and the kidneys are able to better cleanse the body of wastes. Also, good body alignment helps prevent complications of immobility, such as contractures and atrophy. Contractures are the permanent and often painful stiffening of a joint and muscle. Atrophy is the weakening or wasting of muscles.

You first learned about body mechanics in Chapter 7. When you do not move and position residents using good body mechanics, you and residents can be injured. These ten guidelines will help you remember to use proper body mechanics:

1. **Assess the load.** Before lifting, assess the weight of the load to determine if you can safely move the object without help. Know the lift policies at your facility. Never attempt to lift someone you are not sure you can lift.

2. **Think ahead, plan, and communicate the move.** Check for any objects in your path or any potential risks, such as a wet floor. Make sure the path is clear. Watch for hazards, like high-traffic areas, combative residents, or a loose toilet seat. Decide exactly what you are going to do together and agree on the verbal cues you will use before attempting to **transfer**, or move the resident from one place to another.

3. **Check your base of support and be sure you have firm footing.** Use a wide but balanced stance to increase support, and keep this stance when walking. Have enough room to maintain a wide base of support. Make sure you and the resident are wearing non-skid shoes with the laces tied.

4. **Face what you are lifting.** Your feet should always face the direction you are moving. This enables you to move your body as one unit and keeps your back straight. Twisting at the waist increases the likelihood of injury.

5. **Keep your back straight.** Keeping your head up and shoulders back will keep the back in the proper position. Take a deep breath to help you regain correct posture.

6. **Begin in a squatting position, and lift with your legs.** Bend at the hips and knees and use the strength of your leg muscles to stand and lift the object (Fig. 11-1). You will need to push your buttocks out to accomplish this. Before you stand with the object you are lifting, remember that your legs, not your back, will enable you to lift. You should be able to feel your leg muscles as they work. Lift with the large leg muscles to decrease stress on the back.

7. **Tighten your stomach muscles when beginning the lift.** This will help to take weight off the spine and maintain alignment.

8. **Keep the object close to your body.** This decreases stress to your back. Lift objects to your waist. Carrying them any higher can affect your balance (Fig. 11-2).

9. **Do not twist.** Turn and face the area you are moving the object to and then set the object down. Twisting increases the stress on your back and should always be avoided.

10. **Push or pull when possible rather than lifting.** When you lift an object, you must

overcome gravity to balance the load. When you push or pull an object, you only need to overcome the friction between the surface and the object. Use your body weight to move the object, rather than your lifting muscles. Push rather than pull whenever possible. Stay close to the object. Use both arms and tighten your stomach muscles.

Fig. 11-1. To lift an object, you will bend your knees slightly and lift with your legs.

Fig. 11-2. Keeping objects close while carrying them decreases stress on your back.

RESIDENTS' RIGHTS

Safety, not speed!
Repositioning residents can be challenging. The simple act of turning a resident may break a bone, tear fragile skin, or pull on tubing. Be very careful when moving and positioning residents. Moving too quickly can cause serious injury and potential complications. Moving residents in a hasty or rough manner is abusive behavior.

3. Explain why position changes are important for bedbound residents and describe basic body positions

Residents who are bedbound or who spend a lot of time in bed often need help getting into comfortable positions. They also need to change positions periodically. Residents need to be turned often so that pressure on skin surfaces alternates from one side to the other. Too much pressure on one area for too long can cause a decrease in circulation. This increases the risk of pressure sores and other problems like muscle contractures. Constant pressure causes the greatest risk of pressure sores, a major problem in long-term care. To try to prevent these sores from occurring, many facilities have established turning schedules. You will learn much more about pressure sores and prevention in Chapters 12 and 18.

Positioning means helping residents into positions that promote comfort and good health. You will position bedbound residents at least every two hours. Follow posted turn schedules and care plans carefully. You may have several residents who require frequent turning. Every time you position a resident, you must document the position and time. When positioning residents, use proper body mechanics to help prevent injury. Check the resident's skin for whiteness, redness, or warm spots, especially around bony areas, each time you reposition a resident.

You first learned about body positions in Chapter 9. Here are five basic body positions you may use for residents:

1. **Supine**: In this position, the resident lies flat on his back. To maintain correct body position, support the head and shoulders with a pillow (Fig. 11-3). You may also use pillows, rolled towels, or washcloths to support his arms (especially a weak or immobilized arm) or hands. The heels need to be raised so they do not touch the bed. Place a pillow under the calves. Use footboards, padded boards placed against the resident's feet to keep them positioned properly, as needed.

2. **Lateral**/Side: A resident in the lateral position is lying on either side (Fig. 11-4). There are many ways to do this. Pillows can support the arm and leg on the upper side, the back, and the head. Ideally, the knee on the upper side of the body should be flexed. The leg is brought in front of the body and supported on a pillow. There should be a pillow under the bottom foot, and the toes should not touch the bed. If the top leg cannot be brought forward, it should be placed slightly behind the bottom leg, never resting directly on it. Pillows should be used between the two legs to help relieve pressure and avoid skin breakdown.

3. **Prone**: A resident in the prone position is lying on the abdomen, or front side of the body (Fig. 11-5). This is not comfortable for many people, especially elderly people. Never leave a resident in a prone position for very long. In this position, the arms are either placed at the sides, raised above the head, or one raised and one by the side. The head is turned to one side. A small pillow may be used under the head and under the legs. This keeps the feet from touching the bed.

4. **Fowler's**: A resident in the Fowler's position is in a partially-reclined sitting position (45 to 60 degrees) (Fig. 11-6). The head and shoulders are elevated and the resident's knees may be flexed and elevated. Use a pillow or rolled blanket as a support. The feet may be supported using a footboard or other support. The spine should be straight. In a high-Fowler's position, the upper body is sitting nearly straight up (between 65 and 90 degrees). In a semi-Fowler's position, the upper body is not raised as high (30 to 40 degrees).

5. **Sims'**: The Sims' position is a left side-lying position (Fig. 11-7). The lower arm is behind the back. The upper knee is flexed and raised toward the chest, using a pillow as support.

There should be a pillow under the bottom foot so that the toes do not touch the bed.

Fig. 11-3. *A person in the supine position is lying flat on her back.*

Fig. 11-4. *A person in the lateral position is lying on his side.*

Fig. 11-5. *A person lying in the prone position is lying on his abdomen.*

Fig. 11-6. *A person lying in the Fowler's position is partially reclined.*

Fig. 11-7. *A person in the Sims' position is lying on his left side with one leg drawn up.*

The Trendelenburg and Reverse Trendelenburg positions are used with residents who have special needs. For example, Trendelenburg may be used for a resident who has gone into shock and

POSITIONING, MOVING, AND LIFTING

has poor blood flow (Fig. 11-8). Reverse Trendelenburg may be used for a resident who needs a faster emptying of the stomach due to a digestive problem (Fig. 11-9). These positions always require a doctor's order. Some electric beds have buttons or levers that place the bed in these two positions.

Fig. 11-8. The Trendelenburg position. This position is only used with a doctor's order.

Fig. 11-9. The Reverse Trendelenburg position. This position is only used with a doctor's order.

Many positioning devices are available to help make residents more comfortable and safe in different body positions. See Chapter 25 for a list of these devices.

RESIDENTS' RIGHTS

Communicate.

Any time you assist a resident, discuss with them what you would like to do. Promote their independence by allowing them to do what they can. The two of you must work together, especially during transfers!

Locking arms with a resident and raising head and shoulders

1. Identify yourself by name. Identify the resident. Greet the resident by name.

2. Wash your hands.

3. Explain procedure to resident. Speak clearly, slowly, and directly. Maintain face-to-face contact whenever possible. Encourage resident to assist if possible.

4. Provide for the resident's privacy with a curtain, screen, or door.

5. Practice good body mechanics. Adjust the bed to a safe level, usually waist high. Lock the bed wheels.

6. Place pillow at the head of bed against the headboard.

7. Lower the side rail (if bed has one and if it is not already lowered) on side nearest you.

8. Stand at the side of the bed and face the head of bed.

9. Spread feet shoulder-width apart and slightly bend the knees to protect your back.

10. Avoid trauma or pain to the resident throughout the procedure.

11. Gently slide one hand under the resident's closest shoulder.

12. Gently slide the other hand under the resident's upper back.

13. At the count of three, slowly raise the resident's head and shoulders. Give necessary care (Fig. 11-10).

Fig. 11-10.

14. Replace pillow under the resident's head.

15. Make resident comfortable.

16. Return bed to low position if raised. Ensure resident's safety. Return side rails to ordered position. Remove privacy measures.

17. Leave call light within resident's reach.

18. Wash your hands.

19. Be courteous and respectful at all times.

20. Report any changes in the resident to the nurse. Document procedure using facility guidelines.

Use draw sheets under residents who cannot help with turning, lifting, or moving up in bed. A **draw sheet**, or turning sheet, is an extra sheet placed on top of the bottom sheet (Fig. 11-11). Draw sheets help prevent skin damage caused by shearing. **Shearing** is rubbing or friction resulting from the skin moving one way and the bone underneath it remaining fixed or moving in the opposite direction.

Fig. 11-11. A draw sheet is a special sheet (or a regular bed sheet folded in half) used to move residents in bed without causing shearing.

Assisting a resident to move up in bed

1. Identify yourself by name. Identify the resident. Greet the resident by name.

2. Wash your hands.

3. Explain procedure to resident. Speak clearly, slowly, and directly. Maintain face-to-face contact whenever possible. Encourage resident to assist if possible.

4. Provide for the resident's privacy with a curtain, screen, or door.

5. Practice good body mechanics. Adjust the bed to a safe level, usually waist high. Lock the bed wheels.

6. Lower the head of bed. Move the pillow to the head of bed.

7. Lower the side rail (if bed has one and if it is not already lowered) on side nearest you.

8. Stand by bed with feet shoulder-width apart. Face the resident. Point foot closest to the head of the bed towards the head of the bed.

9. Avoid trauma or pain to the resident throughout the procedure.

10. Place one arm under the resident's shoulder blades. Place the other arm under the resident's thighs.

11. Ask resident to bend knees, brace feet on the mattress, and push feet on the count of three.

12. Keep your back straight. At the count of three, shift body weight to move resident while resident pushes with her feet (Fig. 11-12).

Fig. 11-12. Keep your back straight and your knees bent.

13. Replace pillow under the resident's head.

14. Make resident comfortable.

15. Return bed to low position if raised. Ensure resident's safety. Return side rails to ordered position. Remove privacy measures.

16. Leave call light within resident's reach.

17. Wash your hands.

18. Be courteous and respectful at all times.

19. Report any changes in the resident to the nurse. Document procedure using facility guidelines.

Ask a co-worker to help you move residents if one is available. Always get help if you feel it is not safe to move the resident by yourself.

Assisting a resident to move up in bed with assistance (using draw sheet)

Equipment: draw sheet

1. Identify yourself by name. Identify the resident. Greet the resident by name.

2. Wash your hands.

3. Explain procedure to resident. Speak clearly, slowly, and directly. Maintain face-to-face contact whenever possible. Encourage resident to assist if possible.

4. Provide for the resident's privacy with a curtain, screen, or door.

5. Practice good body mechanics. Adjust the bed to a safe level, usually waist high. Lock the bed wheels.

6. Lower the head of bed. Move the pillow to the head of bed.

7. Lower the side rail (if bed has one and if it is not already lowered) on side nearest you.

8. Stand on the opposite side of the bed from your helper. Each of you should be turned slightly toward the head of the bed. For each of you, the foot that is closest to the head of the bed should be pointed in that direction. Stand with feet about 12 inches apart. Bend your knees. Keep your back straight.

9. Avoid trauma or pain to the resident throughout the procedure.

10. Roll the draw sheet up to the resident's side. Have your helper do the same on his side of the bed. Grasp the sheet with your palms up at the resident's shoulders and hips. Have your helper do the same.

11. Shift your weight to your back foot (the foot closer to the foot of the bed). Have your helper do the same (Fig. 11-13). On the count of three, both shift your weight to your forward feet. Slide the resident toward the head of the bed (Fig. 11-14).

Fig. 11-13. *Both workers shift their weight to their back feet and prepare to move.*

Fig. 11-14. *On the count of three, both workers shift their weight to their forward feet and slide the resident toward the head of the bed.*

12. Replace pillow under the resident's head.

13. Make resident comfortable. Unroll the draw sheet. Leave it in place for the next repositioning.

14. Return bed to low position if raised. Ensure resident's safety. Return side rails to ordered position. Remove privacy measures.

15. Leave call light within resident's reach.

16. Wash your hands.

17. Be courteous and respectful at all times.

18. Report any changes in the resident to the nurse. Document procedure using facility guidelines.

Moving a resident to the side of the bed

1. Identify yourself by name. Identify the resident. Greet the resident by name.

2. Wash your hands.

3. Explain procedure to resident. Speak clearly, slowly, and directly. Maintain face-to-face contact whenever possible. Encourage resident to assist if possible.

4. Provide for the resident's privacy with a curtain, screen, or door.

5. Practice good body mechanics. Adjust the bed to a safe level, usually waist high. Lock the bed wheels.

6. Lower the head of bed. Move the pillow to the head of bed.

7. Stand on one side of the bed. Lower the side rail (if bed has one and if it is not already lowered) on side nearest you.

8. Stand with feet about 12 inches apart. Bend your knees. Keep your back straight.

9. Avoid trauma or pain to the resident throughout the procedure.

10. Gently slide your hands under the resident's head and shoulders and move toward you (Fig. 11-15).

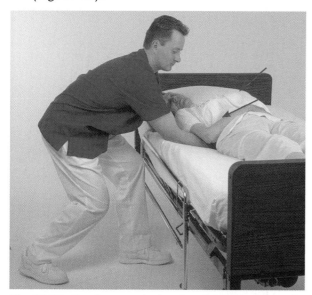

Fig. 11-15. *Gently move the head and shoulders toward you.*

11. Gently slide your hands under the resident's midsection and move toward you.

12. Gently slide your hands under the resident's hips and legs and move toward you (Fig. 11-16).

Fig. 11-16. *Gently move the hips and legs toward you.*

13. Make resident comfortable. Reposition pillow under head.

14. Return bed to low position if raised. Ensure resident's safety. Return side rails to ordered position. Remove privacy measures.

15. Leave call light within resident's reach.

16. Wash your hands.

17. Be courteous and respectful at all times.

18. Report any changes in the resident to the nurse. Document procedure using facility guidelines.

Moving a resident to the side of the bed with assistance (using draw sheet)

Equipment: draw sheet

1. Identify yourself by name. Identify the resident. Greet the resident by name.

2. Wash your hands.

3. Explain procedure to resident. Speak clearly, slowly, and directly. Maintain face-to-face contact whenever possible. Encourage resident to assist if possible.

4. Provide for the resident's privacy with a curtain, screen, or door.

5. Practice good body mechanics. Adjust the bed to a safe level, usually waist high. Lock the bed wheels.

6. Lower the head of bed. Move the pillow to the head of bed.

7. Stand on the opposite side of the bed from your helper. Each of you should be facing each other. Lower both side rails (if bed has them). Stand up straight facing the side of the bed with feet about 12 inches apart. Point feet toward the side of the bed. Bend your knees.

8. Avoid trauma or pain to the resident throughout the procedure.

9. Roll the draw sheet up to the resident's side. Have your helper do the same on his side of the bed. Grasp the sheet with your palms up at the resident's shoulders and hips. Have your helper do the same (Fig. 11-17).

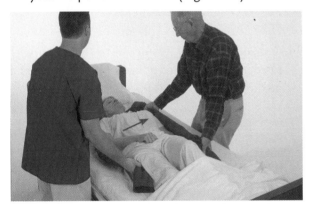

Fig. 11-17. Both workers grasp the draw sheet at the resident's shoulders and hips and prepare to move.

10. On the count of three, slide the resident toward the side of the bed. Your weight should be equal on each foot because you are moving the person to the side of the bed, not the head of the bed.

11. Make resident comfortable. Unroll the draw sheet. Leave it in place for the next repositioning. Reposition pillow under head.

12. Return bed to low position if raised. Ensure resident's safety. Return side rails to ordered position. Remove privacy measures.

13. Leave call light within resident's reach.

14. Wash your hands.

15. Be courteous and respectful at all times.

16. Report any changes in the resident to the nurse. Document procedure using facility guidelines.

Turning a resident away from you

1. Identify yourself by name. Identify the resident. Greet the resident by name.

2. Wash your hands.

3. Explain procedure to resident. Speak clearly, slowly, and directly. Maintain face-to-face contact whenever possible. Encourage resident to assist if possible.

4. Provide for the resident's privacy with a curtain, screen, or door.

5. Practice good body mechanics. Adjust the bed to a safe level, usually waist high. Lock the bed wheels.

6. Lower the head of bed.

7. Stand on side of bed opposite to where person will be turned. The far side rail should be raised (if bed has one).

8. Lower side rail nearest you if it is up.

9. Avoid trauma or pain to the resident throughout the procedure.

10. Move resident to side of bed nearest you using previous procedure.

11. Cross resident's arm over his or her chest. Move arm out of the way on side toward which resident is being turned. Cross leg nearest you over the far leg (Fig. 11-18).

Fig. 11-18. Cross leg nearest you over the far leg.

12. Stand with feet about 12 inches apart. Bend your knees.

13. Place one hand on the resident's shoulder. Place the other hand on the resident's nearest hip.

14. While supporting the body, gently push resident toward other side of bed. Shift your weight from your back leg to your front leg (Fig. 11-19). Make sure resident's face is not covered by the pillow.

Fig. 11-19. *Gently push resident toward other side of bed while shifting your weight from your back leg to your front leg.*

15. Position resident properly in good alignment:

- head supported by pillow

- shoulder adjusted so resident is not lying on arm

- top arm supported by pillow

- back supported by supportive device

- hips properly aligned

- top knee flexed

- supportive device between legs with top knee flexed; knee and ankle supported

16. Cover resident with top linens and straighten. Make resident comfortable.

17. Return bed to low position if raised. Ensure resident's safety. Return side rails to ordered position. Remove privacy measures.

18. Leave call light within resident's reach.

19. Wash your hands.

20. Be courteous and respectful at all times.

21. Report any changes in the resident to the nurse. Document procedure using facility guidelines.

Turning a resident toward you

1. Identify yourself by name. Identify the resident. Greet the resident by name.

2. Wash your hands.

3. Explain procedure to resident. Speak clearly, slowly, and directly. Maintain face-to-face contact whenever possible. Encourage resident to assist if possible.

4. Provide for the resident's privacy with a curtain, screen, or door.

5. Practice good body mechanics. Adjust the bed to a safe level, usually waist high. Lock the bed wheels.

6. Lower the head of bed.

7. Stand on side of bed opposite to where person will be turned. The far side rail should be raised (if bed has one).

8. Lower side rail nearest you if it is up.

9. Avoid trauma or pain to the resident throughout the procedure.

10. Move resident to side of bed nearest you using previous procedure. Put side rail up and go to the opposite side of the bed. Lower the side rail.

11. Cross resident's arm over his or her chest. Move arm out of the way on side toward which resident is being turned. Cross leg furthest from you over the near leg.

12. Stand with feet about 12 inches apart. Bend your knees.

13. Place one hand on the resident's far shoulder. Place the other hand on the resident's far hip.

14. While supporting the body, gently roll the resident toward you (Fig. 11-20). Make sure resident's face is not covered by the pillow.

Fig. 11-20. *Gently roll the resident toward you.*

15. Position resident properly in good alignment:

- head supported by pillow

- shoulder adjusted so resident is not lying on arm

- top arm supported by pillow

- back supported by supportive device

- hips properly aligned

- top knee flexed

- supportive device between legs with top knee flexed; knee and ankle supported

16. Cover resident with top linens and straighten. Make resident comfortable.

17. Return bed to low position if raised. Ensure resident's safety. Return side rails to ordered position. Remove privacy measures.

18. Leave call light within resident's reach.

19. Wash your hands.

20. Be courteous and respectful at all times.

21. Report any changes in the resident to the nurse. Document procedure using facility guidelines.

Logrolling allows you to turn a resident as a unit, while keeping the spine straight. The alignment of the body is not disturbed; the head, back and legs are kept in a straight line. Logrolling may be necessary if the resident has neck or back problems, spinal cord injuries, or has had back or hip surgeries. Use a draw sheet to perform this procedure. Be very careful when logrolling a resident. You will need at least one co-worker to assist.

Logrolling a resident with assistance

Equipment: draw sheet

1. Identify yourself by name. Identify the resident. Greet the resident by name.

2. Wash your hands.

3. Explain procedure to resident. Speak clearly, slowly, and directly. Maintain face-to-face contact whenever possible. Encourage resident to assist if possible.

4. Provide for the resident's privacy with a curtain, screen, or door.

5. Practice good body mechanics. Adjust the bed to a safe level, usually waist high. Lock the bed wheels.

6. Lower the head of bed.

7. Both co-workers stand on the same side of the bed. Lower the side rail (if bed has one and if it is not already lowered) on side nearest you. One person stands at the resident's head and shoulders. The other stands near the resident's midsection.

8. Avoid trauma or pain to the resident throughout the procedure.

9. Place a pillow under the resident's head to support the neck during the move.

10. Place the resident's arms across his or her chest. Place a pillow between the knees.

11. Stand with feet about 12 inches apart. Bend your knees.

12. Grasp the draw sheet on the far side (Fig. 11-21).

Fig. 11-21. Both workers should grasp the draw sheet on the far side.

13. On the count of three, gently roll the resident toward you. Turn the resident as a unit (Fig. 11-22).

Fig. 11-22. On the count of three, both workers should roll the resident towards them, turning the person as a unit.

14. Reposition resident comfortably in good alignment. Place pillow under head. Cover resident with top linens and straighten.

15. Return bed to low position if raised. Ensure resident's safety. Return side rails to ordered position. Remove privacy measures.

16. Leave call light within resident's reach.

17. Wash your hands.

18. Be courteous and respectful at all times.

19. Report any changes in the resident to the nurse. Document procedure using facility guidelines.

Dangling moves the resident into a sitting position on the side of the bed with the legs hanging over the side. This helps residents regain balance before standing up, equalizes blood flow in the body, and returns blood flow to the head. It helps prevent dizziness and lightheadedness that can cause fainting. Residents who cannot walk may have an order to dangle their legs for a few minutes.

Assisting a resident to sit up on side of bed: dangling

1. Identify yourself by name. Identify the resident. Greet the resident by name.

2. Wash your hands.

3. Explain procedure to resident. Speak clearly, slowly, and directly. Maintain face-to-face contact whenever possible. Encourage resident to assist if possible.

4. Provide for the resident's privacy with a curtain, screen, or door.

5. Practice good body mechanics. Adjust the bed to the lowest safe working level. Lock the bed wheels.

6. Avoid trauma or pain to the resident throughout the procedure.

7. Raise the head of bed to sitting position. Fold linen to the foot of the bed. Lower the side rail (if bed has one and if it is not already lowered) on side nearest you.

8. Stand at the side of the bed with feet about 12 inches apart. Bend your knees. Keep your back straight. Help resident slowly move toward the side of the bed on which you are standing.

9. Place one arm under resident's shoulder blades. Place the other arm under resident's thighs (Fig. 11-23).

Fig. 11-23. One arm should be under the resident's shoulder blades, and the other arm should be under the thighs.

10. On the count of three, gently and slowly turn resident into sitting position with legs dangling over the side of bed (Fig. 11-24).

Fig. 11-24. The resident should remain sitting with legs dangling over the side of bed for as long as ordered.

11. Ask resident to sit up straight and push both fists into the edge of mattress. Assist resident to put on robe.

12. Have resident dangle as long as ordered. Place a pillow or other supporting device behind resident's back during dangle. Stay with the resident at all times. Check for dizziness. If resident feels dizzy or faint, help her lie down again and make sure she is secure. Tell the nurse at once.

13. Take vital signs as ordered (Chapter 13).

14. Gently assist resident back into bed. Place one arm around resident's shoulders. Place the other arm under resident's knees. Slowly swing resident's legs onto bed.

15. Make resident comfortable. Cover resident with top linens and straighten. Replace pillow under the resident's head.

16. Return bed to low position if raised. Ensure resident's safety. Return side rails to ordered position. Remove privacy measures.

17. Leave call light within resident's reach.

18. Wash your hands.

19. Be courteous and respectful at all times.

20. Report any changes in the resident to the nurse. Document procedure using facility guidelines.

4. Describe how to safely transfer residents

Transfers allow residents to move from one place to another. Examples of transfers include from bed to chair or toilet, bed to stretcher, or wheelchair to toilet or vehicle.

In transferring, it is important to know that some residents have a strong side and a weak side. The weak side is called the "involved" or "affected" side. You must plan the move so that the strong side moves first and the weak side follows. It is difficult for a resident to move a weak arm and leg first and be able to bear enough weight to allow for the move.

Safety is one of the most important concerns during resident transfers. OSHA has set specific ergonomic guidelines to help avoid injuries during transfers. **Ergonomics** is the science of designing equipment and setting up areas to make them safer and to suit the worker's abilities. One goal of ergonomics is to reduce stress on the body to avoid potential injury.

Certain parts of the body, such as the back, are more prone to injury. OSHA's ergonomic guidelines address ways to help avoid these work-related musculoskeletal disorders, or **MSDs**. OSHA states that manual lifting and transferring of residents should be reduced as much as possible. This means that proper equipment should be available in facilities. Staff should be trained on how to use this equipment and use it whenever possible to avoid injury. Avoid heavy lifting and always have enough help when moving and lifting residents.

When evaluating residents for transfers, staff may determine that residents require a transfer belt or gait belt for safety. A **transfer belt** is a safety device used to transfer residents who are weak, unsteady, or uncoordinated. It is called a **gait belt** when it is used to help residents walk. The belt is made of canvas or other heavy material and it has a strong buckle or handles. It fits around the resident's waist, over his clothes, and then it is secured. The transfer belt gives you something firm to hold onto when assisting with transfers (Fig. 11-25). These belts are generally not used if a resident has fragile bones or recent fractures. A transfer belt may also not be used when a resident has difficulty breathing, has had abdominal surgery, or any type of surgical removal of a part of the intestines. Follow the care plan and the nurse's instructions.

Fig. 11-25. *A transfer belt, or gait belt, is used to help residents who can walk but are weak or unsteady. The belt is made of canvas or other heavy material.*

Applying a transfer belt

Equipment: transfer belt

1. Identify yourself by name. Identify the resident. Greet the resident by name.

2. Wash your hands.

3. Explain procedure to resident. Speak clearly, slowly, and directly. Maintain face-to-face contact whenever possible. Encourage resident to assist if possible.

4. Provide for the resident's privacy with a curtain, screen, or door.

5. Practice good body mechanics. Adjust bed to low, flat position. Lock bed wheels.

6. Supporting the back and hips, assist resident to a sitting position with feet flat on the floor.

7. Put on and properly fasten non-skid footwear on resident.

8. Place the belt over the resident's clothing below the rib cage and above the waist. Do not put it over bare skin.

9. Tighten the buckle until it is snug. Leave enough room to insert three fingers into the belt. The fingers should fit comfortably under the belt. The belt must not interfere with

circulation or breathing.

10. Check to make sure that breasts are not caught under the belt.

11. Position the buckle slightly off-center in the front or back for comfort.

Sliding or transfer boards help residents transfer from one sitting position to another (Fig. 11-26). These boards can be used for transferring from wheelchairs or chairs to beds, vehicles, shower chairs, and other areas. Sliding boards are used for people who have weak legs or cannot bear any weight on their legs. Sliding or transfer boards are made out of sturdy material, such as wood, so they can hold the resident's weight.

Fig. 11-26. *A sliding or transfer board.*

Wheelchairs and Geriatric Chairs

Wheelchairs must always be locked before transferring residents to or from the wheelchair (Fig. 11-27). Here are some general guidelines for wheelchair use:

Fig. 11-27. *You must always lock the wheelchair before a resident gets into or out of it.*

Guidelines
Wheelchairs

- To open a standard wheelchair, pull on both sides to make the armrests separate and the seat flatten. To close the wheelchair, lift the center of the seat and pull upward until the chair collapses.

- To remove an armrest on a standard wheelchair, press a button by the armrest, and lift it off. To attach an armrest, line up the button, and slip into place until the buttons click.

- To remove the footrest, locate the lever, pull back, and pull the footrest off the knobs (Fig. 11-28). To re-attach the footrest, line up the knobs, and slide footrest into place until it clicks.

Fig. 11-28. *To remove footrests, pull back the lever, and pull the footrest off the knobs.*

- To lift or lower footrest, support the leg or foot, squeeze lever and pull up or push down.

- If there is a pocket in the back of the wheelchair, it can be used to temporarily store a resident's chart during the transport.

- When moving down a ramp, go down backwards, with the resident facing the top of the ramp, also going down backwards. The wheelchair could get away from you if the wheelchair heads down first.

- When using an elevator, turn the chair around before entering it, so the resident faces forward in the elevator.

- When positioning a resident in a wheelchair, make sure his hips are at the very back of the chair. To do this, lock the wheelchair wheels.

Stand in front of the wheelchair and ask the resident to grasp the armrests while his feet are flat on the floor. Brace your knees against the resident's knees. On the count of three, ask the resident to push with his feet into the floor and move himself back into the chair. Gently assist with moving him back into the chair. Help him get into a comfortable position.

- An alternate method of positioning a resident properly is to get behind him while he pushes. First go to the back of the chair and reach forward and down under the resident's arms. The resident can put his feet flat on the floor and push up with his feet. Pull the resident up in the chair while the resident pushes. You may need a co-worker to help you do this safely.

A geriatric chair, or geri-chair, is a special chair that reclines. A tray table can be attached to it. This chair helps residents who are mostly bed-bound avoid the need to stay in bed all day. The chair helps keep residents in proper alignment, which reduces pressure on the skin.

When using a geriatric chair, remember to lock the wheels on both sides before moving a resident into or out of the chair. The tray tables on geri-chairs can be heavy. Use caution when raising and lowering this tray table. Do not catch your fingers or the resident's fingers in the tray when attaching or releasing the tray table. When the tray table is attached, geri-chairs are considered restraints. See Chapter 7 for more information on restraints and related care.

HOT TIP

The strong arm transfers.
When transferring a resident with one weak side, remember that the strong arm transfers.

Transferring a resident from bed to a chair or wheelchair

Equipment: wheelchair, transfer belt, non-skid footwear

1. Identify yourself by name. Identify the resident. Greet the resident by name.

2. Wash your hands.

3. Explain procedure to resident. Speak clearly, slowly, and directly. Maintain face-to-face contact whenever possible. Encourage resident to assist if possible.

4. Provide for the resident's privacy with a curtain, screen, or door.

5. Practice good body mechanics.

6. Remove wheelchair footrests close to the bed.

7. Place wheelchair near the head of the bed with arm of the wheelchair almost touching the bed. Wheelchair should be placed on resident's stronger, or unaffected, side. Lower the side rail (if bed has one and if it is not already lowered) on side nearest you.

8. Lock wheelchair wheels.

9. Raise the head of the bed. Adjust bed level. The height of the bed should be equal to or slightly higher than the chair. Lock bed wheels.

10. Avoid trauma or pain to the resident throughout the procedure.

11. Assist resident to sitting position with feet flat on the floor. Let resident sit for a few minutes.

12. Put non-skid footwear on resident and securely fasten.

13. **With transfer (gait) belt**:

   a. Stand in front of resident.

   b. Stand with feet about 12 inches apart. Bend your knees. Keep your back straight.

   c. Place belt below the rib cage and above the waist. Do not put it over bare skin. Grasp belt securely on both sides.

   Without transfer belt:

   a. Stand in front of resident.

   b. Stand with feet about 12 inches apart. Bend your knees. Keep your back straight.

   c. Place your arms around the resident's torso under the arms, but not in the armpits (axilla). Repeated pressure in the axilla may cause nerve damage. Do not allow resident to grasp your shoulders or around your neck. This may cause you to lose your balance.

14. Provide instructions to allow resident to help with transfer. Instructions may include: "When you start to stand, push with your hands against the bed." "Once standing, if you're able, you can take small steps in the direction of the chair." "Once standing, reach for the chair with your stronger hand."

15. With your legs, brace resident's lower legs to prevent slipping (Fig. 11-29).

Fig. 11-29. *Bracing the resident's lower legs with your legs helps prevent slipping.*

16. Count to three to alert resident.

17. On three, slowly help resident to stand.

18. Help resident to pivot to front of wheelchair with back of resident's legs against wheelchair (Fig. 11-30).

Fig. 11-30. *Pivoting is safer than twisting.*

19. Ask resident to put hands on wheelchair armrests if able.

20. Gently lower resident into wheelchair.

21. Reposition resident with hips touching back of wheelchair. See previous guidelines on how to do this. Remove transfer belt, if used.

22. Attach footrests. Place resident's feet on footrests.

23. Make resident comfortable.

24. Remove privacy measures.

25. Leave call light within resident's reach.

26. Wash your hands.

27. Be courteous and respectful at all times.

28. Report any changes in the resident to the nurse. Document procedure using facility guidelines.

TO TRANSFER BACK TO BED FROM WHEELCHAIR, FOLLOW THESE STEPS:

1. Perform steps 1 through 8 above.

2. Adjust bed level to a low position. The height of the bed should be equal to or slightly lower than the chair. Lock bed wheels.

3. Avoid trauma or pain to the resident throughout the procedure.

4. Perform steps 13 through 17 above.

   The resident should be allowed to stand until he feels stable enough to move toward the bed. If the transfer belt is used, do not let go of it during this time.

5. Help resident to pivot to bed with back of resident's legs against bed. When he feels the bed, he should slowly sit down on the side of the bed.

6. Make resident comfortable. Remove transfer belt, if used.

7. Return bed to low position if raised. Ensure resident's safety. Return side rails to ordered position. Remove privacy measures.

8. Leave call light within resident's reach.

9. Wash your hands.

10. Be courteous and respectful at all times.

11. Report any changes in the resident to the nurse. Document procedure using facility guidelines.

Stretchers

Stretchers, also called gurneys, are a way to transport residents from place to place within a facility. They are also used to transfer a resident to a vehicle. Residents who are unable to walk or sit in a wheelchair may need to be moved in a stretcher. People who are severely ill and must be transported by ambulance will need to be moved in a stretcher.

Stretchers have safety straps that are used when the resident is on the stretcher. Nursing assistants must secure the safety belts on the stretcher before moving residents. Lock the brakes on the stretcher when it is not in motion.

Keep residents properly covered at all times for warmth and privacy while on a stretcher. Residents should never be left alone on a stretcher. If riding with a resident who is being transported, make sure to formally transfer the care to the nurse at the new facility. The chart and any equipment or belongings must also be transferred to the nurse.

A draw sheet is used to transfer a resident to a stretcher. The procedure below shows a transfer to a stretcher from a bed using four workers. At least three workers are necessary to safely transfer a resident to a stretcher.

Transferring a resident from bed to stretcher with assistance

Equipment: stretcher, bath blanket

1. Identify yourself by name. Identify the resident. Greet the resident by name.

2. Wash your hands.

3. Explain procedure to resident. Speak clearly, slowly, and directly. Maintain face-to-face contact whenever possible. Encourage resident to assist if possible.

4. Provide for the resident's privacy with a curtain, screen, or door.

5. Practice good body mechanics. Lower the head of bed so that it is flat. Lock bed wheels.

6. Fold linens to foot of the bed. Cover resident with bath blanket. Do not expose resident during the procedure.

7. Lower the side rail on side to which you will move resident (if in use for resident).

8. Avoid trauma or pain to the resident throughout the procedure.

9. Move the resident to the side of the bed. Have your co-workers help you do this. Refer back to the procedure "Moving a resident to the side of the bed" earlier in this chapter.

10. Place stretcher solidly against the bed. Lock stretcher wheels. Bed height should be equal to or slightly above the height of the stretcher. Move stretcher safety belts out of the way.

11. Two workers should be on the side of the bed opposite the stretcher. Two more workers should be on the outside of the stretcher.

12. Each worker should roll up the sides of the draw sheet and prepare to move the resident (Fig. 11-31). Protect the resident's arms and legs during the transfer. If facility policy permits, two workers may actually get up on the bed on their knees to protect their backs.

Fig. 11-31. With two workers on each side, roll up the sides of the draw sheet and prepare to move the resident.

13. On the count of three, the workers should lift and move the resident to the stretcher. All

should move at once (Fig. 11-32). Make sure the resident is centered on the stretcher.

Fig. 11-32. On the count of three, all workers should lift and move at once.

14. Raise the head of the stretcher or place a pillow under the resident's head if allowed. Make sure bath blanket still covers the resident.

15. Place safety straps across the resident. Raise side rails on stretcher.

16. Unlock stretcher's wheels. Take resident to appropriate site. Stay with the resident until another team member takes over.

17. Wash your hands.

18. Be courteous and respectful at all times.

19. Report any changes in the resident to the nurse. Document procedure using facility guidelines.

    TO TRANSFER BACK TO BED FROM STRETCHER: The bed height should be equal to or slightly below the stretcher when transferring the resident back to bed.

Mechanical Lifts

Mechanical lifts are types of equipment that are used to lift and move residents. They help prevent injury and help protect staff and residents. Learn to use the lifts available at your facility. Know how to explain their use to residents to ease their fears of them.

There are many different types of mechanical lifts (Fig. 11-33). Some common names of these lifts include "hydraulic," "power," "standing," "heavy duty," and "pool and bath." You must be trained on the specific lift you will be using.

Fig. 11-33. *There are many different types of lifts for transferring both completely dependent residents and residents who can bear some weight.* (Photo courtesy of VANCARE Inc., 800-694-4525)

This is a basic procedure for transferring a resident using a mechanical lift with the type of sling shown in the photo. Other lifts may have different procedures. If you are unsure how to perform this procedure, ask for more training. Do not operate lifts if you have not been trained in their use. Do not use the lift if it is broken or does not appear to be functioning properly.

Many facilities require two or more people to perform the following procedure. Follow your facility's policy.

Transferring a resident using a mechanical lift with assistance

Equipment: wheelchair or chair, mechanical or hydraulic lift, washcloth

Before performing this procedure, check the weight limit of the lift to make sure the resident

is within the weight limit. Make sure you know how to use this lift.

1. Identify yourself by name. Identify the resident. Greet the resident by name.

2. Wash your hands.

3. Explain procedure to resident. Speak clearly, slowly, and directly. Maintain face-to-face contact whenever possible. Encourage resident to assist if possible.

4. Provide for the resident's privacy with a curtain, screen, or door.

5. Practice good body mechanics. Lower bed to proper position for the move. Lock bed wheels.

6. Remove wheelchair footrests close to the bed.

7. Position wheelchair next to bed. Lower the side rail (if bed has one and if it is not already lowered) on side nearest you. Lock wheelchair brakes.

8. Avoid trauma or pain to the resident throughout the procedure.

9. Help the resident turn to one side of the bed. Pad the sling where the neck will rest with a washcloth for resident's comfort. A sheet may be used over the sling to protect it from soiling. Position the sling under the resident, with the edge next to the resident's back. Fanfold if possible. Fanfolding means folding several times into pleats. Make the bottom of the sling even with the resident's knees (some slings only come to the top of the buttocks). Help the resident roll to his opposite side. Spread out the fanfolded edge of the sling, then roll back to the middle of the bed.

10. Roll the mechanical lift to bedside. Make sure the base is opened to its widest point. Push the base of the lift under the bed. Lock lift wheels.

11. Place the overhead bar directly over the resident. Be careful so the swing does not hit anyone.

12. With the resident lying on her back, attach one set of straps to each side of the sling.

Attach one set of straps to the overhead bar (Fig. 11-34). If available, have a co-worker support the resident at the head, shoulders, and knees while being lifted. The resident's arms should be folded across her chest. If the device has "S" hooks, they should face away from resident. Make sure all straps are connected properly.

Fig. 11-34. *Attach straps to overhead bar.*

13. Following manufacturer's instructions, raise the resident two inches above the bed. Pause a moment for the resident to gain balance.

14. If available, a lifting partner can help support and guide the resident's body (Fig. 11-35). You can then move the lift so that the resident is positioned over the chair or wheelchair.

Fig. 11-35. *Make sure that one person supports and guides the resident's body to help prevent injury.*

15. Slowly lower the resident into the chair or wheelchair. Push down gently on the resident's knees to help the resident into a sitting position.

16. Undo the straps from the overhead bar. Leave the sling in place for transfer back to bed (some slings can be easily removed when resident is seated).

17. Be sure the resident is seated comfortably and correctly in the chair or wheelchair. Put non-skid footwear on resident and fasten. Replace footrests. Cover the resident with a lap cover or robe if he requests it.

18. Remove privacy measures.

19. Leave call light within resident's reach.

20. Wash your hands.

21. Be courteous and respectful at all times.

22. Report any changes in the resident to the nurse. Document procedure using facility guidelines.

Toilet Transfers

The toilet is better than a bedpan or a urinal for eliminating urine. The bladder tends to empty more completely when using the toilet or portable commode because of the position of the person over the toilet. Chapter 15 has more information on bedpan and urinal use.

Ask residents often if they need to use the bathroom. Take them to the bathroom as soon as they request a trip. When a call light is pressed, respond immediately.

For a resident to be able to use a toilet, he must be able to bear some weight on his legs. Falls can occur on the way to the bathroom, during toileting, or on the way back to bed or chair. Use a transfer belt to assist, as it can help prevent injury. Review the transfer belt procedure found earlier in this chapter. Do not leave residents alone if you feel it is unsafe or if residents require assistance.

Transferring a resident onto and off a toilet

Equipment: disposable gloves, toilet tissue, wheelchair, transfer belt, non-skid shoes

1. Identify yourself by name. Identify the resident. Greet the resident by name.

2. Wash your hands.

3. Explain procedure to resident. Speak clearly, slowly, and directly. Maintain face-to-face contact whenever possible. Encourage resident to assist if possible.

4. Provide for the resident's privacy with a curtain, screen, or door.

5. Practice good body mechanics.

6. Position wheelchair at a right angle to the toilet to face the hand bar/wall rail. Place wheelchair on the resident's stronger side, if possible.

7. Remove wheelchair footrests. Lock wheels. Put on and properly fasten non-skid footwear on resident.

8. Avoid trauma or pain to the resident throughout the procedure.

9. Apply a transfer belt around the resident's waist. Grasp the belt. Put one of your hands toward the resident's back and one toward the resident's front.

10. Ask resident to push against the armrests of the wheelchair and stand, reaching for and grasping the hand bar with his stronger arm (Fig. 11-36).

Fig. 11-36. *Ask the resident to push up using the armrests of the wheelchair, stand and grasp the hand bar.*

11. Ask resident to pivot her feet and back up so that she can feel the front of the toilet with the back of her legs (Fig. 11-37).

Fig. 11-37. *Have the resident pivot and feel the toilet with the back of her legs.*

12. Help resident to pull down underwear and pants. You may need to keep one hand on the transfer belt while helping to remove clothing.

13. Help resident to slowly sit down onto the toilet. Remove transfer belt. Allow privacy unless resident cannot be left alone. Ask resident to pull on the emergency cord if she needs help. Close bathroom door. Stay near the door until resident is finished.

14. When the resident is finished, apply gloves. Assist with perineal care as necessary (see Chapters 12 and 16). Reapply transfer belt if removed. Ask her to stand and reach for the hand bar.

15. Use toilet tissue or damp cloth to clean the resident. Make sure he or she is clean and dry before pulling up clothing. Remove and dispose of gloves.

16. Pull up resident's clothing. Help resident to the sink to wash hands. Wash your hands.

17. Help resident back into wheelchair. Be sure the resident is seated comfortably and correctly in the chair or wheelchair. Replace footrests.

18. Help resident to leave the bathroom.

19. Leave call light within resident's reach.

20. Wash your hands.

21. Be courteous and respectful at all times.

22. Report any changes in the resident to the nurse. Document procedure using facility guidelines.

Car Transfers

When a resident is discharged from a facility, you may need to help him or her into a car. The front seat of the car is wider and is usually easier to get into. Remember that your responsibility does not end until the resident is safely inside the car and the door is closed.

Transferring a resident into a car

Equipment: car, wheelchair

1. Identify yourself by name. Identify the resident. Greet the resident by name.

2. Wash your hands.

3. Explain procedure to resident. Speak clearly, slowly, and directly. Maintain face-to-face contact whenever possible. Encourage resident to assist if possible.

4. Practice good body mechanics.

5. Place wheelchair close to the car at a 45-degree angle. Open the door on the resident's stronger side.

6. Lock wheelchair.

7. Ask the resident to push against the arm rests of the wheelchair and stand.

8. Ask the resident to stand, grasp the car or dashboard, and pivot his foot so the side of the car seat touches the back of the legs.

9. The resident should then sit in the seat and lift one leg, and then the other, into the vehicle (Fig. 11-38).

10. Carefully position the resident comfortably in the car. Help secure seat belt.

11. See that door can be safely shut. Shut the door.

12. Return the wheelchair to the appropriate place for cleaning.

13. Wash your hands.

14. Document procedure using facility guidelines.

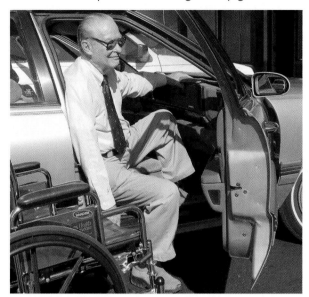

Fig. 11-38. *After resident sits in the car seat, he should put his legs in one at a time.*

For more information on transferring residents recovering from a hip replacement or stroke, see Chapters 21 and 22.

5. Discuss ambulation

Ambulation means walking. A resident who is ambulatory can get out of bed and walk. Residents should ambulate to maintain independence and prevent problems. Regular ambulation and exercise are very important and help to improve these things:

- quality and health of the skin
- circulation
- strength
- sleep and relaxation
- appetite
- elimination
- oxygen level

Residents should only walk for short distances, especially if the person is just starting to ambulate. Over time, the distance may be increased. Residents may require a transfer or gait belt and/or more than one staff member to ambulate safely. Follow the nurse's instructions and the care plan.

Assisting a resident to ambulate

1. Identify yourself by name. Identify the resident. Greet the resident by name.

2. Wash your hands.

3. Explain procedure to resident. Speak clearly, slowly, and directly. Maintain face-to-face contact whenever possible. Encourage resident to assist if possible.

4. Provide for the resident's privacy with a curtain, screen, or door.

5. Avoid trauma or pain to the resident throughout the procedure.

6. Help resident move to a dangling position as described in earlier procedure.

7. Practice good body mechanics. Adjust bed to a low position so that the resident's feet are flat on the floor. Lock bed wheels.

8. Put on and properly fasten non-skid footwear for resident.

9. Stand in front of and face the resident.

10. Brace the resident's lower extremities. Bend your knees. If resident has a weak knee, brace it against your knee.

11. **With transfer (gait) belt**: Place belt around resident's waist. Grasp the belt while assisting resident to stand.

    Without transfer belt: Place arms around the resident's torso under the arms, but not in the armpits (axillae), while assisting resident to stand.

12. **With transfer belt**: Walk slightly behind and to one side of resident for the full distance, while holding onto the transfer belt (Fig. 11-39). If the resident has a weaker side, stand on the weaker side. Ask resident to look forward, not

down at floor, during ambulation. If resident becomes dizzy or faint, help him to a nearby seat and call nurse for help.

Fig. 11-39. *Walk slightly behind, standing on the weaker side, when assisting a resident to ambulate. Hold onto the transfer belt, if used, for the full distance.*

Without transfer belt: Walk slightly behind and to one side of resident for the full distance. Support resident's back with your arm. Ask resident to look forward, not down at floor, during ambulation. If resident becomes dizzy or faint, help him to a nearby seat and call nurse for help.

13. After ambulation, make resident comfortable. Remove transfer belt, if used.

14. Return bed to low position if raised. Ensure resident's safety. Remove privacy measures.

15. Leave call light within resident's reach.

16. Wash your hands.

17. Be courteous and respectful at all times.

18. Report any changes in the resident to the nurse. Document procedure using facility guidelines.

When helping a visually-impaired resident walk, let the person walk beside and slightly behind you, as he rests a hand on your elbow. Walk at a normal pace. Let the person know when you are about to turn a corner, or when a step is approaching. Tell him whether you will be stepping up or down.

For more information on ambulating a resident with a walker, cane, or crutches, see Chapter 25.

CHAPTER REVIEW

1. How is the body helped to function by good body alignment (LO 2)?

2. Why should a nursing assistant face what she is lifting (LO 2)?

3. In what position should a nursing assistant be before lifting an object (LO 2)?

4. Should objects be lifted by using muscles in the legs or the back (LO 2)?

5. Explain why objects should be kept close to the body when carrying them (LO 2).

6. Why should regular turning schedules always be maintained (LO 3)?

7. Briefly describe what each of the following positions are: supine, lateral, prone, Fowler's, and Sims' (LO 3).

8. What is the benefit of using a draw sheet when repositioning (LO 3)?

9. Define "logrolling" (LO 3).

10. During dangling, what should the nursing assistant do if the resident feels faint (LO 3)?

11. For a resident with one weak side and one strong side, which side should move first and why (LO 4)?

12. What is a transfer belt (LO 4)?

13. When moving a resident down a ramp in a wheelchair, in which direction should the resident be facing (LO 4)?

14. Why is it important to use mechanical lifts if they are available (LO 4)?

15. What must a resident be able to do in order to use the toilet (LO 4)?

16. List six factors that regular ambulation helps to improve (LO 5).

12 Personal Care

Public Health and Hygiene

During the fifth century, many people lived in tiny homes with poor ventilation. Since there was no way to keep the streets clean, people were usually filthy. Bathing was done in public bath houses, as well as in the home. Public baths were shared by the people of the community. In later centuries, public baths were still used, but less regularly due to the spread of diseases.

"To get the whole world out of bed and washed and dressed, and warmed, and fed...and back to bed again..."

John Masefield, 1878-1967

"Bid them wash their faces/And keep their teeth clean."

William Shakespeare, 1564-1616

1. Define important words in this chapter

additive: a substance added to another substance, changing its effect.

aspiration: the inhalation of food or drink into the lungs; can cause pneumonia or death.

axilla: underarm or armpit area.

bridge: a type of dental appliance that replaces missing or pulled teeth.

dandruff: excessive shedding of dead skin cells from the scalp.

dentures: artificial teeth.

edema: swelling in body tissues caused by excess fluid.

edentulous: lacking teeth; toothless.

gingivitis: an inflammation of the gums.

grooming: practices to care for oneself, such as caring for fingernails and hair.

halitosis: bad-smelling breath.

hygiene: methods of keeping the body clean.

partial bath: bath that includes washing the face, underarms, and hands, and performing perineal care.

pediculosis: an infestation of lice.

perineal care: care of the genitals and anal area.

plaque: a substance that forms in a brief period of time if oral care is not done regularly.

tartar: hard deposits on the teeth that are filled with bacteria and may cause gum disease and loose teeth if they are not removed.

2. Explain personal care of residents

Good hygiene is important to good health. **Hygiene** is the term used to describe methods of keeping the body clean. Good grooming helps keep a person clean and healthy as well. **Grooming** includes practices like fingernail, foot, and hair care. Hygiene and grooming, along with other personal care tasks, are called activities of daily living (ADLs). ADLs include grooming, dressing, bathing, eating and drinking, transferring, and elimination. Nursing assistants help residents every day with their ADLs.

The type of daily care you provide for residents depends on what shifts you work at the facility. Care will vary according to what time of day it is. Bathing usually happens in the morning; however, it can be done in the evening, depending on residents' preferences and facility policy. Care generally done in the mornings is called "a.m. care" and care done in the evening is "p.m. care."

A.M. care includes:

- Taking resident to the bathroom, offering a bedpan, urinal, or an incontinent brief change and washing resident's hands

- Helping with mouth care or denture care before and/or after breakfast, as the resident prefers

- Assisting with washing face and hands in bed, shower room, or in bathroom

- Changing resident's gown or pajamas or clothing

- Providing breakfast and fluids

- Assisting with bathing, as the resident prefers

- Helping resident with shaving, hair care, hand and fingernail care, foot care, and cosmetics (Fig. 12-1)

- Giving a back massage

- Making the bed and tidying resident's room

Fig. 12-1. *Assisting residents with their ADLs, such as shaving, is part of a.m. care.*

P.M. care includes:

- Taking resident to the bathroom, offering bedpan or urinal, or an incontinent brief change and assisting with handwashing

- Helping with mouth care or denture care after lunch and dinner, as the resident prefers

- Providing lunch, dinner, snacks, and fluids; passing fresh drinking water

- Assisting the resident with bathing, if evening is preferable

- Giving a back massage

- Changing resident's gown or pajamas

- Helping resident with hair care

- Assisting with washing face and removing makeup as needed

- Changing linens as needed and preparing the bed for the resident's return

- Tidying resident's room

The personal care you provide will depend upon the resident's needs and ability to care for himself. The way that you go about providing this care is important to residents' self-esteem and dignity. Promote self-care as much as possible. Encourage residents to perform tasks independently whenever they can. This may make some tasks, such as getting dressed, take longer. Be patient; residents should do as much as they are able to do, no matter how long it takes. In addition to promoting dignity and independence, doing self-care also helps keep the body functioning well.

It is very difficult to give up all or part of independence. Residents may never have needed help with bathing, dressing or eating during their adult lives. Being required to accept help with these activities can cause anger, frustration, and sadness. Residents may be embarrassed by having someone, especially a member of the opposite sex, provide personal care. Be understanding and sympathetic to the emotions residents are experiencing. Explain the care you are going to provide and answer any questions the resident has. Let the resident make as many choices as possible about the care you will be performing (Fig. 12-2). Always provide privacy when giving personal care. Here are additional ways to provide respect and dignity when performing personal care tasks:

Fig. 12-2. Talk with residents about the care you are going to perform. Let them make as many decisions as possible about personal care.

- Allow residents enough time to use the bathroom. Do not rush or interrupt them. It is a good idea to ask if a resident wants to use the bathroom or bedpan before beginning personal care.

- Assist with dressing as needed, but allow as much independence as possible. Provide for personal choice throughout personal care. Residents have the right to choose what they will wear, including jewelry. They can choose to wear cosmetics. Be patient while they make these decisions.

- Be patient while they perform care tasks. Encourage residents to do whatever they can for themselves.

- Be respectful if residents are using the phone or talking with visitors. Leave the room if they want privacy.

- Keep residents covered whenever possible when dressing and bathing.

- Promote residents' safety. Do not leave them alone during bathing. Do not rush them during care, as it may cause falls or other injuries. Always ask for help to perform personal care when you need it.

- Take the time to talk with residents during personal care. Report any changes, concerns, or problems you notice to the nurse.

3. Describe different types of baths and list observations to make about the skin during bathing

There are four basic types of baths: a partial bath, a shower, a tub bath, and a complete bed bath. The type of bath given is determined first by the resident's needs and abilities and then by the resident's preference.

A **partial bath**, also called a set-up bath, includes washing the face, underarms, hands, and the perineal (genitals and anal) area. It is best suited to a resident who:

- has drier, fragile, and more sensitive skin

- should not have daily full baths

- is unable to get up to take a shower or tub bath

- wants a quick bath before a meal and plans on taking a shower or bath later in the day

A shower is best suited to a resident who:

- is able to stand during a shower

- is able to safely sit in a shower chair

A tub bath can take place in a regular bathtub or in a special tub, such as a whirlpool. It is best suited to a resident who:

- is able to transfer into and out of a tub

- has a doctor's order for a special bath using an **additive**—a substance added to another substance, changing its effect—to the tub water; examples of bath additives are bran, oatmeal, sodium bicarbonate, and epsom salts

A complete bed bath is best suited to a resident who:

- is unable to get out of bed to shower or bathe and requires a full bath

The decision on which bath to give a resident rests first with the doctor or nurse, then with the resident. For example, a doctor may write an order for "no shower" until a wound has healed. Some residents are confined to bed, which prevents them from getting up for a tub bath or a shower. Some residents do not shower for personal reasons; they may simply prefer a tub bath because they have always taken baths at home. Discuss residents' preferences and decisions regarding bathing with the nurse prior to giving care.

Personal care and bathing give you the opportunity to carefully observe for changes in residents or their skin (Fig. 12-3). This is especially important in the prevention of pressure sores, a serious skin wound caused by skin breakdown. You will learn more about pressure sores and prevention in Chapter 18.

Fig. 12-3. Every time you bathe residents, closely observe their skin for any changes. Report changes promptly to the nurse.

Residents may discuss health problems and issues during personal care. They may also bring up personal concerns regarding staff, family, or friends. Listen to residents closely and report concerns or observations to the nurse.

Some of the things to observe for and report during personal care and bathing include:

- Change in size of one or both pupils
- Difference in appearance from one eye to another
- Yellow or red color in whites of the eyes
- Drooping on one side of the face
- Weight loss

- Drainage coming from any area including eyes, ears, nipples, or genitals
- Foul odors from any body area
- Pale, blue-tinged (cyanotic), white, reddened, or purple areas on the skin
- Dry, flaky, broken or cracked skin
- Lumps or bumps on the skin
- Moles or spots, especially red, white, yellow, dark brown, gray or black
- Rashes or any skin discoloration
- Bruises
- Blisters
- Cuts, scrapes or scratches
- Open sores, wounds or ulcers on any area of the body
- Changes in open sore, wound or ulcer (color, size, drainage, odor, overall depth of sore)
- Swelling/edema of any area, especially the knuckles, fingers, groin, ankles or feet (**edema** is swelling in body tissues caused by excess fluid)
- Poor condition of fingernails or toenails
- Nails in need of trimming
- Dry, cracked, or broken skin in between toes or toenails
- Change in emotional state
- Change in level of mobility
- Complaints of pain or discomfort
- Changes in vision, ability to hear, and sense of smell
- Stiff neck
- Numbness, burning, warmth or tingling
- Itching or scratching

4. Explain safety guidelines for bathing

Safety must be the highest priority when bathing residents. Many accidents happen in the bathroom or shower room. Assess the area for any risks before bathing a resident. Follow these guidelines for safety:

Guidelines
Safety for Bathing

- Make sure you can perform this procedure alone. If you need help, ask for it. Do not try to bathe a resident alone if you do not believe you can handle the task safely.

- Know any special orders for bathing. Follow the care plan.

- Some facilities have a rule that requires residents to be undressed in their rooms before transporting them to the shower room. If this is the case, cover residents completely before moving them to the shower or tub room. This provides warmth and promotes dignity. If facility policy requires that residents be undressed in the shower room, make sure the door is closed. Residents should be kept covered.

- Clean showers, tubs, and all equipment before and after use, per facility policy.

- Make sure the floor in the shower or tub room is dry. Wipe up any spills or wet areas.

- Place nonslip mats in regular tubs. A slippery tub may cause falls.

- Check to see that hand rails and grab bars are secure and in proper working order. Encourage weak and unsteady residents to use safety bars to get into and out of tubs or showers.

- Gather all needed equipment before entering the shower area. Be organized. Place needed items within easy reach.

- Bath oils and gels can create slippery surfaces and can put residents at risk of falling. Talcum powder also creates slippery surfaces. Avoid using these items.

- Make sure that water temperature is not too hot for residents. Comfortable temperature varies for each person. Water temperature should not be over 105°F. Check water temperature with a bath thermometer or on your wrist. Then have the resident test water himself.

- Put away electrical appliances when they are not in use. Do not use electrical appliances near a water source.

- Do not leave residents alone while bathing or showering.

5. List the order in which body parts are washed during bathing

When bathing a person, it is important to follow a specific order. This reduces the risk of transferring microorganisms from a dirty area to a clean area of the body. The general rule is to wash from cleanest to dirtiest. For example, you will wash the face before washing the buttocks. The correct order of washing parts of the body is listed below and shown in the illustration (Fig. 12-4):

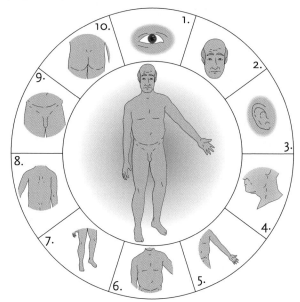

Fig. 12-4. *The parts of the body have corresponding numbers that show the exact order to complete a bed bath. Following this order helps prevent the transfer of microorganisms from a dirty area to a clean area of the body.*

1. eyes
2. face
3. ears
4. neck
5. arms, **axilla** (axillae), and hands
6. chest and abdomen
7. legs and feet

8. back

9. perineal area

10. buttocks

6. Explain how to assist with bathing

Regular bathing provides many benefits. It promotes good health and hygiene. Bathing increases circulation, especially for bed-bound residents. Bathing also provides an opportunity to observe the skin.

The face, underarms, hands and perineal area should be bathed every day. **Perineal care** is care of the genitals and anal area. People with fragile, dry skin may not be bathed every day. Bathing a couple of times per week will help prevent further dryness. In some facilities, complete baths are done on certain days of the week. Follow bathing schedules and care plans carefully. In addition, follow these guidelines:

- Make sure the room is warm enough before starting a bath or shower.

- Make sure the water temperature is comfortable. As stated earlier, the resident should help choose a proper and comfortable water temperature. Comfortable temperature is different for each person.

- Wear gloves if the resident has any broken skin. Always wear gloves when performing perineal care.

- Make sure all soap residue is removed. This prevents further drying and irritation of the skin.

- When preparing to do perineal care, make sure residents understand the care you are going to provide. Get a translator if necessary. More information on perineal care is in Chapter 16.

- If using a tub or shower room for bathing, clean and prepare the room, and gather all equipment before moving the resident there.

During the bath, you will have the chance to observe residents closely. You should check the skin carefully every time you bathe residents.

Review the list of items to observe and report on in Learning Objective 3.

Giving a complete bed bath

Equipment: bath blanket, bath basin, soap, bath thermometer, 2-4 washcloths, 2-4 bath towels, clean gown or clothes, gloves, lotion, deodorant, orangewood stick or emery board

1. Identify yourself by name. Identify the resident. Greet the resident by name.

2. Wash your hands.

3. Explain procedure to resident. Speak clearly, slowly, and directly. Maintain face-to-face contact whenever possible. Encourage resident to assist if possible.

4. Provide for the resident's privacy with a curtain, screen, or door. Be sure the room is at a comfortable temperature and there are no drafts.

5. Practice good body mechanics. Adjust bed to safe working level, usually waist high. Lock bed wheels.

6. Adjust position of side rails (if bed has them) to ensure resident safety at all times.

7. Place a bath blanket or towel over resident. Ask him to hold onto it as you remove or fold back top bedding (Fig. 12-5). Keep resident covered with bath blanket (or top sheet).

Fig. 12-5. *Cover the resident with a bath blanket before removing top bedding.*

8. Fill the basin with warm water. Test water temperature with thermometer or your wrist and ensure it is safe. Water temperature should not be over 105°F. It cools quickly. Have resident check water temperature. Adjust if necessary. Change the water when it becomes too cool, soapy, or dirty.

9. If resident has open wounds, put on gloves.

10. Ask the resident to participate in washing. Help him do this whenever needed.

11. Uncover only one part of the body at a time. Place a towel under the body part being washed.

12. Wash, rinse, and dry one part of the body at a time. Start at the head. Work down, and complete the front first. Fold the washcloth over your hand like a mitt and hold it in place with your thumb (Fig. 12-6).

Fig. 12-6. Fold the washcloth to make a mitt.

Eyes, Face, Ears, Neck: Wash face with wet washcloth (no soap). Begin with the eye farther away from you. Wash inner aspect to outer aspect (Fig. 12-7). Use a different area of the washcloth for each eye. Wash the face from the middle outward. Use firm but gentle strokes. Wash the ears and behind the ears and the neck. Rinse and pat dry with blotting motion.

Fig. 12-7. Wash the eye from the inner part to the outer part.

Arms and Axillae: Remove the resident's top clothing. Cover him with the bath blanket or towel. With a soapy washcloth, wash the upper arm and underarm. Use long strokes from the shoulder to the elbow. Rinse and pat dry. Wash the elbow. Wash, rinse, and dry from the elbow down to the wrist (Fig. 12-8).

Fig. 12-8. Support the wrist while washing the shoulder, arm, underarm, and elbow.

Hands: Wash the hand in a basin. Clean under the nails with an orangewood stick or nail brush (Fig. 12-9). Rinse and pat dry. Make sure to dry between the fingers. Give nail care (see procedure later in this chapter) if it has been assigned. Repeat for the other arm. Put lotion on the resident's elbows and hands if ordered.

Fig. 12-9. Wash the hand in a basin. Thoroughly clean under the nails with a nail brush.

Chest: Place the towel across the resident's chest. Pull the bath blanket down to the waist. Lift the towel only enough to wash the chest. Rinse it and pat dry. For a female resident, wash, rinse, and dry breasts and under breasts. Check the skin in this area for signs of irritation.

Abdomen: Fold the bath blanket down so that it still covers the pubic area. Wash the abdomen, rinse, and pat dry. Cover with the towel. Pull the bath blanket up to the resident's chin. Remove the towel.

Legs and Feet: Expose one leg. Place a towel under it. Wash the thigh. Use long downward strokes. Rinse and pat dry. Do the same from the knee to the ankle (Fig. 12-10). Place another towel under the foot. Move the basin to the towel. Place the foot into the basin. Wash the foot and between the toes (Fig. 12-11). Rinse foot and pat dry. Dry between toes. Give nail care (see Chapter 23) if it has been assigned. Do not give nail care for a diabetic resident. Never clip a resident's toenails. Apply lotion to the foot if ordered, especially at the heels. Do not apply lotion between the toes. Repeat steps for the other leg and foot.

Fig. 12-10. *Use long downward strokes when washing the legs.*

Fig. 12-11. *Washing the feet includes cleaning between the toes.*

Back: Help resident move to the center of the bed. Ask resident to turn onto his side so his back is facing you. If the bed has rails, raise the rail on the far side for safety. Fold the blanket away from the back. Place a towel lengthwise next to the back. Wash the back, neck, and buttocks with long, downward strokes (Fig. 12-12). Rinse and pat dry. Apply lotion if ordered.

Fig. 12-12. *Wash the back with long downward strokes.*

13. Place the towel under the buttocks and upper thighs. Help the resident turn onto his back. If the resident is able to wash his or her perineal area, place a basin of clean, warm water and a washcloth and towel within reach. Leave the room if the resident desires. If the resident has a urinary catheter in place, remind him not to pull on it.

14. If the resident cannot provide perineal care, you must do so. Put on gloves first (if you haven't already done so). Provide privacy at all times.

15. **Perineal area and buttocks**: Change bath water. Wash, rinse, and dry perineal area. Work from front to back (clean to dirty).

    For a female resident: Wash the perineum with soap and water from front to back (Fig. 12-13). Use single strokes. Do not wash from the back to the front, as this may cause infection. Use a clean area of washcloth or clean washcloth for each stroke. First wipe the center of the perineum, then each side. Then spread the labia majora, the outside folds of perineal skin that protect the urinary meatus and the vaginal opening. Wipe from front to back on each side. Rinse the area in the same way. Dry entire perineal area. Move from front to back. Use a blotting motion with towel. Ask resident to turn on her side. Wash, rinse, and dry buttocks and anal area. Clean the anal area without contaminating the perineal area.

Fig. 12-13. *Always work from front to back when performing perineal care.*

For a male resident: If the resident is uncircumcised, pull back the foreskin first. Gently push skin towards the base of penis. Hold the penis by the shaft. Wash in a circular motion from the tip down to the base (Fig. 12-14). Use a clean area of washcloth or clean washcloth for each stroke.

Fig. 12-14. *Wash the penis in a circular motion from the tip down to the base.*

Rinse the penis. If resident is uncircumcised, gently return foreskin to normal position. Then wash the scrotum and groin. The groin is the area from the pubis (area around the penis and scrotum) to the upper thighs. Rinse and pat dry. Ask the resident to turn on his side. Wash, rinse, and dry buttocks and anal area. Clean the anal area without contaminating the perineal area.

16. Remove bath blanket. Remove and dispose of gloves properly.

17. Wash your hands.

18. Provide deodorant.

19. Put clean gown on resident. Assist with brushing or combing resident's hair (see procedure later in the chapter).

20. Replace bedding. Make resident comfortable.

21. Return bed to low position if raised. Ensure resident's safety. Return side rails to ordered position. Remove privacy measures.

22. Empty, rinse, and wipe bath basin. Return to proper storage.

23. Place soiled clothing and linens in proper containers.

24. Leave call light within resident's reach.

25. Wash your hands.

26. Be courteous and respectful at all times.

27. Report any changes in the resident to the nurse. Document procedure using facility guidelines.

Partial Bath

A partial bath is performed on days when a complete bed bath, tub bath, or shower is not done. It usually includes washing the face, underarms, hands, and the perineal area. However, for testing purposes, nursing assistants are often asked to give a partial bath that may include other body parts than those listed here. Follow your facility's guidelines.

Shampooing a resident's hair in bed

Equipment: shampoo, hair conditioner if requested, 2 bath towels, washcloth, bath thermometer, pitcher or handheld shower or sink attachment, waterproof pad, bath blanket, trough, basin, comb and brush, hair dryer

1. Identify yourself by name. Identify the resident. Greet the resident by name.

2. Wash your hands.

3. Explain procedure to resident. Speak clearly, slowly, and directly. Maintain face-to-face contact whenever possible. Encourage resident to assist if possible.

4. Provide for the resident's privacy with a curtain, screen, or door. Be sure the room is at a comfortable temperature and there are no drafts.

5. Practice good body mechanics. Adjust bed to safe working level, usually waist high. Lock bed wheels.

6. Lower the head of bed. Remove pillow.

7. Test water temperature with thermometer or your wrist. Ensure it is safe. Water temperature should not be over 105°F. Have resident check water temperature. Adjust if necessary.

8. Raise the side rail (if bed has one) farthest from you.

9. Place the waterproof pad under the resident's head and shoulders. Cover the resident with the bath blanket. Fold back the top sheet and regular blankets.

10. Place collection container (e.g., trough, basin) under resident's head. Place one towel across the resident's shoulders.

11. Protect resident's eyes with dry washcloth.

12. Use pitcher or attachment to wet hair thoroughly. Apply a small amount of shampoo, usually the size of a quarter.

13. Lather and massage scalp with fingertips. Use a circular motion from front to back (Fig. 12-15). Do not scratch the scalp.

14. Rinse hair until water runs clear. Apply conditioner. Rinse as directed on container.

15. Cover resident's hair with clean towel. Dry his face with washcloth used to protect eyes.

16. Remove trough and waterproof covering.

17. Raise head of bed.

18. Gently rub the scalp and hair with the towel.

19. Dry and comb resident's hair as he or she prefers. See procedure later in the chapter.

20. Make resident comfortable.

21. Return bed to low position if raised. Ensure resident's safety. Return side rails to ordered position. Remove privacy measures.

22. Empty, rinse, and wipe bath basin/pitcher. Return to proper storage.

23. Clean comb/brush. Return hair dryer and comb/brush to proper storage.

24. Place soiled linen in proper container.

25. Leave call light within resident's reach.

26. Wash your hands.

27. Be courteous and respectful at all times.

28. Report any changes in the resident to the nurse. Document procedure using facility guidelines.

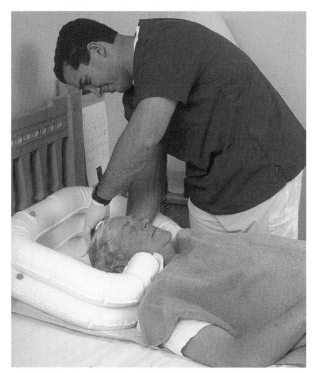

Fig. 12-15. *Use your fingertips to work shampoo into a lather. Be gentle so that you do not scratch the scalp.*

Shampooing

Some residents will have their hair shampooed at a sink. Seat them in a chair that is the correct height for the sink. Pad the edge of the sink so that the neck is comfortable. The resident's head should be tilted back slightly; the head should not be sharply extended beyond its normal range. Carefully spray water over the hair, taking care that the water and shampoo/conditioner do not get into the eyes. Rinse the hair thoroughly.

When assisting a resident on a stretcher with shampooing hair, bring the stretcher to the sink and adjust the height of the stretcher to be even with the sink. Lock the stretcher wheels and fasten safety straps. Raise one side rail on the side farthest from you. Follow the same guidelines as listed above.

Before giving a tub bath or shower, check the room for cleanliness and clean if needed. Pre-fill the tub with warm water and place all needed clean supplies and equipment in the room. Remember not to unnecessarily expose the resident when transporting him or her to the shower or tub room (Fig. 12-16).

Fig. 12-16. *A common style of tub used in nursing homes.* (Photo courtesy of Lee Penner of Penner Tubs.)

Giving a shower or tub bath

Equipment: bath blanket, soap, shampoo, bath thermometer, 2-4 washcloths, 2-4 bath towels, clean gown and robe or clothes, non-skid footwear, gloves, lotion, deodorant

1. Wash your hands.

2. Place equipment in shower or tub room. Clean shower or tub area and shower chair.

3. Wash your hands.

4. Go to resident's room. Identify yourself by name. Identify the resident. Greet the resident by name.

5. Explain procedure to resident. Speak clearly, slowly, and directly. Maintain face-to-face contact whenever possible. Encourage resident to assist if possible.

6. Provide for the resident's privacy with a curtain, screen, or door.

7. Help resident to put on non-skid footwear. Transport resident to shower or tub room.

For a shower:

8. If using a shower chair, place it into position and lock its wheels. Safely transfer resident into shower chair (Fig. 12-17).

Fig. 12-17. *A shower chair must be locked before transferring a resident into it.*

9. Turn on water. Test water temperature with thermometer. Water temperature should be no more than 105°F. Have resident check water temperature.

For a tub bath:

8. Safely transfer resident onto chair or tub lift.

9. Fill the tub halfway with warm water. Test water temperature with thermometer. Water temperature should be no more than 105° F. Have resident check water temperature.

Remaining steps for either procedure:

10. Put on gloves.

11. Help resident remove clothing and shoes.

12. Help the resident into shower or tub. Put shower chair into shower and lock wheels.

13. Stay with resident during the entire procedure.

14. Let resident wash as much as possible on his or her own. Assist to wash his or her face.

15. Help resident shampoo hair. The resident's head should be tilted back slightly for the shampoo. The head should not be sharply extended beyond its normal range. Carefully spray water over the hair, taking care that the water and shampoo/conditioner do not get into the eyes. Rinse the hair thoroughly.

16. Help to wash and rinse the entire body. Move from head to toe (clean to dirty).

17. Turn off water or drain the tub. Cover resident with bath blanket until the tub drains.

18. Unlock shower chair wheels if used. Roll resident out of shower, or help resident out of tub and onto a chair.

19. Give resident towel(s) and help to pat dry. Remember to pat dry under the breasts, between skin folds, in the perineal area, and between toes.

20. Apply lotion and deodorant as needed.

21. Place soiled clothing and linens in proper containers.

22. Remove gloves and dispose of them properly.

23. Wash your hands.

24. Help resident dress and comb hair before leaving shower or tub room (see procedures later in this chapter). Put on non-skid footwear. Return resident to room.

25. Make resident comfortable.

26. Leave call light within resident's reach.

27. Wash your hands.

28. Be courteous and respectful at all times.

29. Report any changes in the resident to the nurse. Document procedure using facility guidelines.

After returning resident to his room, return to shower room, and clean and disinfect the shower or tub area, as well as the shower chair. Wear gloves and follow facility policy. After this is complete, remove and dispose of gloves and wash your hands.

Some residents will have whirlpool baths. These baths are special baths in which the water moves around the tub. The water movement helps clean the body, improve circulation, and promote wound healing. To take a whirlpool bath, the resident must first be covered and kept warm. The resident will need to be safely transported to the whirlpool bath site. The resident will be placed in a chairlift and lowered into the whirlpool bath.

If you assist with this bath, do not leave the resident alone, even for a few seconds. During or after the whirlpool bath, residents may become dizzy or feel faint. If this happens, you may need help to remove the resident from the whirlpool bath. Help the resident as needed. Do not hurry him or her through the bath.

Following a whirlpool bath, safely transport residents back to their rooms, assist with dressing, and make sure they are safe and comfortable. Return to the bath site and clean and disinfect the chair and the whirlpool bath using heavy-duty gloves. Remove and dispose of gloves properly. Wash your hands.

7. Describe how to perform a back rub

Back rubs help relax tired, tense muscles and improve circulation. Residents sometimes request a back massage prior to going to bed in the evening. Back rubs are often given after bathing or prior to going to bed at night. Sometimes back rubs should not be given due to conditions or illnesses. Follow the care plan. If the resident has broken or open skin on his back, apply gloves before giving a back rub.

Giving a back rub

Equipment: bath blanket or towel, lotion

1. Identify yourself by name. Identify the resident. Greet the resident by name.

2. Wash your hands.

3. Explain procedure to resident. Speak clearly, slowly, and directly. Maintain face-to-face contact whenever possible. Encourage resident to assist if possible.

4. Provide for the resident's privacy with a curtain, screen, or door.

5. Practice good body mechanics. Adjust bed to safe working level, usually waist high. Lock bed wheels.

6. Lower the side rail (if bed has one and if it is not already lowered) on side nearest you.

7. Position resident lying on his side or his stomach. Many elderly residents find lying on their stomachs uncomfortable. If so, put him on his side. Cover with a bath blanket. Expose back to the top of the buttocks. Back rubs can also be given with the resident sitting up.

8. Warm lotion by putting bottle in warm water for five minutes. Run your hands under warm water. Pour lotion on your hands. Rub them together. Always put lotion on your hands rather than directly on resident's skin.

9. Place hands on each side of upper part of the buttocks. Use the full palm of hand. Make long, smooth upward strokes with both hands. Move along each side of the spine, up to the shoulders (Figs. 12-18 and 12-19). Circle hands outward. Move back along outer edges of the back. At buttocks, make another circle. Move hands back up to the shoulders. Without taking hands from resident's skin, repeat this motion for three to five minutes.

Fig. 12-18. *A resident on his side.*

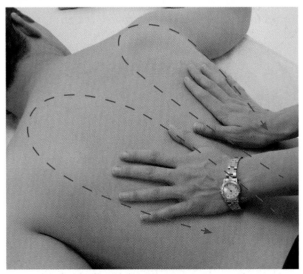

Fig. 12-19. *A resident on his stomach.*

10. Knead with the first two fingers and thumb of each hand. Place them at base of the spine. Move upward together along each side of the spine. Apply gentle downward pressure with fingers and thumbs. Follow same direction as with the long smooth strokes, circling at shoulders and buttocks.

11. Gently massage bony areas (spine, shoulder blades, hip bones). Use circular motions of fingertips. If any of these areas are red, massage around them rather than on them.

12. Finish with some long, smooth strokes.

13. Dry the back if it has extra lotion remaining.

14. Remove bath blanket. Help the resident with getting dressed. Make resident comfortable.

15. Return bed to low position if raised. Ensure resident's safety. Return side rails to ordered position. Remove privacy measures.

16. Store supplies. Place soiled clothing and linens in proper containers.

17. Leave call light within resident's reach.

18. Wash your hands.

19. Be courteous and respectful at all times.

20. Report any changes in the resident to the nurse. Document procedure using facility guidelines.

8. Explain guidelines for performing good oral care

The methods used to care for the mouth, teeth, and gums are called "oral care." Oral care must be provided at least twice a day, but some residents will need or want this care more often. Oral care consists of brushing the teeth and tongue, flossing and caring for dentures (Fig. 12-20). You will learn more about dentures in the next learning objective.

Regular oral care helps prevent gum disease and bad-smelling breath, or **halitosis**. A healthy mouth also promotes a healthy appetite, which can prevent unintended weight loss, a serious problem with the elderly. Quality oral care may also reduce the risk of respiratory infections, such as pneumonia.

Fig. 12-20. *Some supplies needed for oral care.*

Plaque is a substance that forms in a brief period of time if oral care is not done regularly. Plaque can turn into hard deposits, called tartar, if left on the teeth too long. **Tartar** is filled with bacteria and may cause gum disease and loose teeth if they are not removed by a dentist. **Gingivitis** is an inflammation of the gums. This can lead to periodontal disease when the areas supporting the teeth, such as the gums, become diseased. When you give oral care, observe the resident's mouth and teeth to help prevent these and other problems.

Sometimes a problem will be found in the mouth and can be a sign that a bigger problem exists elsewhere in the body. For example, a person who has fruity breath that smells like lemons may have diabetes (see Chapter 23). Observing and reporting signs and symptoms is very important in treating illnesses and preventing them from getting worse.

During oral care, these are observations to note and report to the nurse:

- dry, cracked, bleeding or chapped lips
- cold sores on the lips
- raised areas
- swollen, irritated, red, bleeding or whitish gums
- loose, cracked, chipped, broken or decayed teeth
- yellow-filled or red sores, such as canker sores inside the mouth

- white spots inside the mouth
- infection
- pus or drainage
- coated or swollen tongue
- bad breath or fruity-smelling breath
- change in the resident's ability to drink, suck on a straw, or swallow
- gagging or choking
- resident reports of mouth pain

Always wear gloves when giving oral care. Follow Standard Precautions.

Providing oral care

Equipment: toothbrush, toothpaste, emesis basin, gloves, towel, glass of water

Maintain clean technique with placement of toothbrush throughout procedure.

1. Identify yourself by name. Identify the resident. Greet the resident by name.

2. Wash your hands.

3. Explain procedure to resident. Speak clearly, slowly, and directly. Maintain face-to-face contact whenever possible. Encourage resident to assist if possible.

4. Provide for the resident's privacy with a curtain, screen, or door.

5. Practice good body mechanics. Adjust bed to safe working level, usually waist high. Lock bed wheels. Make sure resident is sitting upright.

6. Lower the side rail (if bed has one and if it is not already lowered) on side nearest you.

7. Put on gloves.

8. Place towel across resident's chest.

9. Wet brush. Put on small amount of toothpaste.

10. Clean entire mouth (including tongue and all surfaces of teeth and the gumline) using gentle strokes. First brush inner, outer and chewing surfaces of the upper teeth, then

do the same with the lower teeth. Use short strokes. Brush back and forth.

11. Hold emesis basin to the resident's chin.

12. Have resident rinse mouth with water and spit into emesis basin (Fig. 12-21).

Fig. 12-21. *Rinsing and spitting removes food particles and toothpaste.*

13. Wipe resident's mouth and remove towel. Make resident comfortable.

14. Return bed to low position if raised. Ensure resident's safety. Return side rails to ordered position. Remove privacy measures.

15. Empty, rinse and wipe emesis basin. Rinse toothbrush. Return supplies to proper storage.

16. Dispose of soiled linen in the proper container.

17. Remove and dispose of gloves properly.

18. Leave call light within resident's reach.

19. Wash your hands.

20. Be courteous and respectful at all times.

21. Report any changes in the resident to the nurse. Report any problems with teeth, mouth, tongue, and lips to nurse. This includes odor, cracking, sores, bleeding, and any discoloration. Document procedure using facility guidelines.

HOT TIP

Edentulous Residents

A resident may not have any teeth. The term for lacking teeth or being toothless is **edentulous**. Giving oral care to an edentulous resident is similar to

caring for a resident who has teeth. You will clean the outside and inside of the mouth, including the lips, top and bottom gums and gumlines, and the inside of the mouth with a moistened swab. Make sure to clean the tongue, too. Change swabs as needed.

A resident who can brush his own teeth will only need a little assistance. The nursing assistant may need to do the following:

- Collect and set up supplies

- Cover the overbed table

- Raise the head of bed

- Provide a bath towel for the chest

- Pour fresh water and mouthwash

- Help with cleaning the face and neck

- Remove the towel, overbed table cover and all supplies

- Empty, clean and store supplies

Encourage the resident to do as much self-care as he is able. Only help the resident with what he cannot do on his own. Wash your hands when you are finished assisting.

Flossing teeth

Equipment: floss, cup with water, emesis basin, gloves, towel

1. Identify yourself by name. Identify the resident. Greet the resident by name.

2. Wash your hands.

3. Explain procedure to resident. Speak clearly, slowly, and directly. Maintain face-to-face contact whenever possible. Encourage resident to assist if possible.

4. Provide for the resident's privacy with a curtain, screen, or door.

5. Practice good body mechanics. Adjust bed to safe working level, usually waist high. Lock bed wheels. Make sure resident is in an upright sitting position.

6. Lower the side rail (if bed has one and if it is not already lowered) on side nearest you.

7. Put on gloves.

8. Wrap the ends of floss securely around each index finger (Fig. 12-22).

Fig. 12-22. *Before beginning, wrap floss securely around each index finger.*

9. Starting with the back teeth, place floss between teeth. Move it down the surface of the tooth. Use a gentle sawing motion (Fig. 12-23).

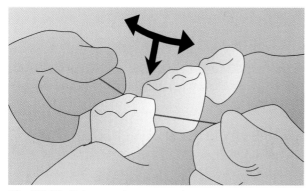

Fig. 12-23. *Being gentle protects the gums.*

Continue to the gum line. At the gum line, curve the floss into a letter C. Slip it gently into the space between the gum and tooth. Then go back up, scraping that side of the tooth (Fig. 12-24). Repeat this on the side of the other tooth.

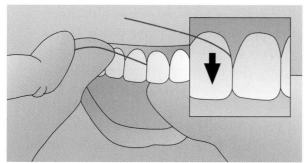

Fig. 12-24. *Floss gently in the space between the gum and tooth. This removes food and prevents tooth decay.*

10. After every two teeth, unwind floss from your fingers. Move it so you are using a clean area. Floss all teeth.

11. Offer water to rinse the mouth. Ask the resident to spit it into the basin.

12. Offer resident a face towel when done flossing all teeth.

13. Return bed to low position if raised. Ensure resident's safety. Return side rails to ordered position. Remove privacy measures.

14. Clean and return supplies to proper storage.

15. Dispose of soiled linen in the proper container.

16. Remove and dispose of gloves properly.

17. Leave call light within resident's reach.

18. Wash your hands.

19. Be courteous and respectful at all times.

20. Report any changes in the resident to the nurse. Report any problems with teeth, mouth, tongue, and lips to nurse. This includes odor, cracking, sores, bleeding, and any discoloration. Document procedure using facility guidelines.

9. Define "dentures" and explain care guidelines

Dentures are artificial teeth. There are different types of dentures. A person may have a full set of dentures, a top or bottom set of dentures, a partial plate, or a bridge. A **bridge** is a type of dental appliance that replaces missing or pulled teeth. A bridge may be permanently placed in the mouth or it may be removable for cleaning.

Dentures are very expensive and time-consuming for a specialist to make. Handle dentures carefully. They are important to residents. Remember, if residents' dentures break, they cannot eat.

Always wear gloves when cleaning dentures. The type of cleaning product used will depend on the resident's preference or facility policy.

After cleaning dentures, store them in a covered denture cup with the resident's name on it. Make sure you match the dentures to the correct resident. Dentures must always be stored in cool water so that they do not dry out and warp. Dentures may crack if left uncovered.

Cleaning and storing dentures

Equipment: denture brush or toothbrush, denture cleanser or tablet, labeled denture cup with cover, 2 towels, gauze squares, gloves, cup with water, emesis basin, denture cream or adhesive (if replacing dentures in mouth)

Maintain clean technique with placement of dentures and the toothbrush throughout procedure.

1. Identify yourself by name. Identify the resident. Greet the resident by name.

2. Wash your hands.

3. Explain procedure to resident. Speak clearly, slowly, and directly. Maintain face-to-face contact whenever possible. Encourage resident to assist if possible.

4. Provide for the resident's privacy with a curtain, screen, or door.

5. Practice good body mechanics. Adjust bed to safe working level, usually waist high. Lock bed wheels. Make sure resident is sitting upright.

6. Lower the side rail (if bed has one and if it is not already lowered) on side nearest you.

7. Put on gloves.

8. Line sink/basin with a towel(s) or fill sink 3/4 full with water. This prevents dentures from breaking if dropped. Handle dentures carefully.

9. If you are allowed to do so, and if a resident cannot remove dentures, you must do it. Ask resident to sit upright.

10. Remove the lower denture first. The lower denture is easier to remove because it floats on the gum line of the lower jaw. Grasp the lower denture with a gauze square (for a

good grip) and remove it. The upper denture is sealed by suction. Firmly grasp the upper denture with a gauze square. Give a slight downward pull to break the suction. Turn it at an angle to take it out of the mouth.

11. Rinse dentures in cool running water before brushing them. Do not use hot water. Hot water may damage dentures.

12. Apply toothpaste or cleanser to toothbrush.

13. Brush the dentures on all surfaces (Fig. 12-25). This includes the inner, outer and chewing surfaces of the upper and lower dentures.

Fig. 12-25. *Brush dentures on all surfaces to properly clean them.*

14. Rinse all surfaces of dentures under cool running water. Do not use hot water.

15. Offer water to rinse the resident's mouth. Ask the resident to spit it into the emesis basin.

16. Rinse denture cup if placing clean dentures inside it.

17. Place dentures in clean denture cup with solution or cool water and cover. Make sure cup is labeled with resident's name. Return denture cup to storage.

18. If replacing dentures in resident's mouth, make sure resident is still sitting upright. Apply denture cream or adhesive to the dentures if needed. When the resident's mouth is open, place upper denture into the mouth by turning it at an angle. Straighten it. Press it onto the upper gum line firmly and evenly (Fig. 12-26). Insert the lower denture onto the gum line of the lower jaw. Press firmly.

Fig. 12-26. *Press upper denture onto the upper gum line firmly and evenly.*

19. Return bed to low position if raised. Ensure resident's safety. Return side rails to ordered position. Remove privacy measures.

20. Clean and return the equipment to proper storage.

21. Dispose of towels in appropriate container or drain sink.

22. Remove and dispose of gloves properly.

23. Leave call light within resident's reach.

24. Wash your hands.

25. Be courteous and respectful at all times.

26. Report any changes in the resident or the appearance of dentures to the nurse. Document procedure using facility guidelines.

10. Discuss guidelines for performing oral care for an unconscious resident

Oral care must be done frequently when a person is unconscious. When a person is unconscious, the mouth becomes dry due to lack of oral fluids, breathing through the mouth, and oxygen therapy. Good oral care keeps the mouth clean and moist.

Crusts called sordes are common on the lips, gums, and teeth of people who are unconscious. These contain microorganisms, certain types of cells, mucus, and food. Quality mouth care can remove sordes and prevent them from developing again.

Aspiration is the primary risk for unconscious residents. **Aspiration** is the inhalation of food or drink into the lungs; it can cause pneumonia or death. Using as little liquid as possible during oral care is the best way to prevent aspiration. Turning unconscious residents on their side before beginning oral care can also help prevent aspiration. In addition, only swabs soaked in tiny amounts of fluid should be used to clean the mouth. Follow the care plan. Chapter 14 has more information on aspiration.

Providing oral care for the unconscious resident

Equipment: sponge swabs, tongue depressor, towel, emesis basin, gloves, lip lubricant, cleaning solution (check the care plan)

1. Identify yourself by name. Identify the resident. Greet the resident by name. Even residents who are unconscious may be able to hear you. Always speak to them as you would to any resident.

2. Wash your hands.

3. Explain procedure to resident. Speak clearly, slowly, and directly. Maintain face-to-face contact whenever possible.

4. Provide for the resident's privacy with a curtain, screen, or door.

5. Practice good body mechanics. Adjust bed to a safe level, usually waist high. Lock bed wheels.

6. Lower the side rail (if bed has one and if it is not already lowered) on side nearest you.

7. Put on gloves.

8. Turn resident's head to the side. Place a towel under his cheek and chin. Place an emesis basin next to the cheek and chin for excess fluid.

9. Hold mouth open with tongue depressor. Do not use your fingers to open the mouth or keep it open.

10. Dip swab in cleaning solution. Wipe inner, outer, and chewing surfaces of the upper and lower teeth, gums, tongue, and inside

surfaces of mouth (Fig. 12-27). Change swab often. Repeat until the mouth is clean.

11. Rinse with clean swab dipped in water.

Fig. 12-27. *Wipe all inside surfaces of the mouth to clean the mouth, stimulate the gums and remove mucus.*

12. Remove the towel and basin. Pat lips or face dry if needed. Apply lip lubricant.

13. Return bed to low position if raised. Ensure resident's safety. Return side rails to ordered position. Remove privacy measures.

14. Clean and return supplies to proper storage.

15. Dispose of soiled linen in the proper container.

16. Remove and dispose of gloves properly.

17. Leave call light within resident's reach.

18. Wash your hands.

19. Be courteous and respectful at all times.

20. Report any changes in the resident to the nurse. Report any problems with teeth, mouth, tongue, and lips to nurse. This includes odor, cracking, sores, bleeding, and any discoloration. Document procedure using facility guidelines.

RESIDENTS' RIGHTS

Unconscious Residents
Even when people are unconscious, they still may be able to hear what is going on around them. Unconscious people have been known to regain consciousness and relate many of the things they heard while they were unconscious. Limit your discussions to appropriate subjects. Speak respectfully and explain what you are doing. Do not talk about anything personal while giving care. Speak to unconscious residents as you would to any resident.

An unconscious resident's eyes usually require special care because they can become dry (Fig. 12-28). The blink reflex is usually absent, leading to drier eyes. The air around the person also contributes to dryness. If you assist in eye care for an unconscious resident, follow these guidelines:

Fig. 12-28. *Unconscious residents may require special eye care. When cleaning the eyes, move from the inner area to the outer area.*

- Use gloves when bathing the eye and use clean washcloths and towels.

- If using a washcloth, rinse the washcloth thoroughly before cleansing the opposite eye. If using cotton balls, always use one cotton ball for one eye and then dispose of it. Do not use the same cotton ball to clean both eyes.

- Wipe from the inner aspect of the eye to the outer canthus of the eye when cleaning. This helps prevent harmful deposits from being pushed into the tear duct at the inner corner of the eye.

- Follow the care plan and special instructions regarding placing moist compresses on the eyes. (More information on compresses is in Chapter 18.)

- Special lubricant may need to be applied to the eyes. Follow the nurse's instructions and the care plan.

11. Explain how to assist with grooming

Grooming is a very important part of the activities of daily living (ADLs). Each day, some residents will require help with brushing and styling their hair, shaving, dressing, caring for fingernails and applying makeup and jewelry.

Appearance has a great deal to do with the way people feel about themselves. Good grooming can have a positive effect on self-esteem, attitude, and independence (Fig. 12-29). A well-groomed person is also likely to feel better physically because she is clean and neatly dressed.

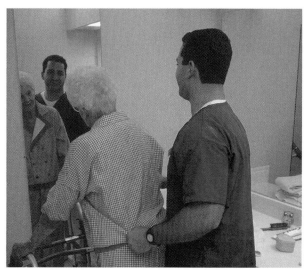

Fig. 12-29. *A well-groomed appearance helps people feel good about themselves.*

When assisting residents with grooming, make sure they do whatever they can for themselves. Promote self-care and independence whenever possible. Follow their preferences and routines, as well as the care plan. Residents may be depressed, angry, or embarrassed about the help they need to perform these tasks. Be sensitive and empathetic.

Shaving

Shaving is a very important part of the daily grooming routine. Wear gloves when shaving residents due to the risk of bleeding. Glove use promotes infection control. Follow Standard Precautions and avoid nicks and cuts.

Guidelines
Shaving

ⓖ Some residents will not want to be shaved. Respect personal preferences for shaving.

ⓖ Wash and comb beards and mustaches every day after asking the resident how he would like it done. Never trim or shave a beard or mustache without the resident's permission.

ⓖ Always wear gloves when shaving.

ⓖ When using safety or disposable razors, soften hair on face first with a warm, wet cloth.

ⓖ Always shave in the direction of the hair growth.

ⓖ Use shaving products, such as after-shave, only with resident's permission.

ⓖ Carefully discard any disposable shaving products in the biohazard container.

Types of razors are electric razors, disposable razors, and safety razors. An electric razor is the safest and easiest type of razor to use. It does not require soap or shaving cream and may help prevent nicks and cuts. Do not use an electric razor near water or any water source, where oxygen is in use, or on a resident who has a pacemaker.

A safety razor requires shaving cream, lotion or soap to be used. These razors are usually very sharp. Safety razors have a special safety casing to help prevent cuts. The blades need to be changed periodically. When changing blades, handle them carefully. Dispose of the old blade in a sharps container.

Disposable razors are used with shaving cream, lotion or soap. They can be extremely sharp and must be used carefully. Discard disposable razors in a sharps container after use. Do not try to reapply the caps on these razors, as it can cause cuts.

Shaving a resident

Equipment: basin, 2 towels, washcloth, bath thermometer, mirror, shaving cream or soap, after-shave (optional), gloves, razor

1. Identify yourself by name. Identify the resident. Greet the resident by name.

2. Wash your hands.

3. Explain procedure to resident. Speak clearly, slowly, and directly. Maintain face-to-face contact whenever possible. Encourage resident to assist if possible.

4. Provide for the resident's privacy with a curtain, screen, or door.

5. Practice good body mechanics. Adjust bed to safe working level, usually waist high. Lock bed wheels.

6. Lower the side rail (if bed has one and if it is not already lowered) on side nearest you.

7. Raise head of bed so resident is sitting up.

Shaving using a safety or disposable razor:

8. Fill bath basin halfway with warm water.

9. Drape towel under resident's chin.

10. Apply gloves.

11. Moisten beard with warm washcloth. Put shaving cream or soap over area.

12. Hold skin taut. Shave beard in downward, short and even strokes on face and upward strokes on neck (Fig. 12-30). Rinse razor often in warm water to keep it clean and wet.

Fig. 12-30. *Shave in downward strokes on face and upward strokes on neck.*

13. Offer mirror to resident.

14. Wash, rinse, and dry face after shave. Apply after-shave lotion if requested.

15. Remove towel.

16. Remove and dispose of gloves properly. Wash your hands.

Shaving using an electric razor:

8. Do not use an electric razor near any water source, when oxygen is in use, or if resident has a pacemaker.

9. Drape towel under resident's chin.

10. Apply gloves.

11. Apply pre-shave lotion as resident wishes.

12. Hold skin taut. Shave with smooth, even movements. Shave beard with back and forth motion in direction of beard growth with foil shaver. Shave beard in circular motion with three-head shaver.

13. Offer mirror to resident.

14. Apply after-shave lotion as resident wishes.

15. Remove towel.

16. Remove and dispose of gloves properly. Wash your hands.

Final steps:

17. Make sure that resident and environment are free of loose hairs. Make resident comfortable.

18. Return bed to low position if raised. Ensure resident's safety. Return side rails to ordered position. Remove privacy measures.

19. For safety razor: Rinse safety razor. For disposable razor: Dispose of a disposable razor in biohazard container. For electric razor: Clean head of electric razor. Remove whiskers from razor. Recap shaving head. Return razor to case.

20. Return supplies and equipment to proper storage.

21. Dispose of soiled linen in the proper container.

22. Leave call light within resident's reach.

23. Wash your hands.

24. Be courteous and respectful at all times.

25. Report any changes in the resident to the nurse. Document procedure using facility guidelines.

If assisting a woman with shaving, do not shave any facial or body hair she wants to keep. For example, some women do not shave their underarms or legs. Do not judge a resident's personal preferences for shaving. When shaving underarms, be gentle. Be careful to avoid nicks and cuts. Shave in the direction of hair growth.

Nail Care

Good grooming includes regular nail care. Fingernails can collect and harbor microorganisms. In addition, long and ragged nails can easily scratch residents, visitors, and staff. Washing and cleaning the nails is a part of the bathing process.

Fingernail care usually requires the use of an orangewood stick. These small sticks are made of wood and help clean under the nails. If you use an orangewood stick, be gentle to avoid injuring the resident. Emery boards are used for filing the nails. Nail files can tear fragile skin around the nail and must be used carefully.

Do not cut a resident's toenails. Problems with circulation can lead to a serious infection if skin is accidentally cut while caring for the nails. For a resident who has diabetes (Chapter 23), an infection can lead to a severe wound or even amputation. Follow the care plan. Never use the same nail equipment on more than one resident.

Providing fingernail care

Equipment: orangewood stick, emery board, lotion, basin, soap, gloves, washcloth, 2 towels, bath thermometer

1. Identify yourself by name. Identify the resident. Greet the resident by name.

2. Wash your hands.

3. Explain procedure to resident. Speak clearly, slowly, and directly. Maintain face-to-face contact whenever possible. Encourage resident to assist if possible.

4. Provide for the resident's privacy with a curtain, screen, or door.

5. Practice good body mechanics. If the resident is in bed, adjust bed to safe working level, usually waist high. Lock bed wheels.

6. Lower the side rail (if bed has one and if it is not already lowered) on side nearest you.

7. Fill the basin halfway with warm water. Test water temperature with thermometer or your wrist. Ensure it is safe. Water temperature should not be over 105°F. Have resident check water temperature. Adjust if necessary.

8. Place basin at a comfortable level for resident. Soak the resident's nails in the basin of water. Soak all ten fingertips for at least five minutes.

9. Remove hands. Wash hands with soapy washcloth. Rinse. Pat hands dry with towel, including between fingers.

10. Put on gloves.

11. Place resident's hands on the towel. Gently use pointed end of the orangewood stick to remove dirt from under the nails (Fig. 12-31).

Fig. 12-31. *Be gentle when removing dirt from under the nails with an orangewood stick.*

12. Wipe orangewood stick on towel after each nail. Wash resident's hands again. Dry them thoroughly.

13. Groom nails with file or emery board. File in a curve.

14. Finish with nails smooth and free of rough edges.

15. Apply lotion from fingertips to wrists. Make resident comfortable.

16. Return bed to low position if raised. Ensure resident's safety. Return side rails to ordered position. Remove privacy measures.

17. Empty, rinse, and wipe basin. Return to proper storage.

18. Dispose of soiled linen in the proper container.

19. Remove and dispose of gloves properly.

20. Leave call light within resident's reach.

21. Wash your hands.

22. Be courteous and respectful at all times.

23. Report any changes in the resident to the nurse. Document procedure using facility guidelines.

HOT TIP

Cosmetics

Cosmetics or makeup are items used to enhance beauty or cleanse and improve the face, skin, hair, and nails. Women usually use them more, although some men use them. Help to apply cosmetics as residents request. The application of makeup, including type and amount, should be based on residents' wishes. However, if staff note too much makeup on a resident, gentle suggestions may be offered.

Information on foot care is in the section on diabetes in Chapter 23.

Hair Care

Daily hair care affects the way residents look and feel about themselves. NAs help keep residents' hair clean and styled. It is important to allow residents to choose their own hairstyles. Use hair ornaments only as requested. Do not comb or brush residents' hair into a childish style.

Be very gentle when handling residents' hair. Hair usually thins as people age. Pieces of hair can be pulled out of the head while combing or brushing the hair. Also, the skin on an elderly person's head is fragile. Be careful when working with hair.

Do not cut residents' hair. Many facilities have a barber, beautician, and/or professional hairstylist available to residents. If residents make a hair appointment, help them get ready to go.

Dandruff is a skin condition in which dry, white flakes appear on the scalp and hair due to shedding of dead skin from the scalp. Itching can accompany the white flakes.

Causes of dandruff include the following:

- climate, especially dry, cold areas
- stress
- excessive sweating
- a type of fungus
- hormonal changes
- some types of dermatitis

Dandruff cannot be stopped but can be controlled by using a medicated dandruff shampoo regularly.

Combing or brushing hair

Equipment: comb, brush, towel, mirror, hair care items requested by resident

Use hair care products that the resident prefers for his or her type of hair.

1. Identify yourself by name. Identify the resident. Greet the resident by name.

2. Wash your hands.

3. Explain procedure to resident. Speak clearly, slowly, and directly. Maintain face-to-face contact whenever possible. Encourage resident to assist if possible.

4. Provide for the resident's privacy with a curtain, screen, or door.

5. Practice good body mechanics. If the resident is in bed, adjust bed to safe working level, usually waist high. Lock bed wheels.

6. Lower the side rail (if bed has one and if it is not already lowered) on side nearest you.

7. Raise head of bed so resident is sitting up. Place a towel under the head or around the shoulders.

8. Remove any hair pins, hair ties and clips.

9. Remove tangles first by dividing hair into small sections. Gently comb out from ends of hair to scalp. Be careful not to break hair or cause any discomfort.

10. After tangles are removed, brush two-inch sections of hair at a time. Brush from roots to ends (Fig. 12-32).

Fig. 12-32. Gently brush hair from roots to ends.

11. Neatly style hair as resident prefers. Avoid childish hairstyles. Each resident may prefer different styles and different hair products. Offer mirror to resident.

12. Make resident comfortable.

13. Return bed to low position if raised. Ensure resident's safety. Return side rails to ordered position. Remove privacy measures.

14. Return supplies to proper storage. Clean hair from brush/comb. Clean comb and brush.

15. Dispose of soiled linen in the proper container.

16. Leave call light within resident's reach.

17. Wash your hands.

18. Be courteous and respectful at all times.

19. Report any changes in the resident to the nurse. Document procedure using facility guidelines.

Pediculosis is the medical term for an infestation of lice. Lice are tiny parasites that attach their eggs to the skin or the hair. Lice are very hard to see with the eye alone. Parts of the body that may have lice infestation include the head, the pubic area and other areas of the body, such as the underarms.

Symptoms of lice include intense itching, scratching, and scratch marks or rashes on the scalp, neck, or body. Lice eggs can be seen on the hair, behind the ears and on the neck. The eggs are small and round. They are brown before they hatch and white to light brown after hatching. Lice droppings may be visible on sheets or pillows. They look like a fine black powder.

If you note any of these symptoms, report them to the nurse immediately. Lice can spread very quickly. The resident's roommates, spouse, partner, and family and friends may also need to be checked for lice.

Lice can be transmitted through sharing personal items, such as combs, brushes and clothing. They can also be transmitted by sexual contact or sleeping in the same bed with someone who has lice. Do not share residents' combs, brushes, clothing, hats, scarves, caps, wigs, and hairpieces. Lice can be eliminated by using special shampoo, creams, lotions and sprays. Hot water must be used on bed linens and clothing to remove lice. Things that cannot be washed may have to be discarded.

Dressing and Undressing

Dressing and undressing residents is an important part of daily care. Residents may have one side of the body that is weaker than the other side due to stroke or injury. This side is called the "weaker," "affected" or "involved" side. Do not refer to it as the "bad side" or use the terms "bad leg" or "bad arm." When dressing residents, always begin with the weaker side of the body to reduce the risk of injury.

The acronym POW can be used to help you remember to put clothing on the weak side first.

Put

On

Weak

Do the opposite when removing clothing. Begin with the stronger, or unaffected, side first when undressing.

Treat residents' clothing carefully when dressing and/or undressing residents. They may have clothing that is very meaningful to them.

Guidelines
Dressing

- Encourage residents to be as independent as possible when dressing and undressing. Dressing and undressing can increase muscle strength, stimulate circulation, and may help promote self-esteem.

- Additional time is needed when residents dress themselves. Do not rush them through this process.

- Make sure all clothing is marked with the resident's name, if policy at your facility.

- Be careful when handling residents' clothing. Request that clothing be mended when rips or tears are noted.

- Allow residents to choose their own clothing. Encourage use of regular clothing, not nightwear or pajamas.

- Clothing should fit the resident well. Report if clothing is too tight or too loose.

- Always provide privacy when dressing or undressing residents. Cover residents at all times. Do not expose any more than what is necessary.

- Apply clothing to the weaker, or affected side first (Fig. 12-33).

- Be gentle with the feet and legs when applying socks or stockings. Report to the nurse if socks are too tight. Smooth both socks to remove wrinkles and twists.

- Bras should fit female residents properly. Breasts should fit inside the bra cups. Assist females with putting on bras if needed. A bra that fastens in the front can be easier for residents to put on by themselves. Bras that fasten in the back can be applied more easily if wrapped around the waist, fastened and then rotated around to the proper position. Put arms through straps last.

- Slacks, pants, and skirts that have elastic waists are easier to get on and off. Waistbands should fit comfortably and not be twisted. Belts, if used, should not be too tight.

- Use special dressing aids, called assistive or adaptive devices, whenever needed. These help residents dress themselves (Fig. 12-34). See Chapter 25 for more information on assistive devices.

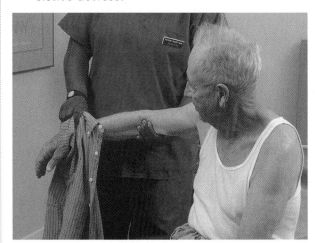

Fig. 12-33. *When dressing residents, start with the affected (weaker) side first.*

Fig. 12-34. *Special dressing aids promote independence by helping residents dress themselves.* (Photo courtesy of North Coast Medical, Inc., www.ncmedical.com, 800-821-9319)

Dressing a resident

Equipment: clean clothes of resident's choice, non-skid footwear

When putting on all items, move resident's body gently and naturally. Avoid force and over-extension of limbs and joints.

1. Identify yourself by name. Identify the resident. Greet the resident by name.

2. Wash your hands.

3. Explain procedure to resident. Speak clearly, slowly, and directly. Maintain face-to-face contact whenever possible. Encourage resident to assist if possible.

4. Provide for the resident's privacy with a curtain, screen, or door.

5. Ask resident what she would like to wear (Fig. 12-35). Dress her in outfit of choice.

Fig. 12-35. *Encourage residents to choose what they want to wear. This promotes their independence, as well as their legal right to choose.*

6. Remove resident's gown. Do not completely expose resident. Take off stronger, or unaffected, side first when undressing.

7. Gather up sleeve to ease pulling over affected arm. Insert your hand through sleeve and grasp resident's hand to support arm while dressing. Assist resident to put the affected/ weak arm through the right sleeve of the shirt, sweater, or slip before placing garment on the unaffected arm.

8. Help resident to put on skirt, pants, or dress. Put the affected/weak leg through skirt or pants first. Raise the buttocks or turn resident from side to side to draw pants over the buttocks up to waist.

9. Place bed at a safe level for resident, usually the lowest position.

10. Apply socks, pulling them up until they are both smooth and without wrinkles. Apply non-skid footwear. Tie laces.

11. Finish with resident dressed appropriately. Make sure clothing is right-side out and zippers/buttons are fastened.

12. Remove privacy measures.

13. Place gown in soiled linen container.

14. Leave call light within resident's reach.

15. Wash your hands.

16. Be courteous and respectful at all times.

17. Report any changes in the resident to the nurse. Document procedure using facility guidelines.

Remember when undressing residents to remove clothing from the stronger, or unaffected, side first.

HOT TIP

Dressing Residents with IVs

When a resident has an IV, you may need to help him or her dress and undress. Remove the clothing starting with the stronger, or unaffected, side. In this case, the unaffected side is the side without the IV. Slowly pull off clothing, sliding it over the tubing. Lift the IV bag off the hook and pull the garment over the bag. Do not pull on or catch the tubing in the clothing. Keep the IV bag above the IV site at all times. Hang the bag back on the hook.

Apply clothing by starting with the weaker, or affected side. In this case the affected side is the side with the IV. Lift the bag off of the hook, and slide the clean clothing over the bag. Hang the bag back on the hook. Gently pull the clothing over the tubing and the arm. Pull the clothing over the other arm and secure clothing. Check to make sure that the tubing is not kinked after you are finished. If you note the IV is not dripping, report to the nurse immediately. Ask the nurse to check the IV if you have concerns.

CHAPTER REVIEW

1. Define the terms "hygiene" and "grooming" (LO 2).

2. List three ways nursing assistants can help promote residents' dignity when performing personal care (LO 2).

3. Explain what a partial bath is and list two reasons why it may be suitable for certain residents (LO 3).

4. Which serious skin wound can nursing assistants help prevent by observing residents' skin closely (LO 3)?

5. List 20 things that are important to observe for and report during personal care and bathing (LO 3).

6. List two reasons residents should be covered before transporting them to the shower room (LO 4).

7. Why should the use of bath oils and gels be avoided when bathing residents (LO 4)?

8. List the correct order of washing parts of the body (LO 5).

9. How often should the perineal area be bathed (LO 6)?

10. Why should residents be involved in choosing a comfortable water temperature (LO 6)?

11. In the procedure "Giving a complete bed bath," step 10 states that nursing assistants should ask the resident to participate in washing. Why (LO 6)?

12. List three benefits of a whirlpool bath (LO 6).

13. What are two benefits of back rubs (LO 7)?

14. How often should oral care be performed (LO 8)?

15. List ten items to observe and report about oral care (LO 8).

16. Why is it important to handle dentures carefully (LO 9)?

17. Explain why hot water should not be used when cleaning dentures (LO 9).

18. What is the best way to prevent aspiration when performing oral care on unconscious residents (LO 10)?

19. Why should nursing assistants explain what they are doing when working with unconscious residents (LO 10)?

20. Should nursing assistants wear gloves when shaving residents? Why or why not (LO 11)?

21. In what circumstances should an electric razor not be used (LO 11)?

22. Why should nursing assistants not cut residents' toenails (LO 11)?

23. Why should nursing assistants be gentle when handling residents' hair (LO 11)?

24. In the section on hair care, it reads, "Do not comb or brush residents' hair into a childish style." Why should nursing assistants not do that (LO 11)?

25. Why is it important not to share personal items with residents who have lice (LO 11)?

26. When dressing and undressing residents, how should nursing assistants refer to the weaker side (LO 11)?

27. When dressing a resident, on which side should a nursing assistant start? When undressing a resident, on which side should a nursing assistant start (LO 11)?

13
Vital Signs

The Invention of the Stethoscope

In 1816, René Théophile Hyacinthe Laënnec had difficulty hearing the heartbeat of a large-sized woman. He solved the problem creatively. Using a rolled-up piece of paper, he placed his ear to one end of the paper and placed the other end over the heart. He realized he could actually hear her heartbeat. This ability to hear the heartbeat so clearly was the beginning of what we now call the stethoscope.

"The same heart beats in every human breast."

Matthew Arnold, 1822-1888

"Once Antigones was told his son was ill, and went to see him. At the door he met some young beauty. Going in, he sat down by the bed and took his pulse. 'The fever,' said Demetrius, 'has just left me.' 'Oh, Yes,' replied the father, 'I met it going out at the door.' "

Plutarch, A.D. 46-120

1. Define important words in this chapter

apical pulse: the pulse on the left side of the chest, just below the nipple.

apnea: the absence of breathing; may be temporary.

BPM: the abbreviation for "beats per minute."

brachial pulse: the pulse inside the elbow; used to measure blood pressure.

bradycardia: a slow heart rate; under 60 beats per minute.

Celsius: the centigrade temperature scale in which the boiling point of water is 100 degrees and the freezing point of water is 0 degrees.

Cheyne-Stokes respiration: type of respiration with periods of apnea lasting at least 10 seconds, along with alternating periods of slow, irregular respirations or rapid, shallow respirations.

diastolic: second measurement of blood pressure; phase when the heart relaxes.

dilate: to widen.

dyspnea: difficulty breathing.

eupnea: normal respirations.

expiration: the process of exhaling air out of the lungs.

Fahrenheit: a temperature scale where the boiling point of water is 212 degrees and the freezing point of water is 32 degrees.

hypertension: high blood pressure.

hypotension: low blood pressure.

hypothermia: a condition in which body temperature drops below the level required for normal functioning; severe sub-normal body temperature.

inspiration: the process of inhaling air into the lungs.

orthopnea: shortness of breath when lying down that is relieved by sitting up.

orthostatic hypotension: a sudden drop in blood pressure that occurs when a person stands up; also called postural hypotension.

prehypertension: a condition in which a person has a systolic measurement of 120–139 mm Hg and a diastolic measurement of 80–89 mm Hg; indicator that the person does not have high blood pressure now but is likely to have it in the future.

radial pulse: the pulse on the inside of the wrist, where the radial artery runs just beneath the skin.

respiration: the process of inhaling air into the lungs (inspiration) and exhaling air out of the lungs (expiration).

sphygmomanometer: a device that measures blood pressure.

stethoscope: an instrument used to hear sounds in the human body, such as the heartbeat or pulse, breathing sounds, or bowel sounds.

systolic: first measurement of blood pressure; phase when the heart is at work, contracting and pushing blood out of the left ventricle.

tachycardia: a fast heartbeat, over 100 beats per minute.

tachypnea: rapid respirations.

thermometer: a device used for measuring the degree of heat or cold.

vital signs: measurements that monitor the function of the vital organs of the body.

2. Discuss the relationship of vital signs to health and well-being

The **vital signs** consist of body temperature, pulse, respirations, blood pressure, and pain level. Vital signs are important readings that monitor the function of the vital organs of the body. They can indicate whether the body is healthy or ill.

Checking residents' vital signs periodically during the day is an important nursing assistant task. Medical providers are always watching for signs of illness. The first sign that a person is ill may be a change in his or her vital signs. When one or more of the vital signs is too high or too low, it signals a potential health problem. This is why it is so important to accurately report changes in vital signs to the nurse.

You will learn more about how to take vital signs and factors that affect vital sign readings later in this chapter. See the box below for a list of normal ranges for vital signs.

Normal Ranges for Adult Vital Signs

Temp. Site	Fahrenheit	Celsius
Oral	97.6° - 99.6°	36.5° - 37.5°
Rectal	98.6° - 100.6°	37.0° - 38.1°
Axillary	96.6° - 98.6°	36.0° - 37.0°

Pulse: 60-100 beats per minute

Respirations: 12-20 respirations per minute

Blood Pressure
Normal
  Systolic: 100-139
  Diastolic: 60-89

High
  140/90 or above

Low
  Below 100/60

RESIDENTS' RIGHTS

Never guess on vital signs.
When measuring vital signs, readings may be difficult to obtain on some residents. If you cannot get a reading, do not guess. If you record a guess, it is illegal and it may put a resident's life in danger. Nurses and doctors make care decisions based on your reports. If you cannot obtain a proper reading, tell the nurse. Always be truthful and accurate in your reporting.

3. Identify factors that affect body temperature

Body temperature is controlled by the hypothalamus in the brain. The hypothalamus regulates body temperature by balancing the amount of heat the body makes with the amount of heat the body loses.

Body temperature averages 98.6°F (Fahrenheit) or 37°C (Celsius). A normal temperature is a sign of well-being. A high or low temperature may indicate a problem or an illness.

There are many factors that affect body temperature, including the following:

- **The person's age**: Elderly people normally have less fat in their bodies, so they may not be able to prevent heat loss and may feel colder. Reduced blood circulation may also cause changes in body temperature (Fig. 13-1).

- **Amount of exercise**: Exercise helps increase body temperature due to the contraction of muscles that produce heat.

- **The circadian rhythm**: You first learned about the circadian rhythm, which is the 24-hour day-night cycle, in Chapter 10. Average temperature readings change during a 24-hour day. People may have lower average temperatures in the morning and higher temperatures in the late afternoon and evening.

- **Stress**: When a person is experiencing stress, certain hormones are released into the body. This hormonal shift may increase body temperature.

- **Illnesses**: Illnesses, such as infections, can increase body temperature. Some infections also cause dehydration, which is a serious condition in which a person does not have enough fluid in the body. When fluid levels are too low, body temperature may increase in response. Other illnesses, like diabetes, cause poor circulation and also affect body temperature.

- **Environment**: The temperature inside and outside influences body temperature. The elderly may become chilled or overheated easily. Drafts in a room also increase the risk of chills. Adjusting the room temperature, layering clothing and using blankets can help.

Fig. 13-1. *Elderly people usually have less fat and decreased circulation, which may make them feel colder.*

People may have body temperatures that are below normal. Sub-normal body temperatures are temperatures below 97°F. Some causes of sub-normal body temperature are infection, alcohol usage, diabetes, problems with the thyroid gland, or exposure to extreme cold. Severe sub-normal body temperature is called hypothermia. **Hypothermia** is a condition in which body temperature drops below the level required for normal functioning. It is a dangerous condition and can lead to death if not treated. Signs and symptoms of hypothermia must be reported to the nurse immediately:

- Shivering
- Numbness
- Quick and shallow breathing
- Slow movements
- Mild confusion
- Changes in mental status
- Pale and/or bluish (cyanotic) skin

Hypothermia is treated with specific warming techniques. Report sub-normal body temperatures to the nurse promptly.

An increase in body temperature may indicate an infection or disease. Signs and symptoms of a fever, in addition to the temperature reading, include headache, fatigue, muscle aches, and chills. Skin may feel warm and look flushed. Residents with darker skin tones who have a fever may show subtle skin color changes. In this case, feel the forehead for warmth when suspecting a fever.

If you suspect a fever, always take a temperature (see next Learning Objective). Fevers develop quickly. It is possible to detect an infection early and prevent complications from occurring. Report fevers to the nurse immediately.

4. List guidelines for taking body temperature

Thermometers measure heat or cold in either degrees **Fahrenheit** (F) or **Celsius** (C). Fahrenheit and Celsius are two different scales that are used to measure temperature. The Fahrenheit scale is more common in the United States. In degrees Fahrenheit (F), each long line represents one degree and each short line represents two-tenths of a degree. In degrees Celsius (C), the long lines represent one degree and the short lines represent one-tenth of a degree (Fig. 13-2). In most other countries, the Celsius scale is used, along with the metric system of measurement.

Fig. 13-2. *This shows a normal temperature reading: 98.6°F and 37°C.*

There are four main sites on the body for measuring a temperature: the mouth (oral), the rectum (rectal), the armpit (axillary), and the ear (tympanic). Taking a temperature orally is most common. A rectal temperature is considered to be the most accurate, while an axillary temperature is considered to be the least accurate.

Common types of thermometers are:

*   mercury-free glass
*   digital
*   electronic
*   disposable
*   tympanic
*   temporal artery thermometer

The mercury-free thermometer can be used to take an oral, rectal, or axillary temperature. Thermometers are usually color-coded to tell you which is an oral and which is a rectal thermometer. Oral thermometers are usually green or blue. Rectal thermometers are usually red (Fig. 13-3).

Fig. 13-3. *A mercury-free oral thermometer and a mercury-free rectal thermometer. (Photos courtesy of RG Medical Diagnostics of Southfield, MI.)*

Digital thermometers can be used to take an oral, rectal, or axillary temperature. This thermometer displays results digitally. A digital thermometer usually takes two to 60 seconds to show the temperature. The thermometer will usually flash or beep when the temperature has registered. These models are battery-operated and require that the battery be replaced periodically. A digital thermometer requires the use of a disposable plastic sheath used to cover the probe (Fig. 13-4). This helps prevent infection. The sheath is used once and then disposed of in a facility-approved container.

Fig. 13-4. *A digital thermometer with a disposable sheath cover.*

The electronic thermometer is battery-operated and is stored in a wall unit for recharging when not in use (Fig. 13-5). It can be used to take an oral, rectal, or axillary temperature. An electronic thermometer registers the temperature digitally in two to 60 seconds. The thermometer flashes or makes a sound when the temperature is displayed. The probe on an electric thermometer must have a probe cover applied before use. The probe cover is used on only one person and is then disposed of properly. The probe cover cannot be used on more than one resident.

Fig. 13-5. *An electronic thermometer.*

A disposable thermometer can be used to take oral or axillary temperatures. This type of thermometer is for single use, meaning it is used once and then disposed of in the proper container. It does not require the use of a disposable sheath. A disposable thermometer helps reduce the risk of infection, since it is only used on one resident. These types of thermometers are often used on residents who are in isolation. The temperature reading registers in approximately 60 seconds. A disposable thermometer is made of rigid plastic and must be removed slowly to avoid causing tears in the mouth.

A tympanic thermometer is used to measure the temperature reading in the ear (Fig. 13-6). It registers the temperature in seconds. When using this thermometer, it is important to follow instructions to get as accurate a reading as possible. Ear wax may cause an inaccurate reading. Ear injury is possible with this thermometer. Hearing aids may need to be removed before taking a temperature this way.

Fig. 13-6. *A tympanic thermometer.*

Another type of thermometer is the temporal artery thermometer (Fig. 13-7). This is an infrared thermometer that measures the temperature of the temporal artery, the artery under the skin of the forehead. The probe on the thermometer is moved straight across the forehead to obtain a reading. It is non-invasive, meaning it does not require a probe to be inserted into the ear, the mouth, under the arm, or in the rectum. Clothing does not need to be removed in order to take a temperature. If temporal artery thermometers are used at your facility, you will be trained how to use them.

Fig. 13-7. *A temporal artery thermometer.* (Photo courtesy of Exergen Corporation, 800-422-3006, www.exergen.com.)

Temperatures are often taken orally. Do not take an oral temperature on a person who:

- is unconscious

- is using oxygen

- is confused or disoriented

- is paralyzed from stroke

- has facial trauma

- is likely to have a seizure

- has a nasogastric or orogastric tube (Chapter 26)

- is younger than six years old

- has sores, redness, swelling, or pain in the mouth

- has an injury to the face or neck

Fig. 13-8. *Shake thermometer down to below the lowest number before inserting in a resident's mouth.*

Measuring and recording oral temperature

Equipment: mercury-free glass, digital, or electronic thermometer, gloves, disposable plastic sheath/cover for thermometers, tissues, pen and paper

Do not take an oral temperature on a resident who has eaten or drank fluids within the last 10–20 minutes.

1. Identify yourself by name. Identify the resident. Greet the resident by name.

2. Wash your hands.

3. Explain procedure to resident. Speak clearly, slowly, and directly. Maintain face-to-face contact whenever possible. Encourage resident to assist if possible.

4. Provide for the resident's privacy with a curtain, screen, or door.

5. Put on gloves.

Using a mercury-free glass thermometer:

6. Hold thermometer by stem.

7. Before inserting thermometer in resident's mouth, shake thermometer down to below the lowest number (at least below 96°F or 35°C). To shake thermometer down, hold it at the end opposite the bulb with the thumb and two fingers. With a snapping motion of the wrist, shake the thermometer (Fig. 13-8). Stand away from furniture and walls while doing so.

8. Put on disposable sheath, if applicable. Gently insert bulb end of thermometer into resident's mouth. Place it under tongue and to one side (Fig. 13-9). Resident should breathe through his or her nose.

Fig. 13-9. *Insert thermometer under the resident's tongue and to one side.*

9. Tell resident to hold thermometer in mouth with lips closed. Assist as necessary. Ask the resident not to bite down or to talk.

10. Leave thermometer in place for at least three minutes.

11. Remove the thermometer. Wipe with tissue from stem to bulb or remove sheath. Dispose of tissue or sheath.

12. Hold thermometer at eye level. Roll thermometer between your thumb and forefinger until the line appears. Read temperature. Remember the temperature reading.

13. Clean thermometer according to facility policy. Return it to plastic case or container. Store it away from any heat source.

Using a digital thermometer:

6. Put on disposable sheath.

7. Turn on thermometer. Wait until "ready" sign appears.

8. Insert end of digital thermometer into resident's mouth. Place under tongue and to one side.

9. Leave in place until thermometer blinks or beeps.

10. Remove the thermometer.

11. Read temperature on display screen. Remember the temperature reading.

12. Using a tissue, remove and dispose of sheath.

13. Clean thermometer according to facility policy. Replace thermometer in case.

Using an electronic thermometer:

6. Remove probe from base unit.

7. Put on probe cover.

8. Insert the covered probe into resident's mouth. Place under tongue and to one side.

9. Leave in place until you hear a tone or see a flashing or steady light.

10. Read the temperature on the display screen. Remember the temperature reading.

11. Remove the probe.

12. Press the eject button to discard the cover (Fig. 13-10).

Fig. 13-10. *Eject the probe cover after use.*

13. Return the probe to the holder.

Final steps for all methods:

14. Remove privacy measures. Make resident comfortable.

15. Remove and dispose of gloves properly.

16. Leave call light within resident's reach.

17. Wash your hands.

18. Be courteous and respectful at all times.

19. Report any changes in the resident to the nurse. Document procedure using facility guidelines. Record resident's name, temperature, date, time, and method used (oral).

HOT TIP

Mercury Glass Thermometers

Using glass bulb or mercury thermometers to take oral, rectal, or axillary temperatures is no longer common because mercury is a dangerous, toxic substance. Many healthcare facilities now discourage the use of mercury, and some states have passed laws to ban the sale of mercury.

If your facility uses mercury glass thermometers, use cool water to rinse it. Do not use hot water because it can heat the mercury and break the thermometer. If a mercury thermometer breaks, tell the nurse immediately. Do not touch the mercury or the broken glass. Specific procedures have to be followed to clean and dispose of mercury safely and properly.

Taking rectal temperatures may be necessary for unconscious residents, residents with poorly-fitting dentures or missing teeth, or residents who have difficulty breathing through the nose, have a seizure disorder or have been vomiting. Rectal thermometers should be lubricated and inserted carefully not more than one inch for adults. Explain clearly what you will be doing before starting this procedure. When taking a rectal temperature you must stay with the resident for the entire time the thermometer is in place. You must also hold the thermometer in place the entire time it is in the rectum. Ask the resident to be very still during this procedure, and explain that it will only take a few minutes.

Measuring and recording rectal temperature

Equipment: rectal mercury-free glass, digital or electronic thermometer, lubricant, gloves, tissue, disposable plastic sheath/cover, pen and paper

1. Identify yourself by name. Identify the resident. Greet the resident by name.

2. Wash your hands.

3. Explain procedure to resident. Speak clearly, slowly, and directly. Maintain face-to-face contact whenever possible. Encourage resident to assist if possible.

4. Provide for the resident's privacy with a curtain, screen, or door.

5. Practice good body mechanics. Adjust bed to safe working level, usually waist high. Lock bed wheels.

6. Lower the side rail (if bed has one and if it is not already lowered) on side nearest you.

7. Help the resident to left-lying (Sims') position (Fig. 13-11).

Fig. 13-11. *The resident must be in the left-lying (Sims') position.*

8. Fold back linens to expose only rectal area.

9. Put on gloves.

10. **Mercury-free glass thermometer**: Hold thermometer by stem. Shake thermometer down to below the lowest number.

    Put on disposable sheath. Apply small amount of lubricant to sheath.

    Digital thermometer: Put on disposable sheath. Apply small amount of lubricant to sheath.

    Turn on thermometer. Wait until "ready" sign appears.

Electronic thermometer: Remove probe from base unit. Put on probe cover. Apply small amount of lubricant to cover.

11. Separate the buttocks. Gently insert thermometer one inch into rectum (Fig. 13-12). Stop if you meet resistance. Do not force the thermometer in the rectum.

Fig. 13-12. *Gently insert a rectal thermometer one inch into the rectum. Do not force it into the rectum.*

12. Replace sheet over buttocks. Hold onto the thermometer at all times.

13. **Mercury-free glass thermometer**: Hold thermometer in place for at least three minutes.

    Digital thermometer: Hold thermometer in place until thermometer blinks or beeps.

    Electronic thermometer: Leave in place until you hear a tone or see a flashing or steady light.

14. Gently remove the thermometer. Wipe with tissue from stem to bulb or remove sheath or cover. Dispose of tissue.

15. Read thermometer as you would for an oral temperature. Remember the temperature reading.

16. **Mercury-free glass thermometer**: Clean thermometer according to facility policy. Return it to plastic case or container.

    Digital thermometer: Discard sheath. Clean thermometer according to facility policy. Return thermometer to storage area.

Electronic thermometer: Discard the cover. Return probe to holder.

17. Remove and dispose of gloves properly. Wash your hands.

18. Make resident comfortable.

19. Return bed to low position if raised. Ensure resident's safety. Return side rails to ordered position. Remove privacy measures.

20. Leave call light within resident's reach.

21. Wash your hands.

22. Be courteous and respectful at all times.

23. Report any changes in the resident to the nurse. Document procedure using facility guidelines. Record resident's name, temperature, date, time, and method used (rectal).

Tympanic thermometers take fast temperature readings. When taking a tympanic temperature, let the resident know that you will be placing the tip of the thermometer in his ear and that it should be painless. The tip of the thermometer will only go into the ear one-quarter to one-half inch. Follow the manufacturer's instructions, as models vary.

Measuring and recording tympanic temperature

Equipment: tympanic thermometer, gloves, disposable probe sheath/cover, pen and paper

1. Identify yourself by name. Identify the resident. Greet the resident by name.

2. Wash your hands.

3. Explain procedure to resident. Speak clearly, slowly, and directly. Maintain face-to-face contact whenever possible. Encourage resident to assist if possible.

4. Provide for the resident's privacy with a curtain, screen, or door.

5. Put on gloves.

6. Put a disposable sheath over earpiece of the thermometer.

7. Position the resident's head so that the ear is in front of you. Straighten the ear canal by pulling up and back on the outside edge of the ear (Fig. 13-13). Insert the covered probe into the ear canal. Press the button.

Fig. 13-13. *Straighten the ear canal by pulling up and back on the outside edge of the ear.*

8. Hold thermometer in place until thermometer blinks or beeps.

9. Read temperature. Remember the temperature reading. (If the reading seems too low, repeat the procedure.)

10. Dispose of sheath. Return thermometer to storage or to the battery charger if thermometer is rechargeable.

11. Make resident comfortable.

12. Remove privacy measures.

13. Remove and dispose of gloves properly.

14. Leave call light within resident's reach.

15. Wash your hands.

16. Be courteous and respectful at all times.

17. Report any changes in the resident to the nurse. Document procedure using facility guidelines. Record resident's name, temperature, date, time, and method used (tympanic).

Axillary temperatures are not as accurate as temperatures taken at other sites. Make sure the axillary area is clean and dry before taking a temperature reading. The arm should be placed over the chest to hold the thermometer in place.

Measuring and recording axillary temperature

Equipment: mercury-free glass, digital or electronic thermometer, gloves, tissues, disposable sheath/cover, pen and paper

1. Identify yourself by name. Identify the resident. Greet the resident by name.

2. Wash your hands.

3. Explain procedure to resident. Speak clearly, slowly, and directly. Maintain face-to-face contact whenever possible. Encourage resident to assist if possible.

4. Provide for the resident's privacy with a curtain, screen, or door.

5. Practice good body mechanics. Adjust bed to safe working level, usually waist high. Lock bed wheels.

6. Put on gloves.

7. Remove resident's arm from sleeve of gown. Wipe axillary area with tissues.

8. *Mercury-free glass thermometer*: Hold thermometer by stem. Shake thermometer down to below the lowest number.

   Put on disposable sheath, if applicable.

   Digital thermometer: Put on disposable sheath. Turn on thermometer. Wait until "ready" sign appears.

   Electronic thermometer: Remove probe from base unit. Put on probe cover.

9. Place the end of thermometer in center of armpit. Fold resident's arm over chest.

10. *Mercury-free glass thermometer*: Hold thermometer in place, with the arm close against the side, for 10 minutes (Fig. 13-14).

    Digital thermometer: Hold thermometer in place until thermometer blinks or beeps.

Electronic thermometer: Leave in place until you hear a tone or see a flashing or steady light.

Fig. 13-14. *After inserting the thermometer, fold the resident's arm over her chest and hold it in place for the required time.*

11. Gently remove the thermometer. Wipe with tissue from stem to bulb or remove sheath or cover. Dispose of tissue.

12. Read thermometer as you would for an oral temperature. Remember the temperature reading.

13. *Mercury-free glass thermometer*: Clean thermometer according to facility policy. Return it to container for used thermometers.

    Digital thermometer: Discard sheath. Clean thermometer according to facility policy. Return thermometer to storage area.

    Electronic thermometer: Discard the cover. Return probe to holder.

14. Put resident's arm back into sleeve of gown. Make resident comfortable.

15. Return bed to low position if raised. Ensure resident's safety. Return side rails to ordered position. Remove privacy measures.

16. Remove and dispose of gloves properly.

17. Leave call light within resident's reach.

18. Wash your hands.

19. Be courteous and respectful at all times.

20. Report any changes in the resident to the nurse. Document procedure using facility guidelines. Record resident's name, temperature, date, time, and method used (axillary).

5. Explain pulse and respirations

When the left ventricle of the heart contracts, it causes a wave of blood to move through an artery. This "pulse" is what you feel at the wrist or other pulse site. The pulse count is the number of times the heart beats per minute. Sometimes the abbreviation **BPM** (beats per minute) is used after a pulse count. The heartbeat or pulse is measured with the fingers or by electronic devices that automatically measure the pulse. There are many areas on the body where a pulse can be felt. Common pulse sites are shown in Figure 13-15.

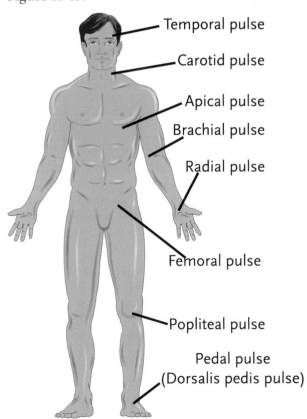

- Temporal pulse
- Carotid pulse
- Apical pulse
- Brachial pulse
- Radial pulse
- Femoral pulse
- Popliteal pulse
- Pedal pulse (Dorsalis pedis pulse)

Fig. 13-15. Common pulse sites.

For adults, the normal pulse rate is 60 to 100 beats per minute. When a pulse is too high, a person has **tachycardia**. If it is too low, a person has **bradycardia**.

The pulse rate is affected by different factors, including the following:

- **Age**: Pulse rate tends to decrease with advanced age.

- **Sex**: Males may have a slightly lower pulse rate than females.

- **Exercise**: Pulse rate normally increases with exercise. However, someone who has exercised regularly for years may have a lower pulse, which can be normal for that person.

- **Stress**: Fear, anxiety, and pain may cause the pulse to increase.

- **Hemorrhage**: The pulse rate will increase when blood is first lost due to the heart trying to work harder to circulate the blood.

- **Medications**: Medications can increase or decrease the heart rate.

- **Fever and illness**: When a person is ill and has a fever, blood vessels may **dilate**, or widen, due to the rise in temperature. A decrease in blood pressure then occurs due to the dilated blood vessels. The heart responds by working harder and increasing the pulse rate.

Respiration is the process of **inspiration** (inhaling air into the lungs) and **expiration** (exhaling air out of the lungs). Each respiration consists of an inspiration and an expiration. The chest rises during inspiration and falls during expiration. The normal respiration rate for adults ranges from 12 to 20 breaths per minute.

Different types of respirations are:

- **apnea**: the absence of breathing; may be temporary

- **dyspnea**: difficulty breathing

- **eupnea**: normal respirations

- **orthopnea**: shortness of breath when lying down that is relieved by sitting up

- **tachypnea**: rapid respirations
- **Cheyne-Stokes respiration**: type of respiration with periods of apnea lasting at least 10 seconds, along with alternating periods of slow, irregular respirations or rapid, shallow respirations (see Chapter 27 for more information)

6. List guidelines for taking pulse and respirations

The **radial pulse** is the most common site for counting pulse beats. This pulse is found on the inside of the wrist on the thumb-side of the body. A pulse may be regular, having the same amount of time between the beats, or irregular, having varying amounts of time between the beats.

You will sometimes use a stethoscope to measure pulse rate. A **stethoscope** is an instrument used for listening to sounds within the body, such as the heartbeat or air in the lungs. Clean the earpieces and diaphragm of the stethoscope with alcohol wipes before and after each use. The diaphragm is the larger, round side of the stethoscope; you will use this side to hear a pulse (Fig. 13-16). The smaller round side of the stethoscope is called the bell side.

Fig. 13-16. Use the diaphragm side of the stethoscope to hear a pulse and to take blood pressure. The diaphragm is the larger, round side of the stethoscope.

When checking a resident's pulse, observe for the following:

- The pulse rate (the number of beats in one minute—normal range is 60 to 100 beats per minute)
- The overall pattern of the pulse: is the pulse regular or irregular?
- The quality or type of pulse: is the pulse strong or weak?

The respiratory rate is usually counted directly after taking the pulse because people tend to breathe more quickly if they know they are being observed. Keep your fingers on the resident's wrist or on the stethoscope over the heart to avoid making it obvious that you are watching her breathing (Fig. 13-17). (Some state testing companies divide the procedure for taking the radial pulse and counting respirations into two separate procedures. In that case, you may need to explain what you are going to do before counting respirations. If so, that is for testing purposes only.)

Fig. 13-17. Count the respiratory rate directly after taking the radial pulse. Keep your fingers on the resident's wrist to avoid making it obvious that you are watching her breathing.

When counting respirations, observe for the following:

- The respiratory rate (the number of times the resident breathes in one minute—normal range is 12 to 20)
- The overall pattern of respirations: is breathing regular or irregular?
- The quality or type of breathing: is shortness of breath or difficulty breathing (dys-

pnea) noted? Does the resident have noisy breathing? Normal breathing is quiet. Is the breathing deep or shallow?

Measuring and recording radial pulse and counting and recording respirations

Equipment: watch with second hand, pen and paper

1. Identify yourself by name. Identify the resident. Greet the resident by name.

2. Wash your hands.

3. Explain procedure to resident. Speak clearly, slowly, and directly. Maintain face-to-face contact whenever possible. Encourage resident to assist if possible.

4. Provide for the resident's privacy with a curtain, screen, or door.

5. Place fingertips on thumb side of resident's wrist to locate pulse (Fig. 13-18).

Fig. 13-18. Take the radial pulse by placing fingertips on the thumb side of the wrist.

6. Count beats for one full minute.

7. Keep your fingertips on the resident's wrist. Count respirations for one full minute. Observe for the pattern and character of the resident's breathing. Normal breathing is smooth and quiet.

8. Remove privacy measures. Make resident comfortable.

9. Leave call light within resident's reach.

10. Wash your hands.

11. Be courteous and respectful at all times.

12. Report any changes in the resident to the nurse. Document procedure using facility guidelines. Record pulse rate, date, time and method used (radial). Record the respiratory rate and the pattern or character of breathing.

The **apical pulse** is heard by listening directly over the heart with a stethoscope. The apical pulse is on the left side of the chest, just below the nipple. This type of pulse is checked on residents who have a weak radial pulse or an irregular pulse. It may also be taken on infants and people with heart disease.

Measuring and recording apical pulse

Equipment: stethoscope, watch with second hand, alcohol wipes, pen and paper

1. Identify yourself by name. Identify the resident. Greet the resident by name.

2. Wash your hands.

3. Explain procedure to resident. Speak clearly, slowly, and directly. Maintain face-to-face contact whenever possible. Encourage resident to assist if possible.

4. Provide for the resident's privacy with a curtain, screen, or door.

5. Practice good body mechanics. Adjust bed to safe working level, usually waist high. Lock bed wheels.

6. Lower the side rail (if bed has one and if it is not already lowered) on side nearest you.

7. Before using stethoscope, wipe diaphragm and earpieces with alcohol wipes.

8. Fit the earpieces of the stethoscope snugly in your ears. Place the flat metal diaphragm on the left side of the chest, just below the nipple. Listen for the heartbeat.

9. Use the second hand of your watch. Count beats for one full minute. Each "lubdub" that you hear is counted as one beat. A normal heartbeat is rhythmic (Fig. 13-19). Leave the stethoscope in place to count respirations.

Fig. 13-19. *Count the heartbeats for one full minute to measure the apical pulse.*

10. Clean earpieces and diaphragm of stethoscope with alcohol wipes. Store stethoscope.

11. Make resident comfortable.

12. Return bed to low position if raised. Ensure resident's safety. Return side rails to ordered position. Remove privacy measures.

13. Leave call light within resident's reach.

14. Wash your hands.

15. Be courteous and respectful at all times.

16. Report any changes in the resident to the nurse. Document procedure using facility guidelines. Record pulse rate, date, time, and method used (apical). Note any differences in the rhythm.

An apical pulse is also taken to compare the apical pulse to a pulse somewhere else in the body, such as the wrist (radial). In some cases, the apical and radial pulse counts differ. This is significant when evaluating circulation or a heart problem.

An apical pulse is normally about the same as a radial pulse. When the radial pulse is less than the apical pulse, it may indicate poor circulation to an extremity. The apical pulse will always be the same or higher than any other pulse on the body. It will never be lower than another pulse.

The pulse deficit is the difference between an apical pulse and another pulse. For example, if the apical pulse is 80 beats in one minute, and the radial pulse is 68 beats in one minute, the pulse deficit is 12 (80 - 68 = 12).

Measuring and recording apical-radial pulse

Equipment: stethoscope, watch with second hand, alcohol wipes, pen and paper

Find a co-worker to assist you.

1. Identify yourself by name. Identify the resident. Greet the resident by name.

2. Wash your hands.

3. Explain procedure to resident. Speak clearly, slowly, and directly. Maintain face-to-face contact whenever possible. Encourage resident to assist if possible.

4. Provide for the resident's privacy with a curtain, screen, or door.

5. Practice good body mechanics. Adjust bed to safe working level, usually waist high. Lock bed wheels.

6. Lower the side rail (if bed has one and if it is not already lowered) on side nearest you.

7. Before using stethoscope, wipe diaphragm and earpieces with alcohol wipes.

8. Fit the earpieces of the stethoscope snugly in your ears. Place the flat metal diaphragm on the left side of the chest, just below the nipple. Listen for the heartbeat.

9. Your co-worker should place her fingertips on the thumb side of resident's wrist to locate the radial pulse.

10. After both pulses have been located, look at the second hand of your watch. When the second hand reaches the "12" or "6," say, "Start," and both people will count beats for one full minute. Say, "Stop" after one minute (Fig. 13-20).

Fig. 13-20. *Use the second hand on your watch to count the beats for one full minute.*

11. Clean earpieces and diaphragm of stethoscope with alcohol wipes. Store stethoscope.

12. Make resident comfortable.

13. Return bed to low position if raised. Ensure resident's safety. Return side rails to ordered position. Remove privacy measures.

14. Leave call light within resident's reach.

15. Wash your hands.

16. Be courteous and respectful at all times.

17. Report any changes in the resident to the nurse. Document procedure using facility guidelines. Record both pulse rates, date, time, and method used (apical-radial). Record pulse deficit if the pulse rates are not the same (subtract radial pulse measurement from apical pulse to get pulse deficit). Note any differences in the rhythm.

7. Identify factors that affect blood pressure

Blood pressure is the measurement of the force of the blood against the walls of certain blood vessels, called arteries. Arteries carry blood away from the heart. The left ventricle of the heart causes the blood to surge out of the heart and travel through the body. The force of this movement of blood is the blood pressure. Blood pressure is measured in millimeters of mercury (mm Hg). A blood pressure reading is recorded as a fraction—for example, 120/80.

The top number in a blood pressure reading is called the **systolic** blood pressure. This is the pressure of the blood on the walls of the arteries when the heart is contracting to pump blood out from the left ventricle into the body. The normal range for systolic blood pressure for an adult is 100–139 mm Hg.

The bottom number is the **diastolic** blood pressure. The lower reading is the pressure of the blood when the heart is relaxed. This relaxation happens when the heart is not contracting, between the heartbeats. The normal range for diastolic blood pressure for an adult is 60–89 mm Hg. The diastolic measurement is always lower than the systolic measurement.

When blood pressure is too high, it is called **hypertension**. People with hypertension have elevated systolic and/or diastolic blood pressures. A blood pressure reading of 140/90 is considered high.

When blood pressure is too low, it is called **hypotension**. Loss of blood or slowed blood flow can cause hypotension, which can be life-threatening. More information on these disorders can be found in Chapter 19. **Orthostatic hypotension**, which is also called postural hypotension, is a sudden drop in blood pressure that occurs when a person stands up. Dizziness, lightheadedness or fainting may accompany orthostatic hypotension.

New, more aggressive high blood pressure guidelines from the Seventh Report of the Joint National Committee (JNC 7) were released in 2003. Under the new guidelines, a definition for prehypertension was added. **Prehypertension** is defined as having a systolic measurement of 120–139 mm Hg and a diastolic measurement of 80–89 mm Hg. Prehypertension means that a person does not have high blood pressure now but is likely to have it in the future. Nursing assistants must report to the nurse if a resident's blood pressure is 140/90 or above.

Blood pressure is affected by different factors, including:

- **Age**: Elderly people with circulatory disorders (Chapter 19) may have higher blood pressure readings.

- **Exercise**: Regular exercise and being active may decrease blood pressure.

- **Stress**: Long-term, chronic stress appears to raise blood pressure.

- **Race**: African-Americans are more likely to have high blood pressure than Caucasians.

- **Heredity**: People whose parents have or have had high blood pressure are more likely to develop it than others.

- **Obesity/unhealthy diet**: Being overweight and eating unhealthy diets increase blood pressure.

- **Alcohol**: Regular, high alcohol intake can raise blood pressure.

- **Tobacco products**: Smoking or chewing tobacco products are contributing factors in high blood pressure.

- **Time of day**: Blood pressure may be lower in the morning and higher later in the day.

- **Illness**: People who have certain diseases, such as diabetes and kidney disease, have a higher frequency of high blood pressure.

8. List guidelines for taking blood pressure

Blood pressure is measured with a device called a **sphygmomanometer**. You will need to gather alcohol wipes, a stethoscope, a blood pressure cuff, and a sphygmomanometer when preparing to take a blood pressure. Some facilities do not allow nursing assistants to take blood pressure readings. Follow facility policy and the care plan.

It is important to choose the correct size cuff to take a blood pressure reading. Available sizes include standard, pediatric, and large. Check with the nurse if you have questions about the size of the blood pressure cuff. The cuff must be the proper size and put on the arm correctly so the amount of pressure on the artery is correct. If not, the reading will be falsely high or low.

Types of sphygmomanometers include:

- **Aneroid sphygmomanometer**. This device has a round gauge that is portable or is attached to the wall (Fig. 13-21). It may also hook onto clothing.

- **Electronic sphygmomanometer**. This device automatically inflates and deflates to

measure blood pressure (Fig. 13-22). The readings are displayed digitally. The use of a stethoscope is not required with electronic sphygmomanometers. Ask for instructions on use if you have not been trained to use this equipment.

- **Non-invasive blood pressure monitoring (NIBP)**. These monitoring devices measure blood pressure faster than other methods. They may also measure other vital signs, as well as perform other measurements. For example, some machines measure the temperature, pulse, and respiration, and have the ability to measure blood oxygen levels. You will receive training for these devices if they are used at your facility. Follow facility policy on the use of these machines.

Fig. 13-21. *An aneroid sphygmomanometer.*

Fig. 13-22. *An electronic sphygmomanometer.*

The **brachial pulse** is used to take a blood pressure reading. This is the pulse inside of the elbow, about one to one and a half inches above the elbow (Fig. 13-23). Both the radial and brachial pulse are used in taking blood pressure.

Fig. 13-23. *The brachial pulse is located on the inside of the elbow, about one to one and a half inches above the elbow.*

Do not take blood pressure on an arm or a side of the body when these situations exist:

- an intravenous line (IV) is present
- an amputation has been performed
- the cuff does not fit the arm properly
- the arm has a cast
- burns or injuries are present
- the arm is being used for dialysis
- the arm or side has had recent trauma
- the arm or side is paralyzed due to stroke
- the side has had a mastectomy (or any breast surgery)

When taking blood pressure, observe for the following:

- The blood pressure reading: The normal reading should be from 100/60 to 139/89 (140/90 or above is high and needs to be reported).

- The quality or type of sounds: Are the sounds you hear when listening with your stethoscope strong or weak?

Different Methods for Taking Blood Pressure

This textbook includes two methods for taking blood pressure: the one-step method and the two-step method. In the two-step method, you will get an estimate of the systolic blood pressure before you start. After getting an estimated systolic reading, you will deflate the cuff and begin again. With the one-step method, you will not get an estimated systolic

reading before obtaining the blood pressure reading. Your state may require that you know one or both of these methods. Follow your facility's policy on which method to use.

Measuring and recording blood pressure (one-step method)

Equipment: sphygmomanometer and blood pressure cuff, stethoscope, watch with second hand, alcohol wipes, pen and paper

1. Identify yourself by name. Identify the resident. Greet the resident by name.

2. Wash your hands.

3. Explain procedure to resident. Speak clearly, slowly, and directly. Maintain face-to-face contact whenever possible. Encourage resident to assist if possible.

4. Provide for the resident's privacy with a curtain, screen, or door.

5. Position resident's arm with palm up. The arm should be level with the heart. Roll up long sleeves approximately five inches above the elbow.

6. With the valve open, squeeze the cuff. Make sure it is completely deflated.

7. Place blood pressure cuff snugly on resident's upper arm. The center of the cuff is placed over the brachial artery (1-1½ inches above the elbow toward inside of elbow) (Fig. 13-24).

Fig. 13-24. *Place the center of the cuff over the brachial artery.*

8. Before using stethoscope, wipe diaphragm and earpieces with alcohol wipes.

9. Locate brachial pulse with fingertips.

10. Place diaphragm of stethoscope over brachial artery.

11. Place earpieces of stethoscope in ears.

12. Close the valve (clockwise) until it stops. Do not over-tighten it (Fig. 13-25).

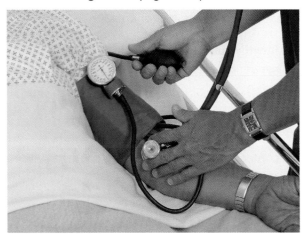

Fig. 13-25. *Close the valve by turning it clockwise until it stops.*

13. Inflate cuff to 30 mm Hg above the point at which the pulse is last heard.

14. Open the valve slightly with thumb and index finger. Deflate cuff slowly.

15. Watch gauge. Listen for sound of pulse.

16. Remember the reading at which the first clear pulse sound is heard. This is the systolic pressure.

17. Continue listening for a change or muffling of pulse sound. The point of a change or the point the sound disappears is the diastolic pressure. Remember this reading.

18. Open the valve. Deflate cuff completely. Remove cuff.

19. Wipe diaphragm and earpieces of stethoscope with alcohol. Store equipment.

20. Make resident comfortable. Remove privacy measures.

21. Leave call light within resident's reach.

22. Wash your hands.

23. Be courteous and respectful at all times.

24. Report any changes in the resident to the nurse. Document procedure using facility guidelines. Record both the systolic and diastolic pressures.

Measuring and recording blood pressure (two-step method)

Equipment: sphygmomanometer and blood pressure cuff, stethoscope, watch with second hand, alcohol wipes, pen and paper

1. Identify yourself by name. Identify the resident. Greet the resident by name.

2. Wash your hands.

3. Explain procedure to resident. Speak clearly, slowly, and directly. Maintain face-to-face contact whenever possible. Encourage resident to assist if possible.

4. Provide for the resident's privacy with a curtain, screen, or door.

5. Position resident's arm with palm up. The arm should be level with the heart. Roll up long sleeves approximately five inches above the elbow.

6. With the valve open, squeeze the cuff. Make sure it is completely deflated.

7. Place blood pressure cuff snugly on resident's upper arm. The center of the cuff is placed over the brachial artery (1-1½ inches above the elbow toward inside of elbow).

8. Locate the radial (wrist) pulse with fingertips.

9. Close the valve (clockwise) until it stops. Inflate cuff slowly, watching gauge.

10. Stop inflating when you can no longer feel the pulse. Note the reading. The number is an estimate of the systolic pressure.

11. Open the valve. Deflate cuff completely.

12. Write down estimated systolic reading.

13. Before using stethoscope, wipe diaphragm and earpieces of stethoscope with alcohol wipes.

14. Locate brachial pulse with fingertips.

15. Place diaphragm of stethoscope over brachial artery.

16. Place earpieces of stethoscope in ears.

17. Close the valve (clockwise) until it stops. Do not over-tighten it (Fig. 13-26).

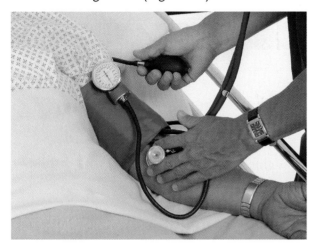

Fig. 13-26. *Close the valve but do not over-tighten it. Tight valves are too hard to release.*

18. Inflate cuff to 30 mm Hg above your estimated systolic pressure.

19. Open the valve slightly with thumb and index finger. Deflate cuff slowly.

20. Watch gauge. Listen for sound of pulse.

21. Remember the reading at which the first clear pulse sound is heard. This is the systolic pressure.

22. Continue listening for a change or muffling of pulse sound. The point of a change or the point the sound disappears is the diastolic pressure. Remember this reading.

23. Open the valve. Deflate cuff completely. Remove cuff.

24. Wipe diaphragm and earpieces of stethoscope with alcohol. Store equipment.

25. Make resident comfortable. Remove privacy measures.

26. Leave call light within resident's reach.

27. Wash your hands.

28. Be courteous and respectful at all times.

29. Report any changes in the resident to the nurse. Document procedure using facility guidelines. Record systolic and diastolic pressures.

HOT TIP

LSS Blood Pressures

LSS blood pressure readings are sometimes ordered for residents. This means that you will take the resident's blood pressure reading three separate times. The reading is first taken while the resident is lying down, then when he is sitting, and then when he is standing. You will report and record all three readings. An example is L=100/80, S=120/82, and S=120/86.

9. Describe guidelines for pain management

It is important to observe and report residents' pain. Some even call pain the "fifth vital sign," because it is as important to monitor pain as it is to monitor the other vital signs.

It can be very difficult to cope with pain. It is uncomfortable and can greatly affect residents' daily lives and their ability to perform ADLs. Pain can swiftly drain energy and hope.

Pain is different for each person; what bothers one person may not bother another. All caregivers are responsible for recognizing pain and taking appropriate action to provide pain management. As the person who is with residents the most, you play a significant role in pain monitoring, management, and prevention. Care plans are made and adjusted based on your reports.

Treat residents' complaints of pain seriously and take action to help them (Fig. 13-27). Ask appropriate questions to help manage the pain, such as the following:

- Where is the pain? Please point to the exact site or area to show me.

- When did the pain start?

- How long does the pain last? Minutes? Seconds? Ask how often it occurs.

- How severe is the pain? To help find out, use available pain scales at your facility. Pain scales are tools that help measure the level of a person's pain. One type is a numerical pain scale. You ask the resident to rate the pain on a scale of 1 to 10, with 10 being the worst. Another is a visual pain scale, which includes drawings of faces with different expressions. Ask the resident to pick the face that most closely resembles the intensity of pain he is experiencing.

- Does the pain come and go?

- Have you experienced this pain before? If so, has anything helped to relieve it?

- What medicine, if any, do you take for the pain?

- Do you remember what you were doing when the pain started?

Fig. 13-27. *Believe residents when they say they are in pain and take quick action to help them. Being in pain is unpleasant. Be empathetic.*

Ask the resident to describe the pain, and using the resident's words, report to the nurse. Take notes if you need to remember the exact words.

Notice signs of pain specific to each resident. Culture plays a role in determining whether or not a resident will be able to express his pain. Some residents will state freely when they are in pain. Others will not feel comfortable reacting in some way to pain or saying that they are in pain.

Some residents will not express pain due to a fear of addiction to pain medication or worry-

ing about constipation or fatigue from the pain medication. Residents may believe that pain is a normal part of aging, although it is not. Other residents may think that staff members are too busy to deal with their pain.

If a resident is not likely to tell staff that he is in pain, watch for body language or other signs that the person is in pain. Signs of pain to observe and report to the nurse include:

- increased pulse, respirations, blood pressure
- sweating
- nausea
- vomiting
- tightening the jaw
- squeezing eyes shut
- holding a body part tightly
- frowning
- grinding teeth
- increased restlessness
- agitation or tension
- change in behavior
- crying
- sighing
- groaning
- breathing heavily
- difficulty moving or walking

Guidelines

Measures to Reduce Pain

- Report complaints of pain or unrelieved pain promptly to the nurse.

- Check on the resident often and ask if the pain has been relieved.

- Monitor the resident's response to pain medication.

- Offer back rubs frequently (Fig. 13-28).

- Assist in frequent changes of position. Be careful when moving, lifting, or transferring a resident in pain. Make sure to have enough help to transfer a resident in pain.

- Offer warm baths or showers.
- Encourage slow, deep breaths if the resident has difficulty breathing.
- Always be patient, caring, gentle, and empathetic.

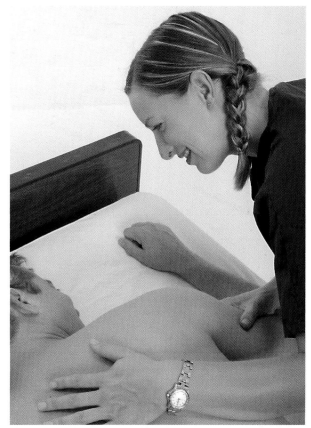

Fig. 13-28. *Back rubs can help reduce pain. Be gentle, kind and caring when residents are in pain.*

CHAPTER REVIEW

1. What are the five vital signs that are regularly monitored (LO 2)?

2. List two reasons a nursing assistant should never document a guess of a resident's vital signs (LO 2).

3. List six factors that affect body temperature (LO 3).

4. What are four symptoms of a fever (LO 3)?

5. List the four main sites on the body for measuring temperature (LO 4).

6. Which site is generally considered to be the most accurate for obtaining temperatures (LO 4)?

7. What color are rectal thermometers usually coded (LO 4)?

8. List ten conditions under which a nursing assistant should not take an oral temperature (LO 4).

9. If a resident has recently eaten or had something to drink, how long must a nursing assistant wait before she can measure his oral temperature (LO 4)?

10. When taking a rectal temperature, how long does a nursing assistant need to hold onto the thermometer while it is in the rectum (LO 4)?

11. Generally, how far should the tip of a tympanic thermometer be inserted into the ear (LO 4)?

12. What is the normal pulse rate for adults (LO 5)?

13. What is the normal respiration rate for adults (LO 5)?

14. What is the most common site for taking the pulse (LO 6)?

15. Where is the apical pulse located (LO 6)?

16. Why is the respiratory rate usually counted directly after taking the pulse, while the fingers are still on the person's wrist (LO 6)?

17. Define the pulse deficit (LO 6).

18. List the two parts of measuring blood pressure and list normal ranges for both (LO 7).

19. What reading is considered to be high blood pressure (LO 7)?

20. List seven factors that affect blood pressure (LO 7).

21. Why must a blood pressure cuff be the proper size and put on the arm correctly (LO 8)?

22. In addition to the radial pulse, what other pulse is involved in taking blood pressure measurements (LO 8)?

23. List six conditions under which a nursing assistant should not take blood pressure on an arm or one side of the body (LO 8).

24. List three reasons why some residents might not express pain openly (LO 9).

25. List 15 signs of pain to observe and report to the nurse (LO 9).

26. What are five ways a nursing assistant can help reduce a resident's pain (LO 9)?

14 Nutrition and Fluid Balance

Pernicious Anemia

A Nobel Prize was awarded to George R. Minot, William P. Murphy, and George H. Whipple for discovering that a serious and fatal disease called pernicious anemia could actually be cured. Minot worked for many years and finally discovered that with a simple change in diet, adding large amounts of liver, the disease could be cured. The three men eventually proved the disease was caused by a lack of vitamin B12. Today many people live long lives with this disease by simply getting periodic B12 shots.

"In general, mankind, since the improvement of cookery, eats twice as much as it requires."
Benjamin Franklin, 1706-1790

"Every tooth in a man's head is more valuable than a diamond."
Miguel de Cervantes, 1547-1616

1. Define important words in this chapter

apathy: a lack of interest.

aspiration: the inhalation of food or fluid into the lungs; may cause pneumonia or death.

dehydration: condition that occurs when a person does not have enough fluid in the body.

diet cards: cards that list residents' names and information about special diets, allergies, likes and dislikes, and any other dietary instructions.

diuretics: medications that reduce fluid volume in the body.

dysphagia: difficulty with swallowing.

edema: swelling in body tissues caused by excess fluid.

fasting: a period of time during which food is given up voluntarily.

fluid balance: taking in and eliminating equal amounts of fluid.

fluid overload: a condition in which the body cannot eliminate the fluid consumed.

force fluids: a medical order for a person to drink more fluids.

glucose: natural sugar.

graduate: a measuring container.

input: the fluid a person consumes; also called intake.

intake: the fluid a person consumes; also called input.

malnutrition: poor nutrition due to insufficient food intake or an improper diet.

metabolism: the process of utilizing all nutrients that enter the body to provide energy, growth, and maintenance.

nutrient: substance in food that enables the body to use energy for metabolism.

nutrition: the taking in and using of food by the body to maintain health.

output: fluid that is eliminated each day through urine, feces, and vomitus, as well as perspiration; also includes suction material and wound drainage.

puree: to chop, blend, or grind food into a thick paste of baby food consistency.

restrict fluids: a medical order that limits the amount of fluids a person takes in.

special diet: a diet for people who have certain illnesses or conditions; also called therapeutic or modified diet.

vegans: vegetarians who do not eat any animal products, including milk, cheese, other dairy items, or eggs; vegans may also not use or wear any animal products, including, wool, silk, and leather.

vegetarians: people who do not eat meat, fish, or poultry for religious, moral, or health reasons; they may or may not eat eggs and dairy products.

2. Describe common nutritional problems of the elderly and the chronically ill

Aging and illness affect **nutrition**, or the taking in and using of food by the body to maintain health. Malnutrition, unhealthy weight loss and dehydration are serious problems among the elderly. **Malnutrition** is the lack of proper nutrition that results from insufficient food intake or an improper diet. Difficulty swallowing, called **dysphagia**, and the inability to chew contribute to a lack of appetite. Fatigue, nausea and pain often accompany certain illnesses, which decrease appetite. Other problems that affect nutritional intake include the following:

- Older people produce less saliva, which affects eating and swallowing. Swallowing problems put people at a high risk for **aspiration**, which is the inhalation of food or fluid into the lungs. You will learn more about aspiration later in the chapter.

- Medications can have side effects for the digestive system, such as diarrhea and con-

stipation, both of which can interfere with appetite.

- A decrease in physical activity and mobility can cause a lack of appetite and constipation.

- The ability to smell and taste food and drink is lessened as people age. Medication can also interfere with the sense of smell and taste. This affects the appetite and the ability to eat (Fig. 14-1).

- The inability to see well can affect the way food looks, decreasing interest in food.

- Problems with teeth, dentures, or poor oral hygiene make chewing difficult.

- Depression and lack of social interaction can decrease appetite.

- Older people may be on special diets that restrict certain foods and drinks, which can lead to poor food and fluid intake. You will learn more about special diets later in the chapter.

Fig. 14-1. Many elderly people are on a variety of medications, which can affect the way food smells and tastes.

Some specific illnesses make eating and swallowing difficult, such as stroke, which can result in paralysis; cancers of the head, neck, or mouth; Parkinson's disease; multiple sclerosis; and Alzheimer's disease. More information on these diseases is found later in the chapter and in Chapters 22 and 24 of the textbook.

3. Describe cultural factors that influence food preferences

A resident's cultural and ethnic background has great impact on his or her food preferences. Traditions in families and cultures influence food choices (Fig. 14-2). The country or the area of the country that a person is from affects his or her food choices. For example, people from the southwestern US are more apt to like spicy foods. People from Asia may prefer rice with their meals, rather than potatoes or bread.

Fig. 14-2. Family traditions influence food likes and dislikes.

Certain people may have foods they cannot eat due to religious reasons. For example, many Jewish people do not eat pork or shellfish, and do not eat meat products at the same meal with dairy products. Some Catholics do not eat meat on Fridays. Muslims may not drink alcohol and may occasionally fast. **Fasting** is a practice during which food is voluntarily given up for a period of time.

Some people may be vegetarians or vegans. **Vegetarians** do not eat meat, fish, or poultry. They may or may not eat eggs and dairy products. **Vegans** are vegetarians who do not eat any animal products, including milk, cheese, other dairy items, or eggs. Vegans may also not use or wear any animal products, including wool, silk, and leather.

Determining a resident's food preferences is first done upon admission to a facility. Periodically these evaluations may need to be redone as a resident's likes and dislikes, as well as nutritional needs, change.

Honoring food preferences is a legal responsibility of the facility. Nursing assistants must report requests for diet substitutions to the nurse right away.

4. Identify six basic nutrients

The human body cannot survive without food and water. Good health requires a daily amount of each of the main nutrients for cells, tissues, organs, and systems to continue to function properly. A **nutrient** is something in food that enables the body to use energy for metabolism. **Metabolism** is the process of utilizing all nutrients that enter the body in order to provide energy, growth, and maintenance. There are six main nutrients required by the body for healthy growth and development:

1. **Water** is the most essential nutrient for life; it is needed by every cell in the body. Water helps move oxygen and other nutrients into the cells and remove the waste products from each of the cells. Without water, a person can only live a few days. Water helps with digestion and absorption of food. It helps to maintain a normal body temperature through perspiration. Keeping enough fluid in the body is necessary for good health (Fig. 14-3).

Fig. 14-3. Water is the most essential nutrient for life. Drinking plenty of water promotes good health.

2. **Fats** protect body organs and help the body store energy. Body fat serves as insulation and helps the body stay warm. Fat also gives flavor to foods. Fat contains many calories and may add cholesterol to the diet. Thus, fat should be used in small amounts. Excess fat in the diet is stored as fat in the body (Fig. 14-4).

Fig. 14-4. *Sources of fat.*

3. **Carbohydrates** supply the body with vital energy. They help the body use fat efficiently. Carbohydrates also add much-needed fiber to diets, which helps with solid waste elimination (Fig. 14-5).

Fig. 14-5. *Sources of carbohydrates.*

4. **Proteins** are needed by every cell in the body. They help the body grow new tissue, enable tissue repair and provide additional energy (Fig. 14-6).

Fig. 14-6. *Sources of protein.*

5. **Vitamins** are substances that are needed by the body to function. The body does not make most vitamins; they can only be obtained by eating certain foods. Some vitamins are fat-soluble, meaning they are carried and stored in body fat. Vitamins A, D, E, and K are examples. Others are water-soluble vitamins, meaning they are broken down by water in the body and cannot be stored. They are eliminated through urine and feces. Vitamins B and C are examples of water-soluble vitamins.

6. **Minerals** help the body function normally. Many minerals are needed daily by the body. Some minerals keep bones and teeth strong, while others help maintain fluid balance. Minerals give the body energy and control body processes. They are found in many foods.

5. Explain the USDA's MyPyramid

In 1980, the The U.S. Department of Agriculture (USDA) developed the Food Guide Pyramid to help promote healthy eating practices. In 2005, in response to new scientific information about nutrition and health, MyPyramid was developed; it replaces the old Food Guide Pyramid.

MyPyramid is a personalized version of the Food Guide Pyramid that offers individual plans based on age, gender, and activity level. Older people do not metabolize food as efficiently as younger people. People over the age of 65 need fewer calories to maintain health than they did when they were younger.

The Pyramid is made up of six bands of different widths and colors (Fig. 14-7). Each color represents a food group—orange for grains, green for vegetables, maroon for fruits, yellow for oils, blue for milk, and purple for meat and beans. The different widths indicate that not all groups should make up an equal part of a healthy diet. The orange band, grains, is the widest. This means that grains should make up the highest proportion of the diet. The smaller bands, such as the purple band representing meat and beans, should make up a smaller part of foods eaten.

The smallest band, the yellow one, represents oils. Oils contain essential fatty acids. However, this band is not emphasized, because as you learned earlier, the body needs fats and oils in smaller quantities.

Fig. 14-7. *MyPyramid was developed by the U.S. Department of Agriculture to help promote healthy eating practices. It offers individual plans based on age, gender and activity level.*

The bands of the Pyramid are wide at the bottom and narrow into a point at the top. This is a reminder that there are a great variety of foods that make up each group. Many choices are available to help meet the daily requirements. Foods low in fat and calories should form the "base" of a healthy diet. Foods that are high in fat and sugar and have less nutritional value are at the narrow top. They should be eaten less often.

The new Pyramid also emphasizes the importance of physical activity, as represented by the figure climbing the stairs. The USDA recommends at least 30 minutes per day of vigorous activity for everyone.

The food groups included on MyPyramid are:

Grains. The grains group includes all foods made from wheat, rice, oats, cornmeal, or barley, such as bread, pasta, oatmeal, breakfast cereals, tortillas and grits. In general one slice of bread, one cup of ready-to-eat cereal, or ½ cup of cooked rice, pasta, or cooked cereal can be considered as one-ounce equivalents from the grains group.

Consuming foods rich in fiber reduces the risk of heart disease and may reduce constipation.

At least half of all grains consumed should be whole grains.

Vegetables. The vegetable group includes all fresh, frozen, canned and dried vegetables and vegetable juices. In general one cup of raw or cooked vegetables or vegetable juice or two cups of raw leafy greens can be considered as one cup from the vegetable group. There are 5 subgroups within the vegetable group, organized by their nutritional content. These are dark green vegetables, orange vegetables, dry beans and peas, starchy vegetables, and other vegetables. A variety of vegetables from these subgroups should be eaten every day. Dark green vegetables, orange vegetables, and dried beans and peas have the best nutritional content.

Vegetables are low in fat and calories and have no cholesterol (although sauces and seasonings may add fat, calories and cholesterol). They are good sources of dietary fiber, potassium, vitamin A, vitamin E, and vitamin C (Fig. 14-8).

Fig. 14-8. *Eating a variety of vegetables every day helps promote good health.*

Fruits. The fruit group includes all fresh, frozen, canned and dried fruits and fruit juices. In general one cup of fruit or 100% fruit juice or ½ cup of dried fruit can be considered as one cup from the fruit group. Most choices should be whole or cut up fruit rather than juice for the additional dietary fiber provided.

Fruits, like vegetables, are naturally low in fat, sodium and calories and have no cholesterol. They are important sources of dietary fiber and many nutrients, including folic acid and vitamin

C. Foods containing dietary fiber help provide a feeling of fullness with fewer calories. Folic acid helps the body form red blood cells. Vitamin C is important for growth and repair of body tissues.

Milk. The milk group includes all fluid milk products and foods made from milk that retain their calcium content, such as yogurt and cheese. Foods made from milk that have little to no calcium, such as cream cheese, cream, and butter, are not part of the group. Most milk group choices should be fat-free or low-fat. One cup of milk or yogurt, one-and-one-half ounces of natural cheese, or two ounces of processed cheese can be considered as one cup from the milk group.

Foods in the milk group provide nutrients that are vital for the health and maintenance of your body. These nutrients include calcium, potassium, vitamin D, and protein. Calcium is used for building bones and teeth and in maintaining bone mass. Milk products are the primary source of calcium in American diets (Fig. 14-9).

Fig. 14-9. *Low-fat yogurt is a good source of calcium.*

Meat and Beans. One ounce of lean meat, poultry, or fish, one egg, one tablespoon peanut butter, ¼ cup cooked dry beans, or ½ ounce of nuts or seeds can be considered as one-ounce equivalents from the meat and beans group. Dry beans and peas can be included as part of this group or part of the vegetable group. If meat is eaten regularly, dry beans and peas should be included with vegetables. If not, they should be included as part of this group.

Most meat and poultry choices should be lean or low-fat. Diets that are high in saturated fats raise "bad" cholesterol levels in the blood.

Fish, nuts, and seeds contain healthy oils (Fig. 14-10). These foods are a good choice instead of meat or poultry. Some nuts and seeds (flax, walnuts) are excellent sources of essential fatty acids. These acids may reduce the risk of cardiovascular disease. Some (sunflower seeds, almonds, hazelnuts) are good sources of vitamin E.

Fig. 14-10. *Fish contains healthy oils and is a good source of protein.*

Vegetarians get enough protein from this group as long as the variety and amounts of foods selected are adequate. Protein sources for vegetarians from this group include eggs (for ovo-vegetarians), beans, nuts, nut butters, peas, and soy products (tofu, tempeh, veggie burgers).

Oils. Oils include fats that are liquid at room temperature, such as canola, corn, olive, soybean and sunflower oil (Fig. 14-11). They come from many different plants and foods. Some foods are naturally high in oils, like nuts, olives, some fish, and avocados. Foods that are mainly oil include mayonnaise, certain salad dressings, and soft margarine.

Fig. 14-11. *Canola oil and olive oil are healthier types of oil to use in cooking or baking.*

Most of the fats you eat should be polyunsaturated (PUFA) or monounsaturated (MUFA) fats. Oils are the major source of MUFAs and PUFAs in the diet. PUFAs contain some fatty acids that are necessary for health. These are called "essential fatty acids."

Most Americans consume enough oil in the foods they eat, such as nuts, fish, cooking oil, and salad dressings.

Activity. Physical activity and nutrition work together for better health. Being active increases the amount of calories burned. As people age, their metabolism slows. Maintaining energy balance requires moving more and eating less. For health benefits, physical activity should be moderate or vigorous and add up to at least 30 minutes a day.

If you would like to know more about MyPyramid, visit www.mypyramid.gov.

6. Explain the role of the dietary department

The dietary department is responsible for providing nutritious meals and snacks to all residents. Each resident is evaluated upon admission in order to create his or her diet plan. The dietary department creates food to match the diet ordered by the doctor, as well as taking into consideration the resident's likes and dislikes and nutritional needs.

In addition to planning and making meals, the dietary department has a responsibility to prepare food in such a way that residents are able to manage. The food must look appetizing to residents. The dietary department also prepares diet cards. **Diet cards** list the resident's name and information about special diets, allergies, likes and dislikes, as well as any other dietary instructions (Fig. 14-12).

For residents who are unable to eat in the dining room, meals arrive on a floor in a warming unit. Each meal comes with a diet card. You must verify that each resident has received the correct meal by checking the resident's identification against the diet card.

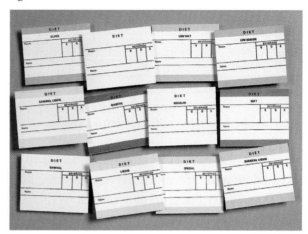

Fig. 14-12. *Sample diet cards. (Reprinted with permission of Briggs Corporation, Des Moines, IA, 800-247-2343.)*

Dietary staff must follow strict infection control guidelines in food preparation. They are periodically surveyed by a local health department for their cleanliness and infection control practices.

Menus

Menus are prepared for different diets and are completed each day at some facilities. If menus are used at your facility, you may be asked to read them to residents and to assist them in completing the menus. Make sure you have the correct diet order menu for each resident. Speak slowly and clearly and answer any questions or concerns the resident may have. Make the selections sound appetizing. Encourage nutritious choices, but allow the resident to make the final decision. Make sure to check one or more items from every category, as well as a beverage. Fill out menus and turn them in promptly. When food arrives, check to see that the resident has received what he or she ordered.

7. Explain the importance of following diet orders and identify special diets

Special diets are often ordered for residents who have certain illnesses or conditions. Sometimes they are ordered to help a resident gain or lose weight (Fig. 14-13). Some diets are ordered for a short time before a medical test or surgery. Doctors prescribe the special diet, also called a "therapeutic" or "modified" diet, and then the dietician plans the diet, along with input from the resident.

Diet Order:	Low fat		
✓ Assist with Feeding			
✓ Limit/Encourage Fluids			

Fig. 14-13. *The care plan specifies the special diet ordered, as well as additional dietary instructions.*

Residents who have orders for specific diets require additional care and supervision. Special diets may restrict or eliminate certain foods or fluids. As stated earlier, it is very important to check resident identification against the diet card before serving meal trays. Also check the food on the tray to see if it matches the diet ordered. Serving a resident the wrong food can cause serious problems, such as allergic reactions and possibly death.

The following information identifies many types of therapeutic diets and abbreviations you are likely to see for these diets on a diet card.

Liquid Diets. Liquid diets are made up of foods that are liquid at body temperature. Liquid diets are usually ordered as "clear" or "full." A clear liquid diet consists of fluids that you can see through, such as clear soups and juices. A full liquid diet includes clear liquids with the addition of cream soups, milk, and ice cream. This diet may be ordered for a short time due to a medical condition or ordered before surgery or a diagnostic test.

Soft Diet and Mechanical Soft Diet. The soft diet is soft in texture. This diet restricts or eliminates foods that are hard to chew and swallow, such as raw fruits and vegetables and some meats. High-fiber foods, fried foods, and spicy foods may also be limited to help with digestion. The soft diet is often used for people who are making the transition from a liquid diet to a regular diet. It is also used for people who are recovering from surgery or a long illness, have dental problems, or extreme weakness.

The mechanical soft diet gets its name from how foods are prepared, such as with blenders, food processors, or cutting utensils. These items are used to chop or blend foods to make them easier to chew and swallow. In contrast to the soft diet, the mechanical soft diet does not limit spices, fat, and fiber. Only the texture of foods is changed. For example, meats can be ground and moistened with sauces or water to ease swallowing. This diet is used for people recovering from surgery, who have difficulty swallowing, or who suffer from dental problems.

Pureed Diet. To **puree** food means to chop, blend, or grind it into a thick paste of baby food consistency. This consistency means the food should be thick enough to hold its form in the mouth, but does not need to be chewed. The pureed diet is used for people who have trouble chewing and swallowing and who cannot tolerate regular or mechanical soft diets.

Bland Diet. In the bland diet, foods that irritate the stomach and digestive tract are eliminated. This includes spicy foods and citrus juices. Some people must also avoid dairy products. This diet is used for people who have intestinal problems or conditions, such as Crohn's disease or irritable bowel syndrome (Chapter 15).

High-Residue or High-Fiber Diet. High-residue or high-fiber diets increase the intake of fiber and whole grains, such as whole grain cereals, bread and raw fruits and vegetables (Fig. 14-14). This diet helps with problems such as bowel disorders, constipation, and other gastrointestinal illnesses (Chapter 15).

Fig. 14-14. *Intake of raw vegetables and fruits will be ordered in a high-residue or high-fiber diet.*

Low-Residue or Low-Fiber Diet. This diet decreases the intake of fiber, grains, seeds, and other foods, such as dairy and coffee. The low-residue diet is used for people with bowel disorders, such as diverticulitis (Chapter 15).

Modified Calorie Diets. A high calorie diet increases the amount of calories to help a person gain weight. This may be necessary due to malnutrition, surgery, or illness. In order to lose weight or to maintain weight, a person is put on a low calorie diet, which decreases calorie intake. Common abbreviations for these diets are "High-Cal" or "Low-Cal."

Low-Sodium Diet. People with heart disease or kidney disease are put on low-sodium diets. When a resident is on a low-sodium diet, salt will be restricted. No salt shakers or salt packets should be on a meal tray. The abbreviations for this diet are "Low Na," which means low sodium, or "NAS" which stands for "No Added Salt."

High-Protein Diet. A high-protein diet is used for people recovering from surgery and for healing serious wounds, such as burns. High-protein foods, such as meat, fish, and cheese or those foods with added protein, such as protein milkshakes, are encouraged.

Low-Protein Diet. This diet is often used for people who have kidney or liver disease. Protein is restricted because the body cannot use the protein properly and it may lead to further damage of these organs. Protein is never completely eliminated from the diet, though, because the body needs protein to function. Vegetables and starches, such as breads, cereals, and pasta, are encouraged.

Low-Fat/Low-Cholesterol Diet. People who have heart disease and artery problems are often placed on this diet. The low-fat/low-cholesterol diet is also used for people who have gallbladder or liver disease. Low-fat and low-cholesterol foods, such as skim milk, white meats of turkey and chicken, fish, and low-fat cottage cheese are usually permitted. A common abbreviation for this diet is "Low-Fat/Low-Chol."

High-Potassium Diet. This diet is used for people who take **diuretics**, which are medications that reduce fluid volume, or for people who take blood pressure medications. Because diuretics increase urine output, a person's body may be low in potassium. Foods high in potassium include bananas, grapefruit, oranges, orange juice, prune juice, prunes, dried apricots, figs, raisins, dates, cantaloupes, tomatoes, potatoes with skins, sweet potatoes and yams, winter squash, legumes, avocados, and unsalted nuts. "K+" is the common abbreviation for this diet.

Fluid-Restricted Diet. People with severe heart disease and kidney disease may have trouble processing fluid and may be on a fluid-restricted diet. You will need to measure and document the amount of fluid a resident consumes. The fluid a person consumes is called **intake**, or **input**. You will learn more about fluid restrictions and documenting intake later in the chapter. Additional fluids or foods that count as fluids, such as soups, ice cream, etc. cannot be offered to a resident on a fluid-restricted diet. The abbreviation for this diet is "RF," which stands for "Restrict Fluids."

Diabetic Diet. Diabetes is a condition in which the pancreas does not produce enough insulin. Insulin converts **glucose**, or natural sugar, into energy for the body. Without insulin to process glucose, these sugars collect in the blood. This causes problems with circulation and can damage vital organs.

People with diabetes must be very careful about what they eat (Fig. 14-15). A registered dietician and the resident will make up a meal plan, including snacks, that must be followed exactly. Calories and carbohydrates are carefully controlled, and protein and fats are also regulated. The foods and the amounts are determined by nutritional and energy needs. Diabetic residents must eat the right amount of the right type of food at the right time, and they must eat everything that is served. This is necessary to maintain blood sugar. Encourage them to eat all of their meals and snacks. Do not offer other foods without the nurse's approval. If a resident will not finish meals and snacks, or throws food away, notify the nurse immediately.

Fig. 14-15. *Diabetics must be very careful about what they eat and must keep their weight in a healthy range.*

A diabetic's meal tray may have artificial sweetener, and low-calorie jelly and maple syrup. When serving coffee or tea to a diabetic resident, use artificial sweeteners rather than sugar. The common abbreviations for this diet on a diet card are "NCS," which stands for "No Concentrated Sweets" or "LCS", which stands for "Low Concentrated Sweets." It may also be listed by showing the amount of calories followed by the abbreviation "ADA," which stands for American Diabetic Association. An example is "1700 calorie ADA." For more information on diabetes, see Chapter 23.

HOT TIP

NPO

The abbreviation "NPO" stands for "Nothing by Mouth." It comes from the Latin "nil per os." This means that a resident is not allowed to have anything to eat or drink. Some residents have a serious problem with swallowing, and it is unsafe to give them anything by mouth. These residents will receive nutrition another way, either through a feeding tube or intravenously (Chapter 26). Some residents may be NPO for a short time before a medical test or surgery. If you see this abbreviation on a diet card or on the resident's care plan, do not offer the resident any food or drink.

8. Explain thickened liquids and identify three basic thickening consistencies

Residents with dysphagia, or difficulty swallowing, are evaluated by speech language pathologists or speech therapists to determine if they should consume thickened liquids to ease swallowing. Thickened liquids have a thickening powder or agent added to them, which improves the ability to control fluid in the mouth and throat. Residents with swallowing problems may require thickened fluids to reduce the risk of choking on fluids. They tend to choke on thinner fluids, such as water or tea. Thickened liquids move down the throat more slowly, reducing coughing and limiting the risk for choking.

After the speech language pathologist assesses a resident, the doctor writes the order for the type of thickening the resident needs. The dietary department then prepares the liquids or the thickening agent is added on the nursing unit before serving. If you have any responsibilities for thickening liquids, you will be properly trained in this task.

Follow instructions carefully for residents who have orders for thickened liquids. These residents are unable to drink any fluid that is not thickened. This means fluids such as soda, water, tea, and coffee are not allowed with their diets. Check with the nurse before serving any fluids to residents with these restrictions.

The three types of thickened consistencies generally used by facilities are:

1. **Nectar Thick**. This consistency is similar to a fruit nectar or other thicker juices, such as tomato juice. A resident can drink this from a cup with or without a straw.

2. **Honey Thick**. This consistency is similar to that of honey. It will pour very slowly, and spoons are usually used to consume these types of liquids.

3. **Pudding Thick**. This consistency is semi-solid, much like the consistency of pudding.

A spoon will stand up straight when put into this thickened liquid. Spoons are used to consume these liquids.

9. List ways to identify and prevent unintended weight loss

Sometimes residents unintentionally lose weight, which is a serious problem for the elderly. The unintended weight loss may be due to a medical condition, such as cancer, HIV, diabetes, or other diseases. It can also be due to an unappetizing diet. Unintended weight loss puts a person at a greater risk for malnutrition. This is why it is important to report any weight loss you notice, no matter how small (Fig. 14-16).

Fig. 14-16. Observing residents for weight loss, no matter how small, is an important part of your job.

When weight loss occurs, staff will look for causes and may re-evaluate special diet orders. This will help them decide whether to modify the diet to encourage the resident to eat more. The resident may be better off eating a less strict diet. If you notice food going uneaten or if a resident complains to you or others about the food, report this to the nurse.

Warning signs for unintended weight loss include the following:

* Resident needs help eating or drinking
* Resident eats less than 70% of meals/snacks
* Resident has mouth pain
* Resident has dentures that do not fit properly

* Resident has difficulty chewing or swallowing
* Resident coughs or chokes while eating
* Resident is sad, cries, or withdraws from others
* Resident is confused, wanders, or paces

If you notice any of these signs, report it immediately to the nurse. Also report if the resident has any of these signs or symptoms, which could indicate the resident is malnourished:

* Feeling of coldness throughout body
* Weight loss
* Abdominal distention
* Abdominal pain
* Constipation
* **Edema** (swelling in body tissues caused by excess fluid)
* Cracks or splits at the corners of the mouth
* Inflammation of the mucous membranes of the mouth
* Dry or peeling skin
* Brittle, easily-cracked nails
* Rapidly thinning hair that breaks off easily; hair that changes or loses color
* Frequent infections
* Muscle weakness
* Fainting
* Fatigue
* Withdrawal or **apathy** (lack of interest)
* Anxiety and irritability
* Problems with sleeping
* Low body temperature
* Slow pulse
* Low blood pressure

In addition, follow these guidelines to help prevent unintended weight loss:

Guidelines

Preventing Unintended Weight Loss

🅖 Report observations and warning signs to the nurse immediately.

- Report any decrease in appetite to the nurse. If a resident has a loss of appetite, ask him or her about it.

- Encourage residents to eat by talking about eating and the food being served in a positive way (Fig. 14-17).

- Check to make sure residents are receiving the correct diet.

- Respond promptly to resident complaints about foods. Serve favorite foods.

- Season the food to the resident's preferences.

- Use special adaptive equipment, as needed, to increase independence with eating.

- Record the meal/snack intake as ordered.

- Ask for a dietician, occupational therapist, or speech language therapist consultation if necessary.

Fig. 14-17. Being positive during mealtime can encourage residents to eat. It helps prevent unintended weight loss.

HOT TIP

Making the Most of Snacks and Nourishments
Residents are usually fed three meals a day, along with additional snacks or nourishments. Supplementary snacks or nourishments include liquids such as milk, juice and specially-formulated nutritional drinks that may contain added protein, vitamins, or other ingredients. Solid snacks include foods like cheese and crackers, peanut butter, sherbet, gelatin, or small sandwiches. These items may be served once or twice or more often per day.
Sometimes snacks or nourishments are required by special diets. For example, a diabetic needs all of her snacks to maintain her blood sugar while on insulin injections. Another resident who is losing too much weight will need to drink all of his nutritional supplements to maintain a healthy weight. Due to

disease and the problem of unintended weight loss, encourage residents to eat all of their snacks or supplements. If a resident does not finish a snack, a family member eats it, or you find it in the trash, notify the nurse.

10. Describe how to make dining enjoyable for residents

Often the most anticipated times of the day for residents are breakfast, lunch and dinner. Meals provide time to see friends and socialize. Mealtimes are also the time for getting proper nourishment. Due to serious problems of weight loss and dehydration, which you will learn more about later in the chapter, nursing assistants are responsible for encouraging eating and promoting healthy appetites. To make mealtimes enjoyable and pleasant, follow these guidelines:

Guidelines
Dining

- Follow a routine for dining. This encourages structure in residents' days.

- Residents may want to look their best. Assist them with their grooming requests. All residents should be neat and clean for meals. Dress residents appropriately for dining.

- Make sure that residents have their eyeglasses, hearing aids, dentures, and any other equipment required for eating comfortably.

- Help to give oral care before meals if they request it.

- Assist them as necessary with washing hands before eating.

- Help with toileting or help them to the bathroom before eating.

- Honor requests to seat residents by their friends. Seat residents with common interests together. Encourage conversation.

- Position residents properly for eating. This position is usually upright at a 90-degree angle, which helps prevent swallowing and choking problems.

- Place residents in appropriate chairs. Wheelchairs should be positioned at the right height for the table. Many tables at facilities are adjustable. These tables should be adjusted to the right height for wheelchairs. Make sure special seats, such as geriatric chairs (geri-chairs), are available if needed for a particular resident. Residents who use geri-chairs must be sitting upright, not reclining, while eating.

- Serve food promptly to maintain the correct temperature of the food.

- Give residents the proper eating tools they will need for their meals. If they need assistive devices, such as special utensils or cups, make sure they are available (Fig. 14-18).

- Cut food into small portions when necessary. Do this before bringing food to the table if possible. This promotes dignity.

- Allow enough time for eating. Do not rush residents through their meals.

- Keep the noise level low. Do not shout or bang trays or plates. Soft music may accompany the meal (Fig. 14-19).

- Remain cheerful and positive during mealtime. Make conversation if residents wish to talk.

- Honor requests regarding food. Residents have the right to ask for and receive different food. They also may be able to have additional food when requested. Check diet orders first before getting any extra food or additive, such as sugar or salt.

Fig. 14-18. Examples of assistive devices that can help with eating. (Photos courtesy of North Coast Medical, Inc., 800-821-9319, www.ncmedical.com.)

Fig. 14-19. The environment is important in promoting appetites. Keep the noise level low.

11. Describe how to serve meal trays and assist with eating

Meals are usually served on trays or are brought from the kitchen. Nursing assistants must work quickly to make sure food is served at the proper temperature and that residents do not have to wait long for their meals. Follow these guidelines for serving meals to residents:

Guidelines
Serving Meal Trays

- Wash your hands before serving any meal trays.

- Check the diet card for special diet orders, and identify each resident before serving a meal tray. Make sure the food looks correct for each person. As you learned earlier, serving a resident the wrong food can cause serious health problems, even death.

- Serve all residents sitting at one table before serving other tables, so the residents will be able to eat together.

- If a resident needs your help to eat, leave the tray on the cart until you are able to do this task. Keep the door to the food cart closed after removing each tray. Maintaining the proper temperature of food helps prevent foodborne illnesses.

- Prepare the food before helping residents eat. Only do what residents cannot do for themselves.

- Open juice or milk cartons, if residents need help. If a resident is able to use a straw and wants one, place it in the container using the wrapper; do not touch straws with your fingers. Pour beverages into cups if residents do not want to use cartons.

- Butter rolls, bread, and vegetables as residents prefer.

- Season food according to what the resident wants, even pureed food. Remember not to season food with salt if a resident is on a low-sodium diet.

- When serving additional snacks or nourishments to residents, follow the same guidelines as for serving regular meal trays. Provide any necessary assistance with snacks and nourishments. Report to the nurse if residents do not finish their supplemental snacks or nourishments.

You may be required to serve meal trays to residents in isolation. Carefully follow Isolation Precautions, in addition to Standard Precautions, ordered for each resident. Apply PPE as needed, and make sure dietary department staff puts on proper PPE as well.

For residents in isolation, food trays may be served using regular dishes and standard utensils. These items are then washed and in some cases, disinfected. Some facilities use disposable serving equipment. Properly dispose of this equipment after use according to facility policy.

Food inside an isolation room must never be shared with visitors, other residents, or staff. Discard uneaten food in the proper container in the isolation room. Apply PPE before entering the room to remove a meal tray.

HOT TIP

Ask before you pass.
When serving meal trays on a unit, ask the nurses before you serve them to learn about any special diet orders and names of residents who are NPO. Check diet cards carefully.

Residents differ in the amount of assistance they need with eating. Good organization on your part will help make the dining experience run smoothly. Prepare residents who require the least assistance first. Make sure everything is ready, such as opening cartons and cutting and seasoning food. When the resident is ready to feed himself, you can move on to the next resident. Continue this process until all residents who can eat on their own are set up and eating. Check back with these residents from time to time to see if they need anything else.

Some residents will be completely unable to feed themselves. When assisting residents with feeding, promote independence by encouraging them to do whatever they can for themselves. For example, if a resident can hold and use a napkin, she should. If she can hold and eat finger foods, offer them. As mentioned earlier, special assistive devices for eating can be helpful, too.

Promoting independence with eating positively affects self-esteem. It is very difficult when a person has to depend on another person for assistance with a basic need such as eating. Empathize with residents and be sensitive to this. Provide privacy as needed when eating.

Eating is a social time, and even residents who must be fed or who get their nutrition via tubes (Chapter 26) may still enjoy being social with others. While assisting with eating, make conversation if the resident wishes, using appropriate topics, such as the news and weather (Fig. 14-20). Pay attention to the person you are helping; do not talk to other staff members while assisting residents with eating. Say positive things about the food being served. For example, "This smells really good," and, "This looks really fresh." Meal time should be a pleasant experience, and cheerful company can actually increase how much a resident eats and drinks. Do not rush residents through their meals.

Fig. 14-20. *Be friendly and social while helping residents with eating. Encourage them to do whatever they can for themselves.*

In addition, follow these guidelines for helping residents at meal time:

- Offer a clothing protector to the resident before assisting with eating. Do not refer to the clothing protector as a "bib." If he refuses to wear one, respect his wishes. Residents have the right to choose whether or not to use a clothing protector (Fig. 14-21).

- Treat the resident with respect. Do not make fun of or judge any food choices.

- Follow all infection control precautions.

- Sit at the resident's eye level and make eye contact. Give the resident your full attention.

- Identify foods and fluids in front of the resident. Call pureed foods and soft foods by their correct names. For example, ask, "Would you like some steak?" rather than asking if they want "some of this brown stuff."

- Ask the resident which foods he wants to eat first and honor his choices.

- Do not mix foods unless the resident requests it.

- If you are concerned that food is too hot, do not touch it to test its temperature. Put your hand over the food to sense the heat. Do not blow on it to cool it if it feels too hot. Offer other foods first while you wait for it to cool down.

- Alternate between food and drink. Offer fluids to the resident throughout the meal.

- If a resident wants different food than what is being served, tell the dietician or the nurse right away.

- If a resident refuses to eat, respect this. Do not insist that he eat the food, but report it to the nurse immediately.

Fig. 14-21. *Residents have the right to choose whether to use a clothing protector. Respect each resident's decision.* (Reprinted with permission of Briggs Corporation, Des Moines, IA, 800-247-2343.)

Feeding a resident who cannot feed self

Equipment: meal tray, clothing protector, 1-2 washcloths

1. Identify yourself by name. Identify the resident. Greet the resident by name.

2. Wash your hands.

3. Explain procedure to resident. Speak clearly, slowly, and directly. Maintain face-to-face contact whenever possible. Encourage resident to assist if possible.

4. Provide for the resident's privacy with a curtain, screen, or door.

5. Pick up diet card. Verify that resident has received the right tray.

6. Help resident to wash hands (and face if needed) if the resident cannot do it on her own.

7. Adjust bed height so you will be able to sit at resident's eye level. Lock bed wheels.

8. Lower the side rail (if bed has one and if it is not already lowered) on side nearest you.

9. Raise the head of the bed. Make sure resident is in an upright sitting position (at a 90-degree angle).

10. Help resident to put on clothing protector, if desired.

11. Sit facing resident. Sit at resident's eye level (Fig. 14-22). Sit on the stronger side if resident has one-sided weakness.

Fig. 14-22. The resident should be sitting upright and you should be sitting at her eye level.

12. Offer drink of beverage. Offer different types of food, allowing for resident's preferences. Do not feed all of one type before offering another type.

13. Offer the food in bite-sized pieces (Fig. 14-23). Report any swallowing problems to the nurse immediately. If resident has one-sided weakness, direct food to the unaffected, or stronger, side.

Fig. 14-23. Offer the food in bite-sized pieces, and direct food to the resident's stronger, or unaffected, side.

14. Make sure resident's mouth is empty before next bite or sip.

15. Offer beverage to resident throughout the meal.

16. Talk with the resident during the meal (Fig. 14-24).

Fig. 14-24. Talking with the resident makes mealtime more enjoyable and may promote her appetite.

17. Use washcloths to wipe food from resident's mouth and hands as needed during the meal. Wipe again at the end of the meal (Fig. 14-25).

Fig. 14-25. Wiping food from the mouth during the meal helps to maintain the resident's dignity.

18. Remove clothing protector if used. Dispose of in proper container.

19. Remove food tray. Check for eyeglasses, dentures, hearing aids, or any personal items before removing tray.

20. Make resident comfortable.

21. Return bed to low position if raised. Ensure resident's safety. Return side rails to ordered position. Remove privacy measures.

22. Leave call light within resident's reach.

23. Wash your hands.

24. Be courteous and respectful at all times.

25. Report any changes in the resident to the nurse. Document procedure using facility guidelines. Record intake of solid food and fluids properly (see Learning Objective 14 for more information).

Residents' Rights and Eating

Residents have the right to refuse food and drink. Residents also have the right to ask for and receive different kinds of food.

12. Describe how to assist residents with special needs

Residents with certain diseases or conditions, such as Parkinson's disease, stroke, dementia, head trauma, blindness, and confusion may need additional help with eating. For example, a resident who has Parkinson's disease may have tremors or shaking and stiffness, which make it very difficult to eat without help. Follow these guidelines for special dining techniques.

Guidelines
Dining Techniques

ⓖ Use assistive or adaptive devices for eating when necessary. They help people feed themselves. Utensils with padded handles and plates with high edges to prevent food from sliding off are two examples of assistive devices for eating.

ⓖ To help maintain independence with eating, use physical and verbal cues. The hand-over-hand approach is an example of a physical cue. The resident lifts a utensil if he is able, and you put your hand over his to help with eating (Fig. 14-26). With your hand placed over the resident's hand, assist in getting food on the utensil. Steer the utensil from the plate to the mouth and back. Repeat this until the resident is done with his meal.

ⓖ Verbal cues must be short and clear so that they are easily understood. After each task is done, give additional prompts one at a time. For example, "Pick up your spoon." "Put some potatoes on your spoon." "Lift the spoon to your mouth." These types of phrases are repeated until the resident has finished eating.

ⓖ For residents who have had a stroke and have a weaker side, always put food into the stronger, or unaffected, side of the mouth.

This helps prevent choking. Make sure food is swallowed before offering more bites.

ⓖ For residents who have Parkinson's disease, dementia, confusion, or trauma, use physical and verbal cues if needed. Allow enough time to chew and swallow. Place food and drinks within the resident's reach.

ⓖ For residents who are visually-impaired or blind, read menus to them if needed. Allow enough time for decision-making on menu items. When assisting with eating, face them when speaking and use a normal tone of voice. Place plate or tray directly in front of residents. Use the face of an imaginary clock to explain the position of what is in front of them (Fig. 14-27). If necessary, let residents know when to open their mouths and what food they are eating.

Fig. 14-26. The hand-over-hand approach is used when a resident can help by lifting utensils. It helps promote independence.

Fig. 14-27. Use the face of an imaginary clock to explain the position of food to visually-impaired residents.

In addition to the above guidelines, use these techniques to handle specific problems with eating:

If the resident eats too quickly, remind him to chew, and set the utensils down between bites. Use smaller cups and plates and put less food on plates.

If the resident bites down on utensils, ask the resident to open his mouth. Wait until the jaw relaxes to pull the utensil out of the mouth. Offer finger foods instead. Use smaller utensils, but do not use plastic utensils. Avoid using forks.

If the resident cannot or will not chew, ask him to chew. Lightly press on the edge of the lips or on the chin to stimulate chewing. You can also show him how to chew by doing it yourself. Serve softer foods that require less chewing; dip meats and other foods in sauce or gravy if allowed.

If the resident will not stop chewing, ask him to stop chewing. Offer smaller bites of food and feed softer foods that do not need as much chewing.

If the resident holds food in his mouth or will not swallow, remind him to swallow after every bite. After feeding a bite of real food, lightly press an empty teaspoon against the lips to encourage the person to swallow the food. This may help stimulate saliva production, along with the swallowing reflex.

If the resident pockets food in his cheek, ask him to chew and swallow the food. Touch the side of the cheek and ask him to use his tongue to get the food. Using your fingers on the cheek near the lower jaw, gently push food toward teeth. Avoid offering food such as rice that can stick inside the mouth or on dentures. Give sips of fluids often. Check the mouth for food often before offering more food, but do not place your fingers inside the mouth. Ask the resident to open his mouth so that you can check for food. Ask residents not to stand up with food in their mouths.

If the resident has poor lip closure, remind him to close his lips. Show him how to close his lips if necessary. A speech language pathologist or a nurse may teach this resident to practice blowing a whistle to help him close his lips.

If the resident has no teeth or is missing teeth, a dentist will do an assessment of oral health. Thickened liquids or soft or pureed diets may be ordered.

If the resident has dentures that do not fit properly, report it to the nurse immediately. A dentist will evaluate the resident as soon as possible for denture replacement. Thickened liquids or soft or pureed diets may be ordered until dentures are replaced.

If the resident has a change in vision causing problems with seeing food clearly and reduced appetite, make sure resident wears glasses and make sure they are clean. Report to the nurse if resident's glasses are damaged or broken. Read menus out loud and describe food in front of the resident using the imaginary clock if necessary.

If the resident has a protruding tongue or tongue thrust, using special straws and cups may help. A tongue thrust is a forceful protrusion of the tongue, often during eating and drinking. The jaw will need to be encouraged to move upward so that the tongue will retract and the lips will close on the eating utensil. A speech language pathologist or a nurse may teach this resident to practice blowing a whistle to help him close his lips.

If the resident will not open his mouth, touch his lower lip to encourage him to open the mouth. Identify each bite of food you offer. Do not feed sticky food such as peanut butter.

If the resident falls asleep while eating, seat him with residents who talk a lot and are very social. Make appropriate conversation while he is eating.

If the resident chokes when drinking, remind him to lift his chin before taking a sip of fluid. Offer fluids when he has no food in his mouth.

Do not distract the resident by talking while he is eating. The resident should be seated, not standing, while drinking.

If the resident is susceptible to choking when eating, avoid foods like cake, hot dogs, peanut butter, nuts, popcorn, raw vegetables and small, shiny fruits, like grapes.

If the resident forgets to eat, remind him to take another bite. Offer praise and encouragement. Do not rush the person.

If the resident drools excessively, make sure he is in an upright eating position, using good posture. A consultation with a speech language pathologist may be ordered to help the resident learn better swallowing techniques. If drooling interferes with basic safety, medications may be ordered to decrease the drooling. Clothing protectors, towels or pads may be used to protect clothing.

If the resident has poor sitting balance, seat him in a regular dining room chair with armrests, rather than a wheelchair. Position him upright at a 90-degree angle. Knees should be flexed and feet and arms should be fully supported. Push the chair under the table and place his forearms on the table.

If the resident tends to lean on one side, ask him to keep his elbows on the table. Using a wheelchair wedge cushion may help.

If resident tends to fall forward, a geriatric chair may help. Using a wheelchair wedge cushion may also help.

If the resident has poor neck control, a soft neck brace may be used to stabilize the head. For a resident in a geriatric chair, a wedge cushion behind the head and shoulders may be used.

For tips on feeding residents who are cognitively impaired, see Chapter 22.

13. Discuss dysphagia and list guidelines for preventing aspiration

Difficulty in swallowing, or dysphagia, can be a serious problem for elderly residents. Causes of dysphagia include: illness (stroke is one example), certain medications, problems with the mouth and throat muscles, weakness, and even food choices. Problems with teeth or dentures also put a person at risk for swallowing problems. The need for proper oral care can affect the ability to eat or drink safely.

Signs and symptoms of swallowing problems must be reported to the nurse immediately. Nurses, doctors, and care team members, such as the speech language pathologist, will determine what steps to take to reduce dysphagia. The following are signs and symptoms of dysphagia to report to the nurse:

- eating very slowly
- avoidance of eating
- spitting out pieces of food
- difficulty chewing food
- difficulty swallowing small bites of food or pills
- swallowing several times when eating a single bite
- dribbling saliva, food or fluid from the mouth
- keeping food inside the mouth or cheeks during and after meals
- vomiting while eating or drinking
- frequent throat clearing
- food or fluid coming up into or out of the nose
- coughing during or after meals
- choking during meals or while drinking
- gurgling sound in voice during or after meals
- problems breathing when eating or drinking
- visible effort to swallow
- watering eyes when eating or drinking

In addition, observing and reporting the following may help the care team assess a resident who has dysphagia:

- type of food or drink that caused the problem
- time of day the problem occurred

- whether or not the resident had dentures in place when the problem happened

- whether or not the resident was talking or laughing when the choking occurred

- how the resident was positioned while eating or drinking

- whether or not the resident was ambulating (walking) while eating or drinking

As you have learned, swallowing problems cause a high risk for choking on food or drink. When a person chokes, mucus, food or fluids, or emesis (vomitus) may move into the lungs. Inhaling food or drink into the lungs is called aspiration, which can cause pneumonia or death. To ensure residents' safety, follow these guidelines to prevent aspiration:

Guidelines

Preventing Aspiration

- Ⓔ Place residents in proper position for eating and drinking. They must sit upright at a 90-degree angle (Fig. 14-28). Do not feed residents in a reclining position.

- Ⓔ Feed residents slowly.

- Ⓔ Avoid distractions while eating.

- Ⓔ Offer small pieces of food or small spoonfuls of pureed food.

- Ⓔ Offer a bite of food, then a liquid. Repeat this.

- Ⓔ Place food in the non-paralyzed, or unaffected, side of the mouth, if one side is paralyzed.

- Ⓔ Make sure food is actually swallowed after each bite before offering more food or fluids. However, do not put your fingers inside a resident's mouth.

- Ⓔ Keep residents sitting upright for at least 30 minutes after eating and drinking.

- Ⓔ Provide quality mouth care after eating.

- Ⓔ Observe residents closely who choke easily during eating and drinking. Report signs of aspiration, such as gagging, vomiting, clutching throat, cyanosis (bluish skin color), darkening skin, unconsciousness, shortness of breath, difficulty breathing, or resident complaints of chest pain or tightness in the chest to the nurse immediately.

Fig. 14-28. Sitting as upright as possible when eating and drinking helps prevent aspiration.

More information on swallowing difficulties and alternative methods of feeding is in Chapter 26.

RESIDENTS' RIGHTS

Take your time when feeding residents.
Feeding residents quickly is dangerous. It increases the risk for choking and aspiration. When you are helping residents eat, take your time. Do not rush residents through the dining process. Be patient, cheerful and positive. Taking your time helps to ensure residents' safety. It can also greatly increase the amount a resident eats and drinks.

14. Describe intake and output (I&O)

As you learned earlier, the fluid a person consumes is called intake, or input. **Output** is the fluid that is eliminated each day that cannot stay in the body. Output includes urine, feces, and vomitus, as well as perspiration, and moisture in the air that a person exhales. It also includes suction material and wound drainage. When a person maintains equal intake and output, or consumes and eliminates equal amounts of fluid, it is called **fluid balance**.

Most people maintain fluid balance naturally. However, residents on special diets or who have certain illnesses may need to have their intake and output (I&O) measured. Measuring I&O means that staff record and add together all of the amounts of food and fluids the resident takes in and eliminates within 24 hours. This is recorded on an Intake/Output (I&O) sheet (Fig. 14-29).

Fluids are usually measured in milliliters (mL). Milliliters are units of measurement in the metric system. One milliliter is 1/1000 of a liter and is equal to one cubic centimeter (cc). Ounces (oz) are converted to milliliters. One ounce equals 30 milliliters, so to convert ounces to milliliters, multiply by 30. **Graduates** are containers that measure fluid in milliliters and may also measure in ounces (Fig. 14-30). It is important to know how to convert ounces to milliliters, as well as other common conversions. See the box at right for information on conversions.

Fig. 14-30. A graduate is a measuring container.

Conversions

One milliliter (mL) is a unit of measure equal to one cubic centimeter (cc). Follow your facility's policies on whether to document using "mL" or "cc".

1 oz. = 30 mL or 30 cc
2 oz. = 60 mL
3 oz. = 90 mL
4 oz. = 120 mL
5 oz. = 150 mL
6 oz. = 180 mL
7 oz. = 210 mL
8 oz. = 240 mL
¼ cup = 2 oz. = 60 mL
½ cup = 4 oz. = 120 mL
1 cup = 8 oz. = 240 mL

For example, a resident has an eight-ounce glass of juice. She consumes about half of the juice, or four ounces. To determine her intake, convert ounces to milliliters. Multiply four ounces by 30; the answer is 120 mL, which is what you document on the intake sheet.

Measuring and recording intake and output

Equipment: I&O sheet, graduate (measuring container), pen and paper to record your findings

1. Identify yourself by name. Identify the resident. Greet the resident by name.

2. Wash your hands.

3. Explain procedure to resident. Speak clearly, slowly, and directly. Maintain face-to-face contact whenever possible. Encourage resident to assist if possible.

INTAKE AND OUTPUT RECORD

Fig. 14-29. A sample intake and output (I&O) form.

4. Provide for the resident's privacy with a curtain, screen, or door.

5. A list of container sizes should be available to help with measuring. For example, a water cup equals 240 mL, a cereal bowl equals 150 mL, and a milk carton equals 240 mL. If amounts are not available, use a graduate to measure how much fluid a resident is served. Note the amount of fluid the resident is served on paper.

6. When the resident has finished a meal or snack, measure any leftover fluids. Note this amount on paper.

7. Subtract the leftover amount from the amount served. If you have measured in ounces, convert to milliliters (mL) by multiplying by 30.

8. Record amount of fluid consumed (in mL) in input column on I&O sheet. Record the time and what fluid was consumed.

9. Wash your hands.

Measuring output is the other half of monitoring fluid balance.

Equipment: I&O sheet, graduate, gloves, additional PPE if required, pen and paper to record your findings

1. Wash your hands.

2. Put on gloves before handling bedpan/urinal.

3. Pour the contents of the bedpan or urinal into measuring container. Do not spill or splash any of the urine.

4. Place container on flat surface. Measure amount of urine at eye level. Keep container level (Fig. 14-31).

***Fig. 14-31.** Keep container level while measuring output.*

5. After measuring urine, empty measuring container into toilet. Do not splash.

6. Rinse measuring container. Pour rinse water into toilet. Clean container using facility guidelines.

7. Rinse bedpan/urinal. Pour rinse water into toilet. Use approved disinfectant.

8. Return bedpan/urinal and measuring container to proper storage.

9. Remove and dispose of gloves.

10. Wash hands before recording output.

11. Record contents of container in output column on sheet. Report any changes to the nurse.

To record food intake, the percentage method is often used. Menus that list the percentage of total calories of each item served may be used. A dietician calculates these percentages. It is important to accurately record how much of the meal the resident has eaten. To do this, observe how much of each item was consumed. Then adjust the percentage of total calories the item provided. Finally, add the adjusted percentages for a total percentage consumed.

For example, egg, toast and milk is on a resident's breakfast tray. The egg is worth 20% of calories needed for her breakfast. If she finishes half of the egg, you would document that she consumed 10% of that food. If the toast is worth 15%, and she eats all of the toast, you would record the full 15% toward the total calories consumed. This is one example of how to document intake using the percentage method. Facilities may document intake in other ways. Follow your facility's policy. Document food and drink intake very carefully. Accuracy is important. Report to the nurse if a resident eats less than 70% of his or her meal.

15. List ways to identify and prevent dehydration

Water is one of the most important nutrients for life. Drinking at least 64 ounces (eight 8-ounce glasses) of water or other fluids per day can help prevent constipation, urinary incontinence and dehydration. **Dehydration** is a serious condition that occurs when a person does not have enough fluid in the body. Proper fluid intake also helps to dilute wastes and flush out the urinary system, which lessens the risk of infection (Fig. 14-32).

Fig. 14-32. *Remember, drinking plenty of water is good for you, too!*

Because the sense of thirst lessens as people age, fluids should be offered to residents often. A "force fluids" (FF) order may be written for a resident who is at risk of being dehydrated. **Force fluids** means to encourage the resident to drink more fluids.

Warning signs of dehydration include the following:

- resident drinks less than six 8-ounce glasses of liquids per day
- resident drinks little or no fluids at meals
- resident needs help drinking from a cup or glass
- resident has trouble swallowing liquids
- resident has frequent vomiting, diarrhea, or fever
- resident is easily confused or tired
- resident is thirsty

- resident has a dry mouth
- resident has a decrease in urinary output

If you notice any of these signs, report it immediately to the nurse. Also report if the resident has any of these symptoms:

- severe thirst
- dry mouth and mucous membranes
- cracked lips
- dry, warm, wrinkled, or clammy skin
- sunken eyes
- flushed face
- decrease in urinary output
- dark urine
- strong-smelling urine
- constipation or weight loss
- weakness, dizziness, lightheadedness, or confusion
- headache
- irritability
- rapid or weakened pulse
- irregular heartbeat
- low blood pressure

Preventing dehydration is an important nursing assistant responsibility. Follow these guidelines to help prevent dehydration:

Guidelines

Preventing Dehydration

- Observe residents carefully for signs and symptoms of dehydration. Report observations and warning signs to the nurse immediately.

- Encourage residents to drink fluids every time you see them, if allowed. Offer fresh water or other fluids often (Fig. 14-33).

- Offer fluids that residents prefer, such as water, juice, or milk. Some residents will prefer fluids without ice. Honor this preference. If the resident wants ice in his drink, use and store the ice scoop properly. Do not let ice touch your hand and then fall back into the container. Place the ice scoop in the proper receptacle after each use. Report if the resident complains about the fluids being offered.

- If drinking water causes a resident to choke, he has the right to have alternative fluids. Discuss this with the nurse.

- Make sure water pitcher and cup are close enough to the resident and light enough for the resident to lift, approximately half-full.

- Offer assistance if the resident cannot drink without help. Use assistive devices as needed.

- Offer ice chips, flavored ice sticks, and gelatin often. These items are considered liquids. Do not offer ice chips or sticks if resident has a swallowing problem.

- Keep accurate I&O records.

- Follow posted schedules for offering fluids.

Fig. 14-33. *Encouraging residents to drink every time you see them can help prevent dehydration.*

One method of encouraging fluids is outlined in the acronym below:

POURR

Post a regular schedule for offering fluids to residents.

Observe residents carefully for signs and symptoms of dehydration.

Use other kinds of fluids, such as flavored frozen ice sticks, to improve fluid balance and increase fluid intake.

Remind all staff, visitors and volunteers as necessary of the importance of following the schedule.

Report changes in fluid balance or any signs and symptoms of dehydration promptly.

RESIDENTS' RIGHTS

A request for a drink must be honored.
When residents are thirsty, they may ask for water, juice, or some other beverage. Respond promptly to these requests. Ignoring a request for a drink is considered abuse. The only time you should not honor this request is when a resident is on a fluid restriction or "NPO." NPO stands for "Nothing by Mouth." In this situation, explain why a drink cannot be given. Report the request to the nurse.

16. List signs and symptoms of fluid overload and describe conditions that may require fluid restrictions

Fluid overload is a condition that occurs when more fluid enters the body than is eliminated from the body. The body cannot eliminate the additional fluid, and fluid gathers in certain areas of the body, such as the ankles. Fluid overload can occur when the heart, kidneys or lungs are not working properly. People can also have this problem after having surgery.

Symptoms of fluid overload to observe and report to the nurse include:

- weight gain (daily weight gain of one to two pounds)
- fatigue
- difficulty breathing or shortness of breath, especially if lying down
- swelling (edema) of the ankles, feet, fingers or hands
- coughing
- less urine output
- increased heart rate
- skin that appears tight, smooth, and shiny
- swollen abdomen due to excess fluid, called ascites

Treating fluid overload usually consists of a reduction in activity, medicine to eliminate the excessive fluid, a change in the number of pillows the person sleeps with, and careful monitoring of weight gain and edema.

Fluid restrictions are ordered when the amount of fluid must be carefully measured and limited due to certain disorders. Examples are congestive heart failure (CHF) (Chapter 19), or chronic kidney failure (Chapter 16). Some residents will have a **restrict fluids** (RF) order, which means the person is allowed to drink, but must limit the daily amount to a level set by the doctor. When a resident has a restrict fluids order, do not give that resident extra fluids or a water pitcher unless the nurse approves it.

Other reasons for fluid restrictions include:

- recent surgery
- illness, such as a gastrointestinal (GI) illness
- special medical test ordered
- feeding done through a special tube (For more information on feeding tubes and related care, see Chapter 26.)

CHAPTER REVIEW

1. List five common nutritional problems that elderly people may experience (LO 2).

2. List two factors that influence food choices (LO 3).

3. List the six basic nutrients and identify which nutrient is the most essential for life (LO 4).

4. Identify what each of the six colored bands of MyPyramid stand for. Which color band is the smallest and why (LO 5)?

5. Why may elderly people need fewer calories to maintain health (LO 5)?

6. How much activity per day does MyPyramid recommend (LO 5)?

7. List the information contained on diet cards (LO 6).

8. Why is it very important to check resident identification against the diet card before serving meal trays (LO 7)?

9. How is the mechanical soft diet different from the soft diet (LO 7)?

10. What is one common abbreviation for a low-sodium diet (LO 7)?

11. What is the difference between a clear liquid diet and a full liquid diet (LO 7)?

12. Why must diabetic residents eat the right amount of the right type of food at the right time, and eat everything that is served (LO 7)?

13. What does the abbreviation "NPO" stand for (LO 7)?

14. Explain three basic thickening consistencies (LO 8).

15. What is the benefit of thickening liquids (LO 8)?

16. List six warning signs for unintended weight loss that should be reported (LO 9).

17. What is the proper position to place a resident for eating (LO 10)?

18. Look at the guidelines for dining in Learning Objective 10. List four that promote residents' dignity (LO 10).

19. When serving meal trays, why should nursing assistants only do what residents cannot do for themselves? Why should residents be encouraged to do whatever they can for themselves (LO 11)?

20. Give two examples, other than those listed in Learning Objective 11, of positive things to say about food being served (LO 11).

21. If a resident refuses to wear a clothing protector, what should the nursing assistant do (LO 11)?

22. How should a nursing assistant properly test the temperature of food if she feels it might be too hot (LO 11)?

23. To which side of the mouth should food be directed if a resident has a weaker side—the weaker (affected) or stronger (unaffected) side (LO 12)?

24. When assisting a resident who is visually-impaired, how should the nursing assistant explain the position of food and objects in front of the resident (LO 12)?

25. For each of the following conditions, list a technique that would help with eating (LO 12):

    The resident bites down on utensils

    The resident will not chew

    The resident pockets food in his cheek

    The resident has poor sitting balance

    The resident has poor neck control

26. List 11 signs and symptoms of dysphagia (LO 13).

27. List eight guidelines for preventing aspiration (LO 13).

28. List four examples of output (LO 14).

29. Define "fluid balance" (LO 14).

30. How many milliliters (mL) equal one ounce (oz.) (LO 14)?

31. How many ounces of water or other liquids should a healthy resident be encouraged to drink every day (LO 15)?

32. List four warning signs of dehydration that should be reported (LO 15).

33. List six ways to prevent dehydration (LO 15).

34. List seven symptoms of fluid overload (LO 16).

35. What is a "restrict fluids (RF)" order (LO 16)?

15
The Gastrointestinal System

1. Define important words in this chapter

absorption: the digestive process in which digestive juices and enzymes break down food into materials the body can use.

anal incontinence: an inability to control the muscles of the bowels, which leads to an involuntary passage of stool or gas; also called fecal incontinence.

anatomy: the study of body structure.

biology: the study of all life forms.

body systems: groups of organs that perform specific functions in the human body.

bowel elimination: the physical process of releasing or emptying the colon or large intestine of stool or feces.

cells: the basic structural unit of all organisms.

chyme: semi-liquid substance made as a result of the chemical breakdown of food in the stomach.

colon: the large intestine.

colostomy: surgically-created opening into the large intestine to allow feces to be expelled; causes stool to be semi-solid.

constipation: the difficult and often painful elimination of a hard, dry stool.

Crohn's disease: a disease that causes the wall of the intestines (large or small) to become inflamed (red, sore and swollen).

defecation: the process of eliminating feces from the rectum through the anus.

diarrhea: frequent elimination of liquid or semi-liquid feces.

digestion: the process of breaking down food so that it can be absorbed into the cells.

diverticulitis: inflammation of sacs that develop in the wall of the large intestine due to diverticulosis.

diverticulosis: a disorder in which sac-like pouchings develop in weakened areas of the wall of the large intestine (colon).

duodenum: the first part of the small intestine where the common bile duct enters the small intestine.

electrolytes: chemical substances that are essential to maintaining fluid balance and homeostasis in the body.

elimination: the process of expelling wastes.

enema: a specific amount of water, with or without an additive, introduced into the colon to eliminate stool.

fecal impaction: a mass of dry, hard stool that remains packed in the rectum and cannot be expelled.

feces: solid body waste excreted through the anus from the large intestine; also called stool.

flatulence: air in the intestine that is passed through the rectum; also called gas or flatus.

fracture pan: a bedpan that is flatter than a regular bedpan; used for small or thin people or those who cannot lift their buttocks onto a standard bedpan.

gastroesophageal reflux disease (GERD): a chronic condition in which the liquid contents of the stomach back up into the esophagus.

gastrointestinal tract: a continuous tube from the opening of the mouth all the way to the anus, where solid wastes are eliminated from the body.

heartburn: a condition that results from a weakening of the sphincter muscle which joins the esophagus and the stomach; also known as acid reflux.

hemorrhoids: enlarged veins in the rectum that can cause itching, burning, pain, and bleeding.

homeostasis: the condition in which all of the body's systems are balanced and are working at their best.

ileostomy: surgically-created opening into the end of the small intestine, the ileum, to allow feces to be expelled; causes stool to be liquid.

ingestion: the process of taking food or fluids into the body.

irritable bowel syndrome (IBS): a chronic condition of the gastrointestinal tract that is worsened by stress.

lactose intolerance: the inability to digest lactose, a type of sugar in milk and other dairy products.

malabsorption: a condition in which the body cannot absorb or digest a particular nutrient properly.

occult: hidden.

organ: a structural unit in the human body that performs a specific function.

ostomy: surgical creation of an opening from an area inside the body to the outside.

pathophysiology: the study of the disorders that occur in the body.

peristalsis: muscular contractions that push food through the gastrointestinal tract.

physiology: the study of how body parts function.

portable commode: a chair with a toilet seat and a removable container underneath.

specimen: a sample, such as of tissue, blood, urine, stool, or sputum, used for analysis and diagnosis.

stoma: an artificial opening in the body.

suppository: a medication given rectally to cause a bowel movement.

tissues: a group of cells that performs similar tasks.

ulcerative colitis: a chronic inflammatory disease of the large intestine.

ureterostomy: a type of urostomy in which a surgical creation of an opening from the ureter through the abdomen is made for urine to be eliminated.

urostomy: the general term used for any surgical procedure that diverts the passage of urine by re-directing the ureters.

2. Explain key terms related to the body

Biology is the study of all life forms. Anatomy and physiology are a part of the science of biology. **Anatomy** is the study of body structure, while **physiology** looks at how body parts function.

The human body is made up of many different kinds of cells. **Cells** are the basic structural unit of all organisms. Living cells divide, grow, and die, renewing the tissues and organs of the body. Each cell looks different and has specific functions. Examples of cells are blood, nerve, and muscle cells.

Tissues are made up of groups of cells. Together, these groups of cells perform specific body functions. Examples of tissues are epithelial, connective, muscle, and nervous.

Groups of tissues come together to form **organs**. Each organ has a specific function to perform to keep the body healthy. The heart is an example of an organ.

Organs in the human body are organized into body systems. **Body systems** are made up of different organs that perform specific functions in the body. Each system in the body has its own unique function. Two examples are the circulatory system, consisting of the heart and blood vessels, and the urinary system, consisting of

the kidneys, ureters, bladder, and urethra. Chapters 15 through 24 discuss body systems and related care. This textbook has organized the human body into these ten systems:

1. Gastrointestinal or Digestive
2. Urinary
3. Reproductive
4. Integumentary, or Skin
5. Circulatory or Cardiovascular
6. Respiratory
7. Musculoskeletal
8. Nervous
9. Endocrine
10. Lymphatic and Immune

Staying healthy and functioning normally is very important. In order to do this, the body must keep certain internal conditions stable, regardless of external factors. This is called homeostasis. **Homeostasis** is the condition in which all of the body's systems are balanced and are working at their best. Keeping body temperature around 98.6° Fahrenheit, regardless of how cold or hot it is outside, is an example of homeostasis.

Pathophysiology is the study of the disorders (conditions or diseases) that occur in the body. You will learn about diseases, along with normal, age-related changes for each body system listed above. Knowing what normal changes of aging are for each body system will help you better recognize any abnormal changes in your residents.

3. Explain the structure and function of the gastrointestinal system

The gastrointestinal (GI) system, also called the digestive system, is made up of two sections: the gastrointestinal tract and the accessory organs (Fig. 15-1). The **gastrointestinal tract** is a continuous tube from the opening of the mouth all the way to the anus, where solid wastes are eliminated from the body.

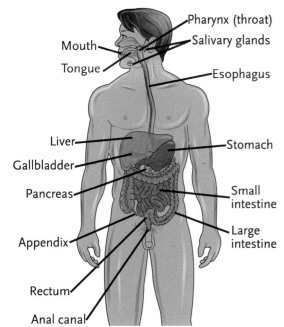

Fig. 15-1. The GI system consists of all the organs needed to digest food and process waste.

Food enters the mouth when a person eats. The tongue begins by moving food around in the mouth. The salivary glands secrete a fluid called saliva, which begins lubricating and dissolving the food. The teeth break up food during a process called mastication (chewing). Food forms into a bolus, a mass of food that is easier to swallow. The bolus moves into the pharynx or throat, where it travels down to the esophagus, a tube about ten inches in length. This occurs as part of the swallowing reflex. Breathing pauses during swallowing because breathing and swallowing cannot occur at the same time. The epiglottis shuts off the larynx during the swallowing process. This blocks food from entering the trachea, or windpipe, and causing choking. Food moves into the stomach from the esophagus because of muscular contractions that push it toward the stomach. This is called **peristalsis**.

When the food reaches the stomach, it mixes with gastric juice. This fluid is capable of killing most microorganisms that enter the stomach. The stomach changes the food into a substance called **chyme**. Food usually stays in the stomach for about two to six hours after eating. From

there, the chyme passes into the first part of the small intestine, called the **duodenum**. The small intestine is about 20 feet long and is approximately an inch in diameter.

The small intestine receives secretions from the liver and the pancreas. The small intestine also secretes intestinal digestive juice from its walls. The liver produces bile, a substance that breaks down fats, and releases bile into the gallbladder. When needed, the gallbladder sends the bile to the small intestine through the common bile duct. The pancreas produces juices that digest carbohydrates, proteins, and fats. These juices are sent to the small intestine through the pancreatic duct, which joins the common bile duct.

The small intestine is lined with villi, tiny finger-like projections that absorb food and fluids. **Absorption** takes place because the food is broken down into tiny molecules that are able to travel through the cells into the blood and lymph. Approximately 90% of food and fluids is absorbed in the small intestine.

The rest of absorption occurs in the large intestine. It is about two and one-half inches in diameter and about five feet long. The large intestine helps regulate water balance by absorbing water and electrolytes and eliminating solid wastes as **feces**. **Electrolytes** are chemical substances that are essential to maintaining fluid balance and homeostasis within the body.

The first part of the large intestine, the cecum, has a valve that prevents the feces from moving backward into the small intestine. The appendix is attached to the cecum. The exact function of the appendix is not known. The rest of the large intestine consists of the ascending, transverse, and descending **colon** along with the rectum and anus. The chyme takes three to ten hours to become feces within the colon. Feces is made up of water, solid waste material, bacteria, and mucus. Feces is eliminated from the body by peristalsis through the anus, the rectal opening. This process is called **defecation**.

The functions of the gastrointestinal system are:

- **ingestion** (taking food or fluids into the body) of food
- **digestion** (breaking down food so that it can be absorbed into the cells) of food
- absorption of nutrients
- **elimination** of waste products from food/fluids

Destination: Homeostasis

Fluid balance is a vital part of the body's ability to maintain homeostasis. A person becomes dehydrated when his output is greater than his intake. The body reacts quickly to try to correct dehydration. One of the primary responses is to stimulate thirst. If the intake of water and other fluids is not increased, the body responds by decreasing sweating and urination. If fluid balance is not restored, other more severe symptoms occur. Eliminating dehydration can be as simple as drinking a glass of water. When fluids are re-introduced into the body, fluid balance and homeostasis are restored.

TRIVIA

Process of Digestion

Lazzaro Spallanzani (1729-1799), an Italian scientist, studied digestion. He performed experiments with birds called kites. In his studies with these birds, he found that gastric juice works to dissolve food in the stomach.

4. Discuss changes in the gastrointestinal system due to aging

For each system in the body, there are normal changes of aging. Knowing these normal changes for each body system will help you better recognize and understand what is abnormal for the body as a person ages.

Normal age-related changes for the gastrointestinal system include the following:

- Ability to taste decreases.
- Difficulty with digestion causes more frequent constipation.
- Difficulty chewing and swallowing may occur.
- Absorption of vitamins and minerals decreases.
- Production of saliva and digestive fluids decreases.

For each body system, there are signs and symptoms that need to be reported to the nurse if observed. You will learn more about important observations that should be reported in Learning Objectives 5 and 7.

5. List normal qualities of stool and identify signs and symptoms to report about stool

Bowel elimination is the physical process of releasing or emptying the colon or large intestine of stool or feces. Feces, or stool, are solid waste products eliminated by the colon. The frequency of bowel movements varies; they can occur as often as one to three times per day or as infrequently as several times a week. Regular bowel movements help keep the gastrointestinal system healthy. It is especially important for elderly people to have regular bowel movements because they help prevent serious problems, such as bowel obstructions, from occurring.

Stool is normally brown in color, and its consistency is soft, moist, and formed (not loose). Certain foods can change its color. For example, red gelatin or large amounts of beets can make stool appear red. Large amounts of green, leafy vegetables can make stool look green. Stool is tubular in shape, which is due to its passage through the colon. The amount of stool produced per day depends upon the food eaten.

Normal bowel elimination means not having any pain with passing stool. Residents should not have accidents with passing stool and should be able to make it to the bathroom without a problem. There should be no blood, pus, mucus, or worms in the stool. A change in the appearance of stool can signal a health problem. Report any of the following signs or symptoms to the nurse:

- abnormally-colored stool (whitish, black [tarry], or bloody)
- hard, dry stools
- liquid stools (diarrhea)
- constipation (inability to have a bowel movement)
- pain when having a bowel movement
- blood, pus, mucus, or discharge in stool
- fecal/anal incontinence (inability to control the muscles of the bowels which leads to an involuntary loss of stool)

6. List factors affecting bowel elimination and describe how to promote normal bowel elimination

There are many things that may affect normal bowel elimination:

Growth and Development: Aging affects the regularity of bowel elimination. Peristalsis slows due to a decrease in muscle tone. Tooth loss and less saliva may make eating less appealing and more challenging. Nutrients are absorbed less, making digestion more difficult.

To promote normal elimination, encourage fluids and nutritious meals. Supplements may be ordered. Encourage regular exercise and activity as allowed. Provide good oral care and make sure dentures are clean, in place, and fit properly.

Psychological Factors: The lack of privacy may affect bowel elimination. Having a roommate for the first time, being in a place that is not home, and needing help with elimination can disrupt normal elimination patterns. Anxiety, stress, fear, or anger can increase the frequency of bowel movements, causing watery, loose stools, and may even cause incontinence. Depression can decrease the frequency of elimination.

To promote normal elimination, always provide privacy and allow plenty of time for elimination. Leave the call light in reach. Respond to call lights and requests for help with toileting immediately. If residents want to talk about their concerns, take the time to listen to them. Report their concerns to the nurse.

Diet: A diet low in fiber may decrease elimination and cause constipation. Foods high in animal fats, such as dairy products, red meat, and eggs may also cause constipation. Chocolate and other foods may increase bowel movements and can cause diarrhea. Other foods are gas-causing, which can increase elimination but may also cause discomfort. Beans, whole grains, apples, cabbage, onions, dairy products, and carbonated drinks are examples of foods that can cause gas.

To promote normal elimination, encourage nutritious meals. Increase fiber intake and decrease fatty, sugary foods if constipation is a problem. Use dietary supplements as ordered.

Fluid Intake: The sense of thirst decreases as a person ages. A decrease in fluids may cause constipation. A lack of strength or coordination can also lower fluid intake. Some beverages, such as orange or prune juice, can cause an increase in bowel elimination.

To promote normal elimination, encourage fluid intake. Generally, a healthy person needs from 64 to 96 ounces of fluid each day. Remind residents to drink often if they are not on a fluid restriction. Make sure pitcher and water are within reach and are light enough for residents to lift. Assist with fluid intake as needed.

Physical Activity and Exercise: A lack of exercise and mobility can weaken muscles and slow elimination. Regular physical activity helps bowel elimination by strengthening abdominal and pelvic muscles. This helps peristalsis (Fig. 15-2).

To promote normal elimination, increase daily exercise. Encourage regular walks and other types of activities that are allowed.

Personal Habits: Certain times of day may be more common for having bowel movements. Drinking hot fluids can increase bowel movements by stimulating peristalsis. Elimination usually occurs after meals. Familiar places, such as the resident's own bathroom, may encourage bowel elimination. Positioning in bed also affects elimination. A resident who is lying flat on his back (supine) will have difficulty with elimination because it is difficult to contract the muscles in this position.

Fig. 15-2. Regular exercise is important. Encourage walks and other types of approved exercise.

To promote normal elimination, make sure residents are helped to the bathroom at the time of day that is best for each person. Use the bathroom the resident prefers or get a portable commode if the resident cannot make it to the bathroom. Raise the head of the bed for residents who use a bedpan. The best position for elimination is squatting and leaning forward.

Medications: Some medications affect bowel elimination. Antibiotics may cause diarrhea; pain relievers may cause constipation.

To promote normal elimination, laxatives may be ordered. Laxatives can help with elimination but may cause diarrhea. Report diarrhea or constipation to the nurse promptly.

Assisting with Elimination

A bedpan is used by residents who cannot get out of bed to go to the bathroom. Women use bedpans for urination and bowel movements.

Men will generally use urinals for urination and bedpans for bowel movements. There are two kinds of bedpans: standard pans and fracture bedpans (Fig. 15-3). A **fracture pan** is flatter than the regular bedpan and is used for small or thin people or those who cannot lift their buttocks onto a standard bedpan.

Fig. 15-3. a) Standard bedpan and b) fracture pan.

Feces and urine are considered infectious wastes. Wear gloves when handling bedpans, urinals, or basins that contain wastes. Wear additional PPE as needed. Use caution in removing bedpans or waste containers from beds; avoid spilling the contents. Do not place this equipment on an overbed table or on top of a side table. Use a bedpan cover or disposable pad to transfer bedpans to the bathroom. Dispose of wastes in the toilet and clean these containers thoroughly after each use. Clean them immediately to avoid odors. Some facilities will want an approved disinfectant used when cleaning bedpans and urinals. Follow facility policy.

When placing a bedpan, position a standard bedpan so that the wider end is aligned with a resident's buttocks. Position a fracture pan with the handle toward the foot of the bed. You may need to warm the bedpan using warm water and dry it completely before placing it under a resident if it is cold to the touch.

Assisting a resident with use of a bedpan

Equipment: bedpan, bedpan cover, disposable bed protector, bath blanket, toilet paper, washcloths or wipes, 2 pairs of gloves

1. Identify yourself by name. Identify the resident. Greet the resident by name.

2. Wash your hands.

3. Explain procedure to resident. Speak clearly, slowly, and directly. Maintain face-to-face contact whenever possible. Encourage resident to assist if possible.

4. Provide for the resident's privacy with a curtain, screen, or door.

5. Before placing bedpan, lower head of bed. Lock bed wheels.

6. Lower the side rail (if bed has one and if it is not already lowered) on side nearest you. Make sure far side rail is raised.

7. Apply gloves.

8. Cover the resident with a bath blanket. Ask him to hold it while you pull down the top covers underneath. Do not expose more of the resident than is needed.

9. Place the disposable bed protector under the resident's buttocks and hips. To do this, have the resident roll away from you. If the resident cannot do this, you must turn him away from you (see Chapter 11). Be sure resident cannot roll off the bed. Place bed protector on the area where the resident will lie on his back. The side of the protector nearest the resident should be fanfolded (folded several times into pleats) and tucked under the resident (Fig. 15-4). Ask resident to roll onto his back, or assist him to roll back if he is unable. Unfold rest of bed protector so it completely covers area under and around the resident's hips (Fig. 15-5).

Fig. 15-4. Fanfold the bed protector near the resident's back.

Fig. 15-5. Unfold the rest of the bed protector so it completely covers area under and around the resident's hips.

10. Ask resident to remove undergarments or help him do so.

11. If resident is able, ask him to raise hips by pushing with feet and hands. Place bedpan correctly under resident's buttocks avoiding trauma or pain:

    Standard bedpan: Position bedpan so wider end of pan is aligned with resident's buttocks (Fig. 15-6).

Fig. 15-6. Wider end of bedpan should be aligned with resident's buttocks.

    Fracture pan: Position bedpan with handle toward foot of bed (Fig. 15-7).

Fig. 15-7. Handle on fracture pan should face the foot of the bed.

    If a resident cannot help you in any way, keep the bed flat and roll the resident away from you. Slip the bedpan under the hips and roll him back onto the bedpan.

12. Raise head of bed after placing bedpan under resident. Raise side rail if bed has one.

13. Put toilet tissue within resident's reach.

14. Leave call light within resident's reach while resident is using bedpan. Ask resident to signal when finished.

15. Remain outside the curtain until called by the resident. When called, return and lower head of bed.

16. Remove bedpan carefully without causing trauma or pain. Cover bedpan.

17. Provide perineal care if assistance is needed. Remember to wipe from front to back.

18. Note color, odor, amount and consistency of contents. Empty contents of bedpan into toilet.

19. Rinse bedpan. Pour rinse water into toilet. Use approved disinfectant if facility policy.

20. Remove and dispose of gloves properly.

21. Wash hands.

22. Put on clean gloves.

23. Return bedpan to proper storage.

24. Assist resident to wash hands after using bedpan. Dispose of soiled washcloth or wipes in proper container. Help resident put on undergarment.

25. Remove and dispose of gloves properly. Wash your hands.

26. Make resident comfortable.

27. Return bed to low position if raised. Ensure resident's safety. Return side rails to ordered position. Remove privacy measures.

28. Leave call light within resident's reach.

29. Wash your hands.

30. Be courteous and respectful at all times.

31. Report any changes in the resident to the nurse. Document procedure using facility guidelines.

Bedpans and urinals are usually kept in the bathroom when they are not being used. If the bathroom is shared, this equipment may need to be labeled. Follow facility policy for storage.

Men generally use a urinal for urinating (Fig. 15-8). You will learn more about urination in the next chapter, Chapter 16.

Fig. 15-8. *Urinals.*

Assisting a male resident with a urinal

Equipment: urinal, disposable bed protector, washcloths or wipes, gloves

1. Identify yourself by name. Identify the resident. Greet the resident by name.

2. Wash your hands.

3. Explain procedure to resident. Speak clearly, slowly, and directly. Maintain face-to-face contact whenever possible. Encourage resident to assist if possible.

4. Provide for the resident's privacy with a curtain, screen, or door.

5. Lock bed wheels. Apply gloves.

6. Place a protective pad under the resident's buttocks and hips.

7. Hand the urinal to the resident. If the resident cannot do so himself, place urinal between his legs and position penis inside the urinal (Fig. 15-9). Replace bed covers.

Fig. 15-9. *Position the penis inside the urinal if the resident cannot do it himself.*

8. Leave call light within resident's reach while resident is using urinal. Ask resident to signal when finished.

9. Remain outside the curtain until called by the resident. When called, return and remove urinal carefully.

10. Note color, odor, amount, and qualities (e.g. cloudy) of contents. Empty contents into toilet.

11. Rinse urinal. Pour rinse water into toilet. Use approved disinfectant if facility policy. Return to proper storage.

12. Remove and dispose of gloves properly. Wash your hands.

13. Assist resident to wash hands after using urinal. Dispose of soiled washcloth or wipes properly.

14. Make resident comfortable.

15. Ensure resident's safety. Remove privacy measures.

16. Leave call light within resident's reach.

17. Wash your hands.

18. Be courteous and respectful at all times.

19. Report any changes in the resident to the nurse. Document procedure using facility guidelines.

Portable commodes are used for people who can get out of bed but who find it difficult to walk to the bathroom. A **portable commode** is a chair with a toilet seat and a removable container underneath (Fig. 15-10). The removable container must be cleaned after each use. Commodes may have wheels. The wheels must be locked before helping residents onto commodes. Once seated, leave the resident alone to use the commode if it is safe to do so.

Fig. 15-10. A portable commode. (Photo courtesy of Nova Ortho Med, Inc.)

Equipment: portable commode with basin, toilet paper, washcloths or wipes, 2 pairs of gloves, non-skid footwear, bath blanket

1. Identify yourself by name. Identify the resident. Greet the resident by name.

2. Wash your hands.

3. Explain procedure to resident. Speak clearly, slowly, and directly. Maintain face-to-face contact whenever possible. Encourage resident to assist if possible.

4. Provide for the resident's privacy with a curtain, screen, or door.

5. Practice good body mechanics. Adjust bed to low position. Lock bed wheels. Lock commode wheels.

6. Help resident out of bed and to portable commode. Make sure resident is wearing non-skid shoes.

7. If needed, help resident remove clothing and sit comfortably on toilet seat. Put toilet tissue within reach.

8. Place bath blanket over resident's legs. Leave call light within resident's reach. Ask resident to signal when finished.

9. When called, return and apply gloves.

10. Give perineal care if help is needed. Wipe residents from front to back.

11. Remove and dispose of gloves properly. Wash your hands.

12. Assist resident to wash hands after using commode. Dispose of soiled washcloth or wipes properly.

13. Assist back to bed. Return bed to proper position. Ensure resident's safety. Remove privacy measures.

14. Remove waste basin. Note color, odor, amount and consistency of contents. Empty into toilet.

15. Rinse container. Pour rinse water into toilet. Use approved disinfectant if facility policy. Return to proper storage.

16. Remove and dispose of gloves properly.

17. Leave call light within resident's reach.

18. Wash your hands.

19. Be courteous and respectful at all times.

20. Report any changes in the resident to the nurse. Document procedure using facility guidelines.

HOT TIP

Be careful when cleaning bedpans and commodes.

Cleaning bedpans can be tricky. If you are using a sprayer to clean and rinse a bedpan, the contents can spray all over you. Be careful not to do this. Urine and stool are considered infectious waste. Use proper PPE when cleaning bedpans and commodes.

7. Discuss common disorders of the gastrointestinal system

Heartburn

Heartburn, also known as acid reflux, occurs when the sphincter muscle which joins the esophagus and the stomach weakens. Normally, this muscle tries to prevent return, or reflux, of stomach contents back into the esophagus. If this is not done, stomach juices will move into the esophagus and cause burning and pain. The esophagus has a delicate lining which can be damaged by these stomach juices. Symptoms include a burning feeling in the esophagus, and pain in the chest, around the breastbone (sternum) or the rib area. The pain may also move into the neck area. Pain usually occurs directly after a eating a meal. Heartburn often causes a bitter taste in the mouth or the feeling of food coming back up into the throat or the mouth. This may worsen when a person is lying down. Treatment includes medication, such as antacids, or other types of medicine. A change in diet or sleep position is often ordered.

Gastroesophageal Reflux Disease (GERD)

Gastroesophageal reflux disease (GERD) is a chronic condition in which the liquid contents of the stomach back up into the esophagus. The liquid can inflame and damage the lining of the esophagus, which can cause bleeding, ulcers, or difficulty swallowing. Frequent heartburn is a common symptom of GERD. Other symptoms are chest pain, hoarseness in the morning, difficulty swallowing or a tightness in the throat. Coughing and foul-smelling breath can also occur with GERD. Possible causes of GERD are hiatal hernia, a weak lower esophageal sphincter, and slow digestion. Other causes may be diets high in acidic and spicy foods, obesity, smoking and alcohol use.

Treatment includes stopping smoking and drinking alcohol, avoiding spicy and acidic foods, and losing weight. Wearing loose-fitting clothing may help. Serving frequent, small meals throughout the day is advised, as well as serving the last meal of the day three to four hours before bedtime. Sitting up for at least two to three hours after eating may help. Elevation of the head of the bed and using extra pillows to keep the body upright help reduce acid reflux while in bed (Fig. 15-11).

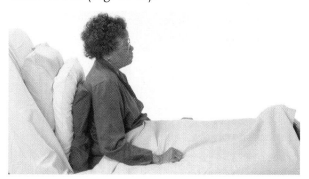

Fig. 15-11. *Sitting upright, elevating the head of the bed, and using extra pillows help reduce acid reflux.*

Ulcers

Ulcers are raw sores in the stomach (peptic or gastric ulcers) and the small intestine (duodenal ulcers). Dull or burning pain occurs from one hour to three or more hours after eating, accompanied by belching or vomiting. Peptic ulcers may cause bleeding, and stool may appear black (tarry). Ulcers are caused by excessive acid secretion. Infection of the stomach by a bacteria called *Helicobacter pylori* may also cause ulcers. Excessive aspirin use may be a factor in the development of ulcers. Treatment includes antacids and medications, as well as a change in diet. Alcohol, caffeine, and cigarette use should be avoided, as they increase the production of gastric acid.

Ulcerative Colitis and Crohn's Disease

Ulcerative colitis is a disorder that causes inflammation of and sores in the lining of the large intestine (colon). It is a form of inflammatory bowel disease (IBD). Symptoms include diarrhea (which may be bloody), abdominal pain, cramping, rectal bleeding, poor appetite, fever, and weight loss. Ulcerative colitis can cause intestinal bleeding and death if not treated.

Crohn's disease is a disease that causes the wall of the intestines (large or small) to become inflamed (red, sore and swollen). Crohn's disease is also a form of inflammatory bowel disease (IBD). Symptoms include diarrhea, abdominal pain, fever, weight loss, and joint pain.

There is no known cause of ulcerative colitis and Crohn's disease. Research has shown that they tend to run in families. The immune system may overreact to normal bacteria present in the intestines and cause inflammation. Bacteria and viruses also may cause the diseases.

Treatment includes medications to stop inflammation; however, medication does not cure ulcerative colitis or Crohn's disease. Surgery may be done if medications do not help these disorders. Surgical treatment may include an ileostomy or colostomy. More information on these types of ostomies can be found in Learning Objective 11 of this chapter.

Diverticulosis and Diverticulitis

Diverticulosis is a disorder of the intestinal wall of the large intestine (colon). Sac-like pouchings of the intestinal wall develop in weakened areas of this wall. A small percentage of people with diverticulosis develop inflammation inside the pouchings called **diverticulitis**. With diverticulitis, stool and bacteria become trapped inside the sacs, causing pain and fever. If the condition worsens, the intestine can tear, causing stool to enter the abdominal cavity and cause peritonitis (inflammation of the lining of the abdominal cavity due to microorganisms). One cause of diverticulitis is a low-fiber diet. The lack of fiber may cause the weakening of the intestinal wall.

Treatment for diverticulitis includes rest, medications to reduce inflammation and treat infection, and special diets. Surgery is sometimes necessary.

Information on hepatitis, a gastrointestinal system disorder, is found in Chapter 6.

Flatulence

Flatulence, also called gas or flatus, is the presence of excessive air in the digestive tract. It is passed through the rectum and may cause cramping or abdominal pain. High fiber foods can cause gas. It can also be caused by eating foods that a person cannot tolerate, such as lactose in dairy products. The inability to digest lactose, a type of sugar in milk and other dairy products, is called **lactose intolerance**. Other causes of flatulence, or gas, are:

- Swallowing air when eating
- Antibiotics
- **Malabsorption**, which means that nutrients from the intestinal tract are not properly absorbed; can also be accompanied by diarrhea.
- **Irritable bowel syndrome (IBS)**, which is a chronic condition of the GI tract that is worsened by stress. IBS causes abdominal pain and discomfort, bloating, and constipation. No exact cause has been identified.

For the relief of flatulence, two positions are used to help reduce gas: the left-side-lying, or left-lateral, position, and the supine (flat on the back) position. Lying on the left side allows gas to escape due to gravity. Placing a resident in this position for at least 20 minutes usually assists in the elimination of gas. The supine position is used with residents who are recovering from surgery. Placing the resident in the supine position allows gas inside the abdomen due to surgery to escape more quickly.

Methods used for the relief of flatulence are the rectal tube and the Harris flush. A rectal tube is placed in the rectum to reduce gas. A Harris flush, also called a return-flow enema or a colonic irrigation, is a special type of enema that reduces gas.

Constipation

Constipation is the difficult and often painful elimination of a hard, dry stool. It occurs when body waste moves slowly through the intestines. As you have learned, constipation is a common problem for elderly people. As people age, digestion takes longer and is less efficient. It can also result from poor diet, lack of exercise, decrease in fluid intake, medications, disease, or ignoring the urge to eliminate. Signs of constipation include abdominal swelling, gas, and irritability. The resident's medical chart may also show no recent bowel movement.

Treating constipation often involves increasing fiber in the diet, as well as physical activity if possible. Medications may be ordered to assist, such as laxatives, enemas, or suppositories. An **enema** is a specific amount of water or other fluid, with or without an additive, introduced into the colon to help eliminate stool. You will learn more about enemas later in this chapter. A **suppository** is a medication given rectally to cause a bowel movement.

Some states allow nursing assistants to give a rectal suppository. A procedure on how to give a suppository is included in your instructor's material.

Diarrhea

Diarrhea is the frequent elimination of liquid or semi-liquid feces. Abdominal cramps, urgency, nausea, and vomiting can accompany diarrhea, depending on the cause. Infections, microorganisms, irritating foods, and medications can cause diarrhea. Treatment is usually medication and a change of diet. A diet of bananas, rice, apples, and tea/toast (BRAT diet) is often suggested.

Fecal/Anal Incontinence

Fecal/**anal incontinence** is an inability to control the muscles of the bowels, which leads to an involuntary passage of stool or gas. Causes of anal incontinence include muscle and nerve damage, disorders of the spinal cord or anus, injuries to the anal muscles during childbirth, injuries due to anal operations, fecal impaction, constipation, and tumors. Treatment for anal incontinence often includes changes in diet, medication, bowel training, and surgery. You will learn more about bowel training in Learning Objective 12 of the chapter.

Fecal Impaction

A **fecal impaction** is a build-up of dry, hardened feces in the rectum that results from unrelieved constipation. A person cannot remove an impaction naturally. Signs and symptoms of a fecal impaction include no stool for several days, cramping, abdominal or rectal pain, abdominal swelling (distention), nausea and vomiting. Another sign is the seeping or oozing of liquid stool, which can be mistaken for diarrhea. Other signs are an increase in urination or the inability to urinate, fever, or confusion or disorientation. When an impaction occurs, the nurse or doctor will insert one or two gloved fingers into the rectum to break the mass into fragments. Usually the stool can then be passed. A fecal impaction can be a serious, even fatal, condition if a complete bowel obstruction occurs and is not immediately treated. Report signs and symptoms promptly to the nurse. Ways to prevent fecal impactions include encouraging fluids, eating a high-fiber diet, following a toileting schedule, and exercising regularly.

Hemorrhoids

Hemorrhoids are enlarged veins in the rectum. They may also be visible outside the anus. Untreated constipation, obesity, pregnancy, chronic diarrhea, overuse of enemas or laxatives, and straining during bowel movements are common causes of hemorrhoids. Rectal itching, burning, pain, and bleeding during bowel elimination are symptoms of hemorrhoids. Treatment includes changing the person's diet, such as adding more fiber and increasing water intake, medications, compresses, and sitz baths (Chapter 18). Surgery may be necessary. Excessive cleaning and wiping of the area should be avoided. When cleaning the anus, be very gentle. Avoid using scented soaps, as these may further irritate the anal area.

8. Discuss how enemas are given

An enema is given when help is needed eliminating stool from the colon. A specific amount of water flows inside of the colon in order to help remove stool. Some facilities allow nursing assistants to give enemas. If your facility allows this, follow facility policies, and make sure you are trained to give enemas. Talk to the nurse if you have any questions or concerns.

Enemas are ordered for these reasons:

- Preparation for a diagnostic test
- Preparation for surgery
- To remove stool that a resident cannot eliminate on his or her own

Doctors will write an enema order. Four different types of enemas are:

- Tap water enema (TWE): 500-1000 mL water from a faucet (nothing added to the water)
- Soapsuds enema (SSE): 500-1000 mL water with 5 mL of mild castile soap added
- Saline enema: 500-1000 mL water with two teaspoons of salt added
- Commercial enema (also called "pre-packaged" enema): 120 mL solution; may have oil or other additive

Tap water, soapsuds, and saline enemas are all considered cleansing enemas. Cleansing enemas require more fluid than commercial enemas do. Equipment needed for cleansing enemas includes an IV pole, the enema solution and tubing and a clamp. Residents should be encouraged to hold in the enema solution as long as possible—at least 10 to 20 minutes for the best results.

Before giving a cleansing enema, remove the air from the enema tubing before inserting the tube into the rectum. Allowing a small amount of water to flow into a bedpan will allow the air to escape.

Provide plenty of privacy for the resident with this procedure. Make sure others cannot see the resident and that he is not unnecessarily exposed in any way.

During an enema, the resident must be in the Sims' position (Fig. 15-12). If the person is positioned on the left side, the water does not have to flow against gravity. Give the enema slowly, holding the enema tubing in place. Enemas are given very slowly to avoid causing cramping. Stop immediately if the resident has pain or if you feel resistance. Be reassuring and gentle during the procedure.

Fig. 15-12. *Place the resident in the Sims' position for an enema, which is a left side-lying position.*

Observe for cramping, pain or discomfort, bleeding, the ability to retain the fluid, and any change in the resident's condition during and following giving an enema.

HOT TIP

Enemas and Vital Signs
Stimulation of the rectal area by a tube may temporarily increase the heartbeat and blood pressure. Residents with heart disease may not be able to have enemas. Follow the nurse's instructions regarding the use of enemas.

Giving a cleansing enema

Equipment: 2 pairs of gloves, bath blanket, IV pole, enema solution, additive (if needed), tubing and a clamp, disposable bed protector, bedpan, bedpan cover, lubricating jelly, bath thermometer, tape measure, toilet paper, two washcloths, robe, non-skid footwear

1. Identify yourself by name. Identify the resident. Greet the resident by name.

2. Wash your hands.

3. Explain procedure to resident. Speak clearly, slowly, and directly. Maintain face-to-face contact whenever possible. Encourage resident to assist if possible.

4. Provide for the resident's privacy with a curtain, screen, or door.

5. Practice good body mechanics. Adjust bed to safe working level, usually waist high. Lock bed wheels.

6. Raise side rail (if bed has one and if it is not already lowered) on far side of bed. Lower side rail nearest you.

7. Help resident into Sims' position. Cover with a bath blanket.

8. Place the IV pole beside the bed. Raise the side rail.

9. Clamp the enema tube. Prepare the enema solution. Add specific additive, if ordered. Fill bag with 500-1000 mL of warm water (105°F) and swish fluid to mix well.

10. Unclamp the tube. Let a small amount of solution run through the tubing to release the air. Re-clamp the tube.

11. Hang bag on IV pole. Make sure bottom of enema bag is not more than 12 inches above the resident's anus (Fig. 15-13).

Fig. 15-13. *Bottom of the bag should not be more than 12 inches above the anus.*

12. Apply gloves.

13. Lower the side rail. Uncover resident enough to expose anus only.

14. Place disposable bed protector under resident. Place bedpan close to resident's body.

15. Lubricate two to four inches of the tip of the tubing with lubricating jelly.

16. Ask resident to breathe deeply. This relieves cramps during procedure.

17. Place one hand on the upper buttock. Lift to expose the anus. Ask the resident to take a deep breath and exhale (Fig. 15-14). Using other hand, gently insert the tip of the tubing two to four inches into the rectum. Stop immediately if you feel resistance or if the resident complains of pain. If this happens, clamp the tube. Tell the nurse immediately.

Fig. 15-14. *Lift the upper buttock to expose the anus. Ask the resident to take a deep breath.*

18. Unclamp the tubing. Allow the solution to flow slowly into the rectum. Ask resident to take slow, deep breaths. If resident complains of cramping, clamp the tubing and stop for a couple of minutes. Encourage him or her to take as much of the solution as possible. Resident should let you know when he cannot accept any more fluid.

19. Clamp the tubing before the bag is empty when the solution is almost gone. Gently remove the tip from the rectum. Place the tip into the enema bag. Do not contaminate yourself, resident, or bed linens.

20. Ask the resident to hold the solution inside as long as possible.

21. Help resident to use bedpan, commode, or get to the bathroom. If the resident uses a commode or bathroom, apply robe and non-skid footwear. Lower the bed to an appropriate level for the resident before the resident gets up.

22. Place call light and toilet paper within resident's reach. If the resident is using the bathroom, ask him not to flush the toilet when finished.

23. Leave the resident if possible. Ask him to signal when he's finished.

24. Discard disposable equipment. Clean area.

25. Remove and dispose of gloves properly. Wash your hands.

26. When resident is done, put on clean gloves. Using washcloths, help with perineal care as needed.

27. Remove bedpan. Cover bedpan. Remove the disposable bed protector.

28. Call the nurse to observe enema results, whether in bedpan or in toilet. Consistency, color, and amount will be observed.

29. Empty and rinse bedpan. Pour rinse water into toilet. Use approved disinfectant if facility policy. Return to proper storage. Dispose of soiled washcloths.

30. Remove and dispose of gloves properly. Wash your hands.

31. Help resident wash hands.

32. Remove bath blanket. Make resident comfortable.

33. Return bed to low position if raised. Ensure resident's safety. Return side rails to ordered position. Remove privacy measures.

34. Leave call light within resident's reach.

35. Wash your hands.

36. Be courteous and respectful at all times.

37. Report any changes in the resident to the nurse. Document procedure using facility guidelines.

Commercial enemas may have oil, such as mineral oil, or other additives. The goals of using an oil-retention enema may include the following: lubricating the intestine to make stool pass more easily; softening stool for ease of elimination; encouraging gentle bowel movements; reducing straining with bowel movements; and eliminating a fecal impaction.

With commercial enemas, no IV pole, tubing, or clamp are needed. They come in a prepackaged kit; no mixing is usually required. The tip of a commercially prepared enema is usually pre-lubricated and should only be inserted about one-and-one-half inches into the rectum. Commercial enemas generally take longer to work than cleansing enemas. Encourage residents to hold in the enema solution as long as possible. For best results, fluid should be retained for at least 20 minutes. Oil-retention enemas should be retained for 30 to 60 minutes.

Giving a commercial enema

Equipment: 2 pairs of gloves, bath blanket, standard or oil retention commercial enema kit, disposable bed protector, bedpan, bedpan cover, lubricating jelly, washcloths or wipes, toilet tissue, robe, non-skid footwear

1. Identify yourself by name. Identify the resident. Greet the resident by name.

2. Wash your hands.

3. Explain procedure to resident. Speak clearly, slowly, and directly. Maintain face-to-face contact whenever possible. Encourage resident to assist if possible.

4. Provide for the resident's privacy with a curtain, screen, or door.

5. Practice good body mechanics. Adjust bed to safe working level, usually waist high. Lock bed wheels.

6. Raise side rail (if bed has one and if it is not already lowered) on far side of bed. Lower side rail nearest you.

7. Help resident into left-sided Sims' position. Cover with a bath blanket.

8. Apply gloves.

9. Place disposable bed protector under resident. Place bedpan close to resident's body.

10. Uncover resident enough to expose anus only.

11. Add extra lubricating jelly to the tip of bottle if needed.

12. Ask resident to breathe deeply to relieve cramps during procedure.

13. Place one hand on the upper buttock. Lift to expose the anus. Ask the resident to take a deep breath and exhale. Using other hand, gently insert the tip of the tubing about one and a half inches into the rectum. Stop immediately if you feel resistance or if the resident complains of pain.

14. Slowly squeeze and roll the enema container so that the solution runs inside the resident. Stop when the container is almost empty.

15. Gently remove tip from the rectum, continuing to keep pressure on the container until you place bottle inside the box upside down (Fig. 15-15).

Fig. 15-15. *Place enema bottle upside-down in the box.*

16. Ask the resident to hold the solution inside as long as possible.

17. Help resident to use bedpan or commode, or get to the bathroom. If the resident uses a commode or bathroom, apply robe and non-skid footwear. Lower the bed to its lowest position before the resident gets up.

18. Place call light and toilet paper within resident's reach. If resident is using the bathroom, ask him not to flush the toilet when finished.

19. Leave the resident if possible. Ask him to signal when he's finished.

20. Discard disposable equipment. Clean area.

21. Remove and dispose of gloves properly. Wash your hands.

22. When resident is done, put on clean gloves. Using washcloths, help with perineal care as needed.

23. Remove bedpan. Cover bedpan. Remove the disposable bed protector. Call the nurse to observe enema results, whether in bedpan or in toilet.

24. Empty bedpan. Rinse bedpan. Pour rinse water into toilet. Use approved disinfectant if facility policy. Return it to proper storage. Dispose of soiled washcloths properly.

25. Remove and dispose of gloves properly. Wash your hands.

26. Help resident wash hands.

27. Remove bath blanket. Make resident comfortable.

28. Return bed to low position if raised. Ensure resident's safety. Return side rails to ordered position. Remove privacy measures.

29. Leave call light within resident's reach.

30. Wash your hands.

31. Be courteous and respectful at all times.

32. Report any changes in the resident to the nurse. Document procedure using facility guidelines.

A follow-up cleansing enema may be ordered after using an oil-retention enema. This helps cleanse the bowels more thoroughly and eliminate remaining oil in the intestine. The resident may ask for a shower or a bath after this procedure and the bowel movements that follow. Assist as needed.

THE GASTROINTESTINAL SYSTEM

9. Demonstrate how to collect a stool specimen

You may be asked to collect a stool specimen from a resident. A **specimen** is a sample, such as tissue, blood, urine, stool, or sputum, used for analysis and diagnosis. Specimens are used for different types of tests. A stool sample may be needed to test for blood, pathogens, and other things. Stool may be collected and tested for ova and parasites (O & P) to detect worms or amoebas. If testing stool for ova and parasites or for the *C. difficile* toxin (Chapter 6), deliver the specimen to the lab immediately. These tests must be done while the stool is still warm. Stool that cannot be sent to the lab immediately may need to be placed in a special refrigerator used strictly for specimens. Never place a specimen in a refrigerator that is used for food or drinks. Check with the nurse or the lab for instructions on proper handling of stool.

When collecting a stool specimen, first show the resident the correct container to use. Ask the resident not to get urine or toilet tissue in the sample because they can ruin the sample and require a new specimen.

A plastic collection container called a "hat" is sometimes inserted into a toilet to collect and measure urine or stool (Fig. 15-16). Hats should be labeled with the resident's name and room number and must be cleaned after each use.

Fig. 15-16. A "hat" is placed under the toilet seat to collect specimens for residents who use the toilet.

Collecting a stool specimen

Equipment: specimen container and lid, completed label, 2 tongue blades, 2 pairs of gloves, bedpan if resident cannot use the bathroom or commode, "hat" if resident uses toilet or commode, 2 plastic bags, toilet tissue, laboratory slip, washcloth or towel, supplies for perineal care, pen

Ask the resident to let you know when he or she can have a bowel movement. Be ready to collect the specimen.

1. Identify yourself by name. Identify the resident. Greet the resident by name.

2. Wash your hands.

3. Explain procedure to resident. Speak clearly, slowly, and directly. Maintain face-to-face contact whenever possible. Encourage resident to assist if possible.

4. Provide for the resident's privacy with a curtain, screen, or door.

5. Practice good body mechanics. Adjust bed to safe working level, usually waist high, if using a bedpan. Lock bed wheels.

6. Lower the side rail (if bed has one and if it is not already lowered) on side nearest you.

7. Put on gloves.

8. When the resident is ready to move bowels, ask him not to urinate at the same time. Ask him not to put toilet paper in with the sample. Provide a plastic bag for toilet paper.

9. Fit hat to toilet or commode, or provide resident with bedpan. Leave the room. Ask the resident to signal when he is finished with the bowel movement. Make sure call light is within reach.

10. After the bowel movement, help as necessary with perineal care. Help resident wash his or her hands. Make the resident comfortable.

11. Using the two tongue blades, take about two tablespoons of stool and put it in the container. Cover it tightly, apply label, and bag the specimen.

12. Wrap the tongue blades in toilet paper and throw them away in the proper container. Empty the bedpan or container into the toilet. Clean equipment. Use approved disinfectant if facility policy. Store equipment.

13. Return bed to low position if raised. Ensure resident's safety. Return side rails to ordered position. Remove privacy measures.

14. Remove and dispose of gloves properly.

15. Leave call light within resident's reach.

16. Wash your hands.

17. Be courteous and respectful at all times.

18. Report any changes in the resident to the nurse. Document procedure using facility guidelines. Take specimen to designated place promptly.

Collecting a specimen from a resident in isolation requires special handling. Some steps are done outside the isolation room. Two labels are completed, leaving one label outside on a biohazard bag. Proper PPE must be put on before entering the room. After collecting the specimen and covering the container, place one completed label on the container. When you are ready to leave the isolation room, complete all actions to safely leave the room. Remove gloves and wash your hands last.

Using a clean paper towel, carefully pick up the specimen container and leave the room. Immediately put the specimen container into the biohazard bag on the isolation cart. Discard the paper towel in the appropriate container. Seal the bag properly and take the specimen to the proper site. Wash hands again.

10. Explain occult blood testing

Hidden, or **occult**, blood is found inside stool with a microscope or a special chemical test. This may be a sign of a serious physical problem, such as cancer. The Hemoccult™ test checks for occult blood in stool. The collecting and testing of stool to check for occult blood is a common procedure. In some facilities, staff members do not perform this test; laboratories do it instead. Follow the care plan and your facility's policy. Specific dietary orders or medi-

cations may be necessary prior to occult blood testing.

Testing a stool specimen for occult blood

Equipment: labeled stool specimen, Hemoccult® test kit (Fig. 15-17), 1 or 2 tongue blades, paper towel, plastic bag, gloves

Fig. 15-17. *A Hemoccult® test kit.*

Check expiration date on blood testing cards before using.

1. Wash your hands.

2. Put on gloves.

3. Open the test card.

4. Pick up a tongue blade. Get small amount of stool from specimen container.

5. Using a tongue blade, smear a small amount of stool onto Box A of test card (Fig. 15-18).

Fig. 15-18. *Smear a small amount of stool onto Box A.*

6. Flip tongue blade (or use new tongue blade). Get some stool from another part of specimen. Smear small amount of stool onto Box B of test card.

7. Close the test card. Turn over to other side.

8. Open the flap.

9. Open developer. Apply developer to each box. Follow manufacturer's instructions.

10. Wait the amount of time listed in instructions, usually between 10 and 60 seconds.

11. Watch the squares for any color changes. Record color changes. Follow instructions.

12. Place tongue blade(s) and test packet in disposable bag.

13. Dispose of plastic bag properly in biohazard container.

14. Remove and dispose of gloves properly. Wash hands.

15. Document procedure using facility guidelines. Report results to the nurse.

11. Define the term "ostomy" and identify the difference between colostomy and ileostomy

An **ostomy** is the surgical creation of an opening from an area inside the body to the outside. The terms "colostomy" and "ileostomy" refer to the surgical removal of a portion of the intestines. In a resident with one of these ostomies, the end of the intestine is brought out of the body through an artificial opening in the abdomen. This opening is called a **stoma**. Stool, or feces, is eliminated through the ostomy rather than through the anus.

An ostomy may be necessary due to bowel disease, such as diverticulitis or Crohn's disease, colon cancer, or trauma. (More information on cancer is in Chapter 24.) An ostomy can be either permanent or temporary; a temporary ostomy allows the intestines to heal from a specific condition.

The terms "colostomy" and "ileostomy" tell what section of the intestine was removed and the type of stool that will be eliminated (Fig. 15-19). A **colostomy** is a surgically-created opening into the large intestine to allow feces to be expelled; it causes stool to be semi-solid. An **ileostomy** is a surgically-created opening into the end of the small intestine, the ileum, to allow feces to be expelled; stool will be liquid and may be irritating to the skin.

Fig. 15-19. *a) A colostomy and b) an ileostomy.*

Residents who have had an ostomy wear a disposable bag, or appliance, that fits over the stoma to collect the feces. The bag is custom-fitted over the stoma to collect the stool (Fig. 15-20). The bag is attached to the skin by adhesive, and a belt may be used to secure the appliance.

Fig. 15-20. *An open and a closed ostomy bag.*

Many people with ostomies feel embarrassed or angry. They often feel they have lost control of a basic bodily function. Ostomies can cause odor, discomfort, and fear of the bag falling off. You can do a great deal to help residents with ostomies feel better about themselves. Be sensitive and supportive and always provide privacy for ostomy care. Do not act uncomfortable with ostomy care, especially with the odor or the changing of the bag. Follow these guidelines when giving ostomy care:

Guidelines

Ostomy Care

- Follow Standard and/or Transmission-Based Precautions, including wearing gloves and any additional PPE needed, when caring for ostomies. Wash your hands carefully.

- Make sure residents with ostomies receive good skin care and proper hygiene.

- Remove ostomy appliances carefully to avoid tearing the resident's skin.

- Before removing appliance, allow a little air out of the bag to remove any built-up pressure. This can prevent the bag from exploding.

- Observe contents of ostomy bag before disposing of used bag. If anything unusual is noted, such as blood or a change in the stool quality or amount, notify the nurse.

- Empty, clean, and replace the ostomy bag whenever stool is eliminated.

- Assist residents with ostomies to wash their hands properly.

- During ostomy care, observe for signs of skin irritation, rashes, swelling, or bleeding around stoma. Report these signs, along with complaints of pain or discomfort, immediately.

- Use skin barriers, such as creams and pastes, as ordered.

- Make sure bottom of appliance/bag is securely clamped before applying it to the stoma.

- Make sure bag is attached securely to the resident before completing ostomy care.

- Make sure the bag is secure before the resident goes to activities or appointments or receives visitors.

- Be supportive, empathetic, and caring. Your support will help the resident's ability to handle this important change in lifestyle.

Caring for an ostomy

Equipment: disposable bed protector, bath blanket, clean ostomy bag and belt/appliance, gauze squares, basin of warm water, mild soap or cleanser, washcloth, skin barrier as ordered, 2 towels, plastic disposable bag, gloves, special deodorant if used

1. Identify yourself by name. Identify the resident. Greet the resident by name.

2. Wash your hands.

3. Explain procedure to resident. Speak clearly, slowly, and directly. Maintain face-to-face contact whenever possible. Encourage resident to assist if possible.

4. Provide for the resident's privacy with a curtain, screen, or door.

5. Practice good body mechanics. Adjust bed to safe working level, usually waist high. Lock bed wheels.

6. Lower the side rail (if bed has one and if it is not already lowered) on side nearest you.

7. Place disposable bed protector under resident. Cover resident with a bath blanket. Pull down the top sheet and blankets. Expose only ostomy site. Offer resident a towel to keep clothing dry.

8. Put on gloves.

9. Undo the ostomy belt if used. Pull gently on one edge of ostomy appliance to release air.

10. Remove ostomy bag carefully. Place it in plastic bag. Note the color, odor, consistency, and amount of stool in the bag.

11. Wipe area around stoma with gauze squares (Fig. 15-21). Discard squares in plastic bag.

Fig. 15-21. Use gauze squares to wipe the area around the stoma.

12. Add small amount of mild soap or cleanser to the warm water. Using a washcloth, wash the area in one direction, away from the stoma. Rinse. Pat dry with another towel. Apply skin barrier as ordered. Temporarily cover stoma opening with gauze squares.

13. Apply deodorant to bag if used. Remove gauze squares, and place in plastic bag. Put the clean ostomy appliance on resident. Hold in place and seal securely. Make sure the bottom of the bag is clamped. Attach to ostomy belt if used.

14. Remove disposable bed protector and discard. Place soiled linens in proper container.

15. Remove bag and gauze squares. Discard bag and squares in the proper container.

16. Remove and dispose of gloves properly. Wash your hands.

17. Make resident comfortable.

18. Return bed to low position if raised. Ensure resident's safety. Return side rails to ordered position. Remove privacy measures.

19. Leave call light within resident's reach.

20. Wash your hands.

21. Be courteous and respectful at all times.

22. Report any changes in the resident to the nurse. Document procedure using facility guidelines.

Other types of ostomies

A **urostomy** is the general term used for any surgical procedure that diverts the passage of urine by re-directing the ureters. A **ureterostomy** is a type of urostomy in which an opening from a ureter is brought through the abdomen for urine to be eliminated.

12. Explain guidelines for assisting with bowel retraining

Residents who have had an illness, injury, or a period of inactivity may need assistance in re-establishing a regular routine and normal bowel function. Retraining is the process of assisting residents to regain control of their bowels.

Taking regular trips to the bathroom at specific times each day will help with bowel retraining. Doctors may order suppositories, enemas, laxatives, or stool softeners to assist. Most care team members will be involved with charting and implementing bowel retraining. Understand and follow the care plan for each resident.

Guidelines
Bowel Retraining

- Follow the plan consistently. Explain the training schedule to the resident. Direct any questions the resident has to the nurse.

- Follow Standard Precautions. Wear gloves when handling body wastes. For residents in isolation, additional PPE may be needed. Follow the care plan.

- Observe your resident's elimination habits. This helps predict when a trip to the bathroom or a bedpan will be necessary.

- Keep a record of elimination, including episodes of incontinence. Keeping accurate records will help establish a routine.

- Offer a bedpan or a trip to the bathroom at specific times each day.

- Answer call lights promptly.

- Provide privacy for elimination and do not rush the resident.

- Help the resident with perineal care as needed. This promotes proper hygiene. Watch for skin changes and report them.

- Encourage fluids throughout the day if allowed.

- Encourage the proper diet.

- Dispose of wastes properly. Wastes, clothing protectors, and incontinence briefs may need to be double-bagged before being placed in the proper container.

- Praise attempts and successes in controlling the bowels.

Never show frustration or anger toward residents who are incontinent. That is abusive behavior, and negative reactions will only make the problem worse. Be positive and patient with the retraining efforts.

RESIDENTS' RIGHTS

Handling Incontinence

Always act professionally when handling bowel incontinence or helping to re-establish routines. Bowel incontinence is difficult enough for residents without them having to worry about your reactions. Be patient when setbacks occur.

CHAPTER REVIEW

1. Define these terms: anatomy, physiology, cells, tissues, organs, body systems and homeostasis (LO 2).

2. How does peristalsis aid in elimination (LO 3)?

3. What is feces (LO 3)?

4. What are four functions of the gastrointestinal system (LO 3)?

5. List five normal age-related changes of the gastrointestinal system (LO 4).

6. List three normal qualities of stool (LO 5).

7. List seven things to observe and report about stool (LO 5).

8. For each of the seven factors that affect bowel elimination listed in Learning Objective 6, describe one way nursing assistants can promote normal elimination (LO 6).

9. When is a fracture pan used for elimination, rather than a standard bedpan (LO 6)?

10. How should a standard bedpan be positioned? How should a fracture pan be positioned (LO 6)?

11. When are portable commodes used (LO 6)?

12. How should a resident who has GERD be positioned after eating (LO 7)?

13. List two types of treatments for ulcerative colitis or Crohn's disease (LO 7).

14. What are five causes of flatulence (LO 7)?

15. List three possible treatments for constipation (LO 7).

16. What are five causes of anal incontinence (LO 7)?

17. List six signs and symptoms of a fecal impaction (LO 7).

18. What should be avoided when caring for a resident who has hemorrhoids (LO 7)?

19. Describe four types of enemas (LO 8).

20. What position must the resident be in for an enema (LO 8)?

21. If a resident feels pain while receiving an enema, what should the nursing assistant do (LO 8)?

22. When giving a cleansing enema, how far above a resident's anus should the bottom of the enema bag be placed (LO 8)?

23. Why does a stool specimen need to be delivered to the lab immediately when testing for ova and parasites (LO 9)?

24. What items should not be included in a stool specimen (LO 9)?

25. What is the term for a plastic collection container that is inserted into a toilet to collect and measure urine or stool (LO 9)?

26. How is occult blood found in stool (LO 10)?

27. Define the term "ostomy" (LO 11).

28. When may an ostomy be necessary (LO 11)?

29. How do colostomies and ileostomies differ (LO 11)?

30. List ten guidelines for bowel retraining (LO 12).

16
The Urinary System

Watching the Kidneys

Galen, 130-200 A.D., wrote a 17-book set entitled *On the Uses of the Parts of the Body of Man*. One portion of the work dealt with the function of the kidneys. To help determine how the kidneys produced urine, Galen tied up the ureters and watched the kidneys swell with urine.

"A human being: an ingenious assembly of portable plumbing."
Christopher Morley, 1890-1957

*"Now is this golden crown like a deep well
That owes two buckets filling one another;
The emptier dancing in the air,
The other down, unseen and full of water"*
William Shakespeare, from *Richard II*

1. Define important words in this chapter

24-hour urine specimen: a urine specimen consisting of all urine voided in a 24-hour period.

calculi: kidney stones.

catheter: tube inserted through the skin or into a body opening; used to add or drain fluid.

chronic renal failure (CRF): progressive condition in which the kidneys cannot filter certain waste products; also called chronic kidney failure.

clean-catch specimen: a urine specimen that does not include the first and last urine that is voided; also called mid-stream.

condom catheter: a catheter that has an attachment on the end that fits onto the penis; also called an external or Texas catheter.

dialysis: a process that cleanses the body of wastes that the kidneys cannot remove due to kidney failure.

end-stage renal disease (ESRD): condition in which kidneys have failed and dialysis or transplantation is required.

indwelling catheter: a catheter that stays inside the bladder for a period of time; urine drains into a bag.

ketones: chemical substances that the body produces when it does not have enough insulin in the blood.

micturition: the process of emptying the bladder of urine; also called urination or voiding.

routine urine specimen: a urine specimen that can be collected any time a person voids.

specific gravity: a test performed to measure the density of urine.

sphincter: a ring-like muscle that opens and closes an opening in the body.

straight catheter: a catheter that does not stay inside the person; it is removed immediately after urine is drained or sampled.

urinary incontinence: the inability to control the bladder, which leads to an involuntary loss of urine.

urinary tract infection (UTI): a disorder that causes inflammation of the bladder; also called cystitis.

voiding: the process of emptying the bladder of urine; also called urination or micturition.

2. Explain the structure and function of the urinary system

The urinary system consists of two kidneys, two ureters, the urinary bladder, the urethra and the meatus (Figs. 16-1 and 16-2). The kidneys are kidney-bean-shaped organs. They lie slightly above the waist against the rear wall of the abdominal cavity and on either side of the spine. Each kidney is about four to five inches in length, one inch thick, and weighs between four and six ounces. The kidneys are partially protected by the back muscles and the lower ribs. The kidneys cleanse and filter waste products and toxic materials from the blood. They regulate the amount of electrolytes within the body. They also help to regulate blood pressure and water balance.

Fig. 16-1. The urinary system consists of two kidneys and two ureters, the bladder, the urethra, and the meatus.

Fig. 16-2. The female urethra is shorter than the male urethra. Because of this, the female bladder is more likely to become infected by bacteria traveling up the urethra.

Substances needed by the body are reabsorbed; the substances not needed—toxins and waste products—stay in the kidney and form urine. The urine is then transferred to the bladder through tubes called the ureters. The ureters are narrow tubes about one foot in length. When a person urinates, the ureters also prevent the backflow of urine into the kidneys.

The urinary bladder temporarily stores the urine. When the bladder has collected about 200 to 400 mL of urine, nerve impulses are transferred to the lower portion of the spinal cord. The spinal cord sends nerve impulses back, causing the muscles of the bladder to contract. This relaxes the internal sphincter. The urine moves into the urethra, the tube that carries the urine out of the body. In males the urethra is approximately seven to eight inches long. In females it is approximately three to four inches long. There is an external sphincter from the body that needs to voluntarily relax in order to pass urine. A **sphincter** is a ring-like muscle that opens and closes an opening in the body. Urine then passes out of the body through the meatus, the opening at the end of the urethra. This is the process of urinating, which is also called **micturition** or **voiding**. When this sphincter is damaged, weakened, or loses contact with the nervous system, it can cause urinary incontinence. **Urinary incontinence** is the inability to control the bladder, which leads to an involuntary loss of urine. You will learn more about urinary incontinence later in this chapter.

The functions of the urinary system are:

- elimination of waste products from the blood
- maintenance of water balance in the body
- regulation of the levels of electrolytes in the body
- assistance in regulation of blood pressure

Destination: Homeostasis

When the body's fluid balance is disturbed, the kidneys work hard to try to continue to remove waste products from the blood. When water intake decreases, the body adjusts by retaining or saving more water. To do this, the kidneys increase the amount of water returned to the bloodstream. This causes less water to be moved into the urine, which temporarily produces a more concentrated form of urine. In this way, the body's water balance remains stable, maintaining homeostasis.

HOT TIP

Tiny stones can be a big pain.

A kidney stone is a hard mass developed from crystals that separate from the urine and build up on the inner surfaces of the kidney. The stones themselves are also called renal calculi. They can block a ureter, which can cause extreme pain. Urine production may be decreased during a blockage because of a reflex that causes tiny vessels in the kidney to constrict, or become smaller. Report symptoms, such as blood in the urine, painful urination, frequent urge to urinate, back pain, or flank pain, that may indicate kidney stones.

3. Discuss changes in the urinary system due to aging

Normal age-related changes for the urinary system include the following:

- The kidneys do not filter the blood as efficiently.
- Bladder muscle tone weakens.
- Bladder holds less urine, which causes more frequent urination.
- Bladder may not empty completely, causing an increased chance of infection.

4. List normal qualities of urine and identify signs and symptoms to report about urine

Urination is the physical process of releasing or emptying the bladder of urine. Urine consists of waste products removed from the blood. Humans must urinate several times daily in order to remain healthy. Regular urination is vital to keep the urinary system, including the kidneys, ureters, bladder, and urethra healthy.

Urine is normally light, pale yellow, or amber in color (Fig. 16-3). Certain medications and some foods change the color of urine. For example, beets, berries, and some food dyes can make urine appear pink or red. Urine should be clear or transparent and have a faint smell. Urine can become cloudy as it stands, but if it is cloudy when freshly voided, it can be a sign of infection. Normal urine output varies with age and the amount and type of liquids consumed. Adults produce approximately 1200 to 1500 mL of urine per day. Elderly adults may produce less urine.

Fig. 16-3. *Urine is normally light or pale yellow in color. It should be clear, not cloudy.*

Normal urine elimination means there is no pain during urination. Residents should be able to make it to the bathroom before urinating. There should be no blood, pus, mucus, protein, bacteria, glucose or other abnormal matter in urine. You will learn more about glucose later in the chapter. A change in the appearance of urine can signal a health problem. Report any of the following signs or symptoms to the nurse:

- cloudy urine
- dark or rust-colored urine
- strong-, offensive-, or fruity-smelling urine
- pain, burning, or pressure when urinating
- blood, pus, mucus, or discharge in urine
- protein, glucose, or bacteria in urine
- episodes of incontinence

5. List factors affecting urination and describe how to promote normal urination

There are many things that may affect normal urination:

Growth and Development: Aging affects the bladder's ability to hold urine. The bladder is not able to hold the same amount of urine as it did when a person was younger. Older people may have to urinate more often. Urination during the night occurs more frequently with the elderly. The bladder may not empty completely, causing a higher risk of infection. In males, an inability to urinate properly may be due to an enlargement of the prostate gland.

To promote normal urination, encourage the intake of fluids. Provide water and other beverages often for residents who are not on a fluid restriction. Offer frequent trips to the bathroom. Follow a schedule, if possible. Respond to call lights and bathroom requests promptly. The best position for women to urinate is sitting, and for men, it is standing. Avoid the flat-on-back (supine) position if possible, as it does not put pressure on the bladder and works against gravity. Promote exercise and activity, as ordered in the care plan. Help with perineal care as needed, wiping from front to back. Good perineal care will help reduce the risk of infection. Assist residents in washing hands.

Encourage Kegel exercises; these exercises use the pelvic floor muscles to strengthen muscle tone. To find your Kegel muscles, stop the flow of urine once or twice while urinating. To do Kegel exercises, squeeze the muscles for five to ten seconds and relax for ten seconds. These can be done many times per day and can be done anywhere in any position.

Psychological Factors: A lack of privacy can affect urination. Having a roommate for the first time, being in a place that is not home, and needing help with elimination can disrupt normal elimination patterns. Stress and fear can affect urination. They can cause a person to void frequent, small amounts of urine. Depression can alter urination patterns. A person may not be motivated to change exercise habits and increase fluid intake. This can make urinary elimination more difficult.

To promote normal urination, always provide plenty of privacy and allow time for urination. Do not rush the resident. Leave the call light in reach. Respond to call lights and requests for help with toileting immediately. If residents want to talk about their concerns, take the time to listen to them. Report their concerns to the nurse.

Fluid Intake: The sense of thirst generally decreases as a person ages. Reduced fluid intake decreases urine production. The body's ability to remove wastes in the urine may be affected. When wastes build up, infections and other problems can occur. Drinking alcoholic beverages and caffeinated beverages increases urine production. Fluids high in sodium decrease urine output.

To promote normal urination, encourage fluid intake. Generally, a healthy person needs from 64 to 96 ounces (1920-2880 mL) of fluid each day. Remind residents to drink often. Be aware of excessive caffeine, sodium, alcohol, or sugar in the resident's diet. Make sure pitcher and water are within reach and are light enough for residents to lift. Offer a straw if the resident prefers using one. Assist with fluid intake as needed.

Physical Activity and Exercise: A lack of exercise lessens sphincter control, which can increase episodes of incontinence. Childbirth can affect a woman's muscle tone. Indwelling catheters (Learning Objective 8) and trauma can affect muscle tone, and increase the risk of infection.

To promote normal urination, increase daily exercise. Encourage regular walks and other types of activities that are allowed.

Personal Habits: If a resident is confined to bed, urination may be more difficult due to his position. As stated before, sitting for women and standing for men are the best positions for urination. Complete emptying of the bladder may be difficult when having to use a bedpan or urinal.

To promote normal urination, raise the head of the bed. Try running water in the bathroom sink to encourage urination.

Medications: Some medications affect urination. Residents who have high blood pressure may be taking diuretics, which are medications that reduce fluid in the body by increasing urine output.

To promote normal urination, offer a trip to the bathroom or bedpan or urinal often. Keep encouraging fluids if allowed, even if this causes more frequent urination.

Disorders: Certain disorders affect urination. Fevers cause increased sweating and may decrease urine production. Diabetes, diseases of the bladder or urethra, infection, congestive heart failure (CHF), and arthritis can affect urination. You will learn more about these diseases later in this chapter and in Chapters 19, 21, and 23 of the textbook.

RESIDENTS' RIGHTS

Help residents promptly.
Do your residents wait to go to the bathroom? This is unhealthy for their urinary systems. Residents should be taken to the bathroom as soon as they need to urinate. They should never have to wait. Accidents are not the only problem with waiting. Holding urine in the bladder for too long can cause bacteria to grow. This leads to infection.

See Chapter 15 for procedures on how to assist residents with bedpans and urinals.

6. Discuss common disorders of the urinary system

Urinary Tract Infection (UTI)

A **urinary tract infection (UTI)**, or cystitis, causes inflammation of the bladder. This usually occurs when bacteria enter the urinary tract through the urethra and then begin to multiply in the bladder. The most common cause of this bacterial infection is from *E. coli* bacteria, which is a form of bacteria commonly found in the gastrointestinal tract. It moves from the anus into the urethra and then the bladder, causing a urinary tract infection.

Women are more susceptible to UTIs than men. This is due to the female urethra being shorter than the male urethra. Bacteria can reach a woman's bladder more easily. Women often develop urinary tract infections after having sexual intercourse. Urinating directly after sexual intercourse can reduce these infections.

Symptoms of UTIs include burning or pain with urination, blood in the urine, and frequency of and urgency with urination.

Drinking plenty of water and other fluids can help prevent UTIs. Cranberry, orange, and blueberry juices, which are rich in Vitamin C, help to acidify urine, which can prevent infection. Wiping from front to back after elimination helps to prevent infection (Fig. 16-4). Taking showers, rather than baths, can help prevent UTIs. Antibiotics are usually prescribed to treat UTIs. Report to the nurse if a resident has cloudy, dark, or foul-smelling urine. Report complaints of burning or discomfort during urination, or if a resident urinates often and in small amounts.

Fig. 16-4. *After elimination, wipe from front to back to prevent infection.*

Chronic Renal Failure

Chronic renal failure (CRF) is a condition in which the kidneys cannot filter waste products from the blood. The kidneys are also unable to perform other life-sustaining duties. Chronic renal failure becomes worse over time. With this disorder, the kidneys slowly become damaged. Waste products and fluid accumulate in the body.

This disease can result from diabetes, high blood pressure (hypertension), chronic urinary tract infections, or inflammation of the kidneys (nephritis). Unfortunately, symptoms may appear only after damage to the kidneys has been done. Initial signs and symptoms of this disorder are:

*   unintended weight loss
*   nausea and vomiting
*   fatigue
*   headache
*   frequent hiccups
*   itching

If kidney function is seriously impaired, dialysis may be necessary. Kidney **dialysis** is an artificial means of removing the body's waste products. It is done when the person's kidneys are no longer able to perform their responsibilities. It can improve and extend life for several years. Dialysis is done regularly and continuously until a kidney transplant is performed or until the person dies. Residents will be on fluid restrictions of different degrees when on dialysis.

End-stage renal disease (ESRD) occurs when the kidneys have failed and dialysis or transplan-

tation is required. Diabetes is the most common cause of ESRD. Dialysis must be performed with people with ESRD.

Urine Retention

Urine retention is an inability to adequately or completely empty the bladder. Retention can be short-term or long-term. Surgical procedures, obstruction, infection, and some disorders, such as multiple sclerosis and diabetes, are common causes of urine retention. You will learn more about these diseases in Chapters 22 and 23 of the textbook. In men, the most common cause of urine retention is enlargement of the prostate gland. Symptoms include the following:

*   lower abdominal pain
*   a painful urge but inability to urinate
*   swollen (distended) bladder
*   abdominal swelling
*   frequent urge to urinate
*   difficulty in starting to urinate
*   weak flow of urine
*   dribbling at the end of urinating and in between urinating

Report to the nurse if you note any of the symptoms listed above. If the condition is not treated, it can lead to UTIs or damage to the urinary tract and kidneys. Urine retention is usually treated with medications and catheterization (use of a tube to drain urine from the bladder).

7. Discuss reasons for incontinence

Urinary incontinence is the inability to control the muscles of the bladder, which leads to an involuntary loss of urine. Incontinence can occur in residents who are confined to bed, ill, or paralyzed. Other physical reasons for incontinence are:

*   Circulatory or nervous system diseases or injuries, such as stroke, dementia, or multiple sclerosis
*   Prostate problems
*   Childbirth

Incontinence is not a normal part of aging. Whatever the reason for incontinence, it is important for nursing assistants to act professionally when handling this problem. Never show anger or frustration toward residents who are incontinent. Residents who are incontinent need reassurance and understanding.

There are different types of incontinence:

- Stress incontinence: loss of urine due to an increase in intra-abdominal pressure; for example when sneezing, laughing, or coughing
- Urge incontinence: involuntary voiding due to an abrupt urge to void
- Mixed incontinence: symptoms of both urge and stress incontinence are present
- Functional incontinence: urine loss caused by environmental, cognitive or physical reasons
- Overflow incontinence: due to overflow or over-distention of the bladder

Incontinence can be very difficult for residents to handle emotionally. Residents may avoid discussing the problem due to embarrassment. It may cause frustration and anger. Family and friends may share these feelings as well. Nursing assistants can help by always being professional and positive when dealing with episodes of incontinence. In addition, follow these guidelines:

Guidelines

Urinary Incontinence

- Know residents' routines and urinary habits. Know their physical signs, such as holding the lower abdomen, which might indicate the need to urinate.
- Follow toileting schedules and the care plan carefully.
- Answer call lights promptly to prevent avoidable accidents.
- Offer a bedpan or take residents to the bathroom often.
- Encourage plenty of fluids, unless residents are on a fluid restriction.

- Walking can stimulate the circulation and the need to go to the bathroom. Take daily walks close to a bathroom.
- Disposable incontinence pads or briefs for adults help keep wastes away from the skin (Fig. 16-5). Change wet or soiled briefs immediately. Always refer to incontinence products as briefs or pads; never call them diapers. Residents are not infants, and this is disrespectful.
- Change bed linens any time they are wet or soiled. Leaving residents in wet linens puts them at risk for pressure sores (Chapter 18). It is also considered abusive or neglectful behavior.
- Use bed protectors or plastic or disposable sheets for residents who are incontinent.
- When residents wear incontinence briefs, check them at least every two hours. Change briefs whenever they are wet or soiled. Observe and report any signs of skin irritation. Tell the nurse if the brief does not appear to fit properly.
- Change wet or soiled clothing immediately.
- Give good skin care and good perineal care. This helps prevent skin breakdown. Urine is irritating to the skin. Bathe residents often.
- Provide privacy for episodes of incontinence. Keep your voice low to keep incontinence a private matter. Never expose more of the resident than is necessary.
- Be calm, patient, and professional.
- Family and friends may watch how you behave to see how they should react to the problem. Be reassuring and remain positive.

Fig. 16-5. One type of incontinence brief.

HOT TIP

Perineal Care

When providing perineal care, change the water if it ever becomes cold or too soapy.

Providing perineal care for an incontinent resident

Equipment: 2 clean bed protectors, 4 washcloths or wipes, towel, gloves, basin with warm water, soap, bath blanket, bath thermometer

1. Identify yourself by name. Identify the resident. Greet the resident by name.

2. Wash your hands.

3. Explain procedure to resident. Speak clearly, slowly, and directly. Maintain face-to-face contact whenever possible. Encourage resident to assist if possible.

4. Provide for the resident's privacy with a curtain, screen, or door.

5. Practice good body mechanics. Adjust bed to safe working level, usually waist high. Lock bed wheels.

6. Lower the side rail (if bed has one and if it is not already lowered) on side nearest you.

7. Lower head of bed. Position resident lying flat on his or her back.

8. Test water temperature with thermometer or your wrist. Ensure it is safe. Water temperature should be 105°F. Have the resident check water temperature. Adjust if necessary.

9. Put on gloves.

10. Cover resident with bath blanket. Move top linens to foot of bed.

11. Remove soiled bed protector from underneath resident by turning resident on his side, away from you. (See procedure Turning a Resident in Chapter 11.) Roll soiled pad into itself with wet side in/dry side out.

12. Place clean bed protector under his or her buttocks.

13. Return resident to lying on his back.

14. Expose perineal area only. Clean perineal area.

For a female resident: Wash the perineum with soap and water from front to back. Use single strokes (Fig. 16-6). Do not wash from the back to the front. This may cause infection. Use a clean area of washcloth or clean washcloth for each stroke. First wipe the center of the perineum, then each side. Spread the labia majora, the outside folds of perineal skin that protect the urinary meatus and the vaginal opening. Wipe from front to back on each side. Rinse the area in the same way. Dry entire perineal area. Move from front to back, using a blotting motion with towel. Ask resident to turn on her side. Wash, rinse, and dry buttocks and anal area. Cleanse the anal area without contaminating the perineal area.

Fig. 16-6. *Using single strokes, wipe from front to back when cleaning.*

For a male resident: If the resident is uncircumcised, retract the foreskin. Gently push skin towards the base of penis. Hold the penis by the shaft. Wash in a circular motion from the tip down to the base (Fig. 16-7). Use a clean area of washcloth or clean washcloth for each stroke. Rinse the penis. If resident is uncircumcised, gently return foreskin to normal position. Then wash the scrotum and groin. The groin is the area from the pubis to the upper thighs. Rinse and pat dry. Ask the resident to turn on his side. Wash, rinse, and dry buttocks and anal area. Cleanse the anal area without contaminating the perineal area.

Fig. 16-7. *Wash the penis in a circular motion from the tip down to the base.*

15. Turn resident on his side away from you. Remove the wet bed protector after drying buttocks.

16. Place a dry bed protector under the resident.

17. Reposition the resident.

18. Remove bath blanket. Replace top covers. Make resident comfortable.

19. Return bed to low position if raised. Ensure resident's safety. Return side rails to ordered position. Remove privacy measures.

20. Empty, rinse, and wipe basin. Return to proper storage.

21. Place soiled linens, clothing and bed protector in proper containers.

22. Remove and dispose of gloves properly.

23. Leave call light within resident's reach.

24. Wash your hands.

25. Be courteous and respectful at all times.

26. Report any changes in the resident to the nurse. Document procedure using facility guidelines.

RESIDENTS' RIGHTS

No shortcuts with resident care.
Residents are sometimes incontinent in bed. Do not take shortcuts when changing bed linen after incontinence. If you replace a disposable pad without changing the wet linen, it may be considered neglect. Remove all wet linen and disposable pads. Replace them with clean ones.

8. Describe catheters and related care

Residents who are unable to pass urine normally may need a urinary catheter. A **catheter** is a tube inserted through the skin or into a body opening that is used to add or drain fluid. Some residents will need straight catheterization. A **straight catheter** is a type of catheter that is inserted to drain urine present in the bladder, and immediately removed after urine is drained. This catheter does not stay inside the resident.

Other residents may require a catheter to stay inside the bladder for a period of time. This type of a catheter is called an **indwelling catheter** (Fig. 16-8). With this catheter, the urine drains into a bag and is held in place by a balloon filled with sterile water.

Fig. 16-8. a) An indwelling catheter (female). b) An indwelling catheter (male).

Another type of catheter that is used for males is called an external, or **condom catheter** (sometimes called a "Texas catheter"). It has an attachment on the end that fits onto the penis and is fastened with special tape. The urine drains through the condom catheter into the tubing, then into the drainage bag. Smaller bags, called "leg bags" collect the urine. They attach to the resident's leg (Fig. 16-9). A condom catheter is changed daily or as needed.

Fig. 16-9. An external or condom catheter.

Catheters are inserted by nurses or doctors. Nursing assistants usually do not insert, irrigate, or remove catheters. However, you may be asked to give daily catheter care, clean the area around the urethral opening and empty the drainage bag. The bag is emptied into a measuring container, called a graduate. You learned about measuring urinary output in Chapter 14.

Following care guidelines for catheters is very important. Serious complications, such as infections, can occur from poor catheter care. These infections can be life-threatening. Follow these guidelines for working with catheters:

Guidelines
Catheters

- Wear gloves when emptying catheter drainage bags.

- When draining the bag, open and close the tubing clamp without touching the tip of the clamp to any other object. If the tip touches other objects, it can transfer pathogens to the inside of the tubing, which can move up into the bladder and cause infection.

- Do not let the catheter drainage spout touch the graduate when draining the catheter bag.

- Make sure the drainage bag hangs lower than the level of the hips or bladder, including when the resident is ambulating. Urine must never flow back into the bladder from the tubing or bag, as it can cause infection.

- Do not hang the drainage bag from the bedrail. The drainage bag can be secured to a non-movable part of the bed frame.

- Keep the drainage bag off the floor.

- Make sure the catheter tubing does not touch the floor.

- Keep tubing as straight as possible. Make sure there are no kinks in the tube and that the resident is not lying on the tubing. The tubing should be over the leg, not underneath it. This can prevent urine from draining properly. Do not place tubing over side rails.

- Keep the genital area clean to prevent infection. Pathogens can enter the bladder more easily with catheters. Daily careful care of the genital area is important.

- When cleaning the urinary meatus, move in one direction, away from the meatus. Use a clean area of the cloth for each stroke.

- Report to the nurse if you notice any of the following: blood in the urine, urine leaking from the catheter, catheter bag fills suddenly or does not fill for several hours. Also report resident complaints of pain or pressure, or odor.

- Secure the tubing properly to the leg with catheter strap.

- Be careful not to disconnect the catheter when positioning or transferring residents with catheters.

- Do not try to re-attach a catheter tube that has disconnected. Inform the nurse immediately so that he or she can re-attach the tube. This is a sterile procedure.

Providing catheter care

Equipment: bath blanket, bed protector, bath basin, soap, bath thermometer, 2-4 washcloths or wipes, towel, gloves

1. Identify yourself by name. Identify the resident. Greet the resident by name.

2. Wash your hands.

3. Explain procedure to resident. Speak clearly, slowly, and directly. Maintain face-to-face contact whenever possible. Encourage resident to assist if possible.

4. Provide for the resident's privacy with a curtain, screen, or door.

5. Practice good body mechanics. Adjust bed to safe working level, usually waist high. Lock bed wheels.

6. Lower the side rail (if bed has one and if it is not already lowered) on side nearest you.

7. Lower head of bed. Position resident lying flat on her back.

8. Remove or fold back top bedding. Keep resident covered with bath blanket.

9. Test water temperature with thermometer or your wrist and ensure it is safe. Water temperature should be 105° F. Have the resident check water temperature. Adjust if necessary.

10. Put on gloves.

11. Avoid contact with clothing and soiled pads or soiled linens throughout procedure.

12. Ask the resident to flex her knees and raise the buttocks off the bed by pushing against the mattress with her feet. Place clean bed protector under her buttocks.

13. Expose only the area necessary to clean the catheter.

14. Place towel or pad under catheter tubing before washing.

15. Apply soap to wet washcloth. Clean area around meatus. Use a clean area of the washcloth for each stroke.

16. Hold catheter near meatus. Avoid tugging the catheter.

17. Clean at least four inches of catheter nearest meatus. Move in only one direction, away from meatus (Fig. 16-10). Use a clean area of the cloth for each stroke.

Fig. 16-10. Hold the catheter near the meatus, so that you do not tug it. Moving in only one direction, away from meatus, helps prevent infection.

18. Rinse area around meatus, using a clean area of washcloth for each stroke. Pat dry with clean cloth.

19. Rinse at least four inches of catheter nearest meatus. Move in only one direction, away from meatus. Use a clean area of the cloth for each stroke.

20. Remove towel or pad from under catheter tubing.

21. Replace top covers. Remove bath blanket. Make resident comfortable.

22. Return bed to low position if raised. Ensure resident's safety. Return side rails to ordered position. Remove privacy measures.

23. Empty, rinse, and wipe basin. Return to proper storage.

24. Dispose of soiled linen in proper containers.

25. Remove and dispose of gloves properly.

26. Leave call light within resident's reach.

27. Wash your hands.

28. Be courteous and respectful at all times.

29. Report any changes in the resident to the nurse. Document procedure using facility guidelines.

Emptying a catheter drainage bag

Equipment: graduate (measuring container), alcohol wipes, paper towels, gloves

1. Identify yourself by name. Identify the resident. Greet the resident by name.

2. Wash your hands.

3. Explain procedure to resident. Speak clearly, slowly, and directly. Maintain face-to-face contact whenever possible. Encourage resident to assist if possible.

4. Provide for the resident's privacy with a curtain, screen, or door.

5. Put on gloves.

6. Place paper towel on the floor under the drainage bag. Place graduate on the paper towel.

7. Open the drain or clamp on the bag. Allow urine to flow out of the bag into the graduate.

Do not let clamp touch the graduate (Fig. 16-11).

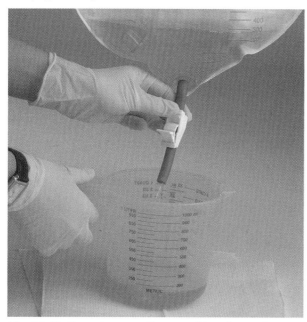

Fig. 16-11. Keep the spout from touching the graduate while draining urine.

8. When urine has drained, close clamp. Using alcohol wipe, clean the drain clamp. Replace the drain in its holder on the bag.

9. Note the amount and the appearance of the urine. Go into the bathroom. Place graduate on a flat surface and measure at eye level. Empty urine into toilet.

10. Clean and store measuring container. Discard paper towel.

11. Remove and dispose of gloves properly.

12. Leave call light within resident's reach.

13. Wash your hands.

14. Be courteous and respectful at all times.

15. Report any changes in the resident to the nurse. Document procedure and amount of urine (output) using facility guidelines.

Applying a condom catheter

Equipment: condom catheter and collection bag, catheter tape (if not a self-adhesive catheter), gloves, plastic bag, bath blanket, bed protector, supplies for perineal care

1. Identify yourself by name. Identify the resident. Greet the resident by name.

2. Wash your hands.

3. Explain procedure to resident. Speak clearly, slowly, and directly. Maintain face-to-face contact whenever possible. Encourage resident to assist if possible.

4. Provide for the resident's privacy with a curtain, screen, or door.

5. Practice good body mechanics. Adjust bed to safe working level, usually waist high. Lock bed wheels.

6. Lower the side rail (if bed has one and if it is not already lowered) on side nearest you.

7. Lower head of bed. Position resident lying flat on his back.

8. Remove or fold back top bedding. Keep resident covered with bath blanket.

9. Put on gloves.

10. Adjust bath blanket to expose only genital area.

11. If condom catheter is present, gently remove it. Carefully disconnect condom from tube and immediately cap tube. Do not allow tube to touch anything. Place condom and tape in the plastic bag.

12. Help as necessary with perineal care.

13. Attach collection bag to leg. Make sure drain stays closed.

14. Move pubic hair away from the penis so it does not get rolled into the condom.

15. Hold penis firmly. Place condom at tip of penis. Roll towards base of penis. Leave at least one inch of space between the drainage tip and glans of penis to prevent irritation. If resident is not circumcised, be sure that foreskin is in normal position.

16. Gently secure condom to penis with special tape provided or use self-adhesive (Fig. 16-12). Apply in a spiral. Never wrap tape all the way around penis because it can impair circulation.

Fig. 16-12. *Gently secure condom to penis with provided tape.*

17. Connect catheter tip to drainage tubing. Do not touch tip to any object but drainage tubing. Make sure tubing is not twisted or kinked.

18. Replace top covers. Remove bath blanket. Make resident comfortable.

19. Return bed to low position if raised. Ensure resident's safety. Return side rails to ordered position. Remove privacy measures.

20. Dispose of plastic bag properly.

21. Remove and dispose of gloves properly.

22. Leave call light within resident's reach.

23. Wash your hands.

24. Be courteous and respectful at all times.

25. Report any changes in the resident to the nurse. Document procedure using facility guidelines.

After a condom catheter is applied, check on it often to make sure urine is draining freely. Reapply condom catheter if it falls off. Report to the nurse if you notice signs that the catheter is interfering with circulation in the penis, such as pale, gray, or blue-tinged skin or if the resident complains of numbness, tingling, or pain.

Continuous Bladder Irrigation (CBI)

Some residents who have an indwelling catheter have an order for continuous bladder irrigation (CBI). This may be needed after surgery on the urinary tract or when a resident has had a catheter for some time and needs to flush out the catheter. The goal of this procedure is to keep the catheter system open and clear of blockage.

When a CBI is ordered, a special type of catheter tubing is needed. A 3-in-1 style is used (Fig. 16-13):

Fig. 16-13. *Bladder irrigation using a three-way catheter.*

- Tube 1 drains the urine.
- Tube 2 allows fluid to be injected to inflate a tiny balloon inside the bladder. This keeps the catheter in place and prevents it from slipping out of the bladder.
- Tube 3 allows the irrigation fluid to flow inside the bladder to flush out the system.

The nurse performs the irrigation procedure. To calculate urine output for a resident with CBI, use this example:

Irrigation fluid used during shift: 750 mL

Fluid output in the catheter drainage bag when emptied: 1250 mL

1250 mL - 750 mL = 500 mL total urine output

9. Explain how to collect different types of urine specimens

Urine specimens are collected for different types of tests (Fig. 16-14). When collecting a urine specimen, make sure that you have the correct resident. The specimen must be put in the proper container and labeled with the resident's name, room number, date, and time. Some urine specimens require special containers.

Fig. 16-14. *Specimens are collected in order to perform tests. Specimens must always be labeled with the resident's name, room number, the date, and time, before being taken to the lab.*

Urine that cannot be sent to the lab immediately may need to be placed in a special refrigerator used strictly for specimens. Never place a specimen in a refrigerator that is used for food.

When collecting a urine specimen, show the resident the correct container to use. The resident should be prepared to give a specimen the next time he or she has to urinate. Ask the resident not to get tissue or stool in the sample because tissue and stool can ruin the sample. Urine specimens must be collected properly in order to obtain accurate results. Take specimen to the lab or designated place after obtaining it.

There are many tests that can be done on urine. A **routine urine specimen** can be collected any time the resident voids. The resident will void into a bedpan, urinal, commode or hat.

Collecting a routine urine specimen

Equipment: specimen container and lid, completed label, 2 pairs of gloves, bedpan or urinal if resident cannot get to the bathroom, "hat" for toilet if resident can get to the bathroom, 2 plastic bags, washcloth, towel, toilet paper, paper towel, supplies for perineal care, pen, completed lab requisition slip

1. Identify yourself by name. Identify the resident. Greet the resident by name.

2. Wash your hands.

3. Explain procedure to resident. Speak clearly, slowly, and directly. Maintain face-to-face contact whenever possible. Encourage resident to assist if possible.

4. Provide for the resident's privacy with a curtain, screen, or door.

5. Put on gloves.

6. Lower the side rail (if bed has one and if it is not already lowered) on side nearest you.

7. Help the resident to the bathroom or commode, or offer the bedpan or urinal.

8. Have resident void into "hat," urinal, or bedpan. Ask the resident not to put toilet paper or stool in with the sample. Provide a plastic bag to discard toilet paper.

9. After urination, help as necessary with perineal care. Help resident wash his or her hands.

10. Remove and dispose of gloves properly. Wash your hands.

11. Replace bed covers. Make resident comfortable.

12. Return bed to low position if raised. Ensure resident's safety. Return side rails to ordered position. Remove privacy measures.

13. Put on clean gloves.

14. Take bedpan, urinal, or commode pail to the bathroom.

15. Pour urine into the specimen container. Specimen container should be at least half full.

16. Cover the urine container with its lid. Do not touch the inside of container. Wipe off the outside with a paper towel and discard. Apply label, and bag the specimen.

17. If using a bedpan or urinal, discard extra urine. Rinse and clean equipment. Use approved disinfectant if facility policy. Store equipment.

18. Remove and dispose of gloves properly.

19. Leave call light within resident's reach.

20. Wash your hands.

21. Be courteous and respectful at all times.

22. Report any changes in the resident to the nurse. Document procedure using facility guidelines. Take specimen and lab slip to designated place promptly.

Urine Straining

Urine is strained to detect the presence of **calculi**, or kidney stones, that can develop in the urinary tract. Urine straining is the process of pouring all urine through a fine filter to catch any particles. Kidney stones can be as small as grains of sand or as large as golf balls. If any stones are found, they are saved and then sent to a laboratory for examination. To strain urine, you will collect a routine urine specimen. In the bathroom, pour it through a strainer or a 4x4-inch piece of gauze into a specimen container. Any stones are trapped in the filter. They are placed in the specimen container and then into a plastic bag for transport to the lab.

A **clean-catch**, or mid-stream (CCMS), **specimen** is collected by first cleaning the perineal area, and then urinating a small amount into the toilet to clear the urethra. After urinating a small amount into the toilet, the sample is then collected mid-stream in a clean or sterile container. The resident stops urinating, if possible, and the container is removed from the stream. Then the resident finishes voiding into the toilet. The specimen is called mid-stream because

the first and last urine that is voided are not included in the sample. This specimen is often collected to detect bacteria in the urine.

Collecting a clean-catch (mid-stream) urine specimen

Equipment: specimen kit with container, completed label, cleaning solution, gauze or towelettes, 2 pairs of gloves, bedpan or urinal if resident cannot use the bathroom, plastic bag, washcloth, toilet paper, paper towel, towel, supplies for perineal care, pen, completed lab requisition slip

1. Identify yourself by name. Identify the resident. Greet the resident by name.

2. Wash your hands.

3. Explain procedure to resident. Speak clearly, slowly, and directly. Maintain face-to-face contact whenever possible. Encourage resident to assist if possible.

4. Provide for the resident's privacy with a curtain, screen, or door.

5. Lower the side rail (if bed has one and if it is not already lowered) on side nearest you.

6. Put on gloves.

7. Open the specimen kit. Do not touch the inside of the container or lid.

8. If the resident cannot clean his or her perineal area, you will do it. Using the towelettes or gauze and cleansing solution, clean the area around the meatus.

   For females, separate the labia. Wipe from front to back along one side. Discard towelette/gauze. With a new towelette or gauze, wipe from front to back along the other side. Using a new towelette or gauze, wipe down the middle.

   For males, clean the head of the penis. Use circular motions with the towelettes or gauze. Clean thoroughly. Change towelettes/gauze after each circular motion. Discard after use. If the man is uncircumcised, pull back the foreskin of the penis before cleaning. Hold it back during urination. Make sure it is pulled back down after collecting the specimen.

9. Ask the resident to urinate into the bedpan, urinal, or toilet, and to stop before urination is complete.

10. Place the container under the urine stream. Do not touch the resident's body with the container. Have the resident start urinating again. Fill the container at least half full. Have resident stop urinating and remove container if possible. Have the resident finish urinating in bedpan, urinal, or toilet.

11. After urination, help as necessary with perineal care. Help resident wash his or her hands.

12. Remove and dispose of gloves properly. Wash your hands.

13. Replace bed covers. Make resident comfortable.

14. Return bed to low position if raised. Ensure resident's safety. Return side rails to ordered position. Remove privacy measures.

15. Cover the urine container with its lid. Do not touch the inside of the container. Wipe off the outside with a paper towel and discard. Apply label, and bag the specimen.

16. If using a bedpan or urinal, discard extra urine. Rinse and clean equipment. Use approved disinfectant if facility policy. Store equipment.

17. Remove and dispose of gloves properly.

18. Leave call light within resident's reach.

19. Wash your hands.

20. Be courteous and respectful at all times.

21. Report any changes in the resident to the nurse. Document procedure using facility guidelines. Take specimen and lab slip to designated place promptly.

A **24-hour urine specimen** tests for certain chemicals and hormones. This specimen collects all the urine voided by a resident in a 24-hour period. Usually the collection begins at 7 a.m. and runs until 7 a.m. the next day. When beginning a 24-hour urine specimen collection, the resident must void and discard the first urine. The collection begins with an empty bladder. All urine must be collected and stored properly. If any is thrown away, spilled, or improperly stored, the collection will have to be done over again.

Collecting a 24-hour urine specimen

Equipment: 24-hour specimen container, completed label, bedpan or urinal for residents confined to bed, "hat" for toilet if resident can get to the bathroom, gloves, washcloth, towel, toilet paper, supplies for perineal care, sign to alert other team members that a 24-hour urine specimen is being collected, lab requisition slip with date and time of first void

1. Identify yourself by name. Identify the resident. Greet the resident by name.

2. Wash your hands.

3. Explain procedure to resident. Speak clearly, slowly, and directly. Maintain face-to-face contact whenever possible. Encourage resident to assist if possible. Emphasize that all urine must be saved. Ask the resident not to put toilet paper or stool in with the sample.

4. Provide for the resident's privacy with a curtain, screen, or door.

5. Place a sign on the resident's bed to let all care team members know that a 24-hour specimen is being collected. Sign may read "Save all urine for 24-hour specimen."

6. When starting the collection, have the resident completely empty the bladder. Discard the urine. Note the exact time of this voiding. The collection will run until the same time the next day (Fig. 16-15).

7. Put on gloves each time the resident voids. Measure I&O each time if needed.

8. Pour urine from bedpan, urinal, or toilet attachment into the container. Container may be stored on ice or in a special refrigerator when not used. The ice keeps the specimen cool. It also prevents components and chemicals in the urine from breaking down, which can prevent proper analysis. Follow facility policy.

INTAKE-OUTPUT RECORD

Resident/Patient Name		Room No.

	FLUID INTAKE	URINE	EMESIS or DRAINAGE
7:00 A.M. to 3:00 P.M.			
8-Hour Total			
3:00 P.M. to 11:00 P.M.			
8-Hour Total			
11:00 P.M. to 7 A.M.			
8-Hour Total			

Form 3039 © Briggs, Des Moines, IA 50306 PRINTED IN U.S.A. R404

DON'T BREAK THE LAW   Save   1-800-247-2343
MAKE THE CALL   **13%**   www.BriggsCorp.com
*savings on buying vs. copying

Fig. 16-15. *One type of form to record urine output over 24 hours.* (Reprinted with permission of Briggs Corporation, 800-247-2343.)

9. After each voiding, help as necessary with perineal care. Help the resident wash his or her hands.

10. Clean equipment after each voiding.

11. Remove gloves.

12. Wash your hands.

13. After the last void of the 24-hour period, add the urine to the specimen container. Remove the sign.

14. Make resident comfortable.

15. Return bed to low position if raised. Ensure resident's safety. Remove privacy measures.

16. Remove and dispose of gloves.

17. Leave call light within resident's reach.

18. Wash your hands.

19. Be courteous and respectful at all times.

20. Report any changes in the resident to the nurse. Document procedure using facility guidelines. Take specimen containers and lab slip to the designated place promptly.

A sterile urine specimen is obtained when a resident cannot urinate on his or her own, or when an infection in the urinary tract may be present. It may also be done when a resident has urinary retention. A nurse will collect this type of specimen. To collect a sterile urine specimen, the nurse will insert a catheter through the urethra into the bladder using sterile technique. The urine is obtained this way to avoid contamination.

A specimen may have to be collected from a resident who has a urostomy. The nurse will remove the urostomy appliance and collect this specimen directly from the stoma. The appliance is then re-sealed over the stoma.

HOT TIP

Five "Rights" of Specimen Collection

Knowing and remembering the five "rights" of specimen collection will help prevent mistakes and ensure that specimens are collected properly:

1. The Right Resident
2. The Right Specimen
3. The Right Container
4. The Right Date/Time
5. The Right Storage/Delivery

Properly collecting specimens helps avoid resident discomfort, and embarrassment, as well as saving time and money.

10. Explain types of tests that are performed on urine

Facilities use different methods to test urine. Your facility may use a dip strip that can test for such things as pH level, glucose, ketones, blood, and specific gravity. These strips, called reagent strips, have different sections that change color when they react with urine (Fig. 16-16).

Fig. 16-16. *Reagent strips change color when they react with urine. The color is then compared to a color chart to determine levels of each chemical factor.* (Photo courtesy of LW Scientific, Inc., www.lwscientific.com, 800-726-7345.)

Testing pH levels: The term "pH" means "parts Hydrogen." The pH scale ranges from 0 to 14. The lower the number, the more acidic the fluid. The higher the number, the more alkaline the fluid. Normal pH range for urine is 4.6–8.0. A disruption of pH may be due to medication, food, or illness.

Testing for glucose and ketones: In diabetes mellitus, commonly called diabetes, the pancreas does not produce enough insulin or does not produce any insulin (see Chapter 23). Insulin is the substance the body needs to convert glucose, or natural sugar, into energy. Without insulin to process glucose, these sugars collect in the blood. Some sugar appears in the urine.

Diabetics may also have ketones in the urine. **Ketones** are chemical substances produced when the body burns fat for energy or fuel. They are produced when there is not enough insulin to help the body use sugar for energy. Without enough insulin, glucose builds up in the blood. Since the body cannot use glucose for energy, it breaks down fat instead. When this occurs, ketones build up in the blood and spill into the urine.

Testing for blood: In normal urine, blood should not be present. Illness and disease can cause blood to appear in urine. Some blood is hidden, or occult. This blood can be detected by testing the urine.

Specific gravity: A **specific gravity** test is done to test urine density. It can be ordered to make sure the kidneys are functioning properly. Density is how much a substance weighs compared to another substance, which in this case is water. Urine can be very dilute, or close to water. It can also be very dense, or concentrated. This test is done to see how the urine compares to water. Normal values are between 1.002 to 1.028.

When you perform urine testing with dip strips, check the expiration date to make sure that the testing strips have not expired. Dip strips that have expired may give inaccurate results. This can prolong the resident's discomfort or problem. Inform the nurse and get a new bottle if the dip strips have expired. Testing strips are usually stored in a light-resistant bottle. Remove strips one at a time when testing a urine specimen. Cap tightly before storing.

The doctor will order the specific type of specimen to be collected and how often urine tests should be done. Follow the care plan and the nurse's instructions.

Testing urine with reagent strips

Equipment: urine specimen as ordered, reagent strip, gloves, paper towel

1. Wash your hands.

2. Put on gloves.

3. Place paper towel on surface before setting urine specimen down.

4. Take a strip from the bottle and recap bottle. Close it tightly.

5. Dip the strip into the specimen.

6. Follow manufacturer's instructions for when to remove strip. Remove strip at correct time.

7. Follow manufacturer's instructions for how long to wait after removing strip. After proper time has passed, compare strip with color chart on bottle. Do not touch bottle with strip.

8. Read results.

9. Discard used items. Discard specimen in the toilet.

10. Remove gloves.

11. Wash your hands.

12. Record and report results. Document procedure using facility guidelines.

HOT TIP

Fresh-fractional Urine Specimen
A fresh-fractional, or double-voided, urine specimen is often used to test for glucose and ketones in urine. The second sample is usually very small. To obtain this specimen, collect a routine urine specimen and test it, as you may not be able to collect a second specimen. Then ask the resident to drink an 8 oz. glass of water. Leave the call light within reach and leave the room. Return in 20-30 minutes or when signaled by resident. Repeat the steps for collecting a urine specimen and test that specimen or take it to the lab for testing.

11. Explain guidelines for assisting with bladder retraining

Illness, injury, or inactivity can cause a loss of normal bladder function. Residents may need help in re-establishing a regular routine and normal bladder function. Incontinence may be a problem when retraining the bladder. Be professional when episodes of incontinence occur. As you have learned, problems with incontinence can be embarrassing or difficult to discuss. Be sensitive to this. Be empathetic and maintain a positive attitude.

Most care team members will be involved with charting and implementing bladder retraining. Accurate charting is very important. Follow the care plan for each resident.

Guidelines

Bladder Retraining

- Follow the plan consistently. Explain the training schedule to the resident. Direct any questions the resident has to the nurse.

- Follow Standard Precautions. Wear gloves when handling body wastes. For residents in isolation, additional PPE may be needed. Follow the care plan.

- Observe your residents' elimination habits. This helps predict when a trip to the bathroom or a bedpan or urinal will be necessary.

- Keep a record of elimination, including episodes of incontinence. Keeping accurate records will help establish a routine.

- Offer a bedpan or urinal or a trip to the bathroom before beginning long procedures and after the procedures have been completed (Fig. 16-17).

- Answer call lights promptly. Residents should never have to wait to go to the bathroom.

- Provide privacy with elimination and do not rush the resident.

- Help the resident with good perineal care as needed. This promotes proper hygiene and helps prevent skin breakdown. Watch for skin changes and report them.

- Encourage plenty of fluids throughout the day if allowed, even if incontinence is a problem. About 30 minutes after fluids are consumed, offer a bedpan, urinal, or trip to the bathroom.

- Ⓔ Have the resident lean forward slightly to put pressure on the bladder. If he or she is having trouble urinating, try running water in the sink.

- Ⓔ Dispose of wastes properly. Wastes, clothing protectors, and incontinence briefs may need to be double-bagged before being placed in the proper container.

- Ⓔ Keep accurate intake and output (I&O) records. Output includes episodes of incontinence.

- Ⓔ Offer praise and positive words for attempts and successes in controlling the bladder.

- Ⓔ Never show frustration or anger toward residents who are incontinent. The problem is out of their control. Be positive and patient with the retraining efforts.

Fig. 16-17. *Offer regular trips to the bathroom, especially before and after performing care.*

RESIDENTS' RIGHTS

Bladder Retraining

Residents have the right to be assisted with their elimination needs as often as necessary. They must be encouraged to ask for help whenever they need it. It is important for them not to feel discouraged or intimidated regarding the frequency of their elimination.

CHAPTER REVIEW

1. What is the name of the tube that carries the urine out of the body (LO 2)?

2. Is a woman's urethra longer or shorter than a man's (LO 2)?

3. List four functions of the urinary system (LO 2).

4. List four normal age-related changes of the urinary system (LO 3).

5. List three normal qualities of urine (LO 4).

6. List seven things to observe and report about urine (LO 4).

7. For each of the six factors (not including disorders) that affect urination listed in Learning Objective 5, describe one way nursing assistants can promote normal urination (LO 5).

8. What is the best position for women to urinate? What is the best position for men (LO 5)?

9. Why are women more susceptible to UTIs than men (LO 6)?

10. List three signs and symptoms of UTIs (LO 6).

11. How should residents wipe after elimination in order to prevent infection (LO 6)?

12. What is dialysis (LO 6)?

13. List eight signs and symptoms of urine retention (LO 6).

14. List five physical reasons for incontinence (LO 7).

15. Define five different types of incontinence (LO 7).

16. List eight guidelines for dealing with incontinence (LO 7).

17. What is the difference between a straight catheter and an indwelling catheter (LO 8)?

18. List ten care guidelines for catheters (LO 8).

19. Why should a drainage bag for a catheter always hang lower than the level of the hips or bladder (LO 8)?

20. What items should not be included in a urine specimen (LO 9)?

21. Explain how a clean-catch urine specimen is obtained (LO 9).

22. What is a 24-hour urine specimen (LO 9)?

23. When is a sterile urine specimen needed (LO 9)?

24. List four things reagent strips can test for in urine (LO 10).

25. About how long after fluids are taken should residents be offered a trip to the bathroom (LO 11)?

26. Why might problems with urinary incontinence be difficult to discuss (LO 11)?

27. What is one way a nursing assistant can promote dignity during bladder retraining (LO 11)?

17
The
Reproductive
System

An Amazing Recovery!

Ephraim McDowell, 1771-1830, a doctor of the Kentucky frontier, was visited in 1809 by a patient with a large ovarian cyst. He asked her to travel 60 miles to his office for an operation which she would probably not survive. She decided to travel the distance on horseback. The physician opened her abdomen without anesthesia while she read from the Bible. He cut out an ovary weighing nearly 20 pounds. After a 25-day recovery, she left the area and returned home. The woman lived another 31 years. McDowell gained international fame for his removal of cysts.

"In the dark womb where I began/My mother's life made me . . . Through all the months of human birth/Her beauty fed my common earth."

John Masefield, 1878-1967

*"Little creature, formed of joy and mirth,
Go, love without the help of any thing on earth."*

William Blake, 1757-1827

1. Define important words in this chapter

benign prostatic hypertrophy: a disorder in which the prostate becomes enlarged, causing problems with urination and/or emptying the bladder.

chlamydia: a sexually-transmitted disease caused by bacteria.

douche: a rinsing of the vagina in order to cleanse the vaginal tract or to introduce medication into the vagina; also called a vaginal irrigation.

genital herpes: a sexually-transmitted disease caused by a virus; cannot be cured.

genital HPV infection: a sexually-transmitted disease caused by human papillomavirus (HPV).

glands: structures that secrete hormones.

gonads: the male and female sexual reproductive glands.

gonorrhea: a sexually-transmitted disease caused by bacteria.

hormones: chemical substances created by the body that control numerous body functions.

impotence: the inability to have or maintain a penile erection.

menopause: the point at which a woman's menstrual periods stop permanently and she can no longer conceive.

menstruation: the shedding of the lining of the uterus that occurs approximately every 28 days; also known as the menstrual cycle or period.

ovum: female sex cell or egg.

sexually-transmitted diseases (STDs): diseases passed through sexual contact; also called venereal diseases.

sexually-transmitted infections (STIs): infections caused by sexual contact; infected person may not show signs or symptoms of disease.

sperm: male sex cells.

syphilis: a sexually-transmitted disease caused by bacteria.

trichomoniasis: a sexually-transmitted disease caused by protozoa (single-celled animals).

vaginal irrigation: a rinsing of the vagina in order to cleanse the vaginal tract or to introduce medication into the vagina; also called a douche.

2. Explain the structure and function of the reproductive system

The reproductive system consists of the reproductive organs, which are different in men and women. This system allows human beings to reproduce, or create new human life. Reproduction begins when male and female sex cells, **sperm** and **ovum**, join. These sex cells are formed in the male and female sexual reproductive glands, called the **gonads**. **Glands** are structures that secrete hormones; **hormones** are chemical substances created by the body that control numerous body functions, including the body's ability to reproduce. You will learn more about glands and hormones in Chapter 23.

The Male Reproductive System

The male reproductive system consists of the penis, testes, scrotum, epididymis, vas deferens, erectile tissue, seminal vesicle, ejaculatory duct, and prostate gland (Fig. 17-1). The testes are found within the sac of skin known as the scrotum. The scrotum supports the testes and regulates the temperature of the testes. The testes produce testosterone, the male hormone needed for the reproductive organs to function properly, and sperm.

Sperm travel from the testes to the epididymis, a coiled tube that can be as long as 20 feet. The epididymis receives and stores sperm. After maturing in the epididymis, sperm move into the vas deferens, the tube that sperm travel through

in order to reach the ejaculatory duct. During their trip, the sperm mix with fluid produced in three glands, the seminal vesicles, the prostate gland, and Cowper's glands.

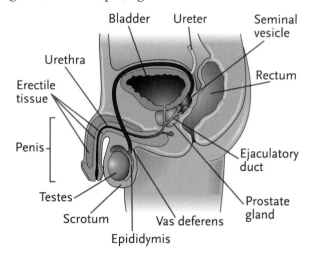

Fig. 17-1. *The male reproductive system.*

From the ejaculatory duct, sperm empty into the urethra, where they are released from the body through the penis. The penis is the sex organ located outside the body, in front of the scrotum. The penis is composed of erectile tissue that becomes filled with blood during sexual excitement. As the penis fills with blood, it becomes enlarged and erect and is able to release semen. Semen is released in small amounts during ejaculation, from about two to five mL at a time. Every milliliter of semen contains 50 to 150 million sperm.

The Female Reproductive System

The female reproductive system is made up of the ovaries, fallopian tubes, uterus, vagina, the external genitals—the vulva—and the mammary glands or breasts (Fig. 17-2). The ovaries produce the female sex cells or eggs (ova) and they produce the female hormones, estrogen and progesterone. Each month from puberty to menopause, ova are released from ovaries (usually alternating ovaries) during the process called ovulation. **Menopause** is the point at which a woman's menstrual periods stop permanently and she can no longer conceive. This monthly cycle is maintained by estrogen and progesterone. The ovum or egg cell then travels into the respective fallopian tube, one of two tubes that open into the uterus.

Fig. 17-2. *The female reproductive system.*

As the ovum reaches the fallopian tube, it may be fertilized by a sperm that will swim its way up into the tube. If it is not fertilized, the ovum will die within about 24 to 48 hours. Sperm usually die within two days. If an ovum is fertilized, it moves into the uterus, or womb. The uterus is a hollow, pear-shaped, muscular organ located within the pelvis. It lies behind the bladder and in front of the rectum.

A fertilized ovum will implant into the lining of the uterus, or the endometrium. This is where the fetus develops. If an ovum is not fertilized, the secretion of female hormones decreases. The endometrium then breaks up and is expelled in a process called **menstruation**.

The vagina is the muscular canal that opens to the outside of the body. It serves as the outlet for the blood during a woman's menstrual cycle. It acts as the receiver of sperm during sexual intercourse and is the birth canal.

The breasts or mammary glands are the glands that nourish a baby. They are responsible for the production of milk within the alveolar glands inside the breast. These glands send the milk into milk ducts that come together at the nipple in the area called the areola. This process is called lactation.

The functions of the reproductive system are:

Male

- manufacture sperm and the male hormone testosterone

Female

- manufacture ova (eggs) and female hormones, estrogen and progesterone
- provide environment for development of fetus
- produce milk (lactation) for the nourishment of a baby after birth

Destination: Homeostasis

Homeostasis can be affected by changes in the reproductive system. For example, a male's testosterone levels can increase due to stressors. This increase in the hormone level causes the brain to send a message to the male reproductive glands to decrease the production of testosterone. The testosterone level then returns to normal, and the body returns to homeostasis.

3. Discuss changes in the reproductive system due to aging

Normal age-related changes for the reproductive system include the following:

Male

- Prostate gland enlarges.
- Number and capability of sperm decreases.
- Sexual response delays; it may take longer to achieve an erection and to reach orgasm.

Female

- Menopause occurs when menstruation ends, usually between the ages of 45 and 55, and ends the female's ability to reproduce.
- Decrease in production of estrogen and progesterone leads to a loss of calcium, causing brittle bones and, potentially, osteoporosis.
- Vaginal walls become drier and thinner; this may cause discomfort during sexual intercourse.

4. Discuss common disorders of the reproductive system

Sexually-Transmitted Diseases (STDs) and Infections (STIs)

Sexually-transmitted diseases (STDs), also called venereal diseases, are diseases caused by sexual contact that show symptoms. However, a term that is becoming more widely used to describe these infections is **sexually-transmitted infection (STI)**. STIs are different in that a person may be infected, and may potentially infect others, without showing signs or symptoms of disease.

STDs and STIs are transmitted through sexual contact, such as sexual intercourse (vaginal and anal), contact of the mouth with the genitals or anus, and contact of the hands with the genital area. Some STDs and STIs can also be transmitted via needles used in IV drug use, as well as through childbirth or breastfeeding.

The transmission of some STDs and STIs can be reduced or stopped by using latex condoms. The human immunodeficiency virus (HIV) can be transmitted sexually, as well. HIV and AIDS are discussed in depth in Chapter 24.

Chlamydia infection is caused by bacteria. Symptoms of chlamydia include burning with urination, yellow or white discharge from the penis or vagina, swelling of the testes, painful intercourse, and abdominal and low back pain. In many cases, no symptoms are apparent. This disorder may cause an eye infection (conjunctivitis, or "pink eye") or pneumonia in babies born to infected mothers. It may also cause infertility and pelvic inflammatory disease (PID) if not promptly and properly treated. Treatment includes the use of antibiotics.

Genital herpes (HSV2) is caused by a virus. It cannot be treated with antibiotics, nor can it be cured. Once infected with genital herpes, a person may have repeated outbreaks of the disease for the rest of his or her life. Symptoms include itching and painful red blisters or open sores. Herpes may also cause a burning sensation while urinating or during intercourse, low-grade fever, headache, and muscle aches. Herpes sores are infectious, and may appear quickly after the sexual contact with an infected partner. However, a person can also spread genital herpes when sores are not present. Treatment consists of anti-viral medications. The medication does not cure the disease, but it can help lessen the frequency of the episodes.

Genital HPV infection is a sexually-transmitted disease caused by human papillomavirus (HPV). These viruses are spread primarily through genital contact and can infect the genital area of both men and women. This includes the penis, vulva, lining of the vagina, cervix, rectum, or anus. Many people have no signs or symptoms of HPV. Some HPV infections cause women to have an abnormal pap test. Genital warts may appear. They may also lead to the development of cervical cancer. Treatment to remove warts is done in a doctor's office or by medications. Treatment for HPV also consists of methods used by doctors to treat changes in the cervix that occur with infection. There is no cure for HPV. However, a new HPV vaccine, licensed by the Food and Drug Administration (FDA), is being offered to girls and women.

Gonorrhea is a sexually-transmitted disease caused by bacteria. It is easier to detect in men because many women with gonorrhea show no early symptoms. Symptoms in men include painful or burning urination, a white, yellow or green cloudy pus-like discharge from the penis, and painful or swollen testes. Symptoms in women include cloudy vaginal discharge, along with vaginal bleeding between periods. Rectal symptoms, such as itching, soreness, bleeding, or painful elimination of stool, can occur in both sexes. This disorder can cause blindness, joint infection, or a serious blood infection in babies born to infected mothers. It can also cause sterility and pelvic inflammatory disease (PID) if not treated. Treatment consists of antibiotics.

Syphilis is caused by bacteria. Syphilis is generally easier to detect in men than in women. The first stage is marked by small, painless sores called chancres that form on the penis soon after infection. In women, these sores may form inside the vagina. If left untreated, the infection progresses to the second stage, in which rashes appear on one or more areas of the body. These rashes do not usually cause itching. A headache and a fever may occur, along with sore throat, weight loss, and muscle aches. The third stage usually take years to develop. During this stage, the symptoms from the second stage disappear. The person will still have the disease, and if not treated with penicillin or other antibiotics, the infection spreads to the heart, brain, and other vital organs. Untreated syphilis will eventually be fatal. The sooner it is treated, the better chance of preventing long-term damage and avoiding infection of others.

Trichomoniasis is a sexually-transmitted disease caused by protozoa (single-celled animals). Men may have no symptoms. However, mild discharge, irritation or a burning sensation after urination or ejaculation may occur. Symptoms of infection in women include a green-yellow vaginal discharge with a strong odor, irritation or itching. The infection may cause discomfort during intercourse or urination. Treatment consists of the administration of the prescription drug metronidazole.

Benign Prostatic Hypertrophy (BPH)

Benign prostatic hypertrophy is a disorder that is quite common in men over the age of 60. Studies show that one-third to one-half of all men over this age show signs of this disorder. When a man has BPH, the prostate becomes enlarged, which causes pressure on the urethra. When the urethra becomes compressed, urination becomes difficult. Other symptoms of BPH are a feeling of incomplete urination, frequent urination, and a weak stream of urine. Dribbling of urine right after urinating, the need to urinate often during the night, and incontinence

are symptoms, too. The cause of BPH is unknown. Medications and surgery are generally used to treat BPH.

Prostate enlargement is not a cancerous condition. However, as men age, they are at increased risk for prostate cancer. A test is available to screen for prostate cancer. This type of cancer is usually slow-growing and responsive to treatment if caught early.

Other Diseases

Other diseases that may be sexually transmitted include bacterial vaginosis (BV), scabies, and pubic lice. For information on these diseases and others, visit the CDC's website, www.cdc.gov.

Hepatitis B is a liver disease transmitted by sexual contact with an infected person. It is also transmitted by sharing infected needles, contact with infected blood, or to a baby from an infected mother during birth. For more information on hepatitis, see Chapter 6.

TRIVIA

The Scourge of Syphilis

The first epidemic of syphilis affected sailors who returned from Columbus' first voyage to The Americas. At that time it was called "Naples Disease" and the "French Disease."

Paul Ehrlich, 1854-1915, doctor and medical scientist, developed a substance called salvarsan in 1910 that was effective in treating syphilis. It was used as a primary drug to treat syphilis until antibiotics became the treatment of choice during the 1940s. Ehrlich won the Nobel Prize for Medicine in 1908.

5. Describe sexual needs of the elderly

Sexual needs continue throughout a person's life. While interest in sex may decline in the elderly, it does not go away. All people regardless of age have sexual needs and desires (Fig. 17-3). The ability to engage in sexual activities, such as intercourse and masturbation, continues unless a disease or injury occurs. You can help by providing privacy whenever necessary for sexual activity and respecting your residents' sexual needs.

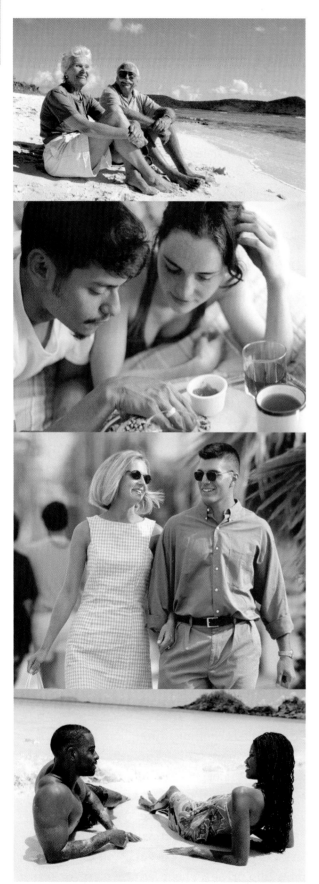

Fig. 17-3. *Sexual needs, behavior and desires are present in all age groups.*

Some things that can affect sexual activity in the elderly include the following:

- illness reducing or affecting the ability of men and women to perform sexually

- erectile dysfunction (ED) (impotence) in males

- vaginal atrophy (weakening or wasting of muscles), pain and dryness in females

- fear of inadequate sexual performance

- depression

- a lack of privacy

- medications

In the past, male impotence was often viewed as a normal response to aging. **Impotence** is the inability to have or maintain an erection. It is not a normal change of aging. Medications can help this problem. Report any resident complaints about impotence to the nurse.

For women, special creams and medications can help with vaginal dryness. Report complaints about dryness or pain to the nurse.

You learned about sexually-transmitted diseases in Learning Objective 4 of this chapter. Nurses and doctors can educate sexually-active older adults about how to reduce the risk of contracting these diseases. Nursing assistants can help by reporting any signs or symptoms of STDs to the nurse immediately.

Remember that older adults are sexual beings like all humans, and they have the right to choose how they express their sexuality. In all age groups, there is a wide variety of sexual behavior. This is also true of residents in nursing homes. An attitude that any expression of sexuality by the elderly is cute, funny, or disgusting deprives residents of their right to dignity and respect. All residents have a right to be treated with dignity and to have their privacy respected.

If you encounter any sexual situation, such as a resident masturbating or two consenting adult residents engaged in sexual activity, provide privacy and leave the area. Do not judge any sexual behavior you see.

6. Describe vaginal irrigation

Vaginal irrigation, or a vaginal **douche**, is a rinsing of the vagina in order to cleanse the vaginal tract prior to surgical procedures or examinations or due to vaginal drainage. It is also performed to introduce medication into the vagina to treat disorders or to reduce discomfort such as itching or redness. These irrigations are only done with a doctor's order.

Vaginal irrigations may be external, internal, or internal and external. Disposable irrigation kits or bags with tubing may be used for this procedure. The solution will run into the vagina through a special vaginal irrigation kit. The solution will run back out of the vagina into a bedpan, toilet, or in the shower due to gravity. Irrigations may be ordered with water and can include any of the following additives:

*   Vinegar

*   Baking soda

*   Medication

Commercial douche kits are also available. The additives are usually already mixed in with the solution. The tip is approximately 2 to 3 inches long and may be pre-lubricated. If using a commercial vaginal douche, attach the tip securely onto the bottle if necessary. Make sure it is secured tightly. If the fluid needs to be mixed more thoroughly, turn the bottle back and forth gently. Do not shake the bottle.

Guidelines
Vaginal Irrigation

*   Always provide plenty of privacy during this procedure.

*   Place the woman in the dorsal recumbent position (flat on her back with knees flexed and slightly separated; feet are flat on bed) (Fig. 17-4).

*   If the irrigation is external only, the fluid will flow over the external vulva. No insertion of tubing is needed.

*   If the irrigation is internal and external, the fluid should first be allowed to flow over the external vulva. Then the tip is inserted into the vagina.

*   Do not force the tip into the vagina. If you are unable to insert the tip, stop, secure the resident and inform the nurse.

*   When giving a vaginal irrigation, observe and report any of the following:

    *   Pain or discomfort

    *   Increase or decrease in vaginal discharge

    *   Bleeding

    *   Itching or burning

    *   Abdominal swelling

Fig. 17-4. *The dorsal recumbent position.*

Many facilities do not allow nursing assistants to perform this procedure. Follow your facility's policy regarding vaginal irrigations.

Giving a vaginal douche

Equipment: vaginal douche, including bag, tubing and tip, lubricating jelly, gloves, bed protector, bath blanket, towel, bedpan and bedpan cover

Assist the resident to urinate before beginning the procedure.

1. Identify yourself by name. Identify the resident. Greet the resident by name.

2. Wash your hands.

3. Explain procedure to resident. Speak clearly, slowly, and directly. Maintain face-to-face contact whenever possible. Encourage resident to assist if possible.

4. Provide for the resident's privacy with a curtain, screen, or door.

5. Practice good body mechanics. Adjust bed to safe working level, usually waist high. Lock bed wheels.

6. Lower the side rail (if bed has one and if it is not already lowered) on side nearest you.

7. Lower head of bed. Position resident lying flat on her back.

8. Apply gloves.

9. Cover the resident with a bath blanket. Ask her to hold it while you pull down the top covers underneath. Do not expose more of her than you have to.

10. Place a bed protector under the resident's buttocks and hips.

11. Hang prepared vaginal irrigation bag on IV pole and lower pole so that bag is 12 inches above resident's perineal area.

12. Remove resident's pants or pajama bottoms, exposing only as much of the resident's body as necessary.

13. Place the bedpan under the resident and make sure she is in the dorsal recumbent position.

14. Open the clamp and allow a little water to run from the tubing into the bedpan to clear air from the tubing.

15. Lubricate tip of tubing if not already lubricated.

16. Insert nozzle slowly and gently into vagina about two to three inches (Fig. 17-5).

Fig. 17-5. *Insert nozzle slowly and gently into vagina about two to three inches.*

17. Begin slow flow of water or fluid by releasing clamp. Before vaginal irrigation bag is empty, clamp tubing.

18. Remove tubing slowly and gently and place tubing tip inside top of bag.

19. Raise the head of the bed so that the resident is in a semi-sitting position on the bedpan so that the solution can drain.

20. Remove bedpan and cover it. Remove the bed protector.

21. Dry perineal area and buttocks and replace clothing or gown. Remove bath blanket and replace top covers.

22. Return bed to low position if raised. Ensure resident's safety. Return side rails to ordered position. Remove privacy measures.

23. Make resident comfortable.

24. Bring bedpan to bathroom and check contents for anything unusual. Empty bedpan.

25. Rinse bedpan. Pour rinse water into toilet. Use approved disinfectant if facility policy. Return to proper storage.

26. Place soiled linens, clothing and bed protector in proper containers.

27. Remove and dispose of gloves properly.

28. Leave call light within resident's reach.

29. Wash your hands.

30. Be courteous and respectful at all times.

31. Report any changes in the resident to the nurse. Document procedure using facility guidelines.

RESIDENTS' RIGHTS

Gynecological Exams

A gynecological examination may be done in the resident's room or in a special examination room. It can also be performed in an emergency room or an urgent care center. When these exams are done, it is important to be sensitive to the resident's feelings and concerns. Gynecological examinations may be embarrassing, uncomfortable, and frightening. Listen to residents who want to talk, and answer any questions that are within your scope of practice. Refer any questions that you cannot answer to the nurse or doctor. Make sure to provide privacy throughout the exam.

CHAPTER REVIEW

1. List the functions of the male and female reproductive systems (LO 2).

2. What is the name of the male hormone needed for the reproductive organs to function properly (LO 2)?

3. What two female hormones help maintain the monthly cycle of menstruation (LO 2)?

4. What are the names of the male sex cells and the female sex cells (LO 2)?

5. List all normal age-related changes of the reproductive system for males and females (LO 3).

6. How are sexually-transmitted diseases (STDs) transmitted from one person to another (LO 4)?

7. How are sexually-transmitted infections (STIs) different from STDs (LO 4)?

8. Which two STDs listed are caused by a virus and cannot be cured (LO 4)?

9. Why does urination become more difficult for men who have BPH (LO 4)?

10. When encountering a sexual situation between consenting residents, what should a nursing assistant do (LO 5)?

11. List seven factors that can affect sexual activity in the elderly (LO 5).

12. Why is it important not to judge residents' sexual behavior (LO 5)?

13. List three reasons that vaginal irrigations are given (LO 6).

14. List five signs and symptoms about vaginal irrigation that must be reported to the nurse (LO 6).

18
The Integumentary System

The Field of Dermatology in its Infancy

Ferdinand Hebra (1816-1880) was one of the first doctors to specialize in the diseases of the skin. He founded a division of dermatology. One of the discoveries he made concerned scabies, a disorder that causes intense itching. Hebra noted that when the itch-mite parasite was destroyed, scabies was cured. He also made the important discovery that scabies was contagious and that it could be passed from one person to another.

"'Tis not a lip or eye we beauty call/But the joint force and full result of all."
Alexander Pope, 1688-1744

"Men should be judged, not by their tint of skin . . . But by the quality of thought they think."
Adela Florence Cory Nicolson, 1865-1904

1. Define important words in this chapter

bony prominences: areas of the body where the bone lies close to the skin.

closed wound: wound in which the skin's surface is not broken.

dermis: the inner layer of the two main layers of tissue that make up the skin.

eczema: a temporary or a chronic skin disorder that results in redness, itching, burning, swelling, cracking, weeping, and lesions; also called dermatitis.

epidermis: the outer layer of the two main layers of tissue that make up the skin.

gangrene: death of tissue caused by infection or lack of blood flow.

integument: natural protective covering.

lesion: an area of abnormal tissue or an injury or wound.

melanin: the pigment that gives skin its color.

melanocyte: cell in the skin that produces and contains the pigment called melanin.

necrosis: the death of living cells or tissues caused by lack of nourishment to tissues.

open wound: wound in which the skin's surface is not intact.

pressure points: areas of the body that bear much of its weight.

pressure sore: a serious wound resulting from skin breakdown; also known as decubitus ulcer or bed sore.

psoriasis: a chronic skin condition caused by skin cells growing too quickly which results in red, white or silver patches, itching and discomfort.

ringworm: a fungal infection that causes red scaly patches to appear in a ring shape, generally on the upper body, or the hands and feet.

scabies: a contagious skin infection caused by mites burrowing into the skin that results in pimple-like irritations, rashes, intense itching, and sores.

shearing: rubbing or friction resulting from the skin moving one way and the bone underneath it remaining fixed or moving in the opposite direction.

shingles: a viral infection caused by the same virus that causes chickenpox; causes pain, itching, rashes, and possibly fever and chills.

sitz bath: a warm soak of the perineal area to cleanse perineal wounds and reduce inflammation and pain.

wart: contagious rough, hard bump caused by a virus.

2. Explain the structure and function of the integumentary system

The integumentary system consists of the following parts: the skin, hair, nails, oil glands, sweat glands, subcutaneous tissue, and nerve endings (Fig. 18-1). The skin is a natural protective covering, or **integument**. The skin is an organ, and it is the largest organ in the human body. It is considered an organ because it has different types of tissues that together function to perform activities of the body. The skin covers and protects the body, provides sensation through nerves, regulates body temperature, and prevents the loss of too much water.

The two basic layers of the skin are the epidermis and the dermis. The **epidermis** is the outer layer of the skin which is composed of dead cells. These cells are continuously shed as new cells move up from the dermis. The epidermis does not contain blood vessels. Keratin is a substance found in the dead skin cells of the epidermis. Keratin has waterproof qualities that protect the inside of the body when we get wet. Beneath the very top of the epidermis lie other types of cells. One is the **melanocyte**, which

contains **melanin**, the substance that gives skin its color. The more melanin your skin produces, the darker your skin color.

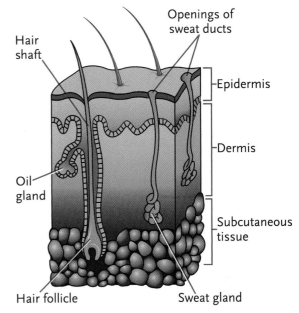

Fig. 18-1. *Cross-section showing the integumentary system.*

The skin is a sense organ. Receptors are found in the skin that give us the ability to feel and touch. One type of receptor is found near the surface of the skin and the other is found within the dermis.

The **dermis** is the inner layer of the skin. Within the dermis lie the structures responsible for unique fingerprints. These ridges are called the dermal-papillae and form before birth. Fingerprints and footprints, which grow as a child becomes an adult, will always have the same pattern and can identify people throughout their lives. Hair and nail follicles, sweat and oil glands, blood vessels, and receptors for touch, temperature, pressure, and pain are also housed in the dermis.

Hair grows from roots located in the dermis. Every hair consists primarily of dead cells, made up of protein called keratin and the pigment that gives hair its color. Hair protects the body. The hair inside the nose protects against inhaling irritants in the air. Hair on the head, underarms, and genitals protect sensitive areas from injuries. Eyebrows and eyelashes help keep objects from getting into the eyes.

Collagen fibers, which make skin tough, are found within the dermis. Elastic fibers are also found in the dermis. They give the skin its elasticity, or ability to stretch.

The subcutaneous layer is positioned immediately underneath the dermis. This is the area of the body where fat, or adipose, tissue lies. This adipose tissue also serves as a cushion over bone and provides some protection as it insulates the body from cold weather. Humans' fat layer is thinner than the fat layer in some other animals.

The functions of the integumentary system are:

* Protects internal organs from injury
* Protects the body against bacteria
* Prevents the loss of too much water
* Regulates body temperature
* Responds to heat, cold, pain, pressure, and touch
* Excretes waste products in sweat
* Helps with production of Vitamin D

Destination: Homeostasis

When cells die or become damaged, homeostasis is disturbed. When the surface of the skin is opened, such as by a cut, the inflammatory response begins. Blood flow increases to the area. Signs of inflammation, such as redness, swelling, heat and pain, occur. Platelets, along with a substance called fibrin, form a clot. White blood cells, called phagocytes, travel to the area and start cleansing the wound of bacteria. A scab, which is a hard protective structure, forms over the area. Normal tissue eventually develops and, over time, the scab is pushed off of the area leaving new skin. When normal tissue repair is complete, the injured area returns to homeostasis.

HOT TIP

Observing Residents' Skin: It Is a Daily Duty!

Every time you help residents bathe and/or dress, carefully and closely observe their skin. This helps identify any changes in the skin which need to be

reported immediately. Pressure sores, skin cancer, and contagious skin diseases can pose serious health risks if not caught early and treated. You will be the person who sees residents the most on a daily basis. Your careful observations can help prevent serious illnesses.

3. Discuss changes in the integumentary system due to aging

Normal age-related changes for the integumentary system include the following:

* Amount of fat and collagen decreases, causing skin to sag.
* Elastic fibers lose elasticity, causing wrinkles.
* Hair and nail growth slows.
* Skin becomes drier due to decreased production of perspiration and oil.
* Skin becomes thinner and more fragile, causing more frequent skin injuries, tearing, and infections.
* Protective fatty tissue layer thins, so person feels colder.
* Hair thins and turns gray, due to a decrease in the melanocyte activity (Fig. 18-2).
* Brown spots on the skin may appear due to an increase in the production of certain melanocytes in areas exposed to the sun.

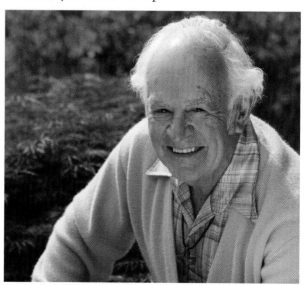

Fig. 18-2. Hair growth slows, and hair thins and turns gray as a person ages.

Be careful with fragile skin.

Have you ever removed a bandage too quickly and caused pain? If this is done to an elderly person, it may not only cause pain, but a piece of skin may come off along with the dressing or bandage. An elderly person's skin is extremely fragile; dressings, tape, and bandages must be removed carefully and gently.

4. Discuss common disorders of the integumentary system

Pressure sores, a major disorder of the integumentary system, are discussed in Learning Objective 5 of this chapter.

Burns

You first learned about how to prevent burns and scalds in Chapter 8. Burns can be caused by fire, hot liquids, warm water applications, such as warm moist compresses, electrical equipment, such as hair dryers and heaters, hot objects, or certain chemicals.

When a burn occurs, there is a varying degree of skin damage (Fig. 18-3). The different degrees of burns are:

Degree	Layer of Skin	Damage Involved
First Degree	Epidermis (Outer layer)	Redness and pain.
Second Degree	Dermis (Deeper layer)	Some skin damage; redness, pain, swelling, and blistering.
Third Degree	Epidermis, dermis and underlying tissue	Serious scarring; muscle and bone may be affected; white or charred skin, pain, swelling, peeling skin.

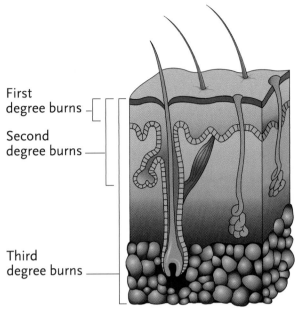

First degree burns

Second degree burns

Third degree burns

Fig. 18-3. Different degrees of burns.

Burns and scalds are very painful and can require surgery. They can cause a resident's condition to deteriorate quickly. When caring for a resident who has burns, be careful not to cause additional pain. Prior to care it may be necessary to arrange with the nurse to have the resident's pain medication given. That way it takes effect before you begin the care. Be gentle when moving and positioning residents to reduce pain and the chance of damaging dressings. Use special protective devices, such as pads or special mattresses or beds, as ordered. Encourage fluids and follow diet instructions closely. Measure intake and output (I&O) as ordered (Chapter 14).

Report to the nurse if you notice pus or other fluids around burn areas or if the resident complains of pain. Report any decrease in appetite or in intake and output.

You may be asked to assist the nurse with dressing care, which you will learn more about later in the chapter.

Scabies

Scabies is a skin infection that causes pimple-like irritations to form on the skin. These irritations are caused by tiny mites that burrow into the skin to lay eggs. A rash, intense itching, and sores can occur, and the sores may become infected. The symptoms may take a month or more to appear.

Scabies is contagious and is usually transmitted by direct person-to-person contact. Using an infected person's towel, washcloth, clothing or bedding can also spread scabies. The elderly and others with weakened immune systems are at a higher risk of acquiring scabies.

Treatment consists of the use of special lotions. Follow instructions on handling and washing clothing and linens. Use caution when touching areas that have been treated.

Even after treatment, the itching may continue for a while. Anyone who may have been infected with scabies should be treated at the same time, such as residents, their families and friends, and their roommates.

Shingles

Shingles is a viral infection that causes a painful rash. Shingles is also called "herpes zoster" or "zoster." It is caused by the same virus that causes chickenpox. This virus is called varicella-zoster virus (VZV). The disease can occur in anyone who has had chickenpox. The start of the infection begins with pain or itching at the site where the rash will appear. The person may have fever or chills. Severe pain can occur after the rash is gone; this happens in about 20% of the people and is more commonly seen in the elderly. The pain may last for many years.

Shingles cannot be transmitted through person-to-person contact. However, the VZV virus can spread to someone who has not had chickenpox, and that person may then develop chickenpox. The virus is spread when the disease is in its blister form (Fig. 18-4). When the blisters have crusts, the disease is no longer contagious.

Fig. 18-4. *Shingles in blister form. (Photo courtesy of Dr. Jere Mammino, DO.)*

A shingles rash must remain covered at all times. Infected people should wash their hands frequently. Medication is used to treat shingles. If the medication is started immediately, it can reduce the severity of the disease and shorten the length of the illness. A doctor should be contacted when shingles first appears. Waiting to treat this infection reduces the effectiveness of the medication.

Wounds

Wounds fall into two categories: open and closed. Skin that is not intact is considered an **open wound**. A **closed wound** is a wound where the skin's surface is not broken, such as bruises or internal bleeding. Types of open wounds include:

- An abrasion is a tearing or wearing away of the surface skin due to friction. Another word for abrasion is "scrape" or "excoriation." There is usually not a lot of bleeding from this type of wound, but the area must be kept clean to help prevent infection.

- An avulsion is a tearing away of tissues during a violent act or accident, such as a gunshot wound or an explosion. A dog bite is another example. Bleeding in this type of wound is usually heavy.

- An incision is a cut caused by a sharp-edged object, such as glass, a knife or a razor. Bleeding in this type of wound is generally rapid and heavy; when an incision is made during surgery however, the bleeding is usually controlled.

- A laceration is an irregular or jagged wound that is caused by blunt tearing of soft tissue. For example, it can result from the tearing of skin that occurs during childbirth. A laceration may cause rapid and extensive bleeding.

- A puncture wound is a wound from a sharp object that causes a small hole in the tissues. For example, a needle or a nail can cause a puncture wound. Bleeding may be slight or heavy.

A common type of a closed wound is a contusion. A contusion is also called a bruise. Trauma to the outside of the body can cause a contusion. The skin's surface remains intact, but internal damage and bleeding can occur.

Symptoms of wounds are pain, tissue damage, discoloration, and light or heavy bleeding. Fever, chills or trouble breathing may occur. If any of these symptoms are observed, report to the nurse immediately. New wounds require immediate medical attention and assessment and monitoring by a nurse.

Treatment includes stopping bleeding and cleaning the wound. A dressing will need to be applied to the wound. Stitches or special bandages may be needed. In some cases, a tetanus shot may be required. A bite from an animal may require rabies shots.

Skin Lesions

There are different types of lesions that can occur on the skin. A **lesion** is an area of abnormal tissue or an injury or wound.

Macules are the most simple skin lesion. Macules are flat spots that can be seen but not felt. They are visible because they change the color of the skin. Freckles are an example.

Papules are skin lesions that are raised, little round bumps on the skin. Papules can be felt. They do not contain pus. Contact dermatitis is an example.

Pustules are raised spots filled with pus, such as acne or infected boils.

Vesicles are small blisters that contain fluid. They can occur on the skin or inside the mouth. Chickenpox is an example.

Wheals are large raised, irregular areas, that are usually itchy (Fig. 18-5). Hives from an allergic reaction are an example.

Fig. 18-5. *An example of wheals.* (Photo Courtesy of Dr. Jere Mammino, DO.)

Hematoma is a collection of blood in one area. The spot can be visible as a bruise, but may also occur on internal organs. Hematomas can become larger over time. They may also change color.

Purpura are small, purplish spots caused by bleeding under the skin. In elderly people, these spots are called senile purpura. Senile purpura occurs because blood vessels become more fragile with age.

Gangrene

Gangrene means death of tissue. Gangrene is caused by infection or lack of blood flow. It must be treated immediately. Causes of gangrene include burns, diabetes, injuries, circulatory disorders, a weakened immune system, and complications from surgery.

Symptoms of gangrene include discoloration of the skin (usually black or blue), sores that do not heal, pain, loss of feeling, and foul-smelling discharge. The person may experience chills or have a change in vital signs.

Be familiar with residents' normal ranges for vital signs. Report elevated temperature, pulse or respiration rate, change in blood pressure, or difficulty breathing.

Treatments consist of antibiotics, surgery, amputation, and hospitalization to treat serious gangrene.

Eczema (Dermatitis)

Eczema, or dermatitis, is a general term for a variety of skin problems. Dermatitis means inflammation of the skin. Eczema can be a temporary or a chronic skin disorder in which redness, itching, burning, swelling, cracking or weeping (oozing fluid) of the skin, and lesions can occur.

Causes of eczema include stress, allergies, family history, and irritating agents in the environment. Some people who have eczema also have asthma or other allergies.

Treatment of eczema includes protecting the skin surfaces from worsening. Topical steroid creams and soothing or drying lotions prescribed by a dermatologist (a physician specializing in conditions of the skin) may help treat the problem.

Discouraging scratching the skin can help healing. Certain types of oral medications can reduce the itching. With contact eczema (contact dermatitis), avoiding the irritating agent can help prevent the problem from occurring again. Follow orders for limiting harsh soaps and other products. Monitor vital signs, especially temperature. If eczema worsens, the resident develops severe itching or pain, or if signs of infection occur, notify the nurse. Signs of infection are warmth, redness, swelling in the affected area or a change in vital signs, especially fever.

Psoriasis

Psoriasis is a chronic skin condition in which cells of the skin grow too fast, causing red, white or silver patches to form. The patches can be small or large and usually occur on the arms,

elbows, lower back, knees, or feet. Psoriasis can be mild or severe. Larger patches can cause itching and discomfort, along with embarrassment. People with psoriasis can also have arthritis and pain.

Psoriasis is usually inherited. It may also be caused or aggravated by a dry climate, cold weather, stress, and a weakened immune system.

Treatment includes topical creams, shampoos and lotions. Oral medication may also help. Phototherapy, which is special ultraviolet light treatments for the skin, may be performed. Some people with psoriasis make dietary changes and use sun therapy to treat the disorder.

Fungal Infections

Fungal and yeast (one type of fungus) infections can occur anywhere on the body. However, they most commonly occur in moist areas, such as the toes, under the breasts, and the groin area. Red, scaly patches appear, accompanied by itching, rawness, and pain. Jock itch, vaginal yeast infections, and athlete's foot are all examples of fungal infections. **Ringworm** is a fungal infection that causes red scaly patches to appear in a ring shape, generally on the upper body, or the hands and feet (Fig. 18-6).

Fig. 18-6. *Ringworm is a fungal infection that causes red scaly patches to appear in a ring-like shape. (Photo courtesy of Dr. Jere Mammino, DO.)*

Perspiration usually causes fungal infections. These infections usually worsen in the summer, when perspiration increases. Tight-fitting clothing may also cause fungal infections.

Treatment includes topical antifungal creams and medications. The earlier the treatment begins, the faster the infection heals. Report any skin changes, skin abrasions, flaking, redness, sores, and scratching to the nurse.

Warts

A **wart** is a rough, hard bump (Fig. 18-7). The bump or bumps may be spongy-looking with red, yellow, brown, or black spots. Warts are contagious, and are caused by a virus that invades the skin, usually through a cut or tear. They may spread to other areas of the body if not treated. People are more prone to developing warts if they have a weakened immune system.

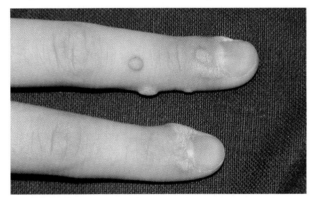

Fig. 18-7. *Warts on the fingers.* (Photo courtesy of Dr. Jere Mammino, DO.)

Treatment includes medication and/or removal with a laser or a special instrument. Wash your hands frequently to help prevent the spread of warts to other parts of the body.

5. Discuss pressure sores and identify guidelines for preventing pressure sores

When a person is confined to bed for long periods of time, the amount of blood that circulates to the skin is reduced. The risk of skin breakdown increases. This breakdown usually occurs at the points of the body that bear much of the body's weight. These points are called **pressure points** and there are many on the human body.

They are mainly located at **bony prominences**, which are areas of the body where the bone lies close to the skin. These areas include the elbows, shoulder blades, sacrum (tailbone), hips and knees (inner and outer parts), ankles, heels, toes, and the back of the neck and the head. Other areas at risk for skin breakdown include the ears, the area under the breasts or scrotum, between the folds of the buttocks or abdomen, and between the legs (Fig. 18-8).

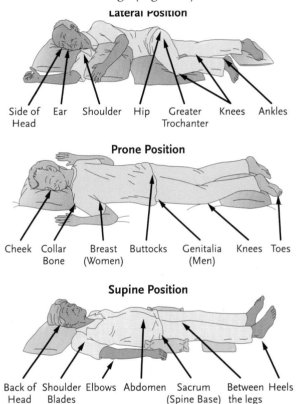

Lateral Position

Side of Head | Ear | Shoulder | Hip | Greater Trochanter | Knees | Ankles

Prone Position

Cheek | Collar Bone | Breast (Women) | Buttocks | Genitalia (Men) | Knees | Toes

Supine Position

Back of Head | Shoulder Blades | Elbows | Abdomen | Sacrum (Spine Base) | Between the legs | Heels

Fig. 18-8. *Pressure sore danger zones.*

When skin breaks down due to poor circulation, the amount of oxygen the cells receive is reduced and necrosis results. **Necrosis** is the death of living cells or tissues caused by lack of nourishment to tissues. This is due to prolonged pressure on an area or any other cause that interferes with circulation. Moisture and warmth also contribute to skin breakdown. Once skin has broken down and is weakened, sores can occur and may become infected, causing damage to the underlying tissue. The sores or wounds that result from skin deterioration and shearing are called **pressure sores**. **Shearing** is rubbing or friction resulting from the skin moving one way and the bone underneath it remaining fixed or moving in the opposite direction. Pressure sores are also called pressure ulcers, decubitus ulcers, or bed sores.

The first signs of skin breakdown include pale, white or reddened skin. Darker skin may look purple. The skin may be dry, cracked, or torn. Blisters, bruises, or rashes may be visible.

Pressure sores are a common, serious problem in long-term care. If caught early, a break or tear in the skin can heal fairly quickly without other complications. However, once a pressure sore forms, it can become bigger, deeper, and infected. Pressure sores are painful and difficult to heal, and can lead to life-threatening infections. Prevention of pressure sores is very important. Pressure sores are much easier to prevent than to cure.

There are four stages of pressures sores (Fig. 18-9):

Fig. 18-9. *Pressure sores are categorized by four stages.* (Photos courtesy of Dr. Tamara D. Fishman and The Wound Care Institute, Inc.)

Stage 1: Skin is intact, but reddens or appears blue or gray. In darker-skinned people, the area may appear purple or darker than the skin surrounding the area. People with darker skin may also have skin that is swollen, or feels warm

or firm. In this stage, redness or discoloration is not relieved within 15 to 30 minutes after removing pressure. Stage 1 can be reversed if discovered promptly and treated. If not treated promptly, the pressure sore will worsen and progress into other stages.

Stage 2: There is partial thickness skin loss involving the epidermis and the dermis. The ulcer is superficial and looks like a blister or shallow crater. It is accompanied by pain, and the skin around the pressure sore may be discolored. There is no dead (necrotic) tissue in the site at this stage.

Stage 3: There is full thickness skin loss (both the epidermis and dermis will be gone), and the ulcer looks like a deep crater. The wound may have necrotic tissue in it. The damage may extend to the muscle. Stage 3 pressure sores require weeks or months to fully heal.

Stage 4: There is full thickness skin loss extending through all layers of the skin, tissue, and possibly, muscle, bone, and other structures, such as joints or tendons. The ulcer will look like a deep crater. The healing process extends over months. Serious infections can result. Stage 4 pressure sores may require a skin graft.

Nursing assistants are in the best position to observe for signs of pressure sores since they see residents' skin on a daily basis. Inspect each resident's skin every time you provide care. Notify the nurse if you observe any of these signs:

- Pale, white, reddened, gray or purple skin
- Dry, cracked, or flaking skin
- Torn skin
- Blisters, bruises or wounds on the skin
- Rashes or any skin discoloration
- Tingling, warmth or burning of the skin
- Itching or scratching
- Swelling of the skin
- Wet skin
- Broken skin anywhere on the body, including between the toes or around the toenails

- Changes in existing wounds or ulcers, including size, depth, drainage, color, odor

In addition to immobility, there are other risk factors for pressures sores. Wrinkled linens that do not lie flat under residents, as well as crumbs or other irritating objects in the bed can increase the risk for pressure sores. Malnutrition and dehydration increase the risk, too. Urinary incontinence is also a major risk factor for pressure sores. Follow these guidelines to help prevent pressure sores from occurring:

Guidelines
Preventing Pressure Sores

- Report any changes in a resident's skin.

- Perform regular skin care and closely observe residents' skin each time it is performed. Check areas closely that can be irritated by an IV, oxygen delivery device, or bandages.

- Keep skin clean and dry. Give skin care immediately after episodes of incontinence. Change clothing and bed linens as needed.

- Assist immobile residents to change position as ordered, but at least every two hours.

- Ask every resident in a wheelchair or any other chair to change position frequently. Follow facility policy on frequency of this practice.

- Be careful during transfers. Avoid rubbing skin against linen or other surfaces. Be gentle so that you do not tear fragile skin.

- Keep linens dry, clean and wrinkle-free.

- Perform range of motion exercises as ordered.

- Massage the skin often if allowed. This increases circulation. Do not massage any white, red, or purple areas or put any pressure on them. Massage healthy skin around the areas.

- Use special positioning devices (Chapter 25) to help reduce pressure as ordered (Fig. 18-10).

- Use pillows to separate skin surfaces.

- Follow diet and fluid orders carefully; encourage fluids and good nutrition.

- Use moisturizers as ordered on unbroken skin. Follow the care plan. Do not use creams, lotions, soaps, or other products on non-intact skin.

Fig. 18-10. *Heel protectors and footboards help prevent pressure sores. (Reprinted with permission of Briggs Corporation, 800-247-2343)*

HOT TIP

Incontinence and Pressure Sores
The Minimum Data Set (MDS) guidelines state to count any time that a resident's skin, pad, brief, or underwear is wet from urine as an episode of incontinence. This is true even if it is a small amount of urine. Document this carefully, following your facility's policy. This is important to help prevent pressure sores.

6. Explain the benefits of warm and cold applications

Applications of heat or cold can have beneficial effects on injuries, infections, fevers, and other conditions. The body responds to heat and cold in different ways.

Heat helps relieve pain and muscular tension and decreases swelling. It elevates the temperature in the tissues, increases waste removal from the area, and increases blood flow due to dilated blood vessels. Increased blood flow brings more oxygen and nutrients to the tissues for healing. However, there are risks associated with warm applications, too. Heat can cause burns, make bleeding worse, and cause confusion, dizziness, or fainting due to a reduction of blood to the brain. The elderly are at an increased risk for burns and other complications because they have thinner and more fragile skin.

With cold applications, blood flow decreases due to the constriction of the vessels. The movement of oxygen and nutrients into the tissues decreases. Cold applications help stop bleeding, prevent swelling and reduce pain. Cold helps bring down high temperatures. Risks of cold applications include cyanosis or pale skin, chills, and shivering. Lack of blood flow to the application area and the cold temperature may damage tissue.

Warm or cold applications can be either moist or dry. Moisture strengthens the effect of heat and cold, which means that moist applications are more likely to cause injury. Be careful when using these applications. Know how long it should be performed, and use the correct temperature listed in the care plan. Check on the application often.

Types of moist applications include:

- Compresses (warm or cold)
- Soaks (warm or cold)
- Tub baths (warm)
- Sponge bath (warm or cold)
- Sitz bath (warm)
- Ice packs (cold)

Types of dry applications include:

- Aquamatic K-pad® (warm or cold)
- Electric heating pad (warm)

- Warming blankets (warm)
- Cooling blankets (cold)
- Disposable warm pack (warm)
- Ice bag (cold)
- Disposable cold pack (cold)

Some facilities do not allow nursing assistants to prepare and apply warm and cold applications. Only perform procedures that are assigned to you and that you are trained to do. If your facility does allow you to perform this care, carefully follow the procedure manuals and the care plan.

Provide privacy when giving warm and cold applications. If you note any of the following, stop the application and report to the nurse immediately. These signs may indicate that the application is causing tissue damage:

- Excessive redness
- Pain
- Blisters
- Numbness

Remember, if the resident has non-intact skin or open sores, wear gloves when applying warm or cold applications. You should always wear gloves when assisting with a sitz bath. A **sitz bath** is a warm soak of the perineal area to clean perineal wounds and reduce inflammation and pain.

HOT TIP

Hot opens; cold closes.

When using warm and cold applications, it helps to remember what happens with each kind of application. The following tip may help you remember the body's response to heat and cold:

Hot opens (blood vessels) and cold closes (blood vessels).

Applying warm moist compresses

Equipment: washcloth or compress, plastic wrap, towel, basin, bath thermometer

1. Identify yourself by name. Identify the resident. Greet the resident by name.

2. Wash your hands.

3. Explain procedure to resident. Speak clearly, slowly, and directly. Maintain face-to-face contact whenever possible. Encourage resident to assist if possible.

4. Provide for the resident's privacy with a curtain, screen, or door.

5. Fill basin one-half to two-thirds with warm water. Test water temperature with thermometer or your wrist. Ensure it is safe. Water temperature should be no more than 105°F. Have resident check water temperature. Adjust if necessary.

6. Soak the washcloth in the water. Wring it out. Immediately apply it to the area needing a warm compress. Note the time. Quickly cover the washcloth with plastic wrap and the towel to keep it warm (Fig. 18-11).

Fig. 18-11. Cover compresses to keep them warm.

7. Check the area every five minutes. Remove the compress if the area is red or numb or if the resident has pain or discomfort. Change the compress if cooling occurs. Remove the compress after 20 minutes.

8. Commercial warm compresses are also available. If you are using these, follow the package directions and the nurse's instructions.

9. Remove privacy measures. Make resident comfortable.

10. Empty, rinse, and wipe basin. Return to proper storage. Discard plastic wrap.

11. Place soiled clothing and linens in appropriate containers.

12. Leave call light within resident's reach.

13. Wash your hands.

14. Be courteous and respectful at all times.

15. Report any changes in the resident to the nurse. Document procedure using facility guidelines.

Administering warm soaks

Equipment: towel, basin, bath thermometer, bath blanket

1. Identify yourself by name. Identify the resident. Greet the resident by name.

2. Wash your hands.

3. Explain procedure to resident. Speak clearly, slowly, and directly. Maintain face-to-face contact whenever possible. Encourage resident to assist if possible.

4. Provide for the resident's privacy with a curtain, screen, or door.

5. Fill the basin half full of warm water. Test water temperature with thermometer or your wrist, and ensure it is safe. Water temperature should be no more than 105°F. Have resident check water temperature. Adjust if necessary.

6. Immerse the body part in the basin. Pad the edge of the basin with a towel if needed (Fig. 18-12). Use a bath blanket to cover the resident if needed for extra warmth.

Fig. 18-12. Pad the edge of the basin for comfort.

7. Check water temperature every five minutes. Add warm water as needed to maintain the temperature. Never add water warmer than

105°F. To prevent burns, tell the resident not to add warm water. Observe the area for redness. Discontinue the soak if the resident has pain or discomfort.

8. Soak for 15-20 minutes, or as ordered.

9. Remove basin. Use the towel to dry the resident.

10. Remove privacy measures. Make resident comfortable.

11. Empty, rinse, and wipe basin. Return to proper storage.

12. Place soiled clothing and linens in appropriate containers.

13. Leave call light within resident's reach.

14. Wash your hands.

15. Be courteous and respectful at all times.

16. Report any changes in the resident to the nurse. Document procedure using facility guidelines.

Applying an Aquamatic K-Pad®

Equipment: K-Pad® and control unit (Fig. 18-13), covering for pad, distilled water

Fig. 18-13. *An Aquamatic K-Pad®.*

1. Identify yourself by name. Identify the resident. Greet the resident by name.

2. Wash your hands.

3. Explain procedure to resident. Speak clearly, slowly, and directly. Maintain face-to-face contact whenever possible. Encourage resident to assist if possible.

4. Provide for the resident's privacy with a curtain, screen, or door.

5. Make sure the surface on the bedside table is dry. Place the control unit on the bedside table. Make sure cords are not frayed or damaged. Check that tubing between pad and unit is intact.

6. Remove cover of control unit to check level of water. If it is low, fill it with distilled water to the fill line.

7. Put the cover of control unit back in place.

8. Plug unit in. Turn unit on. Temperature should have been pre-set. If it was not, check with the nurse for proper temperature. If you need to set the temperature, you must remove the key after doing so. Place key in proper place.

9. Place the pad in the cover. Do not pin the pad to the cover.

10. Uncover area to be treated. Place the covered pad. Note the time. Make sure the tubing is not hanging below the bed. It should be coiled on the bed. Make sure tubing has no kinks.

11. Return and check area every five minutes. Remove the pad if the area is red or numb or if the resident reports pain or discomfort.

12. Check water level. Refill with distilled water to the fill line when necessary.

13. Turn off unit and remove pad after 20 minutes.

14. Remove privacy measures. Make resident comfortable.

15. Return K-pad® to proper storage.

16. Place used linen in appropriate container.

17. Leave call light within resident's reach.

18. Wash your hands.

19. Be courteous and respectful at all times.

20. Report any changes in the resident to the nurse. Document procedure using facility guidelines.

Sitz baths cause circulation to be increased to the pelvic area. Residents with perineal swelling (such as hemorrhoids) may have sitz baths ordered. During sitz baths, blood flow to other parts of the body decreases. This is because the bath causes increased blood flow to the pelvic area. Residents may feel weak, faint, or dizzy after a sitz bath. Stop the bath if the resident complains of feeling dizzy or faint. Sitz baths may cause the need or urge to void. Always wear gloves when helping with a sitz bath.

A disposable sitz bath fits on the toilet seat. It is attached to a rubber bag containing warm water (Fig. 18-14).

Fig. 18-14. *A disposable sitz bath.*

Assisting with a sitz bath

Equipment: disposable sitz bath, bath thermometer, towels, gloves

1. Identify yourself by name. Identify the resident. Greet the resident by name.

2. Wash your hands.

3. Explain procedure to resident. Speak clearly, slowly, and directly. Maintain face-to-face contact whenever possible. Encourage resident to assist if possible.

4. Provide for the resident's privacy with a curtain, screen, or door.

5. Put on gloves.

6. Fill the sitz bath two-thirds full with warm water. Place the disposable sitz bath on the toilet seat. Water temperature should be no more than 105°F. If the sitz bath is ordered for pain and to stimulate circulation, the water temperature may need to be higher.

Follow the care plan. Check the water temperature using the bath thermometer.

7. Help the resident undress and get seated on the sitz bath. A valve on the tubing connected to the bag allows the resident or you to fill the sitz bath again with warm water.

8. You may be required to stay with the resident during the bath for safety reasons. If you leave the room, check on the resident every five minutes to make sure he or she is not dizzy or weak. Make sure resident knows how to use the emergency pull cord in the bathroom if it is needed.

9. Help the resident out of the sitz bath in 20 minutes. Provide towels. Help with dressing if needed.

10. Empty, rinse, and wipe sitz bath container. Return to proper storage.

11. Place soiled clothing and linens in appropriate containers.

12. Remove privacy measures. Make resident comfortable.

13. Remove and dispose of gloves properly.

14. Leave call light within resident's reach.

15. Wash your hands.

16. Be courteous and respectful at all times.

17. Report any changes in the resident to the nurse. Document procedure using facility guidelines.

Commercial warm or cold packs may be used. There are different types of commercial packs. Follow the manufacturer's instructions and the procedure manual on using these packs. Some packs are used once and disposed of, while others are cleaned and re-used. To activate the warm or cold pack, you may need to squeeze the package. Apply a cover before applying the pack to the skin. Follow instructions on cleaning non-disposable packs. Check the site every five minutes and remove the pack after 20 minutes or as ordered. Report to the nurse if you note any of the following: pale skin, burning, numbness and tingling, or pain.

This procedure teaches you how to apply a non-commercial ice pack.

Applying ice packs

Equipment: ice pack or sealable plastic bag and crushed ice, towel or cover for pack or bag

1. Identify yourself by name. Identify the resident. Greet the resident by name.

2. Wash your hands.

3. Explain procedure to resident. Speak clearly, slowly, and directly. Maintain face-to-face contact whenever possible. Encourage resident to assist if possible.

4. Provide for the resident's privacy with a curtain, screen, or door.

5. Practice good body mechanics. Lock bed wheels.

6. Fill plastic bag or ice pack one-half to two-thirds full with crushed ice. Seal bag. Remove excess air. Cover bag or ice pack with towel or cover (Fig. 18-15).

Fig. 18-15. *Seal the bag filled with ice and cover it with a towel.*

7. Apply bag to the area as ordered. Note the time. Use another towel to cover bag if it is too cold.

8. Check the area after five minutes for blisters or pale, white, or gray skin. Stop treatment if resident reports numbness or pain.

9. Remove ice and water after 20 minutes or as ordered.

10. Remove privacy measures. Make resident comfortable.

11. Empty and store ice pack.

12. Place used linen in appropriate container.

13. Leave call light within resident's reach.

14. Wash your hands.

15. Be courteous and respectful at all times.

16. Report any changes in the resident to the nurse. Document procedure using facility guidelines.

Residents with high temperatures may need to have a cooling or tepid sponge bath. Sponge baths can reduce body temperature. Serious side effects from high fevers can occur, such as convulsions and confusion.

Prior to the bath, vital signs, including temperature, will need to be taken. During the procedure, vital signs will need to be taken at specific intervals. Follow your facility's procedure to perform the sponge bath. Possible complications of sponge baths are chills, shivering, a sudden change in vital signs, or breathing problems. If any of these occur, stop the bath, cover the resident completely, and immediately call for the nurse.

Warming and Cooling Blankets

Warming blankets, also called hypothermia blankets, may be used when a resident has severe sub-normal body temperature.

Cooling blankets, also called hyperthermia blankets, may be used when a resident has a high fever.

Warming or cooling blankets are plugged into an electrical socket, and then the resident is placed on the blanket to try to raise or lower his body temperature. Ice bags or commercial ice packs may be used along with a cooling blanket.

The nurse is responsible for this procedure. He or she will apply it, adjust the setting, and monitor the procedure. Cover the blanket with a sheet before the resident lies down on it if needed. You may be asked to take vital signs before, during, and after the warming/cooling blanket procedure.

Notify the nurse if you observe pale or cyanotic skin or nailbeds, sudden changes in vital signs, breathing difficulties, numbness or tingling, or pain. If you note any damage to the blanket, leakage, or sparking, turn the blanket off and get the nurse.

The 20-minute Rule

Warm and cold applications should not be applied for too long. When they are on for too long, the opposite effect of what is intended occurs. This means that if you leave an ice bag on for longer than 20 minutes, the blood vessels may start to open again. This could increase bleeding and swelling at the injury site. Remember to limit warm or cold applications to 20 minutes at a time.

7. Discuss non-sterile and sterile dressings

Open wounds increase the risk of infection because breaks in the skin are a way for bacteria and other microorganisms to enter the body. In order to protect wounds from bacteria, dressings are applied. Dressings can be either non-sterile or sterile. Non-sterile dressings are applied to dry wounds that have less chance of infection. Sterile dressings are required when the wound is new, open, or draining. They are also required when there is a higher risk of infection.

Nursing assistants may help with non-sterile and sterile dressing changes. It is important to know the correct method to perform each procedure. When giving any type of dressing care, it is important not to further damage the wound area or damage the dressing or tape. Be careful not to cause pain to the resident. Ask the nurse if pain medication is needed prior to changing the dressing. Notify the nurse if the resident tells you that he is allergic to latex.

Assisting the nurse with changing a non-sterile dressing

Equipment: package of square gauze dressings, adhesive tape, scissors, 2 pairs of gloves, plastic bag

1. Identify yourself by name. Identify the resident. Greet the resident by name.

2. Wash your hands.

3. Explain procedure to resident. Speak clearly, slowly, and directly. Maintain face-to-face contact whenever possible. Encourage resident to assist if possible.

4. Provide for the resident's privacy with a curtain, screen, or door.

5. The nurse will prepare a clean, flat, dry surface for the dressing materials. Keep the plastic bag close by for immediate disposal of old dressing materials.

6. You may be asked to open packages for the nurse or cut strips of tape. Cut pieces of tape long enough to secure the dressing. Open gauze square packages without touching the insides or the gauze. If asked to set package down, place the opened package on a clean, flat surface.

7. Put on gloves.

8. Only expose the area where the dressing will be changed. The nurse will remove soiled dressing. Dispose of used dressing in proper container.

9. Remove and dispose of gloves in plastic bag.

10. Wash your hands.

11. Put on new gloves. The nurse will observe the wound and then apply the fresh gauze over the wound and tape it in place (Fig. 18-16). Assist as directed.

Fig. 18-16. *The nurse will affix the dressing securely in place.*

12. Remove privacy measures.

13. Remove and dispose of gloves properly.

14. Leave call light within resident's reach.

15. Wash your hands.

16. Be courteous and respectful at all times.

17. Report any changes in the resident to the nurse. Document procedure using facility guidelines.

Sterile gloves will be used for sterile dressing care. A sterile field—the area that is kept sterile—is created with sterile dressing care. You may need to assist the nurse with sterile dressing care. Examples of supplies that are considered sterile are sterile dressings, sterile drapes or pads, and tubing and catheters. Packages are generally marked in some way to indicate whether the supply is sterile or non-sterile.

Make sure not to contaminate the sterile field or the sterile gloves. If any part of the sterile field becomes contaminated, the entire process must be re-started.

Applying sterile gloves

Equipment: 2 pairs of sterile gloves in correct size

1. Wash your hands.

2. Using a clean, flat, dry surface, remove outer wrapper from gloves. Place inner wrapper on the clean surface. The word "Left" should be on your left side and the word "Right" should be on your right side.

3. Slowly open the inner wrapper, only touching the small flaps of the wrapper.

4. The gloves will have been placed palm-side up with cuffs in place. Pick up the first glove by the bottom end of the cuff.

5. Slip your fingers into the glove, without touching the outside of the glove (Fig. 18-17). If you touch the gloves on the outside, it will be contaminated, and you will have to start over. Wait to adjust the glove until the second glove is on your other hand.

Fig. 18-17. *Touching the bottom end of the cuff, slip your fingers into the glove, without touching the outside of the glove.*

6. Slip your gloved hand into the second glove in the area under the cuff.

7. Slowly slip the fingers of your ungloved hand into the second glove, and pull it completely over your hand and wrist (Fig. 18-18).

Fig. 18-18. *Touching the area under the cuff of the second glove, slip the fingers of your ungloved hand inside.*

8. With your gloved second hand, finish pulling the first glove up and over the wrist. Adjust the fingers now if any adjustment is necessary.

9. If either glove has a tear in it, stop and start again with the second set of sterile gloves.

10. Keep your gloved hands in front of you and above the level of your waist at all times during the procedure.

11. Assist the nurse with sterile procedure.

TRIVIA

The History of the Rubber Glove

In the early 20th century, William Halsted developed rubber gloves to protect his nurse's (and future wife's) hands. A student suggested that surgeons adopt them. The gloves were very thick, though, and many surgeons would not wear them. Some surgeons wore cloth gloves over the rubber ones. Over the years, rubber gloves became thinner and easier to wear. Today's gloves are made of different materials, such as nitrile or latex.

CHAPTER REVIEW

1. What are the two basic layers of the skin (LO 2)?

2. List four functions of the integumentary system (LO 2).

3. List eight normal age-related changes of the integumentary system (LO 3).

4. Briefly describe the damage and/or symptoms caused by first-, second-, and third-degree burns (LO 4).

5. How is scabies usually transmitted (LO 4)?

6. What causes shingles (LO 4)?

7. Give one example each of an open and a closed wound (LO 4).

8. Where does skin breakdown most often occur (LO 5)?

9. List the first signs of skin breakdown (LO 5).

10. Why is prevention of pressure sores so important (LO 5)?

11. List four risk factors for pressure sores (LO 5).

12. How often should immobile residents be helped to change position (LO 5)?

13. What are some benefits of applying heat to the body? What are some benefits of applying cold to the body (LO 6)?

14. What signs may indicate that a warm or cold application is causing tissue damage (LO 6)?

15. Generally speaking, for how long should warm or cold applications be applied (LO 6)?

16. Under what circumstances are non-sterile dressings usually used? When are sterile dressings used (LO 7)?

19
The Circulatory or Cardiovascular System

Discovering the Pathways of the Blood

William Harvey (1578-1657), an English physician, wrote *On the Movement of the Heart and Blood in Animals*, which was published in 1628. He noted that blood moves throughout the body in a closed system. He came to the conclusion that the blood recycles itself and moves inside the body in a single direction, not back and forth.

Harvey also identified that the heart is a pump and that it works by using the force of muscle. He found the heart has two phases: systole, when the heart contracts and empties itself of blood, and diastole, when the chambers of the heart are filled with blood.

> *". . . It ennobled our hearts and enriched our blood . . ."*
>
> **Richard Leveridge, 1670-1758**

> *". . . So in my veins red life might stream again . . ."*
>
> **John Keats, 1795-1821**

1. Define important words in this chapter

anemia: a condition in which the red blood cells or the hemoglobin in red blood cells is very low.

angina pectoris: chest pain.

anti-embolic stockings: special stockings used to help prevent swelling and blood clots and aid circulation; also called elastic stockings.

artery: vessel that carries blood away from the heart.

atria: the upper two chambers of the heart.

capillaries: tiny blood vessels in which the exchange of gases, nutrients, and waste products occurs between blood and cells.

cardiomyopathy: a condition in which the heart muscle is diseased and no longer pumps effectively.

congestive heart failure (CHF): a condition in which the heart muscle is damaged and does not pump effectively; blood backs up into the heart instead of circulating; can occur on one or both sides of the heart.

coronary artery disease (CAD): a condition in which blood vessels in the coronary arteries narrow, lowering blood supply to the heart and depriving it of oxygen and nutrients.

diastole: phase when the heart muscle relaxes.

dyspnea: difficulty breathing.

heart: four-chambered pump that is responsible for the flow of blood in the body.

heart attack: a condition in which all or part of the blood flow to the heart is blocked and muscle cells die; also called a myocardial infarction.

hypertension: a condition in which blood pressure consistently measures 140/90 or higher; also known as high blood pressure.

hypoxia: a condition in which the body does not receive enough oxygen.

ischemia: a lack of blood supply to an area.

myocardial infarction (MI): a condition in which all or part of the blood flow to the heart is blocked and muscle cells die; also called a heart attack.

myocardial ischemia: a condition in which the heart muscle does not receive enough blood and lacks oxygen; can cause angina pectoris.

nitroglycerin: medication that relaxes the walls of the coronary arteries.

occlusion: a complete obstruction of a blood vessel.

orthopnea: shortness of breath when lying down that is relieved by sitting up.

peripheral vascular disease (PVD): a condition in which the legs, feet, arms or hands do not have enough blood circulation.

phlebitis: inflammation of the veins in the lower extremities.

pulmonary edema: a condition in which there is an accumulation of fluid in the lungs; usually due to heart failure.

sequential compression device (SCD): special stockings used to improve circulation and prevent blood clots; may be applied during or after surgery.

stable angina: chest pain that occurs when a person is active or under severe stress.

systole: phase where the heart is at work, contracting and pushing blood out of the left ventricle.

unstable angina (USA): chest pain that occurs while a person is at rest and not exerting himself.

vein: vessel that carries blood to the heart.

ventricles: the lower two chambers of the heart.

2. Explain the structure and function of the circulatory system

The circulatory, or cardiovascular, system is made up of the heart, blood vessels, and blood

(Fig. 19-1). The **heart** is the pump of the circulatory system. It is positioned between the lungs, slightly to the left of the middle of the chest. The heart muscle is made up of three layers: the pericardium, the myocardium and the endocardium.

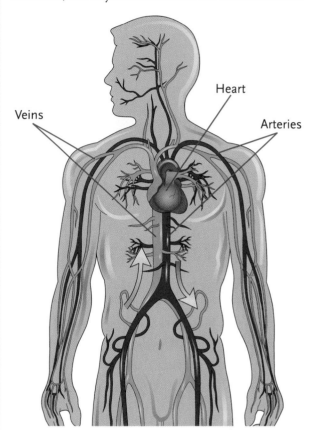

Fig. 19-1. The heart, blood vessels, and blood are the main parts of the circulatory system.

The heart is composed of four main chambers: the **atria** (the upper left and right chambers) and the **ventricles** (the lower left and right chambers). The right atrium receives de-oxygenated blood from the body. It is delivered via the superior vena cava from the head and upper extremities and the inferior vena cava, which delivers blood from the rest of the body (Fig. 19-2).

The heart functions in two phases: systole and diastole. During **systole**, the lower chambers of the heart, the ventricles, contract. This contraction causes blood to move out of the ventricles of the heart and into the arteries. The ventricles relax after contraction, and fill up with blood again. This part of heart function is known as **diastole**. This is the relaxation phase of the heart, or when the heart rests.

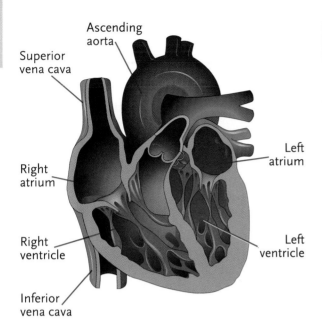

Fig. 19-2. *The four chambers of the heart connect to the body's largest blood vessels.*

Blood is pumped from the right atrium to the right ventricle. The right ventricle pumps the de-oxygenated blood into the lungs via the pulmonary arteries. These are the only arteries in the body that carry de-oxygenated blood; the other arteries carry oxygen-rich blood. The exchange of carbon dioxide for oxygen is made during this process. The blood then travels back into the heart through the pulmonary veins. These are the only veins in the body that carry oxygen-rich blood.

While in the lungs, carbon dioxide is removed when we exhale, or breathe out, and oxygen is added when we inhale, or take a breath. This exchange of gases returns oxygen-rich blood to the left ventricle. The left ventricle then pumps the oxygen-rich blood out of the heart via the largest **artery** in the body, the aorta. The blood is delivered to all of the arteries in the body through the arterial system (Fig. 19-3).

With the exception of the pulmonary arteries, the arteries carry oxygen-rich blood away from the heart to deliver the oxygen to the cells. When blood arrives at the cell level, it moves into arterioles, the tiniest of the arterial vessels. The arterioles deliver the blood to the tiny blood ves-

sels called **capillaries**. Gas, nutrient, and waste exchanges happen within capillaries. Capillaries have very thin walls, allowing blood to move in and out of the tiny vessels. During capillary exchange, oxygen and nutrients move from the blood into the tissues, and tissue cells and waste products move from the tissues into the blood.

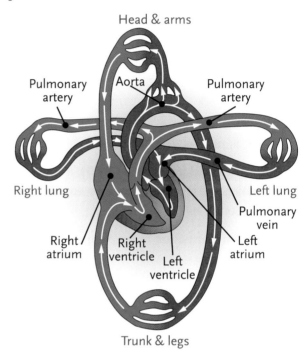

Fig. 19-3. *The flow of blood through the heart.*

Capillaries connect to the venules, small veins. The venules collect the de-oxygenated blood from the capillaries and then drain this blood into the veins. The **veins** carry the de-oxygenated blood back to the heart, and the whole process begins again.

Blood is made up of solids and liquids: cells and plasma. Plasma makes up about 55% of blood; blood cells make up the remaining 45%. Blood is composed of three different types of blood cells: red blood cells, or erythrocytes; white blood cells, or leukocytes; and platelets, or thrombocytes.

Red blood cells (erythrocytes) contain hemoglobin, which carries oxygen through the blood vessels. Red blood cells also transport carbon dioxide from the cells through the heart to the lungs. The lungs are responsible for the elimination of carbon dioxide from the body via exhaling. Red blood cells are produced by bone marrow, a substance found inside hollow bones. Iron, found in bone marrow and red blood cells, is essential to blood. It gives blood its red color. Iron in the diet allows bodies to produce new red blood cells. Red blood cells function for a short time, and then they die. They are filtered out of the blood by the liver and spleen.

White blood cells (leukocytes) protect our bodies from bacteria and viruses and other foreign substances. When the body becomes aware of these invaders, white blood cells rush to the site of infection and multiply rapidly. The bone marrow, spleen, and thymus gland produce white blood cells.

Platelets (thrombocytes) cause the blood to clot, which prevents excess bleeding. Platelets are also produced by the bone marrow.

Plasma, the liquid portion of the blood, is made up mostly of water. The plasma carries nutrients, waste products, hormones, salts, antibodies, and the substance necessary for the blood to clot.

The functions of the circulatory system are:

The heart:

- Pumps blood through blood vessels to every cell in the human body

The blood:

- Transports oxygen, food, and hormones to cells
- Removes carbon dioxide and other waste products from the cells
- Controls pH level and body temperature
- Clots the blood and fights pathogens and poisons

Destination: Homeostasis

A sudden decrease in blood pressure, possibly due to shock (decrease in amount of blood to organs and tissues) or a severe hemorrhage (loss of blood), causes an imbalance in homeostasis. One of the body's responses to this change is to trigger the sympathetic nervous system to increase the heart rate, along with the force of the contraction of the heart. This increases the output of blood from the heart. The change in the output of blood increases blood pressure. The heart tries to restore an adequate volume of blood to all body tissues. When blood volume is back to normal levels, the body has returned to homeostasis.

3. Discuss changes in the circulatory system due to aging

Normal age-related changes for the circulatory system include the following:

- Heart pumps less efficiently.
- Blood vessels narrow and become less efficient.
- Blood vessels become less elastic.
- Blood flow decreases.

4. Discuss common disorders of the circulatory system

Hypertension (HTN) or High Blood Pressure

When blood pressure consistently measures 140/90 or higher, a person is diagnosed as having **hypertension**, or high blood pressure. The major cause of hypertension is a hardening and narrowing of the blood vessels. Hypertension can also result from kidney disease, tumors of the adrenal glands, pregnancy, extreme stress or pain, and certain medications. Arteries may become hardened, or narrower, because of a buildup of plaque on the walls of the blood vessels, and this can cause hypertension (Fig. 19-4).

Prehypertension is a condition in which a person's systolic blood pressure measurement is between 120–139 mm Hg and diastolic measurement is between 80–89 mm Hg. Prehypertension means that a person does not have hypertension now, but is likely to have it in the future.

Artery wall　　　Plaque

Fig. 19-4. *Arteries may harden or narrow because of a build-up of plaque. Hardened arteries cause high blood pressure.*

Hypertension can develop in persons of any age. Signs and symptoms of hypertension are not always obvious, especially in the early stages of the disease. Often the illness is only discovered when a blood pressure measurement is taken by a healthcare provider. Persons with the disease may complain of headache, blurred vision, and dizziness.

Hypertension can lead to a myocardial infarction (heart attack). This is often caused by fatty deposits completely blocking off a coronary artery. This is called an occlusion or a coronary occlusion. An **occlusion** is an obstruction of a blood vessel. Occlusions cause damage to a part of the heart muscle from the lack of blood supply. **Ischemia** is a lack of blood supply to an area. If hypertension is not treated promptly, it can also result in a cerebrovascular accident (CVA), or stroke. This is due to the force causing a rupture in a vessel in the brain. Hypertension can also lead to kidney disease or blindness.

Medication is usually ordered to treat hypertension. This helps to keep hypertension under control and can prevent the complications listed above. Diuretics may also be prescribed. Diuretics are medications that reduce fluid in the body. Extra fluid can increase blood volume and weight, which increases the workload on the heart. Residents may have a prescribed exercise program or be on special low-fat, low-sodium diets. Reducing the intake of sodium (salt) in the diet helps reduce extra fluid in the body. Stopping smoking can increase the size of the blood vessels, increasing the flow of blood. Nicotine

constricts (closes) blood vessels. Lowering stress levels can also help people with hypertension.

Nursing assistants may be asked to measure blood pressure often. You can also assist by encouraging residents to follow their prescribed diets and exercise programs.

HOT TIP

The Silent Killer

Signs of hypertension include nosebleeds, eye hemorrhages (blood showing up in the white of an eye), dizziness, trembling, shortness of breath, and headaches. Hypertension puts a person at high risk for a heart attack or stroke. If you notice any of these signs and symptoms, report them to the nurse.

Coronary Artery Disease (CAD)

The coronary arteries supply blood to the heart. **Coronary artery disease (CAD)** occurs when the coronary arteries narrow, causing reduced blood supply to the heart. This deprives the heart muscle of oxygen and nutrients. Over time, a build-up of fats forms and blocks the arteries. These fatty deposits can partially or completely block the arteries.

When the blood supply to the heart is reduced, myocardial ischemia occurs. **Myocardial ischemia** is a condition in which the heart muscle does not get enough blood, and therefore lacks enough oxygen. When the heart is deprived of oxygen, chest pain can occur. However, myocardial ischemia can occur without causing pain or discomfort. Chest pain or other discomfort due to CAD is known as **angina pectoris** (Fig. 19-5). Angina pectoris is a symptom of myocardial ischemia.

Different forms of angina pectoris are stable angina and unstable angina. **Stable angina** is chest pain that occurs when a person is active or under severe stress. **Unstable angina (USA)** is chest pain that occurs while a person is at rest and not exerting himself.

The pain of angina can be mild or severe. Angina is usually described as intense pressure in the chest, a tightness in the chest, or pain in the back, neck, jaw, or shoulder. Some people have pain that radiates down the inside of the left arm. The person may sweat or look pale and have trouble breathing. Cyanosis of the lips, nail-beds and mucous membranes may develop. Dizziness may occur. To help residents with angina, follow these guidelines:

Area of hardening or blockage

Fig. 19-5. *Angina pectoris is chest pain that results from the heart not getting enough oxygen.*

Guidelines

Angina

- Reduce emotional distress as much as possible. Stress can cause or worsen angina.

- Residents will need to take their medication as ordered. Nitroglycerin is usually ordered for angina. **Nitroglycerin** is medication that relaxes the walls of the coronary arteries.This medication comes in various forms, such as in pill form or in a patch. If the pill is used, the resident places it under his tongue as soon as chest pain occurs. Nitroglycerin pills must be kept nearby at all times, even when residents leave a facility. Notify the nurse immediately if the resident needs help taking this medication. Nursing assistants are not allowed to give medication. Notify the nurse if a nitroglycerin patch falls off. Do not remove nitroglycerin patches.

- Make sure residents get enough rest. Rest is very important for people suffering from

angina pectoris. It reduces the heart's need for extra oxygen. However, rest may not help people who are suffering from unstable angina.

- Residents will need to avoid big meals, especially right before bedtime. People with angina should not overeat.

- Encourage residents to follow their exercise plan as ordered by the doctor. During exercise, observe for chest pain. Report to the nurse if a resident has pain or difficulty during exercising.

- Climate can affect the pain associated with coronary artery disease. During humid weather, some people are unable to breathe properly. Residents may need to avoid hot and humid weather.

- Be encouraging if residents have quit or are trying to quit smoking.

Cardiomyopathy

Extensive CAD can cause **cardiomyopathy**, or a diseased heart muscle that no longer pumps effectively. Cardiomyopathy can also be caused by a virus, diabetes, thyroid problems, drug and alcohol use, a birth defect, or unknown causes. The prognosis for cardiomyopathy is not good. This condition is the most common reason for heart transplants.

HOT TIP

Laughter—The Best Medicine?

Studies have shown that laughing may actually relax the arteries, which in turn, may help people with CAD or other illnesses. Be positive with residents and share in appropriate humor when the situation is right. It may be "just what the doctor ordered."

HOT TIP

Healthy Gums and CAD

There may be a link between poor health of the mouth, specifically the gums, and having heart disease. Without proper oral care, bacteria can tunnel into the gum tissue and cause inflammation. This inflammation may put a person at risk for developing fatty deposits on the arteries. This is another good reason to give excellent oral care to all of your residents, as well as yourself!

Myocardial Infarction (MI) or Heart Attack

When all or part of the blood flow to the heart muscle is blocked, oxygen and nutrients fail to reach the cells in that area. Waste products are not removed and muscle cells die. This is called a **myocardial infarction (MI)** or a **heart attack** (Fig. 19-6). When a clot (thrombosis) causes an MI by blocking the blood supply to an area of the heart, it is called a coronary thrombosis.

Area affected by complete lack of blood flow

Fig. 19-6. *A heart attack occurs when all or part of the blood flow to the heart is blocked.*

After a myocardial infarction, the area of the heart that has been damaged can no longer function and usually turns into scar tissue. The undamaged heart muscle must then compensate (take over) for the part of the heart that has died. This can increase the workload on the part of the heart that is still able to function. See Chapter 8 for warning signs of an MI.

After a myocardial infarction, cardiac rehabilitation is usually ordered. Cardiac rehabilitation may continue for a period of a few months up to six months or more. This comprehensive program consists of a variety of components, including the following:

- A low-cholesterol, low-fat, and low-sodium diet may be ordered. A dietician or nutritionist helps plan the diet.

- Most residents will be placed on a regular exercise program. The exercise program usually starts slowly, advancing to a higher level of exercise. The person's cardiac system, including the pulse and blood pressure, will be closely monitored during these exercise sessions. In some cases, the person's heart will have to be monitored during the exercise sessions.

- Medications to regulate the heart rate and blood pressure may be prescribed by the doctor.

- Stopping smoking will be encouraged.

- A stress management program may be initiated to help reduce stress levels.

- Residents recovering from MIs may be told to avoid cold temperatures.

Peripheral Vascular Disease (PVD)

Peripheral vascular disease (PVD) is a condition in which the blood supply to the legs, feet, arms, or hands is decreased due to poor circulation. This is due to fatty deposits in the blood vessels that harden over time. Peripheral vascular disease refers to diseases of the blood vessels; it does not include the vessels of the heart and brain. Other causes of PVD are a reduction in cardiac output (amount of blood being pumped out of the heart with each contraction) and inflammation of the veins in the lower extremities, called **phlebitis**. When the blood supply is reduced, the oxygen supply is reduced, causing damage to tissues.

The most common type of PVD is peripheral arterial disease (PAD). It is similar to coronary artery disease. A blockage is created by fatty deposits that build up in the artery walls. Blood circulation decreases, mostly in the arteries leading to the kidneys, stomach, arms, legs and feet. The pain associated with PAD occurs because there is not enough blood supply to the muscles during exercise. This decreased blood flow causes the pain or cramping in the legs that is the most common symptom of PAD.

Signs and symptoms of peripheral vascular disease include:

- Painful cramping in the hips, thighs or calves when walking, climbing stairs or doing other exercise
- Painful cramping in the legs that does not go away when exercise stops
- Cyanotic (blue or gray-tinged) hands or feet
- Bluish nailbeds
- Arms and/or legs that feel cold or cool to the touch
- Edema (swelling) in the hands or feet
- Ulcers on the legs or feet, especially sores that do not heal
- Gangrene (see Chapter 18)

Identifying and managing the cause of peripheral vascular disease is done to improve circulation to the peripheral blood vessels. For example, if the cause is fatty deposits, a low-cholesterol diet may be ordered to try to prevent further deposits from forming. Many people do not show symptoms of PAD.

Nursing assistants can help by carefully observing residents for signs and symptoms or changes that might signal poor circulation. Following orders for weighing residents daily and measuring intake and output (I&O) is important. Residents must be encouraged to follow any ordered fluid restrictions and/or special diets. Be positive if the resident has quit smoking.

Report any of the following signs and symptoms to the nurse:

- Resident complaints of pain or discomfort in his hands, legs or feet
- Any change in the hands, legs or feet
- Change in any vital sign, especially in pulse or blood pressure
- Increase in edema
- Weight gain
- Intake or output change
- Headache or any pain in the head or neck area

- Complaints about the inability to see clearly
- Any type of chest, back, jaw, or shoulder pain or discomfort
- Disorientation, dizziness, or confusion

For some cases of poor circulation, special stockings are ordered to help prevent swelling and blood clots. These stockings increase blood circulation and help reduce fluid retention. They are called **anti-embolic** or elastic **stockings**. They should only be used with a doctor's order. Some residents should not use these stockings.

Anti-embolic stockings increase blood circulation by causing smooth, even compression of the legs so that the blood moves better through the vessels. Measurements are taken for these stockings so that the person is given the correct size. There are two styles: thigh-high and knee-high.

Each stocking has a seamed hole in the fabric around the toe or underneath the foot. This allows the skin color of the feet and toes to be observed. Cyanosis can be seen without taking the stockings all the way off. Carefully observe the toes for cyanosis throughout the day.

Using these stockings poses some risks. If the stocking is turned over at the top, the compression can double, causing the blood flow in the leg to be blocked. These stockings should be applied in the morning when legs are at their smallest size. It is more difficult to apply them later in the day. These stockings should be put on while feet are still elevated, before the resident gets out of bed. Follow the manufacturer's instructions and illustrations on how to put them on. Avoid trauma or pain to the resident throughout the procedure.

Putting knee-high elastic stockings on a resident

Equipment: elastic stockings

1. Identify yourself by name. Identify the resident. Greet the resident by name.

2. Wash your hands.

3. Explain procedure to resident. Speak clearly, slowly, and directly. Maintain face-to-face contact whenever possible. Encourage resident to assist if possible.

4. Provide for the resident's privacy with a curtain, screen, or door.

5. Practice good body mechanics. Adjust bed to safe working level, usually waist high. Lock bed wheels.

6. Lower the side rail (if bed has one and if it is not already lowered) on side nearest you.

7. Expose no more than one leg at a time. Take one stocking and turn it inside-out at least to the heel area (Fig. 19-7).

Fig. 19-7. *Turning the stocking inside-out allows stocking to roll on gently.*

8. Gently place foot of stocking over toes, foot, and heel (Fig. 19-8).

Fig. 19-8. *Being gentle promotes resident's comfort and safety. It avoids force and over-extending joints.*

9. Gently pull top of stocking over foot, heel, and leg.

10. Make sure there are no twists or wrinkles in stocking after it is on the leg. It must fit smoothly (Fig. 19-9). The opening in the stocking that allows observation of skin color should be either on the top or the bottom of the toe area, depending upon the manufacturer. Check toes for possible pressure from stocking and adjust as needed.

Fig. 19-9. *Make stocking smooth and twist- and wrinkle-free. Twists or wrinkles cause the stocking to be too tight, which reduces circulation.*

11. Repeat steps 6 through 9 for the other leg.

12. Make resident comfortable.

13. Return bed to low position if raised. Ensure resident's safety. Return side rails to ordered position. Remove privacy measures.

14. Leave call light within resident's reach.

15. Wash your hands.

16. Be courteous and respectful at all times.

17. Report any changes in the resident to the nurse. Document procedure using facility guidelines.

A **sequential compression device (SCD)** is a stocking used to improve circulation and prevent blood clots. The stocking can be applied during or after surgery. This stocking is a plastic, air-filled, sleeve-like device that is applied to the legs and hooked to a machine with an on/off switch. The machine inflates and deflates the stockings on its own, causing alternating compression of the legs. It acts in the same way that the muscles usually do during normal activity (Fig. 19-10).

Fig. 19-10. A sequential compression device.

This method of therapy is sometimes used with anti-embolic stockings. A measurement is needed to order the correct size of sequential compression stockings. As always with any electrical equipment, report to the nurse if you notice damage to any part of this equipment.

Congestive Heart Failure (CHF)

Coronary artery disease, myocardial infarction, hypertension, heart valve problems, or other disorders may damage the heart. When the heart muscle has been damaged, it fails to pump effectively. Blood backs up into the heart instead of circulating. When one or both sides of the heart stop pumping blood effectively, it is called **congestive heart failure (CHF)**. CHF occurs when the normal cardiac output cannot meet the needs for activities of daily living (ADLs).

Signs and symptoms of CHF include:

* fatigue
* reduction in the ability to exercise or be active
* difficulty breathing, or **dyspnea**
* shortness of breath, or **orthopnea** (shortness of breath when lying down that is relieved by sitting up)
* increased pulse
* irregular heartbeat
* chest pain
* dizziness
* confusion

* weight gain
* lack of appetite
* edema, especially in the feet or ankles
* swelling in the abdomen (abdominal distention)
* abdominal pain
* increased urination, especially at night

Other symptoms may occur, depending on the side of the heart that is affected. In right-sided failure, the blood build-up causes swelling of the feet and ankles and can cause the liver and the abdomen to retain fluid. In left-sided heart failure, the build-up of fluid in the lungs causes shortness of breath. Symptoms of CHF associated with a specific side of the heart are:

* Left-sided failure: fatigue, orthopnea, coughing, rapid pulse, weight gain
* Right-sided failure: fatigue, weakness, edema of the extremities (especially the ankles), bulging neck veins, irregular heartbeat and fainting

Congestive heart failure may be treated and controlled through medication and a care plan that encourages rest. Diuretics help reduce excess fluid built up inside the body, thereby reducing edema. Other medications may also help the heart contract more effectively, which increases the movement of blood through the body. Certain medications improve the flow of blood, which help reduce the workload of the heart. Nursing assistants can help residents with CHF by doing the following:

Guidelines

Congestive Heart Failure

Ⓖ Encourage rest and limited activity as ordered. Have the resident sit or lie down if dizziness or fainting (syncope) occur.

Ⓖ Measure daily weight and intake and output accurately.

Ⓖ Encourage residents to follow orders for fluid restrictions and low-sodium diets.

Ⓖ Use special stockings as ordered.

Ⓔ Extra pillows may help residents who have trouble breathing while lying flat in bed.

Ⓔ Assist with personal care and ADLs as needed.

Ⓔ Range of motion exercises improve muscle tone when activity is limited (Fig. 19-11). Chapter 25 has more information on range of motion exercises.

Ⓔ Report any of the following signs and symptoms to the nurse:

- dizziness, confusion, or fainting
- fatigue
- increased respiratory rate, pulse, or blood pressure
- irregular heartbeat
- palpitations
- dyspnea
- coughing
- wheezing
- chest tightness or chest pain
- lack of appetite
- abdominal swelling or pain
- edema
- weight gain from fluid retention
- bulging neck veins
- change in urinary output

Fig. 19-11. *Range of motion exercises improve muscle tone and help circulation.*

Pulmonary Edema

In left-sided heart failure, fluid builds up in the lungs, which presses on the air sacs, that, in turn, causes shortness of breath. This causes **pulmonary edema**. Pulmonary edema is a life-threatening condition that can be caused by an infection or a complication of CHF or an MI.

Symptoms of pulmonary edema include shortness of breath, wheezing, coughing, gurgling when breathing, anxiety and restlessness. A person may feel like he is drowning. Emergency treatment is necessary with acute pulmonary edema. Oxygen will be ordered and a ventilator may be necessary to help the person breathe. Other follow-up treatments include medication and cardiac rehabilitation.

HOT TIP

Never ignore shortness of breath or chest pain. If you are walking with a resident, and she complains of shortness of breath or chest pain, stop and help her sit down. Report this to the nurse immediately. Also report any instances of a resident stopping periodically when walking. Do not assume the resident is just fatigued. Report these signs to the nurse right away.

Blood Disorders

Anemia is a condition in which the red blood cells or the hemoglobin in red blood cells is very low. This prevents adequate oxygen from reaching the organs and tissues, a condition called **hypoxia**. Anemia is the most common blood disorder. It is diagnosed by a simple blood test.

Symptoms of anemia include fatigue, weakness, pale skin, problems with the tongue, brittle nails, and difficulty concentrating. A deficiency of iron (iron-deficiency anemia) is the most common form of anemia. Treatment includes a diet of foods rich in iron, vitamins, iron supplements, and methods to treat constipation that can occur with added dietary iron. If excess bleeding is the suspected cause of the anemia, other tests may be performed.

Pernicious anemia is a form of anemia caused by a lack of a substance that absorbs the vitamin B12 from the digestive tract. This type of anemia is common in people over the age of 60. Symptoms include bleeding gums, problems with the tongue, rapid pulse, unsteadiness, shortness of breath, pale skin, diarrhea, and numbness and tingling in the hands and feet. Treatment includes monthly vitamin B12 injections, B12 given through the nose, and/or vitamin B12 pills, along with a well-balanced diet.

HOT TIP

"The Gift of Life"

Have you ever considered donating blood to help others? The process does not take long, and this act can actually save a life. Think about calling the American Red Cross or another agency and donating blood. You'll be glad you did.

CHAPTER REVIEW

1. What is the largest artery in the body (LO 2)?

2. What are the three different types of blood cells that make up blood (LO 2)?

3. What gives blood its red color (LO 2)?

4. What is the main component of plasma? (LO 2)?

5. List four functions of blood (LO 2).

6. List three normal age-related changes of the circulatory system (LO 3).

7. What four conditions can result from hypertension (LO 4)?

8. List three ways that hypertension is treated (LO 4).

9. How is the pain of angina pectoris commonly described (LO 4)?

10. List three care guidelines for a resident with angina pectoris (LO 4).

11. What are five components that may be included in a cardiac rehabilitation program after a person has had an MI (LO 4)?

12. What is the most common form of PVD (LO 4)?

13. List six signs and symptoms of PVD (LO 4).

14. List three ways nursing assistants can help a resident who has PVD (LO 4).

15. How do anti-embolic stockings help prevent swelling and blood clots (LO 4)?

16. When should anti-embolic stockings be applied (LO 4)?

17. List eight signs and symptoms of CHF that must be reported to the nurse (LO 4).

18. List six ways nursing assistants can help a resident who has CHF (LO 4).

19. List three common symptoms of anemia (LO 4).

20
The Respiratory System

Respiration and the "Vapours" of the Heart

Galen, an early physician and author of many medical works, studied the process of respiration. He formed a belief that respiration actually cooled a person's heart. Galen also thought that chest movement added air that helped get rid of certain "vapours" of the heart. Much later, William Harvey, a doctor and researcher, developed the primary theory that the lungs change venous blood to arterial blood.

". . . Full of sweet dreams, and health, and quiet breathing."
John Keats, 1795-1821

"Nothing to breathe but air.
Quick as a flash 'tis gone . . ."
Benjamin Franklin King, Jr., 1857-1894

1. Define important words in this chapter

alveoli: tiny, grape-like sacs in the lungs where the exchange of oxygen and carbon dioxide occurs.

asthma: a chronic and episodic inflammatory disease that makes it difficult to breathe and causes coughing and wheezing.

bronchi: branches of the passages of the respiratory system that lead from the trachea into the lungs.

bronchiectasis: a condition in which the bronchi become permanently dilated (wider) and damaged.

bronchitis: an irritation and inflammation of the lining of the bronchi.

chest percussion: clapping the chest to help lungs drain with the force of gravity.

chronic obstructive pulmonary disease (COPD): a chronic, progressive, and incurable lung disease that causes difficulty breathing.

emphysema: a chronic, incurable lung disease in which the alveoli in lungs become filled with trapped air; usually results from smoking and chronic bronchitis.

expiration: the process of exhaling air out of the lungs.

hemoptysis: the coughing up of blood from the respiratory tract.

inspiration: the process of breathing air into the lungs.

lungs: main organs of respiration responsible for the exchange of oxygen and carbon dioxide.

multidrug-resistant TB (MDR-TB): disease that occurs when the full course of medication is not taken for tuberculosis (TB).

oxygen therapy: the administration of oxygen to increase the supply of oxygen to the lungs.

pneumonia: acute inflammation in the lung tissue caused by a bacterial, viral, or fungal infection and/or chemical irritants.

respiration: the process of breathing air into the lungs and exhaling air out of the lungs.

sputum: mucus coughed up from the lungs.

trachea: an air passage that goes from the throat (pharynx) to the bronchi; also called the windpipe.

tuberculosis: a contagious lung disease caused by a bacterium that is transmitted through the air; causes coughing, difficulty breathing, fever, and fatigue.

2. Explain the structure and function of the respiratory system

The respiratory system is composed of the nose, nasal cavity, pharynx, larynx, trachea, bronchi, lungs, and alveoli (Fig. 20-1). The nose serves as the front line of the body's air filtration. Air enters the nose and moves through the nasal cavity. Nasal hairs are located in the nasal cavity, which has a mucous membrane lining. The hairs and mucus work to filter particles such as bacteria and other microbes, dust, smoke and pollen from the air as it moves through the cavity. These particles are then moved by the cilia, fine, threadlike projections that work to sweep away particles and fluid, to the pharynx, or throat, to be eliminated from the body.

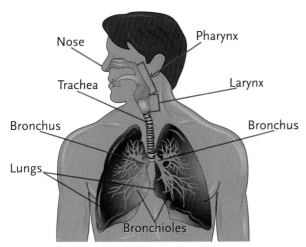

Fig. 20-1. An overview of the respiratory system.

The nasal cavity also warms and humidifies the cooler inhaled air before it continues along toward the pharynx. The pharynx allows for the passage of air and food. The air then moves through the pharynx down to the larynx, or voice box. The larynx is made up of nine pieces of cartilage, including the thyroid cartilage (often called the "Adam's apple") and the epiglottis. The epiglottis acts like a lid, shutting off the larynx during the swallowing process. This blocks food from entering the **trachea**, or windpipe, which can cause choking.

The larynx enables humans to speak. Exhaled air passes over the vocal cords and causes them to vibrate. Males have lower voices because they have thicker and longer vocal cords than females. This causes their vocal cords to vibrate more slowly, which lowers the overall pitch of their voices.

The trachea transfers air to the lungs. The trachea is lined with a mucous membrane. During the movement through the trachea, more foreign particles attach to the mucus, and the cilia there move the particles up toward the pharynx for elimination from the body.

From the trachea, the air travels into the **bronchi**, the branches of the respiratory system that enter into the lungs. It is often said that the trachea and its branches resemble an upside-down tree. The bronchi turn into the tiniest branches, called the bronchioles. These tiny branches end in the grape-like clusters called **alveoli**. These are known as the air sacs of the lungs. The exchange of oxygen and carbon dioxide occurs in the alveoli.

The **lungs** are large organs in the chest cavity. They are covered by a membrane called the pleura, which covers and protect the lungs. The pleura is made up of two layers that have a small amount of fluid in between them. This fluid allows the pleura to move easily without rubbing together as the lungs expand and contract.

The lungs contract and expand the chest cavity when we breathe in (**inspiration**). Inspiration is an active process. Expiration is a passive process. The lungs relax and the chest cavity gets smaller when we breathe out (**expiration**). The process of inspiration uses more energy than the process of expiration. **Respiration**, the body taking in oxygen and removing carbon dioxide, involves inspiration (breathing in) and expiration (breathing out).

Oxygen is a colorless, odorless and tasteless gas that makes up about 21% of the atmosphere. Oxygen nourishes cells, aids in respiration, and provides energy for cell metabolism. Carbon dioxide is a colorless, odorless, and tasteless gas that makes up about 1% of the atmosphere. Carbon dioxide is a waste product produced by the cells.

There are two oxygen and carbon dioxide gas exchanges that occur in the lungs and in the cells. The exchange in the lungs is called external respiration. During external respiration, oxygen moves into the blood, and carbon dioxide moves into the alveoli. The carbon dioxide is transported from the alveoli when we exhale out through the nose and the mouth.

The second exchange of gases inside the cells is called internal respiration. During internal respiration, oxygen moves into the cells and carbon dioxide moves into the blood. The second exchange is now complete. The cells have oxygen, and carbon dioxide is headed to the lungs to be exhaled. This process of breathing air in and out is continuous; it never stops. Cells must constantly be filled with a fresh supply of oxygen.

The functions of the respiratory system are:

- serving as an air filter, cleansing the inhaled air
- supplying oxygen to body cells
- removing carbon dioxide from the cells
- producing the sounds associated with speech

Destination: Homeostasis

When the blood carbon dioxide level increases due to a stressor, the area in the brain responsible for respiratory control, the medulla, sends out nerve impulses. These impulses cause the diaphragm and the other respiratory muscles to contract more forcefully and more often. This is known as hyperventilation, or rapid and deep breathing. This increase in breathing blows off the excess carbon dioxide, thereby increasing the oxygen to meet cellular needs. When the carbon dioxide level returns to normal, homeostasis is restored.

3. Discuss changes in the respiratory system due to aging

Normal age-related changes for the respiratory system include the following:

- Lung strength decreases.
- Air sacs (the alveoli) become less elastic and decrease in number.
- Airways become stiff and less elastic.
- Lung capacity decreases.
- Rib cage changes and chest muscles become weaker.
- Cough reflex becomes less effective and cough becomes weaker.
- Oxygen in the blood decreases.
- Decreased lung capacity causes voice to weaken.

4. Discuss common disorders of the respiratory system

Chronic Obstructive Pulmonary Disease (COPD)

Chronic obstructive pulmonary disease (COPD) is a chronic, progressive disease. Progressive means that the disease gets worse. COPD leads to difficulty breathing due to the obstruction of the airways, especially during exhalation. Many people live with COPD for years. It is not a reversible condition and it cannot be cured, but treatment may slow its progression. Two chronic lung diseases are grouped under COPD: chronic bronchitis and emphysema.

Bronchitis is an inflammation of the lining of the bronchi. There are two types of bronchitis:

acute and chronic. Acute bronchitis is caused by an infection. It is often associated with severe colds and usually lasts a brief period of time. Symptoms include coughing, yellow or green **sputum** (mucus coughed up from the lungs), and trouble breathing. Acute bronchitis is generally treated with antibiotics and/or anti-inflammatory medications.

Chronic bronchitis is a condition that occurs when the lining of the bronchial tubes becomes inflamed. This later causes scarring of the lining of the bronchial tubes. The irritation of these tubes continues for a long period of time, which then causes excessive mucus production. A long-lasting, mucus-producing cough occurs. Air flow may be restricted and the lungs become scarred. Lung infections can occur more easily when this happens. Chronic bronchitis is caused by cigarette smoking, severe air pollution, or other irritants in the air.

Treatment usually consists of reducing the triggers that cause irritation. Quitting smoking is encouraged. Medications may be ordered.

Emphysema is a chronic condition in which the walls between the alveoli (air sacs) in the lungs become over-stretched. The air sacs weaken and break. Air is trapped in the air sacs and normal breathing is impaired. Emphysema usually results from cigarette smoking and chronic bronchitis. Symptoms of emphysema include shortness of breath, coughing, and difficulty breathing.

There is no cure for emphysema. Treatment focuses on providing comfort and relieving symptoms. Quitting smoking is very important. Oxygen may be ordered to assist with breathing. Medication and regular respiratory therapy, including breathing exercises, may reduce discomfort.

General symptoms of COPD include:

- Coughing or wheezing
- Dyspnea (difficulty breathing)
- Shortness of breath, especially during activity
- Cyanosis
- Chest pain or tightness
- Confusion
- Weakness
- Weight loss or loss of appetite
- Fear and anxiety

Guidelines
COPD

- COPD causes difficulty breathing. Residents may be constantly anxious or fearful about not being able to breathe. They may fear suffocation. Be supportive and calm. Be empathetic. Not being able to breathe properly is very frightening.

- Use pillows to help residents sit upright or lean forward. This may help them breathe more comfortably (Fig. 20-2).

Fig. 20-2. *Using pillows to help a resident with COPD sit upright can ease breathing.*

- Be supportive of residents who are quitting smoking.

- Encourage a healthy diet.

- Offer plenty of fluids as long as resident does not have a fluid restriction.

- Encourage periods of rest. Try to get residents to save their energy for important tasks.

- Use proper infection control practices. Wash your hands often and help residents do the same, if help is needed. Dispose of used tissues properly.

- Colds can make COPD worse. Report signs and symptoms of colds or the flu immediately to the nurse.

- Medications that relax the air passages may be prescribed. These may be taken orally or given directly into the lungs with sprays or an inhaler. It is important for residents to take medications as ordered.

- Oxygen must be supplied to the resident exactly as ordered. Follow safety guidelines for oxygen therapy (see Chapter 7).

- Report any of the following signs and symptoms to the nurse:

  - Fever

  - Confusion or changes in mental state

  - Refusal to take ordered medications

  - Change in breathing patterns, especially shortness of breath

  - Change in color or consistency of mucus or sputum

  - Chest pain

  - Inability to sleep due to anxiety or fear

HOT TIP

Oxygen

When oxygen has been ordered for a resident, be alert for fire hazards, such as smoking materials, flammable liquids, open flames, or wool or synthetic clothing, which can spark and cause fire. Remove fire hazards. Never remove an oxygen delivery system or adjust oxygen levels. That is the nurse's responsibility.

Asthma

Asthma is a chronic, episodic disorder in which irritants, allergens, such as pollen or dust, infection, and cold air cause inflammation and swelling in the air passages in the lungs (Fig. 20-3). Exercise and stress can also cause or worsen asthma. When the bronchi become irritated due to any one of these conditions, they constrict, making it difficult to breathe. Thick mucus is produced by the mucous membranes, which further inhibits breathing. Air is trapped in the lungs, which causes heavy wheezing, coughing, and a tight feeling in the chest.

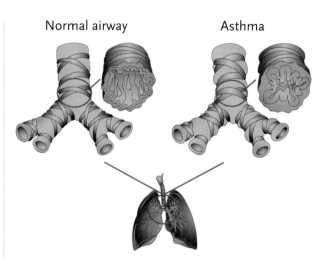

Normal airway   Asthma

Fig. 20-3. *When a person has asthma, air passages in the lungs become inflamed and swollen.*

The cause of asthma is unknown. Medications are usually ordered to treat asthma. Residents may need an inhaler with them at all times (Fig. 20-4). Encourage residents to carry their inhalers. Help residents avoid the triggers that cause asthma attacks. For example, a resident with asthma should not be exposed to strong-smelling cleaning agents or heavy perfume. Smoking and second-hand smoke should be avoided as much as possible. Because stress is a trigger for asthma attacks, reducing stress levels can help. Talking with and listening to residents may help decrease stress levels.

Fig. 20-4. *Encourage residents with asthma to carry their inhalers at all times.*

Report any of the following signs and symptoms to the nurse:

- changes in vital signs, especially respiratory rate or pulse

- wheezing, shortness of breath, or dyspnea

- cyanosis

- chest pain or tightness

- refusal to use inhaler when needed

Bronchiectasis

Bronchiectasis is a condition in which the bronchi become permanently dilated (wider) and damaged. A person may be born with this disorder, or may develop it later. Bronchiectasis is caused by an infection of the airways. Cystic fibrosis is a cause of bronchiectasis. The presence of tumors or the act of inhaling foreign bodies can also cause this problem.

Bronchiectasis is a serious illness that can result in chronic coughing, shortness of breath, wheezing, weight loss, cyanosis, and coughing up blood. Respiratory infections may occur. Over time, foul-smelling sputum may cause halitosis, or bad breath.

Treatment includes proper positioning for drainage (postural drainage) and **chest percussion** (clapping the chest to help the lungs drain with the force of gravity). Recognizing infections early can reduce the severity of the condition. Report fever, chest pain and a change in mucus or phlegm production to the nurse right away. Prompt treatment of infections will reduce the risk of complications.

Pneumonia

Pneumonia is an inflammation of the lungs caused by a viral, bacterial, or fungal infection and/or chemical irritants. The air sacs in the lungs fill with pus and other liquid.

The person usually develops a high fever, chest pain, especially when inhaling, coughing, difficulty breathing, shortness of breath, chills, and a rapid pulse. Thick secretions may be coughed up from the lungs.

People with weaker immune systems, such as young children and the elderly, are at a higher risk of developing pneumonia. Pneumonia can be a serious and potentially fatal disease, especially for the elderly, who may take longer to recover. Treatment may include antibiotics and other medications, along with an inhaler. A special diet and increased fluid intake may be ordered.

Report to the nurse if a resident says he is not taking his prescribed medication. Encourage proper diet and fluid intake. Provide support for periods of coughing and pain.

Tuberculosis (TB)

Tuberculosis, or TB, is a highly contagious lung disease caused by a bacterium that is carried on mucous droplets suspended in the air. TB is an airborne disease. People can be exposed to TB when they spend time with a person who is infected with TB. The infected person can spread the disease by coughing, breathing, singing, sneezing, or even laughing.

TB usually infects the lungs, causing coughing, difficulty breathing, fever, and fatigue. TB can be cured by taking all prescribed medication. However, if left untreated, TB may cause death.

There are two types of TB: latent TB, also called TB infection, and active TB, also called TB disease. Someone with latent TB (TB infection) carries the disease but does not show symptoms and cannot infect others. A person with active TB (TB disease) shows symptoms of the disease and can spread TB to others. Latent TB can progress to active TB. Signs and symptoms of TB include:

- Fatigue
- Loss of appetite
- Weight loss
- Slight fever and chills
- Night sweats
- Prolonged coughing
- Coughing up blood (**hemoptysis**)
- Chest pain
- Shortness of breath
- Dyspnea

Tuberculosis is more likely to be spread in areas with poor ventilation or small, confined spaces.

People are more likely to get active TB (TB disease) if their immune systems are weakened by illness, malnutrition, cancer, HIV/AIDS, alcoholism, or drug abuse.

Multidrug-resistant TB (MDR-TB) is a form of tuberculosis that can develop when a person infected with TB does not take all of his prescribed medication. When the full course of proper medication is not taken, bacteria that is resistant to medication remains in the body. This means that this bacteria is less likely to be killed by medication used to treat TB. The disease then becomes more difficult to cure.

Residents who have active TB are often isolated in an airborne infection isolation room (AIIR). Air within the room is carefully controlled so that the air in the room flows directly into the outside air or is directed through special HEPA filters before being returned to the air-handling system.

Doors to an airborne infection isolation room must remain closed, except when people are entering and leaving the room. It is important to prevent contaminated room air from entering the hallways. You will be instructed on how to properly enter and exit this type of isolation room. A sign will be placed outside the room that identifies the room as an AIIR and the need for Airborne Precautions. If you believe that an AIIR system is not working properly, inform the nurse immediately.

Guidelines
Tuberculosis

- Follow Standard Precautions and Airborne Precautions.

- Wear personal protective equipment (PPE) as instructed during care. Use a N-95, PFR-95, or HEPA respirator mask to provide care (Chapter 6) (Fig. 20-5).

- Be careful when handling sputum.

- Resident must take all of the medication prescribed. Failure to take all medication is a major factor in the spread of TB.

a)   b)

Fig. 20-5. a) an N-95 respirator mask and b) a PFR-95 respirator mask.

TRIVIA

The History of the Mask
Masks were first regularly used when practicing medicine during the 1940s and 1950s. It is hard to believe, but many surgeons left their noses uncovered, wearing masks over their mouths only. If only they had known . . .

5. Describe oxygen delivery

Every living cell in the human body needs oxygen to survive. The oxygen level in the air is adequate for most people. However, when a person has low oxygen levels, supplemental oxygen is required. **Oxygen therapy** is the administration of oxygen to increase the supply of oxygen to the lungs.

You learned about safety guidelines for oxygen use in Chapter 7. There are different ways to deliver additional oxygen to a person. Oxygen may be piped into a room at a healthcare facility from a wall outlet. Compressed oxygen comes in large cylinders or smaller, portable cylinders, which do not require electricity. Liquid oxygen in special reservoirs can be used in facilities and is also supplied in special containers for use in the home and the community. The liquid oxygen warms and becomes a gas that the person can then breathe. Oxygen concentrators are machines that run by electricity, remove oxygen from the air and store it for use.

The doctor determines which oxygen delivery device is the best for a resident who needs additional oxygen. Oxygen is considered a drug and cannot be applied or adjusted by nursing assistants. Common types of oxygen delivery devices include the following:

Nasal cannula: This device has a set of two prongs which are placed into the nostrils, and a plastic tube that fits behind the ears (Fig. 20-6). The tubing is attached to the oxygen delivery source, which is generally a wall outlet. A small plastic piece moves up and down on the tubing below the chin and adjusts it for comfort and stability. A nasal cannula is the simplest oxygen delivery device. It is a low-flow oxygen delivery system. This is the device you will see most often in long-term care.

Fig. 20-6. *A nasal cannula.*

Simple face mask: This plastic device is shaped to fit over the nose and mouth. It is held in place with an elastic band that slides over the head and above the ears. The band can be adjusted for comfort and stability. The person breathes in through the nose and mouth, and oxygen is delivered. Plastic tubing connects the mask to the oxygen source. Simple face masks deliver low-flow oxygen. These masks can irritate the skin and may feel hot and claustrophobic. Masks can prevent normal talking and eating.

Oxygen concentrator: An oxygen concentrator filters out oxygen from normal room air. It delivers low-flow oxygen. It is generally used in conjunction with a nasal cannula. The cannula is placed on the person and is then attached to the oxygen concentrator. Oxygen concentrators are quiet and efficient. They can be either larger units that remain in a room, or smaller, portable

ones that can be used when leaving the facility or the home. Oxygen concentrators plug in to electrical sockets and are not usable during power outages.

Guidelines
Care of the Resident using Oxygen

- Perform frequent skin care on areas of the face where the oxygen device rests, such as by the nose, behind the ears and around the mouth.

- Observe for redness, sores, bruising or discomfort in ear, nose, mouth, or chin area.

- Lubricate sensitive areas on the nose and mouth using water-based lubricants. Do not use any petroleum products on the tubing; oil-based lubricants can be a fire hazard.

- Take vital signs as ordered.

- Check the oxygen delivery device often for proper fit and comfort.

- Notify the nurse if the oxygen equipment does not seem to be working. Tell the nurse if the tubing is clogged or dirty and/or if the tank level drops to the point where replacement is needed.

- Post "No Smoking" and "Oxygen in Use" signs. These should be posted on each door and over the resident's bed. Do not allow smoking or open flames anywhere around oxygen equipment.

- Know the location of the fire alarms and fire extinguishers.

- Add pillows as needed to improve breathing.

- Encourage activity as permitted so resident does not withdraw or feel isolated.

- Provide emotional support; some oxygen delivery devices can be claustrophobic and difficult to use.

- If you notice any of the following, notify the nurse:

  - Sores or crusts on nasal area

  - Dry and/or reddened areas on the skin by the ears, nose, mouth or chin

- Complaints of discomfort or pain
- Shortness of breath
- Changes in vital signs, especially respiratory rate or pulse
- Cyanosis
- Chest pain or tightness

Residents who are using oxygen will need it either continuously or periodically. Continuous oxygen means the oxygen must be on at all times.

6. Describe how to collect a sputum specimen

It is sometimes necessary to collect a specimen of mucus that comes from inside the respiratory system for testing. Sputum is not the same as saliva, which comes from the salivary glands inside the mouth. Sputum may show evidence of cancer or bacteria. The lab will study the sputum, looking for abnormal cells, microorganisms, or blood.

Some facilities allow nursing assistants to collect sputum specimens. Early morning is the best time to collect sputum. When people are flat on their backs for an entire night, mucus tends to collect inside the respiratory passages. This makes it easier to collect the sputum specimen.

The resident should rinse her mouth with water before you obtain the sputum specimen. This removes any leftover food and any excess saliva. The resident should not rinse with mouthwash before a sputum specimen collection. Mouthwash kills certain kinds of bacteria and other

organisms that are helpful in analyzing the sputum.

Collecting a sputum specimen

Equipment: specimen container with cover, completed label, tissues, plastic bag, gloves, mask, emesis basin

1. Identify yourself by name. Identify the resident. Greet the resident by name.

2. Wash your hands.

3. Explain procedure to resident. Speak clearly, slowly, and directly. Maintain face-to-face contact whenever possible. Encourage resident to assist if possible.

4. Provide for the resident's privacy with a curtain, screen, or door.

5. Put on mask and gloves. If the resident has known or suspected TB or another infectious disease, wear the proper mask when collecting a sputum specimen.

6. Ask the resident to rinse her mouth with water. Assist as necessary. Have her spit rinse water in the emesis basin if she does not use the sink.

7. Ask the resident to cough deeply, so that sputum comes up from the lungs. To prevent the spread of infectious material, give the resident tissues to cover his or her mouth. Ask the resident to spit the sputum into the container.

8. When you have obtained a good sample (about two tablespoons of sputum), cover the container tightly. Wipe any sputum off the outside of the container with tissues. Discard the tissues. Apply label and bag the specimen.

9. Remove and dispose of gloves and mask properly.

10. Leave call light within resident's reach.

11. Wash your hands.

12. Be courteous and respectful at all times.

13. Report any changes in the resident to the nurse. Document procedure using facility

guidelines. Take specimen container and lab slip to the designated place promptly.

7. Describe the benefits of deep breathing exercises

Deep breathing exercises help expand the lungs, clearing them of mucus and preventing infections (such as pneumonia). Residents who have had abdominal surgery are instructed to do deep breathing exercises to expand the lungs regularly. The care plan may include using a deep breathing device called an incentive spirometer (Fig. 20-7). Incentive spirometry encourages the resident to take long, slow, deep breaths. The spirometer provides residents with visual or other positive feedback when they inhale. Usually a goal volume is set and this rate is attempted for a minimum of three seconds. Regular use can increase the capacity of the lungs and strengthen the breathing muscles. It also helps clear the lungs. Do not assist with these exercises if you have not been trained.

Fig. 20-7. Incentive spirometers are used for deep breathing exercises.

When assisting with an incentive spirometer, use only the resident's personal device. Do not share incentive spirometers between residents. The resident's name should be labeled on the spirometer.

Make sure both you and the resident wash your hands prior to using the spirometer. Residents may need encouragement from you to use this device. Be encouraging, but do not force the resident to use the spirometer.

Wear proper PPE for assisting with this procedure, and for cleaning the device. The mouthpiece will need to be rinsed and cleaned after each use. The unit may have its own storage bag. Follow the care plan and the nurse's instructions.

CHAPTER REVIEW

1. What is the function of the epiglottis (LO 2)?

2. What does the larynx enable a person to do (LO 2)?

3. What is the process of breathing in and out called (LO 2)?

4. List three functions of the respiratory system (LO 2).

5. List six normal age-related changes of the respiratory system (LO 3).

6. Why might a person with COPD be fearful or anxious (LO 4)?

7. List eight care guidelines for a resident who has COPD (LO 4).

8. What are three ways a nursing assistant can help a resident with asthma (LO 4)?

9. Which populations are at a higher risk for developing pneumonia (LO 4)?

10. How is tuberculosis spread (LO 4)?

11. What is the difference between TB infection and TB disease (LO 4)?

12. List seven signs and symptoms of TB (LO 4).

13. Why is it important for a resident to take all prescribed medication if he has TB (LO 4)?

14. List ten guidelines for caring for a resident using oxygen (LO 5).

15. List five signs and symptoms that must be reported to the nurse when a resident is using oxygen (LO 5).

16. What time of day is best to collect a sputum specimen (LO 6)?

17. What conditions can require a resident to perform deep breathing exercises (LO 7)?

21
The Musculoskeletal System

Roentgen and the Discovery of the X-ray

On November 8, 1895, Wilhelm Konrad Roentgen (1845-1923) passed electric current through a tube and noted afterward that a special-coated cardboard material nearby was glowing. He discovered that the glow came from the radiation coming out of the tube. He named the radiation "X-rays." One of his early X-rays was of his own wife's hand. The tremendous impact of this discovery was felt throughout the entire world. An amazing method to be able to see fractures and diseases of the bones had at last been found.

"And the muscular strength. . . has lasted the rest of my life."
Lewis Carroll, 1832-1898
from Alice's Adventures in Wonderland

"His bones ache with the day's work that earned it."
Ralph Waldo Emerson, 1803-1882

1. Define important words in this chapter

abduction: moving a body part away from the midline of the body.

adduction: moving a body part toward the midline of the body.

amputation: the surgical removal of an extremity.

arthritis: a general term that refers to inflammation of the joints.

atrophy: the wasting away, decreasing in size, and weakening of muscles from lack of use.

bones: rigid connective tissue that make up the skeleton; lend support to body structures, allow the body to move, and protect the organs.

bursae: tiny sacs of fluid that are located near joints and help reduce friction.

bursitis: a condition in which the bursae become inflamed and painful.

cartilage: the protective substance that covers the end of bones and makes up the discs that are found between vertebrae.

contracture: the permanent and painful stiffening of a muscle.

flexion: bending a body part.

fracture: a broken bone.

full weight-bearing (FWB): the ability to support full body weight on both legs.

joints: the points where two bones meet; provide movement and flexibility.

ligaments: strong bands of fibrous connective tissue that connect bones and support the joints and joint movement.

muscles: groups of tissues that contract and relax, allowing motion, supporting the body, protecting organs, and creating heat.

muscular dystrophy: an inherited, progressive disease that causes a gradual wasting of muscle, weakness and deformity.

non-weight-bearing (NWB): the inability to support any weight on one or both legs.

osteoarthritis: a type of arthritis that usually affects weight-bearing joints, especially the hips and knees; also called degenerative joint disease (DJD).

osteoporosis: a condition in which the bones become brittle and weak; may be due to age, lack of hormones, not enough calcium in bones, or lack of exercise.

partial weight-bearing (PWB): the ability to support some body weight on one or both legs.

phantom limb pain: pain in a limb (or extremity) that has been amputated.

phantom sensation: itching or tingling feeling from a body part that has been amputated.

prosthesis: a specially-fitted artificial body part that replaces a missing limb or extremity.

rheumatoid arthritis: a type of arthritis in which joints become red, swollen, and very painful; movement is restricted and deformities of the hands are common.

tendons: tough fibrous bands that connect muscle to bone.

total hip replacement (THR): a surgery that replaces the head of the femur (long bone of the leg) where it joins the hip.

total knee replacement (TKR): a surgery that replaces a damaged or painful knee with artificial parts.

2. Explain the structure and function of the musculoskeletal system

The musculoskeletal system is composed of muscles, bones, joints, tendons, and ligaments. The musculoskeletal system gives the body shape and structure. It allows the body to move and support itself. It also provides protection for the body and creates heat.

Muscles are made up of groups of tissues that help the body move by contracting and relaxing. They support the body, protect organs, and create heat. There are over 600 muscles in the human body. There are three types of muscles:

1. Skeletal muscles, also called voluntary muscles, control body movements by contracting and relaxing. A voluntary muscle is a muscle that can be controlled voluntarily, or at will. Skeletal muscles work together—one muscle moves the bone in one direction, and another moves it back.

2. Smooth muscles, also called involuntary muscles, make up the walls of organs, such as the bladder and uterus. Involuntary muscles are controlled automatically and are not under a person's conscious control. This type of muscle has the ability to stretch without putting a lot of stress on the muscle.

3. Cardiac muscle is an involuntary muscle that is found only in the heart. The cardiac muscle contracts and relaxes anywhere from 60 to 100 times each minute.

Bones are the rigid connective tissue that make up the skeleton, which is the framework of the human body (Fig. 21-1). Bones lend support to body structures, allow the body to move, and protect the organs. The outer layer of bone is hard or compact, while the inner layer at the end of a long bone is soft and spongy. Bone marrow lies within the spongy area of long bones. Bone marrow is responsible for the production of red and white blood cells and platelets. There are 206 bones in the human adult skeleton. There are four types of bones:

1. Long bones: the humerus (upper arm bone), the femur (upper leg or thigh bone)

2. Short bones: carpals (wrist bones), tarsals (ankle bones)

3. Flat bones: the sternum (breastbone) and scapula (shoulder blade)

4. Irregular bones: bones of the vertebrae (spine)

Fig. 21-1. *The skeleton is composed of 206 bones that help movement and protect organs.*

Ball-and-socket joint

Tendon

Bone

Muscle

Hinge joint

Fig. 21-2. *Muscles are connected to bones by tendons. Bones meet at different types of joints. Examples of the ball-and-socket joint and the hinge joint are shown here.*

Joints are found at the places where two bones come together (articulate). The joints or articulations are structures that hold bones together and provide movement and flexibility. Joint movements depend on the way in which the joint is formed. There are three types of joints: immovable, slightly movable, and movable.

Examples of immovable joints are the bones of the cranium (skull). The joints of the skull bones are called sutures. An example of a slightly movable joint is the joint between the pubic bones. The joint between the scapula and the humerus is an example of a freely movable joint. Other types of movable joints are the hip and shoulder joints, which are ball-and-socket joints, and the elbow and knee joints, which are types of hinge joints (Fig. 21-2).

Joints are found within a cavity or "capsule" that is lined with a synovial membrane. This membrane produces a fluid called synovial fluid that aids in joint lubrication. The ends of movable bones are covered with a flexible, protective substance called **cartilage** that allows free joint movement. Cartilage is also found in other parts of the body, such as the nose. **Bursae** are tiny sacs of fluid located near joints. They reduce friction during body movement.

Tendons are tough bands of connective tissue that anchor or connect muscles to bones. **Ligaments** are strong, fibrous bands that connect bones and help support the joints and joint movement. Ligaments can become injured during sports or other strenuous activity. Torn ligaments can take a long time to heal following an injury.

The functions of the musculoskeletal system are:

- Gives shape and form to the body
- Maintains posture
- Permits movement

- Protects internal organs
- Stores calcium and phosphorus
- Produces heat
- Produces some blood cells

Destination: Homeostasis

The musculoskeletal system helps to regulate the calcium levels in the blood. Bones serve as a calcium storage area. When blood calcium decreases to abnormally low levels, bones are alerted to release some of the stored calcium back into the blood. The calcium level then returns to normal range and homeostasis is restored.

HOT TIP

No swinging by the arms!
Pulling too hard on a person's arm can easily dislocate shoulder joints. Because of this, never jerk a resident's arm or attempt to lift or reposition a resident by pulling on the arm. Dislocations can cause extreme pain and may cause permanent damage.

3. Discuss changes in the musculoskeletal system due to aging

Normal age-related changes for the musculoskeletal system include the following:

- Muscles weaken and lose tone.
- Bones lose calcium, causing them to become porous and brittle (easily broken).
- Height is gradually lost due to space between the vertebrae in the spine shrinking.
- Loss of muscle mass in the body causes weight loss.
- Joints are less flexible and stiffer, which slows normal body movements and decreases range of motion.

4. Discuss common disorders of the musculoskeletal system

Muscular Dystrophy (MD)

Muscular dystrophy is a hereditary, progressive disease that causes various disabilities. With this disease muscle tissue is destroyed, and the mus-

cles atrophy. Muscle **atrophy** means the muscle wastes away, decreases in size, and weakens. MD causes muscle weakness, stiffness, and twitching of the hands and arms. People with this disorder may be confined to a wheelchair.

Muscular dystrophy is a genetic disorder caused by a specific gene. It generally appears at birth or during childhood. Duchenne's muscular dystrophy is a type of MD that is more common in males. Currently there is no cure for muscular dystrophy.

Guidelines

Muscular Dystrophy

- Allow enough time for the person to move about with braces or in wheelchair.
- Give frequent skin care to prevent pressure sores.
- Reposition resident often as ordered to help prevent pressure sores or **contractures**, which are the permanent and painful stiffening of a muscle.
- Perform range of motion exercises as directed.
- Assist with ADLs as needed. Encourage independence with ADLs so functioning muscles will not atrophy.
- If any of the following occurs, notify the nurse:
  - red skin, pale skin, or signs of the beginning of a pressure sore
  - stiffening of muscles
  - pain, swelling, or burning in a leg, especially the lower leg and the calf
  - symptoms of a urinary tract infection
  - signs of pneumonia, such as fever, chills, cough and chest pains

Osteoporosis

Osteoporosis is a condition in which the bones lose mass, which causes them to be brittle and easily broken. Osteoporosis is caused by a lack of calcium in the diet, the loss of estrogen, a lack of regular exercise or reduced mobility, and age. Osteoporosis is more common in women, especially after menopause. Signs and symptoms of osteoporosis are low back pain, loss of height and stooped posture (Fig. 21-3).

Fig. 21-3. *Stooped posture, or "dowager's hump," is a common sign of osteoporosis. (Photos courtesy of Jeffrey T. Behr, MD.)*

Osteoporosis is treated with medication and exercise. Taking calcium supplements, starting a doctor-approved exercise program, or taking medication, such as estrogen hormone pills, may help control osteoporosis. Some osteoporosis medications need to be taken once a week. The nurse may ask you to stay with the resident after she takes this medication to make sure she stays upright for the prescribed period of time.

Be patient and allow residents enough time to move. Reposition and transfer residents with osteoporosis very carefully. Follow special diet orders. Encourage ambulatory residents to walk; keep canes or walkers close by if they are used. Report to the nurse if you notice any decline in activity or movement.

HOT TIP

Fragile bones mean fragile residents!
When a person has osteoporosis, bones are weak and fragile. Bones can break with a simple move-

ment. It is important to understand how fragile bones can be. Movements that you take for granted, such as turning in bed, sitting down, or standing, can cause fragile bones to break. Be very careful when moving residents.

Arthritis

Arthritis is a general term for the inflammation of the joints that can cause pain, stiffness and swelling. Decreased mobility may also result. Two common types of arthritis are osteoarthritis and rheumatoid arthritis.

Osteoarthritis, also called degenerative arthritis or degenerative joint disease (DJD), is a condition in which the cushiony cartilage that rests between the bones and pads the ends of the bones begins to slowly erode. The cartilage also loses its elasticity. Without the padding of the cartilage, the bones begin to rub together causing pain, redness, swelling, stiffness, and limited motion. If the condition worsens, the area may eventually become deformed. Osteoarthritis generally occurs with aging and may also be due to a joint injury. It usually affects weight-bearing joints, especially the hips and knees. Joints in the fingers, thumbs, and spine can also be affected. Cold, damp weather can increase pain and stiffness caused by osteoarthritis.

Rheumatoid arthritis is a form of arthritis that may become crippling (Fig. 21-4). It affects a special membrane that lines the joint capsule, called the synovial membrane, causing stiffness, swelling, severe pain and deformities which can be severe and disabling. Fever, fatigue and weight loss are also symptoms of rheumatoid arthritis. The synovial membrane may eventually be completely destroyed. When this occurs, the joint becomes fixed and unable to move. It usually affects smaller joints first, before progressing on to larger ones. Often rheumatoid arthritis develops early in middle age, but it can affect people of any age.

Fig. 21-4. *Rheumatoid arthritis. (Photo courtesy Frederick Miller, MD.)*

The cause of rheumatoid arthritis is not known, but it may be an autoimmune illness. An autoimmune illness occurs when the body's immune system attacks normal tissue in the body. A type of virus or bacteria acts as a trigger, which causes the body to turn on itself.

Treatment for arthritis includes rest and controlled exercise. Range of motion exercises may be ordered. Anti-inflammatory medications, such as ibuprofen, as well as other medications are used to relieve pain. Weight loss can help reduce stress on the joints. Heat applications are often useful to lessen inflammation and pain. With a serious deformity, joint replacement can help.

Guidelines
Arthritis

- Assist with the exercise program as needed. Encourage gentle activity and ambulation as ordered. Keep canes or walkers close by if needed.

- Perform range of motion exercises as directed.

- Let the nurse know about 30 minutes prior to exercise if pain medication is supposed to be given beforehand.

- Assist with ADLs as needed. Using assistive devices for bathing, dressing, and eating can promote residents' independence (Fig. 21-5).

- Encourage the use of handrails and safety bars in the bathroom.

- Be positive and supportive. Listen to residents when they want to talk.

- If any of the following occurs, notify the nurse:
  - stiffness
  - swelling
  - pain
  - reduced ability to perform range of motion exercises
  - decline in activity

Fig. 21-5. *Special equipment can help a person with arthritis be independent. (Photo courtesy of North Coast Medical, Inc., www.ncmedical.com, 800-821-9319.)*

Bursitis

Bursitis is a condition in which the bursae (tiny sacs of fluid found near joints) become inflamed. The tissues around the joint may become painful, swollen and tender. The shoulder, elbow, hip, and knee are joint areas that are commonly affected. Bursitis may also occur in the foot. Treatment for bursitis includes application of ice, immobilization to rest the joint, and the use of anti-inflammatory and pain medications. Removing fluid from the joint with a needle may be necessary. Cortisone injections may be administered. If the area becomes infected, antibiotics will be ordered.

Amputations

An **amputation** is the surgical removal of an extremity, such as a hand, foot, leg, or arm. Amputations are necessary due to disease, such as diabetes, which can cause severe circulatory problems. They are also performed due to cancer or injuries. Traumatic amputations are due to car accidents or an accident involving some type of machinery or equipment. Amputations are performed either above or below the knee or elbow joint.

A person who has had an amputation may have a prosthesis. A **prosthesis** is an artificial body part that is specially-fitted to replace a missing limb or extremity (Fig. 21-6). Improvements have been made to prostheses in recent years. Prostheses are much more lifelike and give greater movement and flexibility. People can walk, exercise and do other activities, such as dancing or writing, with a prosthesis.

Fig. 21-6. *A type of prosthetic arm. (Motion Control Utah Arm. Photo by Kevin Twomey.)*

Transplants of certain body parts are done on some amputees. One serious complication of transplants is rejection of the surgically-attached part. The person must take medication for the rest of his life to prevent rejection of the transplanted body part.

After an amputation, a person may feel that the amputated limb is still a part of his body. Three conditions that can occur following an amputation are phantom limb pain, phantom sensation and stump pain. With **phantom sensation**, the person may feel discomfort such as itching or a tingling sensation in the area where the limb existed. **Phantom limb pain** occurs when the person feels pain in a limb (or extremity) that has been amputated. There are a variety of possible causes for phantom sensation and phantom limb pain. Reasons include the level of pain the person had prior to the amputation, changes in the weather, surgery that was not performed correctly, stress, infections and colds, and inactivity. Phantom sensation and limb pain are real and should not be ignored or ridiculed. Medication or physical therapy may be used to treat these conditions.

Stump pain is pain felt in the area of the part of the limb that is still there. With stump pain, the prosthesis may need to be altered for a better fit.

Guidelines
Amputation and Prosthesis Care

- A resident may have difficulty adjusting physically and emotionally to a new prosthesis. Residents may be depressed, sad, angry, or frustrated. Be supportive during the continued process of adjustment.

- Carefully follow orders for bed elevation and positioning.

- Carefully follow orders for positioning of the leg. Flexion may be restricted, as well as elevation of the knee. **Flexion** is bending a body part.

- Assist resident as needed with ADLs. Occupational therapists may work with the resident to help with ADLs.

- Encourage activity as ordered. Check with the nurse 30 minutes prior to exercising to see if pain medication is needed.

- Follow the exercise program exactly as ordered. Perform range of motion exercises as directed.

- Physical therapists will assist the resident in learning how to bear weight on the prosthesis.

- Be very careful when handling prostheses. They are very expensive. Many prostheses cost tens of thousands of dollars.

- The nurse will demonstrate how to apply a prosthesis. Follow instructions to apply and remove the prosthesis. Assist the resident as needed.

- Follow the care plan and the manufacturer's instructions on caring for the prosthesis and the stump.

- Give careful skin care to the area under a prosthesis. Make sure the skin is always clean and dry.

THE MUSCULOSKELETAL SYSTEM

- Use special stockings as indicated in the care plan. They are used to cover and protect the stump before the prosthesis is applied.

- Provide support for phantom pain, phantom sensation or stump pain. These are real types of pain and should be treated that way.

- Do not react negatively to the stump or the prosthesis during care.

- If any of the following occur, notify the nurse:
  - redness or swelling of stump or extremity
  - drainage, bleeding, or sores of any kind on the stump or extremity
  - stump pain, phantom pain, or phantom sensation
  - reduced ability to move extremity
  - cyanosis of any portion of the extremity
  - problems with the prosthesis

TRIVIA

An Early Method of Amputation

Amputation was a very difficult procedure prior to the discovery of anesthesia. People requiring amputations experienced intense pain during the surgeries. Patients were often given alcohol to drink prior to the procedure to help them manage the pain. The surgical staff would hold the patient down while the amputation was being performed. The use of anesthesia allowed these surgeries to be performed with much less pain.

Fractures

A **fracture** is a broken bone. Fractures are usually caused by some sort of trauma or accident. Fractures can occur spontaneously with diseases such as osteoporosis. Elderly people are more prone to falling, which is a common cause of fractures. Falling also contributes to other serious physical problems, including head injuries and soft tissue injuries. A fractured hip is a very serious problem that can occur with a fall.

Common signs and symptoms of fractures are pain, swelling, and bruising. The pain can be severe, and the area may be painful to touch. Pain may increase if treatment is not obtained soon after the injury. Movement may be limited.

Bleeding can occur with some fractures. There are different types of fractures, including the following:

- Closed or simple fracture: Skin is closed. Bone is in proper position, and has not dislocated.
- Hairline fracture: Skin is closed. Bone has fine-line crack noted on X-ray, and has not dislocated.
- Open or compound fracture: Skin is open. Bone may come through the skin. Person has an increased risk of infection.
- Greenstick fracture: Skin is usually closed. The fracture is incomplete. Only one side of the bone is broken; the other side is bent. Greenstick fractures are more common in children.
- Comminuted fracture: Skin is open or closed. Bone has fractured in two or more places.
- Compression fracture: Fracture occurs in the spine. Skin is usually closed. Bone may break with trauma or without significant trauma. This fracture can be due to osteoporosis, tumor or other condition. It is commonly seen in the elderly.

Preventing Falls

You first learned about fall prevention in Chapter 7. In addition to causing fractures, falls can contribute to other problems related to physical injuries, such as immobility, dehydration, and pressure sores. Falls can have psychological consequences as well, such as triggering fear, anxiety and depression. If a resident is less confident, he may be unwilling to perform routine activities.

As the person who often spends the most time with residents, you play an important role in preventing falls. Make sure that pathways are clear and that there is proper lighting in rooms. Keep hearing aids clean and encourage residents to use them.

Remind residents to wear eyeglasses. Reduce background noise when possible. Encourage properly-fitting clothes (not too long) and make sure non-skid shoes or slippers are worn. Fasten straps and tie shoelaces. Assist with ambulation and encourage use of assistive devices when needed. Problems related to falls are often long-lasting and costly. Elderly residents take longer to heal from complications from falls. Preventing falls is very important.

Fractures are generally diagnosed with an X-ray. During the healing process, X-rays can be used to check on the success of healing. Fractures are treated by specialists. The bones must be set and allowed to heal in normal alignment. The joints above and below the fracture are immobilized. New bone develops to heal a fractured bone. The ends of the broken bones need to be snugly set in order for them to heal properly. Bone healing can take four to eight weeks or longer. However, fractures can take even longer to heal in the elderly. When bones heal properly, there is a greater chance the area of the fracture will return to normal function.

Some fractures require a cast. Casts keep the fractured bones in place so that they may heal. Casts are generally made of fiberglass. Fiberglass casts dry very rapidly. The edges of the cast may need to be padded to reduce sharp edges. Special material may be used for this padding. The stocking under the cast can also be used to help pad the rough edges. Padding the cast helps avoid skin injury from the cast. Never put sharp objects inside a cast because they can pierce the skin. This increases the chance of infection in the area under the cast.

Guidelines
Cast Care

- Allow enough time for the person to move.
- Follow orders exactly on moving and repositioning. Tell the nurse prior to moving if pain medication is needed.
- Help with range of motion exercises as ordered.
- The extremity in a cast may need to be elevated to stop swelling. Use pillows to assist with elevation (Fig. 21-7).

- Pad the cast edges as needed; ask the nurse for help with this.
- Assist with the use of cane, walker, or crutches as needed.
- Do not get the cast wet. Wet casts can lose their shape. If showers are allowed, cover the cast with a plastic bag before showering.
- Use bed cradles to reduce pressure from the bed linens.
- Keep cast clean. Protect the cast from soiling during elimination.
- If any of the following occur, notify the nurse:
  - numbness, tingling or increased swelling
  - cyanosis or pale skin
  - redness, drainage, bleeding, or sores of any kind
  - changes in temperature of the skin (hot or cold skin)
  - resident complains cast feels too tight
  - pain, burning, or pressure
  - wetness in or around a cast
  - odor around the cast
  - resident places sharp object inside the cast

Fig. 21-7. *Elevating the extremity in a cast helps to stop swelling.*

A person may require physical therapy following a fracture, especially if he has had a cast. When the cast is removed, the extremity may have muscle atrophy and can feel weak. It may be necessary to have treatment by a physical therapist to return the limb to normal strength and function.

Sometimes a sling will be ordered to support an injured or broken arm in a cast. A sling is a piece of material that wraps around the neck and is secured. A sling holds and protects the arm. It also helps reduce swelling by keeping the arm elevated. When a resident has a sling, make sure the arm is positioned comfortably and properly elevated.

Fractured Hip

Older people, especially those who have osteoporosis or a specific type of arthritis, are at risk for hip fractures. Hip fractures can result from falls or even from simple movements. If the bones are already weak, they can fracture easily (Fig. 21-8).

Fig. 21-8. An example of a fractured hip.

Surgery is often performed on fractured hips. **Total hip replacement (THR)** is surgery that replaces the head of the long bone of the leg (femur) at the joint where it joins the hip. THR may be performed due to a fractured hip that does not heal properly, a weakened hip due to age and decreased bone strength, or a hip that is painful and stiff and no longer able to bear weight. Once surgery has been performed, the resident will have an order restricting weight-bearing on that leg while the hip heals. The order will be written as partial weight-bearing or non-weight-bearing. **Partial weight-bearing (PWB)** means the resident is able to support some body weight on one or both legs. **Non-weight-bearing (NWB)** means the resident is unable to support any body weight on one or both legs. Once the person can bear full weight again, the order will be for full weight-bearing. **Full weight-bearing (FWB)** means the resident can bear full weight on both legs.

One of the goals of care for a post-operative hip replacement is to avoid dislocating the operated hip. To accomplish this, the affected hip may need to be kept in **abduction**, which means moving a body part away from the midline of the body. The hip that was replaced cannot be in **adduction**, which means moving a body part toward the midline of the body. If the hip is adducted, or moved toward the midline, it can dislocate, which can cause serious complications. A second surgery may be required, and each surgery an elderly person has to undergo can further weaken the person.

An abduction pillow may be used to maintain proper position of the hip. This pillow will need to be in place whenever the resident moves or turns in the bed. For directions on the proper use of an abduction pillow, ask the nurse. You will learn more about abduction and adduction in Chapter 25.

Guidelines

Total Hip Replacement (THR)

- Keep often-used items, such as call light, telephone, tissues, and water, within easy reach.

- Follow the care plan exactly. If the resident wants to do more than is ordered, inform the nurse. Follow orders for weight-bearing.

- Follow care plan regarding positioning and elevation of the head of the bed. There may be limits on how much the head can be elevated.

- Assist with dressing the resident starting with the weaker, or affected, side first.

- Adaptive devices, such as a raised toilet seat, may be helpful for elimination (Fig. 21-9).

- Ask resident to use available handrails when moving into or out of a shower.

- Encourage fluids, if allowed, to prevent complications of immobility, such as urinary tract infections and constipation. Using a fracture pan rather than a regular-sized bedpan may be easier for elimination.

- Assist with coughing and deep breathing exercises as ordered (see Chapter 20 for more information on these exercises).

- Apply anti-embolic stockings as ordered.

- Never rush the resident. Use praise and encouragement often.

- Never perform range of motion exercises on a leg on the side of a hip replacement unless directed by the nurse.

- Caution the resident not to cross legs in bed or in a chair or turn toes inward or outward. The hip cannot be bent or flexed more than 90 degrees (Fig. 21-10). The hip cannot be turned inward or outward.

- Ask the nurse to give pain medication prior to moving and positioning if needed.

- If any of the following occur, notify the nurse:
  - incisions that are red, draining, bleeding, or warm to the touch
  - numbness or tingling
  - cyanosis or pale skin
  - an increase in pain or a burning sensation, especially on the operated side or in the calves of the legs
  - edema (swelling) of the legs
  - fever or other change in vital signs
  - constipation
  - problems with appetite
  - resident is not following the doctor's orders for exercise and activity

Fig. 21-9. *A raised toilet seat helps prevent excess hip flexion after a THR.*

Fig. 21-10. *The hip cannot be bent or flexed more than 90 degrees.*

Total Knee Replacement

Total knee replacement (TKR) is a type of surgery that replaces a knee with artificial parts. This may be necessary due to damage from injuries or arthritis or to help stabilize a knee that buckles repeatedly. The person may also need a knee replacement due to severe knee pain.

Care of a resident recovering from TKR is similar to that for the total hip replacement. However, the recovery time is usually shorter. Residents may be better able to care for themselves. Promote self-care as much as possible.

Guidelines

Total Knee Replacement

- To prevent blood clots, apply special stockings, such as anti-embolic stockings or sequential compression devices (SCD) as ordered (see Chapter 19).

- Special exercises may be ordered for the resident who has had a TKR. A physical therapist may perform these exercises. If you are asked to assist with these exercises, make sure you have been trained to perform them properly. Do not perform range of motion exercises unless ordered.

- Assist with coughing and deep breathing exercises as ordered.

- Encourage fluids, if allowed, to prevent complications of immobility, such as urinary tract infections and constipation.

- Ask the nurse to give pain medication prior to moving and positioning if needed.

- If any of the following occur, notify the nurse:
  - incisions that are red, draining, bleeding, or warm to the touch
  - numbness or tingling
  - cyanosis or pale skin
  - an increase in pain or a burning sensation, especially in the operated side or in the calves of the legs
  - reduced mobility in the extremity
  - fever or other change in vital signs
  - constipation
  - problems with appetite
  - resident is not following the doctor's orders for exercise and activity

A device called a Continuous Passive Motion (CPM) machine may be used for people who have had a TKR (Fig. 21-11). A CPM machine passively moves a specific joint repetitively through its normal range of motion. It helps to prevent stiffness and swelling that can occur post-operatively. It aids in increasing circulation. By continuously cycling through the knee's normal range of motion, it also helps prevent scar tissue and contractures from developing.

Fig. 21-11. *One type of CPM machine. (Photo courtesy of the medcom group, ltd., 800-231-4276, www.medcomgroup.com)*

A nurse or physical therapist will position the leg, set the machine rate and turn on the machine. You may be asked to stay with the resident until the resident is comfortable with the movement of the machine. Notify the nurse if the resident complains of pain or discomfort or if the extremity moves out of proper position in the machine. The nurse or therapist will turn off the machine and remove the leg when the therapy has been completed.

Traction

Traction is a method of treating fractures that keeps bones in place. Traction is also used to reduce pain and pressure or to relieve muscle spasms. Traction is used to treat a fracture by using weights and pulleys to keep the broken bones in proper position in order for the injury to heal. Careful observation of the body is required to prevent complications.

Do not disconnect the traction assembly. Keep the resident in proper body alignment at all times. Make sure the weights are not touching the floor (Fig. 21-12). Do not adjust the weights on a traction unit.

Fig. 21-12. *Make sure weights on a traction unit are not touching the floor, and do not adjust the weights.*

If any of the following occur, notify the nurse:

- numbness or tingling

- cyanosis or pale skin

- wetness on sling

- odor around sling or boot

- sling or boot becomes loose or comes off or weights come off, touch the floor, or move

- pain, burning, pressure, swelling

- changes in skin temperature

- redness, drainage, bleeding, or sores

- resident moves to the side or slides down in bed

HOT TIP

The Trapeze

The trapeze is a triangular piece of equipment that attaches to the bed frame of a person in traction or a person who requires help with movement in bed. Residents grasp the trapeze with their hands and are able to lift themselves more easily. This helps caregivers change bed linens, pads, and gowns and perform other tasks. Make sure the trapeze is secure before the resident uses it. The resident must be shown how to use the trapeze. Ask for help if you are not sure how the trapeze is used.

5. Describe elastic bandages

Elastic bandages, also called non-sterile or self-adhering bandages, are stretchy bandages that are wrapped around an injured body part. They are also referred to as "ACE® bandages," which is a common brand name for these bandages. Elastic bandages are used to keep dressings in place, hold splints in place, and provide protection, compression, and support for body parts (Fig. 21-13). These bandages are also used to decrease swelling from injuries and may be used to keep ice bags in place.

Fig. 21-13. *One type of elastic bandage.*

Elastic bandages must be wrapped snugly enough so that the proper amount of compression and support is provided. These bandages must be wrinkle-free and without twists to avoid too much compression to the area.

It is important that the bandage is not applied too snugly, which can interfere with circulation. Check on a resident 10 to 15 minutes after the bandage has been applied to make sure it is not interfering with circulation. After that, check with the resident periodically. Ask the resident to notify you if the bandage feels too tight.

Signs and symptoms of poor circulation to watch for include the following:

- Pale, gray, cyanotic, or white skin

- Skin that is cold to the touch

- Indentation marks on the skin

- Swelling

- Resident complains of the bandage feeling too tight

- Pain or discomfort

- Numbness or tingling

RICE

When a person is injured, steps can be taken immediately to reduce pain, swelling and further injury until emergency help arrives. The acronym "RICE" stands for rest, ice, compression and elevation. Utilize these steps to help prevent further injury and support the healing process:

Rest: Rest is important for helping an injury heal properly. Putting any weight on the injury could cause more harm.

Ice: Ice helps to prevent or reduce swelling. The skin should always be protected when using ice. (See Chapter 18 for more information on using ice.)

Compression: As you have learned, elastic bandages are used to compress the injured area, hold the extremity in place, and reduce discomfort. In addition, elastic bandages help decrease tissue swelling that occurs with an injury.

Elevation: Elevating the extremity also helps prevent or reduce swelling. When an extremity is elevated above the level of the heart, swelling may decrease.

Applying elastic bandages

Equipment: elastic bandage in the correct size, clip, safety pin, or tape (if using self-adhering bandage, these are not needed)

1. Identify yourself by name. Identify the resident. Greet the resident by name.

2. Wash your hands.

3. Explain procedure to resident. Speak clearly, slowly, and directly. Maintain face-to-face contact whenever possible. Encourage resident to assist if possible.

4. Provide for the resident's privacy with a curtain, screen, or door.

5. Practice good body mechanics. Adjust bed to safe working level, usually waist high. Lock bed wheels.

6. Lower the side rail (if bed has one and if it is not already lowered) on side nearest you.

7. Avoid trauma or pain to the resident throughout the procedure.

8. Assist resident to get into the supine (flat on the back) position.

9. Expose only the part to be bandaged.

10. Hold the rolled bandage with one hand and with the other hand put the loose end on top of the extremity.

11. Wrap extremity beginning at the spot furthest from the heart. Circulation returns toward the heart and this allows extra fluid to flow to the heart and leave the area. (For the wrist, begin wrapping at the hand. For the ankle, begin at the foot.)

12. Wrap bandage once around the beginning spot and turn over the tip so that an anchor is made (Fig. 21-14).

Fig. 21-14. Make an anchor at the beginning spot.

13. Wrap one more time around the spot where anchor lies and then begin slowly wrapping in overlapping spirals up the extremity.

14. Smooth out entire bandage, removing any wrinkles.

15. Secure bandage with self-closure, clip, safety pin, or tape. If using a pin, be careful not to pierce the resident's skin.

16. Straighten all of the linens.

17. Remove and re-apply bandage as directed. Wash and dry bandages as necessary.

18. Make resident comfortable.

19. Return bed to low position if raised. Ensure resident's safety. Return side rails to ordered position. Remove privacy measures.

20. Leave call light within resident's reach.

21. Wash your hands.

22. Be courteous and respectful at all times.

23. Report any changes in the resident to the nurse. Document procedure using facility guidelines.

CHAPTER REVIEW

1. List the three types of muscles that are found in the human body (LO 2).

2. What are three functions of bones (LO 2)?

3. What are two functions of joints (LO 2)?

4. List five normal age-related changes of the musculoskeletal system (LO 3).

5. What happens when a muscle atrophies (LO 4)?

6. List three physical problems that muscular dystrophy can cause (LO 4).

7. List three causes of osteoporosis (LO 4).

8. What can happen to bones when they become brittle (LO 4)?

9. List three problems that arthritis can cause (LO 4).

10. List four treatments for arthritis (LO 4).

11. What are phantom sensation and phantom limb pain? Are they real (LO 4)?

12. List eight care guidelines for amputations and prostheses (LO 4).

13. What is a fracture (LO 4)?

14. Why is preventing falls for elderly residents so important (LO 4)?

15. Why should a sharp object never be placed inside a cast (LO 4)?

16. List three reasons why total hip replacement may be performed (LO 4).

17. What is the difference between partial weight-bearing (PWB) and non-weight-bearing (NWB) (LO 4)?

18. List ten guidelines for caring for a resident who has had a total hip replacement (LO 4).

19. List eight signs and symptoms to observe and report to the nurse about a resident who has had a total hip replacement (LO 4).

20. A person recovering from a total hip replacement should not bend or flex the hip more than ____ degrees (LO 4).

21. List two reasons why a total knee replacement is performed (LO 4).

22. Why should fluids be encouraged when a resident has had a total knee or total hip replacement (LO 4)?

23. List two reasons that traction is ordered (LO 4).

24. List eight signs and symptoms to observe and report to the nurse about a resident who is in traction (LO 4).

25. List six signs and symptoms to observe and report to the nurse about poor circulation due to elastic bandages (LO 5).

26. In regard to a muscle injury, what does the acronym "RICE" stand for (LO 5)?

22
The Nervous System

Galen and the Persian Patient

Galen was a physician who lived and worked in ancient Rome. He treated a man from Persia who had a loss of sensation only in certain parts of his hand. Galen determined the patient had fallen on his back and that caused the injury. He believed nerve damage caused the loss of sensation. Galen was amazed that the man could still move his hand. To him, this meant that different nerves controlled different parts of the body. In addition, Galen thought that an injury could affect feeling, but perhaps not always movement. This was a new and exciting idea at the time.

"The harvest of old age is the recollection and abundance of blessings previously secured."
Marcus Tullius Cicero, 106-43 B.C.

"He that wrestles with us strengthens our nerves and sharpens our skill . . ."
Edmund Burke, 1729-1797

1. Define important words in this chapter

age-related macular degeneration (AMD): a condition in which the macula degenerates, gradually causing central vision loss.

agitated: the state of being excited, restless, or troubled.

Alzheimer's disease (AD): a progressive, degenerative, and irreversible disease that is a form of dementia; there is no cure.

bipolar disorder: a type of depression that causes a person to have mood swings, changes in energy levels and the ability to function; also called manic depression.

brain: the part of the nervous system housed in the skull that is responsible for motor activity, memory, thought, speech, and intelligence, along with regulation of vital functions, such as heart rate, blood pressure, and breathing.

burnout: mental or physical exhaustion due to a prolonged period of stress and frustration.

cataract: a condition in which the lens of the eye becomes cloudy, causing vision loss.

catastrophic reaction: reacting to something in an unreasonable, exaggerated way.

central nervous system: part of the nervous system made up of the brain and spinal cord.

cerebrovascular accident (CVA): a condition caused when the blood supply to the brain is cut off suddenly by a clot or a ruptured blood vessel; also called a stroke.

cognition: the ability to think clearly and logically.

concussion: a head injury that occurs from a banging movement of the brain against the skull.

delirium: a sudden state of severe confusion due to a change in the body; also called acute confusional state or acute brain syndrome.

delusion: a belief in something that is not true, or is out of touch with reality.

dementia: a serious, progressive loss of mental abilities such as thinking, remembering, reasoning, and communicating.

disruptive behavior: any behavior that disturbs others.

elopement: the act of wandering away from the facility in which a resident with Alzheimer's disease lives.

epilepsy: a general term used to describe a pattern of repeated seizures.

farsightedness: the ability to see distant objects more clearly than objects that are near; also called hyperopia.

generalized anxiety disorder (GAD): an anxiety disorder characterized by chronic anxiety, excessive worrying, and tension, even when there is no cause for these feelings.

glaucoma: a condition in which the pressure in the eye increases, damaging the optic nerve and causing blindness.

hallucinations: seeing or hearing things that are not really there.

hearing aid: a battery-operated device that amplifies sound.

hemianopsia: loss of vision on one-half of the visual field, due to CVA, tumor or trauma.

hoarding: collecting and putting things away in a guarded way.

intervention: a way to change an action or development.

irreversible: term used to refer to a disease or condition that cannot be cured.

mental health: refers to the normal function of emotional and intellectual abilities.

mental illness: a disease that disrupts a person's ability to function at a normal level in the family, home, or community.

multiple sclerosis (MS): a progressive disease in which the protective covering for the nerves, spinal cord, and white matter of the brain breaks down over time; without this covering, nerves cannot send messages to and from the brain in a normal way.

nearsightedness: the ability to see objects that are near more clearly than distant objects; also called myopia.

neuron: the basic nerve cell of the nervous system.

obsessive-compulsive disorder (OCD): a disorder characterized by repetitive behavior used to cope with anxiety.

pacing: walking back and forth in the same area.

panic disorder: an anxiety disorder that causes repeated episodes of intense fear for no known reason.

paranoid schizophrenia: a form of mental illness characterized by hallucinations and delusions.

paraplegia: a loss of function of lower body and legs.

Parkinson's disease: a progressive disease that causes a portion of the brain to degenerate; causes rigid muscles, shuffling gait, pill-rolling, mask-like face, and tremors.

peripheral nervous system: part of the nervous system made up of the nerves that extend throughout the body and connect to the spinal cord.

perseveration: the repetition of words, phrases, questions, or actions.

pillaging: taking things that belong to someone else; not considered stealing.

post-traumatic stress disorder (PTSD): anxiety-related disorder caused by a traumatic experience.

progressive: something that continually gets worse or deteriorates.

quadriplegia: loss of function of legs, trunk, and arms.

reality orientation: type of therapy that uses calendars, clocks, signs, and lists to help people with Alzheimer's disease remember who and where they are.

reminiscence therapy: type of therapy that encourages people with Alzheimer's disease to remember and talk about the past.

remotivation therapy: type of therapy that promotes self-esteem, self-awareness, and socialization in groups for people with Alzheimer's disease.

rummaging: going through items that belong to other people.

schizophrenia: a form of chronic mental illness that may have acute episodes; affects a person's ability to think, communicate, make decisions, and understand reality.

social anxiety disorder: a disorder in which a person has excessive anxiety about social situations; also called social phobia.

spinal cord: the part of the nervous system inside the vertebral canal that conducts messages between the brain and the body and controls spinal reflexes.

substance abuse: the use of legal or illegal substances in a way that is harmful to oneself or others.

sundowning: a condition in which a person gets restless and agitated in the late afternoon, evening, or night.

trigger: a situation that leads to agitation.

validating: giving value to or approving.

validation therapy: a type of therapy that lets people with Alzheimer's disease believe they are living in the past or in imaginary circumstances.

violent: word to describe actions that include attacking, hitting, or threatening someone.

wandering: walking around a facility without any known goal or purpose.

withdrawal: the physical and mental symptoms caused by ceasing to use a particular addictive substance.

2. Explain the structure and function of the nervous system

The nervous system controls and coordinates all body functions. It sends messages throughout the body and senses and interprets information from outside the body.

The **neuron**, or nerve cell, is the basic working unit of the nervous system. Neurons send and receive nerve impulses from the receptors through the spinal cord to the brain. Neurons are also involved in thought processes, directing the functioning of glands and the movement of muscles. The neuroglia hold together, support and protect the neurons.

The nervous system is divided into two main parts: the central nervous system (CNS) and the peripheral nervous system (PNS). The brain and the spinal cord make up the **central nervous system**. The nerves connected to the spinal cord that extend throughout the body are classified as the **peripheral nervous system** (Fig. 22-1).

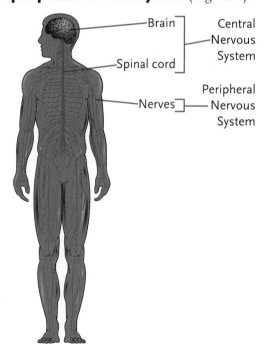

Brain — Central Nervous System

Spinal cord

Nerves — Peripheral Nervous System

Fig. 22-1. The brain, spinal cord, and nerves throughout the body make up the nervous system.

The Central Nervous System (CNS)

The **brain** is housed within the cranium. It weighs approximately three pounds, which makes it one of the largest organs in the human body. The brain controls speech, motor and sensory activity, intelligence, reasoning, coordination, reflexes, breathing, emotions, and heart rate. It is responsible for memory and regulation of certain glands, such as the adrenal gland. The brain is divided into three main parts: the cerebrum, the cerebellum, and the brainstem (Fig. 22-2).

Fig. 22-2. The three main sections of the brain are the cerebrum, the brainstem, and the cerebellum.

The cerebrum is the largest section of the brain; it is the center of the brain where thought and intelligence exist. There are two sides, or cerebral hemispheres, in the brain. The right side of the brain, or right hemisphere, controls the motor activity on the left side of the body. The left side, or left cerebral hemisphere, controls the motor activity on the right side of the body (Fig. 22-3). The cerebellum is the center of coordination. It regulates the movements of the body and controls balance.

The cerebrum and cerebellum are connected to the spinal cord by the brainstem. The midbrain, pons and the medulla oblongata rest within the brainstem. The medulla controls several major functions of the body, including breathing, opening and closing of blood vessels, and heart

rate. The medulla controls swallowing, gagging, coughing, and vomiting.

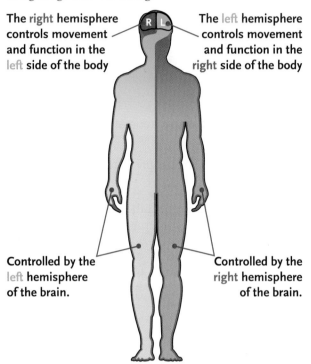

Fig. 22-3. The right hemisphere controls movement and function in the left side of the body. The left hemisphere controls movement and function in the right side of the body.

The **spinal cord** is located inside the vertebral canal in the spinal cavity of the body. It is about 18 inches long and is connected to the brain. The spinal cord conducts messages between the brain and the body within its pathways. The spinal cord is also the center that controls the body's reflex activities. An example of a reflex activity is when you blink your eye because a particle of dirt has touched it.

The brain and the spinal cord are protected by the cerebrospinal fluid (CSF). This fluid cushions the brain and the spinal cord from shocks, serves as a delivery system for certain types of nutrients, and eliminates waste products and toxins. Protective membranes called the meninges cover the brain and spinal cord.

The Peripheral Nervous System (PNS)

The peripheral nervous system (PNS) consists of the cranial and spinal nerves. Nerves carry the messages to and from the brain from the rest of the body. There are 12 pairs of cranial nerves; each set of cranial nerves relates to one side of the body. Cranial nerves direct aspects of the senses, such as taste, smell, and vision, deal with hearing and balance, and control certain muscles in the body.

There are 31 pairs of spinal nerves that emerge out of the spinal cord. Spinal nerves carry messages back and forth from the brain to the spinal cord and to and from areas of the body to the spinal cord.

The peripheral nervous system is divided into the somatic nervous system (SNS) and the autonomic nervous system (ANS). The SNS helps with conscious movement of the skeletal muscles. The ANS has two parts: the parasympathetic and sympathetic nervous systems. The parasympathetic nervous system works to conserve the body's energy and provide for relaxation of the body. The parasympathetic nervous system is responsible for slowing body functions, such as heart rate and blood pressure.

The sympathetic nervous system activates the "fight-or-flight" response. This response occurs when a person faces excessive stress and must act quickly. The body prepares for "fight or flight," or fighting or running away, by increasing blood pressure and heart rate, creating a surge in adrenaline (epinephrine), and increasing the blood glucose (sugar) to be used for the needed energy.

HOT TIP

The 3 Rs vs. Art
The left hemisphere of the brain is usually involved in a person's ability to do the "3 Rs," reading, writing and 'rithmetic, or mathematics. The right hemisphere of the brain is more involved in artistic and creative abilities.

The Sense Organs

The skin, tongue, nose, eyes, and ears are the body's sense organs. They receive impulses from the environment and relay these impulses to the brain.

The sense of touch exists in the nerve endings in the dermis. The touch receptors are responsible for the ability to feel and touch. Taste buds are found on papillae on the tongue. These papillae make the tongue bumpy. The nasal cavity is the receptacle of smell. Within the upper part of the nasal cavity, there is an area called the olfactory area. That area begins the process of sensing odors. It then sends messages to the brain where the odors are identified.

The eye is about an inch in diameter and is located in a bony socket in the skull (Fig. 22-4). The socket protects the eye and is surrounded by muscles that control eye movements. Within the eye are the receptors that function to allow the ability to see. The thickest layer and outer part of the eyeball is called the sclera, which is the white of the eye. The front part of the sclera is called the cornea, and it is transparent. It appears colored because it is positioned over the iris. The iris is the part of the eye that is genetically colored and gives the eyes their unique appearance. The pupil is the circular opening in the center of the iris, which dilates (opens) and constricts (closes) to adjust the amount of light coming into the eye. Inside the back of the eye is the retina. It contains cells that respond to light and send messages to the brain, where the picture is interpreted so you can "see."

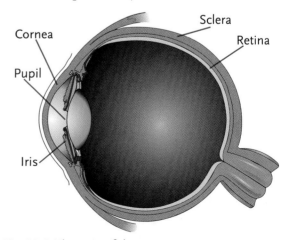

Fig. 22-4. *The parts of the eye.*

The ear is the sense organ that provides balance and hearing. It is divided into three sections: the outer, middle and the inner ear (Fig. 22-5). The outer ear collects sound waves and directs them inward through the external auditory canal toward the middle ear. Hairs and earwax (cerumen) in the outer ear help protect the ear from foreign particles. The eardrum, or tympanic membrane, separates the outer ear from the middle ear. The middle ear amplifies and transfers sound waves to the inner ear. Tiny hair cells within the inner ear send nerve impulses to the brain.

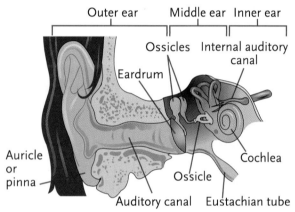

Fig. 22-5. *The outer ear, middle ear, and inner ear are the three main divisions of the ear.*

Hearing occurs when the sounds enter the ear canal and vibrations are transferred by the structures of the middle ear into the inner ear. This happens when the eardrum vibrates. The three tiny bones within the middle ear, known as the ossicles, pick up these vibrations and send impulses to the brain.

The functions of the nervous system are:

• Controls and coordinates mental processes and voluntary movements

• Provides reflex centers of heartbeat and respiration

• Senses and responds to changes occurring both inside and outside of the body

Destination: Homeostasis

To maintain homeostasis the human body has to respond quickly to sudden changes in the environment. A reflex is a rapid, automatic response to a specific change in a person's environment. The body does not formally initiate its response; it is simply automatic. A reflex arc is the path different types of neurons (nerve cells) travel to make the body respond to a sudden change, or a stimulus. For example, if a finger touches a hot stove, the finger immediately withdraws from the intense heat. This is called a withdrawal reflex. Neurons send the message to the spinal cord that the surface is hot. Following the reflex, neurons return to their normal state until they are needed again. Homeostasis is restored.

3. Discuss changes in the nervous system due to aging

Normal age-related changes for the nervous system include the following:

• Responses and reflexes slow.

• Some memory loss occurs, especially short-term memory loss.

• Sensitivity of nerve endings in skin decreases, resulting in weakened sense of touch.

• Some hearing loss occurs.

• Senses of vision, smell, and taste weaken.

4. Discuss common disorders of the nervous system

Cerebrovascular Accident (CVA)

A **cerebrovascular accident (CVA)**, or stroke, is caused by an obstruction (occlusion) inside a blood vessel or the rupture of a blood vessel. This cuts off the blood supply to the brain (Fig. 22-6). Without blood, part of the brain does not receive oxygen. Brain cells will begin to die, and additional damage can occur due to leaking blood, clots, and swelling of the tissues. Swelling can also cause pressure on other areas of the brain.

A transient ischemic attack (TIA), is a warning sign of a CVA. It occurs when the brain loses a portion of its blood supply. The attack is usually quite sudden, and symptoms may last only a few minutes or up to 24 hours. Signs and symptoms that a TIA or CVA is occurring are listed in Chapter 8.

Fig. 22-6. *A cerebrovascular accident (CVA) is caused by an obstruction or rupture of a blood vessel, which cuts off the blood supply to the brain.*

CVAs occur on either the right or left side of the body. Blood flow is affected during a CVA and can cause brain damage and a variety of symptoms. Symptoms differ, depending on which side of the brain is affected. Strokes that occur on the right side of the brain affect functioning on the left side of the body. Strokes that occur on the left side of the brain affect functioning on the right side of the body.

These problems can result from right side or left side brain damage from a CVA:

* hemiparesis (weakness on one side of the body)

* hemiplegia (paralysis on one side of the body)

* one-sided neglect (tendency to ignore a weak or paralyzed side of the body)

* loss of ability to tell where affected body parts are

* aphasia (inability to speak or speak clearly)

* expressive aphasia (inability to express needs to others through speech or writing)

* receptive aphasia (inability to understand what others are communicating through speech or written words)

* trouble understanding spoken or written words

* emotional lability (inappropriate or unprovoked emotional responses including crying, laughing, and anger)

* loss of sensations, such as temperature or touch

* loss of bowel or bladder control

* cognitive impairments, such as poor judgment, memory loss, loss of problem-solving abilities and confusion

* changes in personality

* loss of thinking and learning abilities

* dysphagia (difficulty swallowing) or the total inability to swallow

* vision impairments or blurred vision

* **hemianopsia** (loss of vision on one-half of the visual field due to CVA, tumor or trauma)

Guidelines

Residents Recovering from CVA

* Encourage independence and self-esteem. Use assistive devices when needed to promote self-care.

* Be patient with self-care and communication. Problems with speech and thinking abilities may make tasks take longer. Never rush residents.

* Assist with range of motion exercises as ordered to prevent contractures and to strengthen muscles.

* Carefully assist with shaving, grooming, and bathing. Diminished sensation or one-sided paralysis cause a lack of awareness about such things as water temperature and sharpness of razors. Take care so that injury does not occur.

- Encourage fluids and proper nutrition to prevent unintended weight loss, constipation, and dehydration.

- Residents who have hemiplegia or hemiparesis will have a weaker, or affected, side of the body. Do not refer to weaker sides as "bad," such as the "bad leg" or "bad arm." When referring to a weaker side, use the terms "weaker," "affected," or "involved" instead.

- When assisting with eating, always place food in the unaffected, or stronger, side of the mouth.

- Assist with guidelines from the speech therapist, as directed. Observe for swallowing problems.

- Break instructions down into short, simple sentences. Use communication boards or cards to help make communication easier.

- For one-sided neglect, remind residents often about the weaker side of the body.

- Assist with ambulation to prevent falls. When transferring, stand on and support the weaker side of the body. Lead with the stronger side. Use a gait or a transfer belt as needed (Fig. 22-7).

- Reposition often to help prevent pressure sores and contractures. Position in proper alignment using special positioning devices when necessary.

- With emotional lability, a resident can cry for no apparent reason. Redirect the resident's attention, which will often stop the emotional outburst. Try asking a question or pointing out something in the room. Be patient and supportive.

- Observe resident closely around dangerous objects like space heaters or radiators; these things could harm a resident with decreased sensation.

- Use praise often, even for small successes. Encourage the resident's progress.

- Prevent withdrawal and feelings of isolation. Listen to resident if he/she wants to talk.

Fig. 22-7. *When helping a resident transfer, support the weak side. Lead with the stronger side.*

Many people have trouble with communication after having a stroke. The level of difficulty a person has depends on the severity of the stroke and speech loss or confusion. Use these guidelines to help communicate with a resident post-CVA:

- Speak clearly when communicating.

- Do not rush the resident.

- Use special methods as directed, such as communication boards (Fig. 22-8).

- Use signals, such as nodding the head and pointing, to assist with communication.

- Keep questions and directions simple.

- Use questions that can be answered with a "yes" or "no," such as "Would you like to eat your vegetables first?"

Parkinson's Disease

Parkinson's disease is a progressive disorder that causes a part of the brain to degenerate. **Progressive** means that the disease gets worse with time. Neurons in the brain that produce the substance called dopamine, a neurotransmitter, begin to break down and die. This causes symptoms, such as tremors or shaking, that are uncontrollable. Tremors can make it difficult for a person to eat and perform other ADLs. This disease also causes a mask-like face, pill-rolling (moving the thumb and first finger together like rolling a pill), rigid muscles, and a shuffling gait, or walk. Speech may be affected, causing words to be slurred. Other symptoms are mood swings and gradual behavior changes.

Parkinson's disease usually begins after the age of 40. Drug therapy is one way to treat Parkinson's disease. Some people are candidates for surgery that helps direct the course of this disorder.

A	B	C	D	E	F	G	H	I	J	K	L	M
N	O	P	Q	R	S	T	U	V	W	X	Y	Z
1		2		3		4		5		6		
7		8		9		10		11		12		
13		14		15		16		17		18		
19		20		21		22		23		24		
25		26		27		28		29		30		

CALL BELL — BED UP — BED DOWN — UP IN CHAIR
DOCTOR — NURSE — HUSBAND/SON — WIFE/DAUGHTER
ICE/WATER — MILK — BATHROOM — BEDPAN
RAZOR/SHAVE — GLASSES — MEDICINE — WATCH/TIME
WHEELCHAIR — BACK TO BED — TOO HOT — TOO COLD
CLERGY — HUNGRY — DRINK — TEA/COFFEE
URINAL — BRUSH TEETH — TISSUES — COMB/BRUSH
PEN/PAPER — TELEPHONE — RADIO/TV — MAGAZINE/NEWSPAPER

Fig. 22-8. *Communication boards can help make communication easier for post-CVA residents.*

Guidelines
Parkinson's Disease

- Residents are at a high risk for falls. Assist with ambulation to prevent falls due to shuffling walk or gait.

- Encourage resident to stand as straight as possible when ambulating.

- Encourage self-care. Be patient with self-care and communication. Allow the resident time to do and say things. Listen.

- Assist with ADLs as necessary.

- Assist with range of motion exercises as ordered to prevent contractures and to strengthen muscles (Fig. 22-9).

- Encourage fluids and proper nutrition to prevent weight loss, constipation, and dehydration.

- Help prevent depression. Listen to resident if he/she wants to talk.

- If the following occur, notify the nurse:
  - severe trembling
  - severe muscle rigidity/contractures
  - mood swings
  - sudden incontinence
  - constipation
  - dehydration
  - weight loss
  - signs of depression

Fig. 22-9. *Range of motion exercises help prevent contractures, strengthen muscles and increase circulation.*

Multiple Sclerosis (MS)

Multiple sclerosis (MS) is a progressive nervous system disorder that affects the way impulses are transmitted to and from the brain. When a person has MS, there is a loss of myelin, the protective covering that covers the nerves and spinal cord. Without this covering, nerves cannot send messages to and from the brain in a normal way.

MS progresses in an unpredictable way. A person with MS will have varying abilities and symptoms, such as the following (Fig. 22-10):

Fig. 22-10. MS is an unpredictable disease that causes varying symptoms and abilities. MS can cause a range of problems, including fatigue, poor balance and trouble walking.

- numbness and tingling
- muscle weakness
- extreme fatigue
- tremors
- vertigo (a spinning feeling)
- reduced sensation
- blurred or double vision, along with jerky eye movements
- poor balance
- difficulty walking
- incontinence of bladder and bowel
- paralysis in advanced cases

Multiple sclerosis generally occurs in young adulthood. The exact cause of multiple sclerosis is not known. It may be an autoimmune disease triggered by a type of virus. There is no cure for this disease at this time. Interferon is a substance that has shown some promise with these patients. New therapies are being tested all the time.

Guidelines

Multiple Sclerosis

- Assist with ambulation to prevent falls due to lack of coordination, fatigue, and vision impairments.
- Be patient with self-care and movement. Allow the resident time to do things. Assist with ADLs as needed.
- Offer rest periods as necessary.
- Give frequent skin care to prevent pressure sores.
- Assist with range of motion exercises as ordered to prevent contractures and to strengthen muscles.
- Do not rush the person regarding communication. MS residents may have difficulty communicating their thoughts.
- Stress can worsen the effects of MS. Be calm. Listen to residents, and try to provide a stress-free environment as much as possible.
- Encourage proper nutrition and fluid intake.
- Symptoms of MS sometimes change from day to day; offer support and encouragement.
- Prevent depression. Listen to resident if she wants to talk.
- If the following occur, notify the nurse:
  - red skin, pale skin, or the start of a pressure sore
  - the start of a contracture
  - urinary tract infection symptoms, such as frequency of or burning during urination, increased incontinence or cloudy urine
  - signs of depression

Head and Spinal Cord Injuries

Accidents, such as motor vehicle accidents (MVA), sporting injuries, gunshot wounds (GSW), stab wounds, or falls may cause head or spinal injuries. Head injuries are injuries that occur to the scalp, skull or the brain. They can be open or closed injuries. A head injury that occurs from a banging movement of the brain against the cranium is classified as a **concussion**. A head injury that is a bruise on the brain is called a contusion.

A person can have a head injury and show few or no symptoms initially. Head injuries can cause confusion or disorientation, along with serious complications like coma and death. Other symptoms are headaches, drowsiness, loss of consciousness, seizures, noticeable fractures, drainage from the ears, nose or mouth, irritability, poor coordination, slurred speech, blurred vision, vomiting, a stiff neck and a decreased sense of smell.

When a person sustains a spinal cord injury, it means that the spinal cord is cut or damaged in some way. Symptoms include paralysis and loss of function, depending on where the spine is injured. The higher the injury, the greater the loss of function. **Paraplegia** is the loss of function of the lower body and legs. It is caused by injuries in the thoracic or lumbar area of the spinal cord. **Quadriplegia** is the loss of function of the arms, trunk, and legs. It is caused by injuries in the cervical area of the spine (Fig. 22-11).

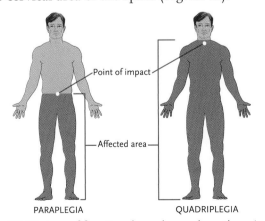

Point of impact
Affected area
PARAPLEGIA   QUADRIPLEGIA

Fig. 22-11. *Loss of function depends on where the spine is injured.*

Spinal cord injuries are treated with some success if the cord is not completely cut or severed. The results of these injuries range from spasms, weakness, and difficulty coordinating movements to complete paralysis. In time, with rehabilitation, some, or in certain cases all, of the former movement is regained. There is no current method to regenerate or regrow spinal cord tissue. Research is being conducted that may prove successful in the future in the treatment of spinal cord injuries.

Guidelines

Head or Spinal Cord Injuries

- Give frequent skin care to prevent pressure sores. A lack of sensation will prevent awareness that a pressure sore is developing. Change position every two hours or more often if ordered.

- Be gentle when turning and repositioning.

- Perform passive range of motion exercises as ordered to prevent contractures and to strengthen muscles.

- Allow as much independence as possible with ADLs.

- Offer rest periods as necessary.

- Help resident with bladder and bowel training as directed.

- Immobility leads to constipation. Encourage fluids and proper diet, high in fiber.

- Loss of control of urination can lead to the need for a catheter. Urinary tract infections are common. Give careful catheter care and encourage a high intake of fluids. Juices high in Vitamin C, such as orange juice and cranberry juice, help prevent UTIs.

- Protect residents from harm due to lack of sensation. Residents with paralysis are at a higher risk for injury from heat, cold, and sharp objects. Keep residents away from space heaters, radiators, or any other source of heat.

- Check water temperature carefully to prevent burns due to lack of sensation. Make sure hot drinks have cooled enough before offering.

Ⓖ Lack of activity can lead to poor circulation and fatigue. Use special stockings to help increase circulation as ordered.

Ⓖ Difficulty coughing and shallow breathing can lead to pneumonia. Encourage deep breathing exercises as ordered.

Ⓖ Male residents may have involuntary erections that may be embarrassing to them. Provide for privacy and be sensitive if this happens.

Ⓖ Listen to the resident. Residents will need emotional support, as well as physical assistance. Anger, irritation, and frustration are some emotions they may experience while dealing with these injuries. Try not to take it personally, and be supportive.

Ⓖ If the following occur, notify the nurse:

- red skin, pale skin, or the start of a pressure sore

- start of a contracture

- urinary tract infection symptoms

- shortness of breath

- constipation

- dehydration

- weight loss

- depression

Seizures (Convulsions)

Seizures are involuntary contractions of muscles. They can involve a small area or the entire body. Seizures are caused by an abnormality in the brain. **Epilepsy** is a general term used to describe a pattern of repeated seizures. A seizure disorder is another term for this pattern of seizures.

Some of the known causes of seizures are tumors, head injuries, injuries to the brain during birth, high fevers, or alcohol and drug abuse. They can occur in young children who have a high fever. Older children and adults who have

a serious illness, fever, or head injury may also have seizures. In many cases, the cause for a seizure disorder (epilepsy) cannot be determined.

Treatment for seizures, if the cause is known, includes medication. Surgery may be performed. For seizures caused by drug and alcohol abuse, rehabilitation can help. See Chapter 8 for more information on types of seizures and how to care for a resident who is having a seizure.

Vision Impairment

Vision changes can affect people of all ages. **Nearsightedness** (myopia) is the ability to see objects that are near more clearly than distant objects. **Farsightedness** (hyperopia) is the ability to see distant objects more clearly than objects that are near. Eyeglasses, contact lenses, or surgery can be used to correct these eye problems (Fig. 22-12).

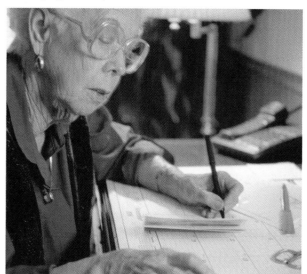

Fig. 22-12. *Nearsightedness and farsightedness are often corrected by the use of eyeglasses.*

Other vision problems include cataracts and glaucoma. A **cataract** develops when the lens of the eye, which is normally clear, becomes cloudy. Light is prevented from entering the eye, which causes decreased vision (Fig. 22-13). The first symptom is blurred vision. Other symptoms are glare when driving at night or a yellowing of vision. A cataract can eventually cause blindness in one or both eyes.

Fig. 22-13. When a cataract develops, the lens of the eye becomes cloudy and light is prevented from entering the eye.

Cataracts may be inherited. They can be caused by diabetes or an eye injury, or they may just be a result of normal aging.

Treatment depends upon the level of maturity of the cataract. Surgery is usually performed to remove the cataract. The lens that has turned cloudy is removed, and an artificial lens, or lens implant, called an intraocular lens (IOL), is placed and remains there. The implanted lens is made of plastic or silicone. The eye must be carefully measured for the lens implant prior to the surgery. This implant is permanent; it rarely has to be removed. It is only removed when inflammation occurs or the implant moves out of place.

Glaucoma is an eye disorder which is the leading cause of blindness in the U.S. The pressure inside the eye, called intraocular pressure, increases, causing damage to the optic nerve. This increase in the intraocular pressure can ultimately cause a loss of vision and blindness if left untreated.

There are many forms of glaucoma. The majority of people have primary glaucoma, which has no known cause. However, glaucoma can be hereditary. All people with a family history of glaucoma should have their intraocular pressure checked regularly. Secondary glaucoma is caused by an eye injury or eye disease and makes up a small percentage of the people who have glaucoma.

Symptoms of glaucoma may be absent with the most common form, open angle glaucoma. The

person may show a decrease in vision, especially in the peripheral vision. Symptoms include pain, nausea, vomiting, seeing a halo around lights, and blurred vision. If not treated immediately, it can cause blindness within a day.

Treatment of glaucoma includes eye drops and other medications. Regular or laser surgery may be used to try to correct the problem. The surgery does not work on every patient.

Age-related macular degeneration (AMD) is a condition in which a part of the retina called the macula, the area of the eye that allows people to see detail, degenerates. Central vision is gradually destroyed, which can affect a person's ability to drive, read, write, and do other tasks. Side vision, called peripheral vision, is not affected. AMD is the most common cause of vision loss in those 60 and older. There is no pain with this disorder, and it may evolve slowly. Vision problems may be different for each eye.

The two forms of this condition are wet and dry AMD; the dry form is more common. The exact cause of AMD is unknown. Risk factors include aging, smoking, sun exposure, heredity, gender, and race. Treatments for wet AMD include laser surgery and injections. Dry AMD may be treated with zinc and antioxidants to slow its progression. When dry AMD reaches the advanced stage, it cannot be treated, and vision loss results.

Guidelines

Vision Impairment

- Encourage the use of eyeglasses if worn.
- Keep eyeglasses clean and safe. If glasses are damaged or do not fit well, notify the nurse.
- Encourage the use of contact lenses, also called "contacts," if used. Report to the nurse if the resident requires help handling contact lenses (Fig. 22-14).
- Always identify yourself as you enter the room. Do not touch the resident until you have done so. When leaving the room, let the resident know you are going.

- Keep doors completely open or closed, so that the resident does not walk into a partially-opened or partially-closed door.

- Leave furniture in place; never move furniture without the nurse's or the resident's permission.

- Use the face of an imaginary clock as a guide to explain the position of objects in a room.

- Make sure there is enough lighting in every room. Lighting should allow the resident to read in comfort without eye strain. Harsh, overly-bright lighting should not be used, however. It can put a strain on the eyes.

- Walk a little ahead of a visually-impaired resident while he touches your arm. This allows you to guide the person and warn him of steps, curbs, etc.

- Walk at the resident's pace, not yours.

- Assist residents who need help completing menus. Set up meal trays, cut meat and vegetables, and open beverage containers as needed. Use the imaginary clock face to explain the position of food and drink on the tray.

- Use special large-print books and magazines if available. Audio books can be used if available.

- Read to residents as often as time permits if they desire it. Volunteers and visitors can also help with this.

- Assist nurses or doctors with vision screenings as needed.

Fig. 22-14. *Contact lenses are made of many types of plastic. Some can be worn and disposed of daily. Others are worn for longer periods. Residents usually insert contact lenses themselves.*

HOT TIP

Using Braille

Braille is a system of touch reading for blind people that uses tiny, raised dots (Fig. 22-15). Braille was developed in the 1800s by Louis Braille when he was a teenager. It was based on a code used to help soldiers communicate in the dark. Braille is composed of an alphabet of "cells" that consists of dots. It takes time and special training to be able to read Braille.

Fig. 22-15. *Examples of words in Braille.*

For more information about visual impairment, see Chapter 4.

Caring for eyeglasses

Equipment: emesis basin, special cleaning fluid, 2 lens cloths, towel

1. Identify yourself by name. Identify the resident. Greet the resident by name.

2. Wash your hands.

3. Explain procedure to resident. Speak clearly, slowly, and directly. Maintain face-to-face contact whenever possible. Encourage resident to assist if possible.

4. Provide for the resident's privacy with a curtain, screen, or door.

5. Gently remove eyeglasses and place in emesis basin.

6. Line sink with towel.

7. Clean eyeglasses over lined sink. Wash glass lenses in lukewarm water and rinse. Clean plastic lenses with cleaning fluid and a lens cloth. While cleaning, observe for loose screws or loose or broken lenses.

8. Dry with soft, 100% cotton cloth or special lens cloth. Do not dry with tissues as they may scratch eyeglasses.

9. Gently assist resident to replace eyeglasses on face. Place over the ears and position comfortably. Observe for proper fit.

10. Remove privacy measures. Make resident comfortable.

11. Leave call light within resident's reach.

12. Wash your hands.

13. Be courteous and respectful at all times.

14. Report any changes in the resident to the nurse. Document procedure using facility guidelines.

The artificial eye is a type of prosthesis necessary for people who have lost an eye to cancer, disease or an injury such as a gunshot wound. Artificial eyes can be made of plastic or glass; however, most artificial eyes are made from a special kind of plastic. Plastic eyes can be adapted to the changing of the eye socket as a person ages, while a glass eye cannot be changed once it is produced. Plastic eyes do not require replacement very often, and they can be cleaned and polished repeatedly.

An artificial eye is held in place by suction. Some artificial eyes do not require frequent removal, unless the eye becomes uncomfortable. Other artificial eyes may need daily removal and cleaning. Each eye specialist will give individual instructions to their artificial eye patients. Carefully follow the instructions for your residents regarding care for their artificial eyes.

If the artificial eye has been removed, clean or rinse the resident's eye socket carefully using cotton balls and water or a special saline solution. Clean empty socket from the inner canthus (inner part of the eye) toward the outer canthus (outer part of the eye). Cleanse the eyelid.

If the artificial eye is in place in the eye socket, clean the area moving in the opposite direction. Clean from the outer part of the eye toward the inner part of the eye. Cleaning in this direction helps prevent accidental movement and dislodging of the eye.

When removing the artificial eye and transporting it, use an eyecup or a small basin. Follow manufacturer's instructions regarding cleaning and storing of the artificial eye. Do not use rubbing alcohol to clean or soak the artificial eye. Do not use abrasives such as cleansers or toothpaste. The artificial eye can be permanently damaged with improper cleaning. The eye will usually be stored in water or saline solution. Always cover the eye completely with any solution used.

It is important not to appear uneasy when cleaning eye sockets or caring for an artificial eye. Act professionally when performing this task.

Hearing Impairment

There are many different kinds of hearing loss. A person may be born with a hearing impairment or it may happen gradually. A person who is hearing-impaired may read lips, use sign language to communicate, or use a hearing aid. A **hearing aid** is a battery-operated device that amplifies sound.

There are many different kinds of hearing aids. Follow the manufacturer's or your facility's directions for cleaning them. In general, they need to be cleaned daily using a special cleaning solution or alcohol and a soft cloth. Do not submerge the hearing aid in water or allow the section that houses the battery to get wet. When cleaning a hearing aid, observe for wax buildup.

Hearing aids are expensive; handle them carefully. Turn it off and keep it in a safe place when it is not being worn. Be gentle when inserting it. Turn the volume down before inserting the hearing aid. Make sure it sits snugly in place before turning it on. The hearing aid should feel comfortable when in place. If you see any sores or abrasions in the ear, report it to the nurse.

Guidelines
Hearing Aids

- Be careful when handling a hearing aid. Hearing aids are very expensive and should be treated carefully.

Turn off the hearing aid when not in use. This helps save the battery life. Store the hearing aid in a container labeled with the resident's full name, room and bed number. It should be stored in a cool, dry area. Hot, sunny areas can damage the device.

Check the batteries often. Replace batteries as needed. Follow directions carefully when replacing batteries. Proper size batteries must be used and they need to be firmly in place in the hearing aid.

If the hearing aid does not work, check the batteries. If this does not solve the problem, ask the nurse to have the hearing aid checked for damage.

Do not get the batteries wet. When cleaning a hearing aid earmold, carefully clean using a soft cloth and mild cleanser and water. Never place the hearing aid in water.

Remove hearing aids before bathing, showering, or shampooing hair.

Do not spray hair care products near a hearing aid.

Check for hearing aids before removing and changing bed linen.

Make sure that residents who use these devices have them inserted and turned on (Fig. 22-16). If the hearing aid does not fit properly, notify the nurse.

Fig. 22-16. *Hearing aids should sit snugly in place and feel comfortable in the ear.*

For more information about hearing impairments, see Chapter 4.

Delirium

Confusion is a temporary or permanent state in which a person is unable to think clearly and logically. It interferes with the ability to make decisions and may change a person's personality. It may be due to a physical problem, such as a stroke or a seizure. It has many other causes, including medication and fever. See Chapter 4 for more information on confusion.

Delirium, also called acute confusional state or acute brain syndrome, is a sudden state of severe confusion due to a change in the body. Severe dehydration or malnutrition, fever, pain, poisons, alcohol and drug use, and prescribed medications can cause delirium. Other causes are hypoxia (low blood oxygen), head injuries, and illnesses such as cancer or diabetes. Infections such as pneumonia and urinary tract infections can also cause delirium.

Signs and symptoms of delirium include:

*   Disorganized thinking
*   Inability to concentrate
*   Problems with speech
*   Agitation
*   Anger or irritability
*   Drowsiness or sleep disturbances
*   Decrease in short-term memory
*   Lack of attention span, especially around familiar people
*   Disorientation
*   Changes in consciousness
*   Decrease in the normal ability to move about
*   Pulling out tubing, such as a nasogastric tube or a urinary catheter
*   Hallucinations

Some effects of delirium are easily treatable with medication, which will reverse or control the delirium. Other causes require emergency care or a hospital stay. If you note any of these signs and symptoms, report them to the nurse immediately.

5. Discuss dementia and related terms

Cognition is the ability to think clearly and logically. A person with a cognitive impairment has a reduced ability to perform these mental tasks. Focus and memory, as well as self-awareness and judgment, may be impaired. Some loss of cognitive ability is a result of normal changes of aging in the brain (Fig. 22-17).

Dementia is a general term for a more serious loss of mental abilities, such as thinking, remembering, reasoning, and communicating. It interferes with normal functioning, and a person may lose the ability to perform activities of daily living (ADLs). Social skills may be affected. Dementia is not a normal part of aging.

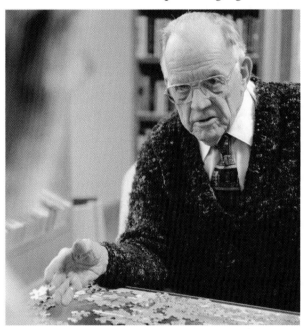

Fig. 22-17. Some loss of cognitive ability is normal; however, dementia is not a normal part of aging.

Alzheimer's disease is the most common form of dementia, which you will learn about later in this chapter. Dementia may also be caused by these disorders:

- Vascular dementia, or multi-infarct dementia
- Lewy body dementia
- Parkinson's disease
- Acquired immunodeficiency syndrome (AIDS) (Chapter 24)
- Huntington's disease

- Excessive alcohol or drug use
- Head injuries
- Thyroid disorders
- Nutritional deficiencies, especially of the B vitamins

Some forms of dementia may be treated. Dementia caused by thyroid disorders or vitamin deficiencies can often be reversed with proper treatment. However, many forms of dementia are **irreversible**, meaning the disease cannot be cured. With those types of dementia, symptoms are managed with specific care techniques and different medications.

Diagnosing dementia is difficult. Physical and mental tests may be performed to rule out other causes. Testing may be started after a person develops two or more problems with brain functioning. Loss of speech or language ability, math skills, or memory skills are examples of problems that may occur.

Dementia and Delirium

Dementia is not the same thing as delirium. Delirium is a sudden state of severe confusion due to medical conditions and other causes. Dementia is a serious loss of cognitive abilities that is not a result of the aging process. However, people who have dementia may develop delirium.

6. Discuss Alzheimer's disease and identify its stages

Alzheimer's disease (AD) is a nervous system disorder that is both progressive and irreversible. Tangled nerve fibers and protein deposits form in the brain, eventually causing this disease. People with Alzheimer's disease lose memory, have behavioral changes, and eventually are completely unable to care for themselves. There is no known cause of Alzheimer's disease.

Alzheimer's disease was first identified by Alois Alzheimer in 1907. The Alzheimer's Association estimates that in 2007 there are more than 5 million people living in the U.S. with Alzheimer's disease. Most of these people are over the age of 65. The disease affects people from all races, backgrounds, socio-economic statuses, and cultures.

Alzheimer's disease generally progresses in three stages. In each stage, the symptoms become progressively worse. All victims are eventually completely dependent on others for care.

Alzheimer's disease progresses differently in different people. One person may show symptoms from two or more stages at once and may never have other symptoms at all. For example, one person may continue to read, but not be able to recognize a family member. Another can play a musical instrument, but does not know how to use the television controls. Skills a person has used over a lifetime are usually retained longer (Fig. 22-18).

Fig. 22-18. *A person with AD may continue to have skills she has used her whole life.*

Three general stages of Alzheimer's disease are:

Stage I (Early/Mild)

- recent (short-term) memory loss
- disorientation to time
- lack of interest in doing things, including working, dressing, and recreation
- inability to concentrate and decreased attention span
- mood swings with anxiety, depression and agitation
- petulance: bad-tempered, ill-humored, rude behavior
- tendency to blame others
- poor judgment

- carelessness in personal habits and safety awareness

Stage II (Middle/Moderate)

- increased disorientation
- increased memory loss; may forget family members and friends
- slurred speech
- difficulty finding the right word, finishing thoughts, or following directions
- tendency to make illogical statements
- inability to read, write, or do math
- inability to care for self or perform ADLs without assistance
- inability to recognize common items, such as combs and eating utensils
- incontinence
- dulled senses (for example, cannot distinguish between hot and cold)
- restlessness, wandering, pacing, and/or agitation (increase of these in the evening is called "sundowning")
- sleep problems
- lack of impulse control (for example, swears excessively or is sexually aggressive or rude)
- obsessive repetition of movements, behavior, or words
- exaggerated behavior, like a temper tantrum
- hallucinations or delusions

Stage III (Late/Severe)

- total disorientation to time, place, and person
- apathy
- total dependence on others for care
- total incontinence
- verbally unresponsive, inability to speak or communicate, except for grunting, groaning, or screaming
- total immobility/confined to bed
- inability to recognize family members or self
- increased sleep disturbances

- difficulty swallowing, which produces the risk of choking
- seizures
- coma
- death

Regardless of what symptoms a person with AD has, it is important to continue to encourage independence for as long as possible. Helping residents keep their minds and bodies active may even help slow the progress of the disease (Fig. 22-19).

Fig. 22-19. Continue to encourage independence and activity for residents with AD.

HOT TIP

ADRD

You may see this abbreviation used to identify Alzheimer's disease and related dementias: ADRD.

---

7. List strategies for better communication with residents with Alzheimer's disease

Many things can be done to improve communication with residents who have Alzheimer's disease. Some general communication guidelines follow:

- Always identify yourself and use the resident's name when greeting him. (Never touch first; this may upset the person.)
- Look at the resident the entire time you are speaking with him.
- Speak slowly and quietly. Be calm. Using a lower tone of voice than normal can be calming and easier to understand.

- Reduce background noise (Fig. 22-20).
- Use touch and gestures if appropriate.
- Only talk about one subject at a time. Be patient. Use simple, short sentences.
- Repeat directions and answers as many times as needed.
- Use pictures.
- Praise often.

Fig. 22-20. Try to find a room with little background noise and distraction when communicating with residents with AD.

Communication with residents with AD can be helped by following these specific techniques:

If the resident is frightened or anxious:

- Move and speak slowly.
- Speak in a quiet area with few distractions.
- Try to see and hear yourself as they might. Always describe what you are going to do.
- Use simple language and short sentences. If performing a procedure or assisting with self-care, simplify and list steps one at a time.
- Check your body language; make sure you are not tense or hurried.

If the resident forgets or shows memory loss:

- Repeat yourself. Use the same words if you need to repeat an instruction or question. However, you may be using a word the resident doesn't understand, such as "tired." Try other words like "nap" or "lie down."
- Repetition can also be soothing for a resident with AD. Alzheimer's disease may

cause a resident to repeat words, phrases, questions, or actions. This is called **perseveration** or repetitive phrasing. Do not try to stop a resident who is perseverating. Answer the questions each time, in the same way. Even though responding over and over may frustrate you, it communicates comfort and security.

- Keep messages simple.
- Break complex tasks into smaller, simpler steps.

If the resident has trouble finding words or names:

- Suggest a word that sounds correct. If this upsets the resident, learn from it and try not to correct. As communicating with words (written and spoken) becomes more difficult, smiling, touching, and hugging can help show love and concern. But remember that some people find touch frightening or unwelcome.

If the resident seems not to understand basic instructions or questions:

- Ask the resident to repeat your statements. Use short words and sentences, allowing time to answer.
- Pay attention to the communication methods that are effective and use them.
- Watch for nonverbal cues as the ability to talk lessens. Observe body language—eyes, hands, facial expressions.
- Use signs, pictures, gestures or written messages. For example, a picture of a toilet on the bathroom door can help remind a person where the bathroom is.

If the resident wants to say something but cannot:

- Encourage the resident to point, gesture, or act it out.
- If he is obviously upset but cannot explain why, offer comfort with a hug or a smile, or try to distract him.

If the resident is disoriented to time and place:

- Post reminders, such as calendars, activity boards, pictures, and signs on doors. Prior to the later stages of dementia, signs and labels can help with orientation. However, these techniques do not help and may only frustrate a person in the late stages of Alzheimer's disease.

If the resident does not remember how to perform basic tasks:

- Help by breaking each activity into simple steps. For instance, "Let's go for a walk. Stand up. Put on your sweater. First the right arm..." Always encourage residents to do what they can.

If the resident insists on doing something that is unsafe or not allowed:

- Try to limit saying "don't." Instead, redirect activities toward something else.

If the resident hallucinates (sees or hears things that are not really happening), is paranoid, or accusing:

- Do not take it personally.
- Try to redirect behavior or ignore it. Because attention span is limited, this behavior often passes quickly.

If the resident is depressed or lonely:

- Take time, one-on-one, to ask how the resident is feeling. Really listen.
- Try to involve the resident in activities. Always report signs of depression to the nurse.

If the resident is verbally abusive or uses bad language:

- Remember it is the dementia speaking and not the resident.
- Try to ignore the language. Redirect attention to something else.

If the resident has lost most verbal skills:

- Use nonverbal communication. As speaking abilities decline, people with AD will still understand touch, smiles, and laughter for much longer (Fig. 22-21). However, remember that some people do not like to be touched. Approach touching slowly. Be gentle, softly touching the hand or placing your arm around the resident. A hug can express affection and caring. A smile can say you want to help.

- Even after verbal abilities are lost, signs, labels, and gestures can reach people with dementia.

- Assume that residents with AD have insight and are aware of the losses in their abilities. Do not talk about them as though they were not there or treat them like children.

Fig. 22-21. *Touch, smiles, hugs, and laughter will be understood longer, even after a resident's speaking abilities decline.*

8. Identify personal attitudes helpful in caring for residents with Alzheimer's disease

The attitude of caregivers can make a big difference when caring for residents with AD. These attitudes will help you give the best care for your residents with Alzheimer's disease:

Do not take it personally. Alzheimer's disease is a devastating mental and physical disorder that affects everyone who surrounds and cares for the one with AD. People with AD do not always have control over their behavior. They may not be aware of what they say or do. If a resident with AD insults you, ignores you, or accuses you, remember that it is the disease causing the behavior. These actions are not within the person's control.

Put yourself in their shoes. Think about what it would be like to have Alzheimer's disease. Imagine being unable to perform your ADLs. Be understanding and compassionate. Assume that residents with AD have insight and are aware of the changes in their abilities. Provide security and comfort.

Work with the symptoms and behaviors you see (Fig. 22-22). Each person with Alzheimer's disease is an individual. AD does not progress the same way in everyone. Each resident will do some things that others will never do. Take an interest in each individual. Work with what you see today. For example, a resident may be able to make it to the bathroom today, but yesterday, he could not walk to the door of his room. Notice changes in behavior, mood, and independence and report your observations to the nurse.

Fig. 22-22. *Treat each resident with AD as an individual and work with symptoms you see.*

Work as a team. Part of AD care is noticing changes in behavior, or physical and emotional health. When you work as a team, more subtle changes will be noticed. Share observations with the care team. Being with residents often allows you insights that others may not have. Make the most of this opportunity. People with AD may not distinguish between nursing assistants, nurses, or administrators, so be prepared to help when needed.

Take care of yourself. Caring for someone with dementia can be both emotionally and physically demanding. Take care of yourself to be able to continue to give the best care (Fig. 22-23). Be aware of your body's signals to slow down, rest, or eat better. Remember that your feelings are real and you have a right to them. Share your feelings with others, especially those experiencing similar situations. Do not worry about mistakes. Use them as learning experiences.

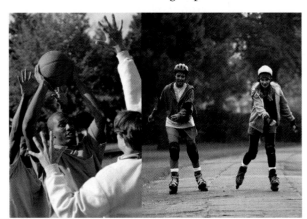

Fig. 22-23. In order to give the best care, you need to take care of yourself. Regular exercise is an important part of taking care of yourself.

Work with family members. Family members can be a great resource. They may know things you would have to learn by trial and error. Family can be of great comfort to victims of AD, helping you provide quality care.

Remember the goals of the care plan. Along with practical tasks, the care plan will call for maintaining residents' dignity and self-esteem. Provide security and comfort. Promote independence for as long as possible.

HOT TIP

Burnout

Caregivers of residents with AD have a tendency to experience burnout. **Burnout** is mental or physical exhaustion due to a prolonged period of stress and frustration. Burnout can include feelings of failure about the work you do. If you feel this is happening to you, ask your supervisor for assistance. She can refer you to people or support groups who can help.

9. Describe guidelines for problems with common activities of daily living (ADLs)

The following guidelines are strategies for making care for a resident with AD easier. These are general tips and may not apply to every resident. Each resident with Alzheimer's disease is an individual. Remember to encourage as much independence as possible during care. Promote self-care. Help residents to care for themselves as much as possible. Residents with AD tend to do better if the staff follow a routine. Be consistent with routines if possible.

Bathing

- Schedule bathing when the resident is least agitated.

- Prepare the resident before bathing. Hand him the supplies, such as soap or towels, which can serve as a visual aid.

- Be organized so the bath can be quick. Give sponge baths if a shower or tub bath is resisted.

- Make sure the bathroom is well-lit.

- Provide for resident's privacy at all times.

- Check that the temperature of the room is comfortable.

- Confusion and frustration during bathing can be reduced by calmly explaining the procedure in the same way every time. Use simple words and short sentences (Fig. 22-24).

- Offer the resident a washcloth to hold, which can help distract him while you finish the bath.

- Ensure safety by using non-slip mats, tub seats, shower chairs and handholds.

- Do not try to force the resident to bathe. Be flexible and try again later in the day.

- Be relaxed during the bath and allow the resident to enjoy the bath.

- Be encouraging and positive. Offer praise and support.

- Observe the skin for any signs of breakdown or irritation during bathing.

Fig. 22-24. *A resident with AD may be frightened or not understand what you are going to do. Stay calm. Gently explain the procedure using simple words.*

Grooming and Dressing

- Assist with grooming. Help residents you care for feel attractive and dignified.

- Choose clothing ahead of time. Mention that you are going to help the person get dressed. If resident is able, allow him to help with choice of clothing. Use clothing that is easy to put on.

- Lay out clothes in the order in which they should be put on (Fig. 22-25). Choose clothes that are simpler to put on. For example, use Velcro™ instead of buttons, slip-on instead of lace-up shoes, pants or skirts instead of dresses.

- Provide for privacy at all times.

- Do not rush the resident.

- Praise and encourage the resident often.

Toileting

- Encourage fluids. Do not withhold or discourage fluids because a resident is incontinent.

- Mark the restroom with a sign as a reminder to residents of its location and that they should use it. Ensure that lighting is adequate.

- Check the resident often for episodes of incontinence. Be matter-of-fact about cleaning resident after an episode of incontinence. Show respect.

Fig. 22-25. *Lay out clothes in the order to be put on.*

- Take the resident to the bathroom after drinking fluids; make sure resident actually urinates.

- Follow the toileting schedule carefully.

- Take resident to bathroom before meals and bedtime.

- If you know the resident's bathroom time, take him to the bathroom prior to and as near to this time as possible.

- If the resident has nighttime incontinence, take him to the bathroom as near to bedtime as possible. Use incontinence briefs as needed.

- Check skin regularly for signs of irritation.

- Cover garbage cans or waste baskets if the residents tries to urinate or defecate in them.

- Document bowel movements.

- Support family or friends who are upset by incontinence.

Nutrition

Nutritional problems are common among people with AD. It is very important to offer nutritious snacks and encourage food and fluid intake. In addition, here are ideas for improving nutritional intake:

- Schedule meals at the same time each day and serve familiar foods.

- Remind the resident when it is mealtime.

- Encourage independence with eating and drinking.

- Make the dining area as pleasant and calm as possible. Use smaller dining areas and tables if needed to reduce distractions. The dining area should be well-lit.

- Make sure residents with AD are seated with other residents to encourage socialization. Adjust seating to allow for any eating problems.

- Foods should look and smell appealing.

- Food and drink should not be too hot.

- Plain plates without patterns or colors work best. Use a simple place setting with a single eating utensil (Fig. 22-26). Remove other items from the table.

- Use a variety of foods that the resident enjoys to stimulate appetite; consider cultural preferences.

- Ask resident which food he would like to eat first, giving him a choice of two or three dishes. Residents in later stages of AD may not be able to make this choice.

- Finger foods may work well because they are easier to eat and allow residents to choose what they want (Fig. 22-27). Bite-sized pieces of food may also work well.

- During meals, offer one bite at a time.

- Offer fluids often. Have different types of fluids available, such as gelatin or popsicles.

- Obtain assistive devices for eating if needed.

- Give resident simple instructions when eating. Ask the resident to open his mouth and place a spoon to the lips, if needed.

- Use the hand-over-hand method to help the resident eat.

- Allow residents plenty of time to eat and drink fluids.

- If your resident needs to be fed, do so slowly, offering small pieces of food.

- Sit directly in front of residents when helping with eating, and make simple conversation during the meal.

- Keep nutritious snacks close by, especially favorites.

- If restlessness or wandering prevents getting through an entire meal, try smaller, more frequent meals.

- Observe and report changes or problems in eating habits. Observe for swallowing problems.

- Promptly report changes in intake or output. In addition, monitor weight accurately and frequently to discover potential problems.

Fig. 22-26. *Simple place settings with white plates on a solid-colored place mat may help avoid confusion and distraction during eating.*

Fig. 22-27. *Finger foods are often easier to eat and promote independence for residents with AD.*

See Chapter 14 for more information on nutrition.

Physical Health

- Prevent infections; they are the leading cause of death in people with Alzheimer's. Follow Standard Precautions.

- Help residents wash their hands frequently.

- Observe physical health and report any potential problems. People with dementia may not recognize their own health problems.

- Reduce the risk of falls; fractures can occur and cause severe pain.

- Provide excellent skin care to reduce the risk of pressure sores.

- Take action to manage pain. Recognize nonverbal signs of pain, such as grimacing or clenching fists (Fig. 22-28). Promptly report possible signs of pain to the nurse. See Chapter 13 for symptoms of pain and ways to manage pain.

- Special pain management techniques will be used for residents with AD who are close to death. See Chapter 27 for more information.

Fig. 22-28. *Be aware of nonverbal signs of pain, such as holding or rubbing a body part. Report these signs to the nurse immediately.*

Mental and Emotional Health

- Maintain self-esteem by encouraging independence in activities of daily living. Assistance with personal grooming will increase self-esteem.

- Provide a daily calendar to encourage activities.

- Share in enjoyable activities, looking at pictures, talking, etc.

- Reward positive and independent behavior with smiles, hugs, and warm touches.

Environmental Issues

Environmental changes can be made to make surroundings safer and more secure for residents with AD. They also can make the environment easier for the person to move around in. General tips for making the environment safer include the following:

- Use pictures or photos to identify each room, such as the dining room and the bathroom.

- Mark stairs and windows with brightly colored tape or signs.

- Use handrails in the bathroom, along with non-skid mats.

- Do not keep shampoos, cleaning agents, toxic substances, plants, or other potentially dangerous items within reach of confused or disoriented residents.

- Provide a safe area for pacing or wandering.

RESIDENTS' RIGHTS

Resident Rights and Alzheimer's Disease
Because people with Alzheimer's disease may not be aware of what they are doing, it is especially important to protect their dignity. For example, if a resident lifts up her skirt often, dress her in pants. If a resident is a messy eater, provide privacy when he is eating. Actively protect residents' privacy and promote their dignity and self-esteem, even if it seems that they are not aware of this.

10. Describe interventions for common difficult behaviors related to Alzheimer's disease

People with Alzheimer's disease can show different behaviors that may be difficult to deal with. By knowing interventions, you can give better responses to these behaviors. An **intervention** is a way to change an action or development.

Nursing assistants may receive special training on cognitive impairment. Sensitivity training can be included to help you understand the needs of residents with physical and/or cognitive impairment.

Agitation: A resident who is excited, restless, or troubled is said to be **agitated**. Feeling insecure or frustrated, encountering new people or places, and changes in routine can all trigger this behavior. A **trigger** is a situation that leads to agitation. Even watching television can cause agitation as a person with AD may lose his ability to distinguish fiction from reality. Try to recognize the triggers and eliminate them. Keep a regular routine and avoid frustration. If a resident becomes agitated, a calm response and slow soothing tone can help minimize the behavior. Reduce noise and distractions. Focusing on a familiar activity may help. Listen carefully and ask gentle questions. Reassure the resident that he is safe.

Catastrophic Reactions: When a person with AD reacts to something in an unreasonable, exaggerated way, it is called a **catastrophic reaction**. Many situations can cause this reaction, and they differ from person to person. It is most often triggered by these conditions:

- fatigue
- change of routine, environment, or caregiver
- overstimulation, including noise, too much activity, difficult choices or tasks
- physical pain or discomfort, including hunger or need for toileting

Respond to catastrophic reactions as you would to agitation. Try to eliminate triggers and help the resident focus on a soothing activity.

Violent Behavior: A resident who attacks, hits, or threatens someone is **violent**. Violent behavior also includes being violent to oneself. For example, a resident may bang his head repeatedly against a wall. Violence may be triggered by many situations. These include frustration, overstimulation, or a change in roommate, caregiver, or routine.

If any residents show violent behavior, notify the nurse immediately. Block blows but never hit back. Step out of reach, and stay calm. Try to remove triggers if possible. Remove other residents or visitors from the area. Use the same techniques as for agitation to try to calm the resident. Do not try to restrain the resident. A care conference may be needed to discuss the behavior, especially if it is new behavior. For

more information about aggressiveness, anger, and combativeness, see Chapter 4.

Hallucinations or Delusions: A resident who is having **hallucinations** is seeing things that are not there (Fig. 22-29). A resident who believes things that are not true is having **delusions** (Fig. 22-30). Most hallucinations and delusions are harmless and can be ignored. Reassure a resident who seems agitated or worried. Do not argue with a resident who is imagining things. Challenging serves no purpose and can make matters worse. Remember that the feelings are real to the resident with AD. Do not tell the resident that you can see or hear his hallucinations. Redirect the resident to other activities or thoughts.

Fig. 22-29. Hallucinating is seeing or hearing things that are not really there. For example, a resident may think he is hearing his mother calling him to dinner. You know that his mother died twenty years ago, but to him this is very real.

Fig. 22-30. A delusion is a belief in something that is not true, or is out of touch with reality. For example, a resident thinks that her long-deceased sister is stealing from her room, like she did when they were young.

Depression: People who become withdrawn, isolated, lack energy, and stop eating or doing things they used to enjoy may be depressed. Losing independence and facing the reality of an incurable disease can cause depression. Feelings of failure and fear are other causes. Chemical imbalances can cause depression. See information in Learning Objective 13 of the chapter for more information on depression and its symptoms.

Report signs of depression to the nurse immediately, as medications may help. Try to note the triggers or events that cause changes in mood. Encourage independence, self-care, and reward activities that improve moods. Find ways to help foster social relationships, such as group activities. Listen to residents if they want to share their feelings. Respect their right to feel sad; offer comfort and concern. Be as pleasant as possible. Use touch to communicate care if it does not bother the person.

Disruptiveness: **Disruptive behavior** is anything that bothers or disturbs others, such as yelling, banging on furniture, slamming doors or other things. Often this behavior is triggered by pain, constipation, frustration, or a wish for attention. When this behavior starts, get the resident's attention. It is important to stay calm and be friendly. Gently try to direct the resident to a quiet area. Ask the resident to tell you the problem, if possible. Try to find out why the behavior is occurring.

Inappropriate Sexual Behavior: Inappropriate sexual behavior, such as removing clothing, touching one's own genitals in public, or being sexually-aggressive can be disturbing to those who see it. When this happens, stay calm and be professional. Do not be judgmental or overreact. Try to determine if the cause is a simple problem, such as a rash or clothing that is too tight or the need to urinate. Gently direct resident to a private area. Distract the resident if possible. Report this behavior to the nurse. Consider appropriate ways to provide physical stimulation, such as holding the resident's hand, giving a back rub, or offering a stuffed animal for him to hold. For more information about inappropriate sexual behavior, see Chapter 4.

Inappropriate Social Behavior: Residents can sometimes show inappropriate social behavior, such as cursing, name calling, or yelling. As with violent or disruptive behavior, there may be a variety of causes. Do not take this behavior personally. When this behavior occurs, try to remove the resident from the area if he is disturbing others. Try to find out what caused the behavior (for example, stress, pain, noise, etc.). Stay calm. Report this behavior to the nurse.

Perseveration or Repetitive Phrasing: Residents with dementia may repeat words, phrases, or questions over and over again. This is called perseveration or repetitive phrasing. They may also repeat an action or task, such as tapping fingers and folding or cleaning things. Be patient with these repetitious behaviors. Remember that the resident is unaware of what he or she is doing. If questions are asked repeatedly, respond each time using the same words. Do not try to silence or stop the resident.

Pillaging, Rummaging, and Hoarding: **Pillaging** is taking things that belong to others. A person with AD may truly believe that something belongs to him, even when it clearly does not. **Hoarding** is collecting and putting items away in a guarded way. **Rummaging** is going through drawers, closets, or personal items that belong to oneself or to other people.

All of these behaviors are not within the control of a resident who has Alzheimer's disease. Pillaging and hoarding should not be considered stealing. These behaviors are not something that is deliberately or consciously planned. It is common for people with AD to wander around collecting items. They may pick items up that catch their attention and leave them somewhere else. This behavior is not intentional.

Steps to take to help this behavior are to label all of the resident's belongings. Note where missing items are located. Remember the hiding places so that you can look there if other things are missing in the future. Notify the family or friends so that they may be aware of this behavior. Enlist the family's help to notify you if they note this behavior. A special drawer for rummaging can be created. This drawer can hold items that are okay and safe for the resident to take with him.

Sundowning: When a resident with AD becomes restless and agitated in the late afternoon, evening or night it is called **sundowning**. Sundowning may be caused by hunger, fatigue, change in routine or caregiver, or any new situation. The best ways to reduce this restlessness are:

- Provide adequate lighting before it gets dark.
- Avoid stressful situations during this time. Limit activities, appointments, trips, and visits.
- Play soft music.
- Try to discourage residents from taking naps during the day.
- Set a bedtime routine and keep it.
- Recognize when sundowning occurs and plan a calming activity just before.
- Serve the evening meal long before bedtime.
- Eliminate caffeine from the diet.
- Give a soothing back rub.
- Try to redirect the behavior or distract the resident with a calm activity like looking at a magazine.
- Maintain a daily exercise routine.

Suspicion: As residents with AD begin to progress in their illness, they often become suspicious. They may accuse caregivers of lying to them or stealing from them. When this occurs, do not argue with them. Arguing just increases defensiveness. Offer calm reassurance. Be understanding and supportive.

Pacing and Wandering: A resident who walks back and forth in the same area is **pacing**. A resident who walks around a facility without any known goal or purpose is **wandering**. Pacing and wandering can have many causes, including the following:

- restlessness
- hunger
- disorientation
- the need to use the bathroom
- constipation
- pain
- forgetting how or where to sit down
- too much daytime napping

Responses to pacing and wandering include:

- Encourage an exercise routine.
- Minimize daytime napping.
- Let residents pace in a safe, locked area. Do not restrain them (Fig. 22-31). Remove clutter and create clear paths. Use only non-skid rugs.
- Redirect attention to something the resident enjoys.
- For nighttime wandering, minimize daytime napping.
- Place stop signs or "closed" signs on doors to remind residents not to exit. Use alarms on exits to indicate the door has been opened. Locks placed either very high or very low may prevent exiting. Remember to keep a key nearby in case of emergency. Never leave a resident alone in a locked room.
- If residents wander away from the enclosed area in which they live, it is called **elopement**. It is very important to keep doors locked when leaving an Alzheimer's unit or area. If a resident wanders away, notify the nurse in charge immediately. Follow all policies for emergency notification of the facility.

Fig. 22-31. *Do not restrain residents who pace. Let them pace or wander in a secure area.*

The Safe Return System

The Alzheimer's Association Safe Return® program can be used in the event a loved one with AD wanders away from home. The program is nationwide, and help is available 24 hours a day, 365 days a year. For a small fee, the family receives an ID bracelet, labels to sew on clothing, and a special wallet-sized card. The identification number matches the registration number with the association. For more information, contact the Alzheimer's Association at 1- 800-272-3900 or at www.alz.org.

Stay calm.

Residents with AD may exhibit frustrating behaviors. These behaviors, such as yelling, hitting, exposing themselves, repeating themselves, and wandering are out of their control. No matter how a resident behaves, it is never appropriate for you to respond with yelling, hitting, or rough handling. Not only is it abusive behavior, it is also grounds for immediate termination. Remain calm when residents demonstrate difficult behaviors. Be empathetic. Try to imagine how you would feel if you were faced with a progressive, incurable, and irreversible disease. Talk to your supervisor if you feel that you cannot respond professionally to residents.

11. Discuss ways to provide activities for residents with Alzheimer's disease

Activities are very important for residents with Alzheimer's disease. Activities residents enjoy help them stay focused and prevent frustration and boredom.

When a person is first diagnosed with Alzheimer's disease or is admitted to the facility, staff should request a detailed biography from family or friends. Information that would be helpful are likes, dislikes, cultural needs, work history, hobbies and interests, and a description of the person's personality. These can all be used to plan the most beneficial types of activities for residents with AD.

There are different types of activities. Meaningful activities help people with Alzheimer's disease maintain or improve their ability to function in daily life. It draws on past skills the resident used throughout his life to help provide a focus. For example, if a resident was a person who filed medical records, giving her papers or folders to file can help her stay focused on a task.

Other activities called "doing" activities keep residents busy (Fig. 22-32). Folding towels can help the resident stay focused. Separating cards into groups can help with motor coordination and keep him focused for a specific period of time.

Fig. 22-32. *Activities that are not frustrating can help keep residents busy and engaged.*

Residents may only be able to stay focused for periods of about 20 to 30 minutes at a time for a given activity. Do not try to push them to continue the activity. Change from one activity to another if a specific activity is not working for a resident.

Some of the things staff can do to provide meaningful activities include the following:

- Encourage family participation in activities.

- Limit some activities to small groups.

- Use quiet areas for activities. Make sure the temperature in activity areas is comfortable.

- Set short time frames for activities to allow for limited attention spans.

- Help plan events that are of interest to residents, based on their interests and past experiences.

- Plan activities at times of the day when residents are feeling their best and are most engaged.

- Encourage residents to exercise in specially-designated areas.

- Plan activities that allow residents to make things that can be utilized.

- Encourage each resident's specific skills, such as playing a musical instrument.

• Immobile residents must not be forgotten; provide opportunities for them to participate in activities as well. Reading to them or playing music in the resident's room are ways to provide activity for bed-bound residents.

In addition to encouraging residents to participate in activities, make sure residents are dressed and ready to go to activities at the designated time. They should be well-groomed, have had a meal or snack, and have been taken to the bathroom. Your responsibility may include taking the resident to the activity site.

12. Describe therapies for residents with Alzheimer's disease

There are different types of therapies that can improve the quality of life for people with Alzheimer's disease. These include the following:

Reality orientation uses calendars, clocks, signs, and lists to reorient the resident to person, place, and time. It can help reduce confusion or disorientation. It is useful in the early stages of Alzheimer's disease, before a person is totally disoriented. Later on, it may only frustrate the resident.

When using reality orientation, always identify yourself and call the resident by name. Ask about family, pictures, or personal items. Inquire about recent meals or activities. Use newspapers, magazines, TV, and radio to help residents know about current events. Point to clocks and calendars to show what time it is and what day of the week it is. Explain why you do things as you do them. For example, "We use your walker, Mrs. Martinez, to help make walking easier." Mention the season or month when selecting clothes or when looking out the window.

Validation therapy is letting residents believe they live in the past or in imaginary circumstances (Fig. 22-33). **Validating** means giving value to or approving and making no attempt to reorient the resident to actual circumstances. It is used for residents with advanced dementia.

Fig. 22-33. *Validation therapy accepts a resident's fantasies. There is no attempt to reorient him to reality. By validating a resident's fantasies, you let him know that you take him seriously.*

For example, Mrs. Montego comes to you and says she is late for prom. Instead of telling her that prom happened many years ago, you quietly ask her about the color of her dress and ask her to describe it. You might ask her who her date is and how late she can stay out. This allows her to work through the memory without forcing her back to reality.

Reminiscence therapy is a form of therapy that encourages the person to remember and talk about past experiences (Fig. 22-34). Explore memories by asking questions. Ask about details and work through feelings. If you trigger a painful past memory, do not hurry the resident through the memory. However, do not dwell on the painful memory. If the resident signals he wants to move on to other memories and thoughts, be ready to do this. Reminiscence therapy can help elderly people remember pleasant times in their past and allow caregivers to increase their understanding of their residents. This therapy can encourage staff to interact more with residents with Alzheimer's disease and other forms of dementia.

Fig. 22-34. *Reminiscence therapy encourages a resident to remember and talk about his past. It helps you show an interest in him as a person, not just as a resident.*

Remotivation therapy promotes self-esteem, self-awareness, and socialization in groups. Residents gather in small groups, and discussion focuses on facts rather than emotion. For example, a group discussion may have participants discuss their former professions in detail. This type of therapy discourages correcting residents and it does not focus on personal problems. The therapy can be in group form. Discussion is based on the cognitive abilities of the people within the small group. Remotivation therapy can be used together with reality orientation and reminiscence therapy.

13. Discuss mental health, mental illness, and related disorders

Mental health is the ability of a person to use cognition and emotion appropriately throughout each day. A mentally healthy person will have successful relationships with family, friends, neighbors, and co-workers (Fig. 22-35). He will perform well in professional and home settings and will meet his responsibilities. He can control his desires and impulses properly. He will be able to deal with difficulties that occur throughout life.

Fig. 22-35. Interacting well with others is a trait of mental health.

Mental illness is a disease, just like any physical disease. It affects a person's ability to function in family, home, work, or community settings. It often causes inappropriate behavior. Certain conditions can affect mental state and may worsen mental illness. Examples include various illnesses, substance abuse, physical

abuse, unstable or traumatic relationships, genetic tendencies toward mental illness, and extreme stress.

Anxiety-Related Disorders

You first learned about anxiety in Chapter 4. Anxiety is uneasiness or fear about a situation or condition. For a mentally ill person, anxiety can exist all the time. If treatment is not sought, the anxiety can get worse. Types of anxiety disorders are as follows:

Generalized anxiety disorder (GAD) is an anxiety disorder characterized by chronic anxiety, excessive worrying, and tension, even when there is no cause for these feelings. Symptoms include headaches, muscle aches, sweating, shaking, difficulty swallowing and irritability. GAD can be treated with medication.

Post-traumatic stress disorder (PTSD) is an anxiety disorder that may develop after a traumatic experience, such as a response to combat while in the military. PTSD can also develop after a crime, tornado, domestic violence, or a severe accident. Symptoms include flashbacks, withdrawal, and sleep disturbances. Flashbacks are experiences in which the person goes through the event again and again. PTSD is generally treated with medication.

Obsessive-compulsive disorder (OCD) is a disorder characterized by repetitive behavior used to cope with anxiety. For example, a person with OCD may wash his hands over and over again, or check repeatedly to make sure the door is locked. A mentally healthy person will not exhibit this behavior, but a person with OCD cannot stop it. OCD is treated with medication and therapy.

Social anxiety disorder, also called social phobia, is a disorder in which a person has excessive anxiety about social situations. It causes extreme self-consciousness in everyday situations, and the person may not want to be around other people at all. The person is unable to manage or control his fears. This phobia can interfere with the ability to attend school, work, social functions, and family events. Symptoms include sweating, shaking, and upset stomach. Medication and therapy are used to treat this disorder.

Panic disorder is an anxiety disorder that causes repeated episodes of intense fear for no known reason. Symptoms include dizziness, rapid heartbeat, chest pain, difficulty breathing, and an upset stomach. The person may have a feeling of doom. Panic attacks may occur infrequently, or may be more frequent and interfere with the ability to function normally. Medication and therapy are used to treat panic disorder.

Depression

Clinical depression is a serious mental illness in which a feeling of overwhelming sadness makes it difficult for a person to function normally. Other symptoms of depression are pain, fatigue, apathy (lack of interest), weight loss, sleep problems, irritability and feelings of worthlessness. A person who is depressed may not be able to perform normal tasks or participate in daily activities (Fig. 22-36).

Fig. 22-36. Signs of depression, such as apathy, sleep problems, irritability and being unable to perform normal tasks are important to report.

Depression is an illness and must be treated as such. A person cannot simply overcome depression through sheer will. Depression is more common in the elderly population. It can

occur along with other illnesses, such as cancer, Alzheimer's disease, HIV or AIDS, and after a heart attack.

Depression may be caused by abnormal levels of chemicals in the brain. Extreme depression can lead to thoughts of death and suicide. If you ever hear a resident make comments, even jokes, about hurting himself, report it immediately to the nurse. Depression is treated with medication and therapy.

Bipolar disorder, or manic depression, is a type of depression that causes a person to have mood swings, changes in energy levels and the ability to function. The mood swings can go from extreme happiness to extreme sadness. The extreme "high" is called mania and the "low" is called depression. High energy, little sleep, high self-esteem and poor judgment are other symptoms of this disorder. Suicide or thoughts of suicide can occur. Bipolar disorder requires long-term treatment with medication.

Schizophrenia

Schizophrenia is a form of chronic mental illness that may have acute episodes. It is a brain disorder that affects a person's ability to think and communicate clearly. Problems with emotions, decision-making, and understanding reality may occur. A person may think she is hearing voices that tell her what to do. Symptoms include hallucinations, delusions, disorganized thinking and speech, and a lack of interest in life and planning activities. The person may have poor hygiene. Problems with memory may develop.

Paranoid schizophrenia is a form of mental illness characterized by hallucinations or delusions. For example, a person may believe that a neighbor is spying on her. She might be afraid that a co-worker is trying to poison her. These types of thoughts are called "delusions of persecution." Treatment of schizophrenia consists of long-term use of anti-psychotic medications.

Guidelines

Mentally Ill Residents

- Encourage self-care.

- Encourage resident independence with ADLs and activities. Watch for any change in a resident's ability to perform the ADLs.

- Know your residents. Observe and watch for changes in behavior, such as episodes of mania in people with bipolar disorder.

- Watch your body language when caring for the resident. He may be sensitive to this.

- Do not treat mentally ill residents like children. Always treat residents like adults.

- Do not yell or use a harsh tone of voice. Never argue with the resident.

- Use eye contact unless it upsets the person.

- Provide support for the resident and family and friends. Do not judge the behavior of the resident or friends or family. Notify the nurse if you become concerned about any specific behavior.

- If you see any of the following, notify the nurse:

  - change in ability to perform ADLs

  - changes in mood

  - change in behavior; behavior that seems extreme or dangerous or frightening to others

  - hallucinations or delusions that upset the person or others

  - any comments about suicide, even jokes

  - concerns that the resident is not properly taking a medication or is hiding medication

  - any person(s), activity, program, telephone call, specific date, object, article of clothing, or place that makes the person's behavior change in some way

14. Discuss substance abuse and list signs of substance abuse to report

Substance abuse is the use of legal or illegal substances in a way that is harmful to oneself or others. Many types of substances are abused, including alcohol, tobacco, legal and illegal drugs, glue, paint, and permanent markers (Fig. 22-37). These substances are also referred to as "mood-altering" substances. An abused substance creates a change in the person's perception or the control of his body. For example, alcohol is a depressant. It can cause the slurred speech, slower reflex response, unsteadiness when walking, irritability, and unsafe driving.

Fig. 22-37. Prescription drugs, cigarettes, and alcohol are examples of legal substances that may be abused.

Risk factors for substance abuse include difficult childhood, unstable home environment, and poor coping skills. Elderly people are more at risk for substance abuse when they have poor or absent relationships with family or friends. Because elderly people are often taking prescribed medication, substance abuse can cause even more problems due to possible drug interactions with their medication.

If you observe any of the following signs, report them to the nurse. Simply report what you see, not what you think the cause may be.

- changes in physical appearance (torn clothing, red eyes, weight loss)
- changes in personality (moodiness, mood swings, odd behavior, lying)
- forgetfulness
- confusion
- loss of appetite
- stealing money or valuables
- smell of alcohol, cigarettes, or other substances in one's room or on clothing
- strong smell of room fresheners
- increased use of breath fresheners
- hiding substances or alcohol
- blackouts or memory loss
- problems with other residents, staff, friends or family
- constricted or dilated pupils
- slurred speech
- thoughts of suicide

When a person stops using an addictive substance, withdrawal can occur. **Withdrawal** is the physical and mental symptoms caused by ceasing to use a particular addictive substance.

Without treatment substance abuse can cause injury or even death. Treatment includes medication, behavioral health therapy, and treatment for any existing mental illness.

CHAPTER REVIEW

1. What is the basic working unit of the nervous system (LO 2)?

2. What makes up the central nervous system? What makes up the peripheral nervous system (LO 2)?

3. What part of the eye gives it its color (LO 2)?

4. What are two functions of the ear (LO 2)?

5. List three functions of the nervous system (LO 2).

6. List four normal age-related changes of the nervous system (LO 3).

7. List 13 problems that can result from a CVA (LO 4).

8. List 12 guidelines for caring for residents who are recovering from a CVA (LO 4).

9. List five care guidelines for residents who have Parkinson's disease (LO 4).

10. List eight care guidelines for residents who have multiple sclerosis (LO 4).

11. List 12 care guidelines for residents who have head or spinal cord injuries (LO 4).

12. What are four possible causes of seizures (LO 4)?

13. List 12 care guidelines for residents who have vision impairment (LO 4).

14. Why is it important not to use rubbing alcohol or abrasives to clean artificial eyes (LO 4)?

15. List seven care guidelines for hearing aids (LO 4).

16. List eight possible causes of delirium (LO 4).

17. What is dementia (LO 5)?

18. What is the most common cause of dementia (LO 5)?

19. Alzheimer's disease is a progressive, degenerative, and irreversible disease. What do each of these descriptions mean (LO 6)?

20. Why is it important for nursing assistants to encourage independence for as long as possible for residents who have AD (LO 6)?

21. Possible communication challenges for residents with AD are listed in Learning Objective 7. They include challenges with a resident who may:

- be frightened or anxious
- forget or show memory loss
- have trouble finding words or names
- seem not to understand basic instructions or questions
- want to say something but cannot
- be disoriented to time and place
- not remember how to perform basic tasks
- insist on doing something that is unsafe or not allowed
- hallucinate, or be paranoid or accusing
- be depressed or lonely
- be verbally abusive, or use bad language
- have lost most verbal skills

For each communication challenge, list one tip that may help.

22. Helpful personal attitudes when working with residents who have AD are in Learning Objective 8. They include the following:

- Do not take it personally.
- Put yourself in their shoes.
- Work with the symptoms and behaviors you see.
- Work as a team.
- Take care of yourself.
- Work with family members.
- Remember the goals of the care plan.

For each attitude, list one example of what nursing assistants can do to express that attitude.

23. List four guidelines for each of the following problems that may occur for a resident who has Alzheimer's disease: bathing, grooming and dressing, toileting, nutrition, physical health, mental and emotional health, and environmental issues (LO 9).

24. List one intervention for each of these problem behaviors related to Alzheimer's disease in Learning Objective 10: agitation; catastrophic reactions; violent behavior; hallucinations and delusions; depression; disruptiveness; inappropriate sexual behavior; inappropriate social behavior; perseveration; pillaging, rummaging, and hoarding; sundowning; suspicion; and pacing and wandering.

25. What is the difference between "meaningful" activities and "doing" activities (LO 11)?

26. Briefly describe each of the four creative therapies for AD (LO 12).

27. What are three characteristics of mental health (LO 13)?

28. What conditions can cause or worsen mental illness (LO 13)?

29. Briefly define each of these anxiety disorders: generalized anxiety disorder, post-traumatic stress disorder, obsessive-compulsive disorder, social anxiety disorder, and panic disorder (LO 13).

30. Does a person usually overcome depression through sheer will (LO 13)?

31. What should a nursing assistant do if a resident makes comments or jokes about suicide (LO 13)?

32. List four symptoms of schizophrenia (LO 13).

33. List six care guidelines for mental illness (LO 13).

34. List 13 possible signs of substance abuse that must be reported to the nurse (LO 14).

23
The Endocrine System

1. Define important words in this chapter

diabetes: a condition in which the pancreas does not produce insulin or does not produce enough insulin; causes problems with circulation and can damage vital organs.

gland: an organ that produces and secretes hormones.

hormones: chemical substances created by the body that control numerous body functions.

hyperthyroidism: a condition in which the thyroid gland produces too much thyroid hormone, which causes body processes to speed up and metabolism to increase.

hypothyroidism: a condition in which the body lacks thyroid hormone, which causes body processes to slow down.

metabolism: the process of burning food for heat and energy.

pre-diabetes: a condition in which a person's blood glucose levels are above normal but not high enough for a diagnosis of type 2 diabetes.

2. Explain the structure and function of the endocrine system

The endocrine system regulates many important body functions. The endocrine system is made up of glands in different areas of the body (Fig. 23-1). The **glands** are organs that produce and secrete chemicals called hormones. **Hormones** are chemical substances created by the body that control numerous body functions. They are vital to survival. Hormones are carried in the blood for delivery to target tissues or organs.

The pituitary gland, also called the "master gland," is located at the base of the brain attached to the hypothalamus. It is called the master gland due to its ability to control the hormone production of other glands. There are two parts, or lobes, of the pituitary gland: the anterior (front) and the posterior (back). The anterior lobe releases the hormones, while the posterior lobe stores hormones for release when needed.

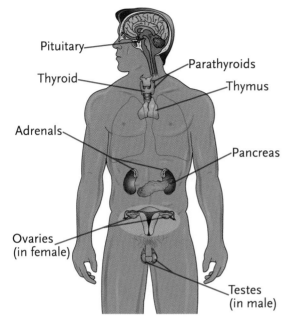

Pituitary

Parathyroids

Thyroid

Thymus

Adrenals

Pancreas

Ovaries
(in female)

Testes
(in male)

Fig. 23-1. *The endocrine system includes glands that produce hormones that regulate body processes.*

The thyroid gland is located in the neck below the larynx or voice box. Thyroid hormones primarily regulate metabolism and growth. **Metabolism** is the burning of food for heat and energy. Thyroid hormones also stimulate the growth of nervous tissue.

Four tiny parathyroid glands are embedded in the thyroid gland. They are responsible for the production of parathyroid hormone. This hormone regulates the levels of calcium and phosphate in the bloodstream.

Two adrenal glands are located on top of the kidneys. They secrete adrenaline (epinephrine) and noradrenaline (norepinephrine), aldosterone, and cortisol. During stressful situations, adrenaline, and the less-potent noradrenaline, increase the efficiency of muscle contractions, increase heart rate and blood pressure, and also increase blood glucose levels to provide extra energy. This is called the "fight-or-flight response." It enhances body performance during stressful or threatening situations. Aldosterone regulates the balance of sodium, potassium, and water. Cortisol

(hydrocortisone) maintains the metabolism by regulating the amount of glucose (natural sugar) in the blood.

The pancreas is a gland located in the back of the abdomen and behind the stomach. The pancreas produces the hormone insulin. Insulin regulates the amount of glucose available to the cells for metabolism. Cells cannot absorb sugar without insulin.

Male and female sex glands, called the gonads, are endocrine glands. The ovaries in the female secrete estrogen and progesterone. The testes in the male secrete testosterone.

The functions of the endocrine system are:

* Maintains homeostasis through hormone secretion
* Influences growth and development
* Regulates levels of calcium in the blood
* Maintains blood sugar levels
* Regulates the body's ability to reproduce
* Determines how quickly cells burn food for energy

Destination: Homeostasis

The parathyroid glands work to maintain calcium levels in the body. If the blood calcium gets too low—for example, possibly due to surgery or cancer—the parathyroid glands increase production of parathyroid hormone (PTH). When the blood calcium reaches the proper level, the parathyroid glands stop the production of PTH. This quick response of the parathyroid glands helps the body return to homeostasis.

HOT TIP

Iodine Allergy and Dye
Iodine is very important for the thyroid gland to function normally. Most people get their daily intake of iodine from common table salt. If you are allergic to iodine, tell your doctor. This allergy must be listed in your medical record. Any test that requires dye to be injected into the body can cause a life-threatening allergic reaction for a person who is allergic to iodine.

3. Discuss changes in the endocrine system due to aging

Normal age-related changes for the endocrine system include the following:

- Levels of hormones, such as estrogen and progesterone, decrease, which signal the onset of menopause in women. Testosterone levels in males usually decrease but production does not stop.

- Insulin production decreases.

- Body is less able to handle stress.

4. Discuss common disorders of the endocrine system

Diabetes

Diabetes mellitus, commonly called diabetes, is a disease that can affect people of any age. **Diabetes** is a condition in which the pancreas does not produce insulin or does not produce enough insulin. Without insulin to process the glucose, or natural sugar, it builds up in the blood. This causes hyperglycemia, or high blood sugar. Because the body is unable to get energy from the sugar in the blood, it has to find energy another way. Usually the energy is obtained by burning fat. Diabetes is common in people with a family history of the illness, in the elderly, and in people who are obese.

Diabetes can cause many complications, including the following:

- Hypoglycemia (insulin reaction) and diabetic ketoacidosis (DKA) are complications of diabetes that can be life-threatening (Chapter 8).

- Decreased blood flow can cause problems with circulation, such as CAD or PVD (Chapter 19). These problems increase the risk of heart attack, stroke, or impaired circulation in the legs. Poor circulation in the legs can increase the risk of infection and the loss of toes, feet, or legs to gangrene.

- Diabetic retinopathy, or damage to blood vessels in the retina, can cause blindness.

- Damage to vital organs, such as the kidneys being unable to properly filter the blood, is another complication of diabetes.

- Diabetic peripheral neuropathy can result from diabetes. It causes numbness, pain, or tingling of the legs and/or feet and nerve damage over time.

There are a few different types of diabetes:

Pre-diabetes is a condition in which glucose levels are elevated, but not high enough to establish a diagnosis of diabetes. Many millions of people in the U.S. have pre-diabetes. They may already have some damage to their vital organs.

In order to be diagnosed with pre-diabetes, a fasting blood sugar level must be above 99 mg/dL. Pre-diabetes can be delayed or prevented with certain lifestyle changes. A change in the diet, along with daily exercise, can reduce weight, and lower the risk of pre-diabetes or diabetes.

Type 1 diabetes is a condition that is usually diagnosed in children and young adults. It was formerly known as juvenile diabetes or insulin-dependent diabetes mellitus (IDDM). In type 1 diabetes, the pancreas does not produce any insulin. This condition will continue throughout a person's life. Daily injections of insulin are needed, but these injections do not always prevent complications of diabetes. Special diets help treat this disorder and must be followed carefully. Blood glucose testing must also be done to monitor the diabetes.

Type 2 diabetes is the most common form of diabetes; it can occur at any age. It was formerly known as adult-onset diabetes or non-insulin-dependent diabetes mellitus (NIDDM). In type 2 diabetes, either the body does not produce enough insulin or the body fails to properly use insulin. This is known as "insulin resistance."

Type 2 diabetes is the milder form of diabetes. It usually develops after age 35. However, the number of children with type 2 diabetes is growing rapidly. This form of diabetes often occurs in obese people or those with a family history of the disease.

Treatment for type 2 diabetes includes careful monitoring of blood glucose levels. It can often be controlled with diet, including weight loss, and medication. Oral medications or injections of insulin will be used to control blood glucose. Smoking will be discouraged. Exercise may be ordered by a doctor to help with weight loss.

People with diabetes may have many different signs and symptoms, including the following:

- Excessive thirst
- Excessive hunger
- Excessive urination
- High blood sugar levels
- Glucose in the urine
- Very dry skin
- Fatigue
- Blurred vision or visual changes
- Slow-healing sores, cuts or bruises
- Tingling or numbness in hands or feet
- Unexplained weight loss
- Increased number of infections

HOT TIP

"The 3 Ps"
There is a trio of symptoms that can signal developing diabetes (Fig. 23-2). "The 3 Ps" are
Polydipsia (excessive thirst)
Polyphagia (excessive hunger)
Polyuria (excessive urination)

Fig. 23-2. *Watch for excessive thirst, hunger, and urination in residents, as these problems can signal diabetes.*

HOT TIP

What is your risk for diabetes?
The American Diabetes Association (ADA) has developed a test to see whether or not a person is at risk for developing pre-diabetes or type 2 diabetes. It is called the "Diabetes Risk Test." You will answer a few questions and your score determines if you are at risk for developing these conditions. For more information, visit www.diabetes.org.

Hypothyroidism (Underactive Thyroid Gland)

Hypothyroidism is a condition in which the body lacks thyroid hormone, which causes body processes to slow down. It is an autoimmune disorder in which the body produces antibodies that attack the thyroid. The antibodies cause the gland to be unable to produce sufficient thyroid hormone.

Hypothyroidism is often caused by Hashimoto's disease, also known as Hashimoto's thyroiditis. Other causes include surgical removal of the thyroid gland, radioactive iodine therapy, and thyroiditis (inflammation of the thyroid). Symptoms of hypothyroidism include:

- fatigue and weakness
- weight gain
- constipation
- intolerance to cold
- dry skin
- thinning hair or hair loss
- brittle hair or fingernails
- slow heart rate
- low blood pressure
- abnormal low temperature
- enlarged thyroid (goiter)
- hoarseness
- heavier than normal menstrual periods or absent menses
- depression

Blood tests and neck examinations diagnose this condition. Treatment is thyroid replacement therapy.

Hyperthyroidism (Overactive Thyroid Gland)

Hyperthyroidism is a condition in which the thyroid gland produces too much thyroid hormone. Body processes speed up, and metabolism increases, causing weight loss, a rapid heartbeat, and sweating. Nervousness and irritability may result.

Hyperthyroidism is primarily caused by Grave's Disease, an autoimmune disorder in which antibodies cause the thyroid gland to produce excessive thyroid hormone. Lumps in the gland, called nodules, thyroiditis, or taking too much thyroid medication can also cause hyperthyroidism. Symptoms of hyperthyroidism include:

- nervousness
- restlessness
- fatigue
- visual problems or eye irritation
- bulging or protruding eyes (exophthalmos)
- trembling, especially of the hands
- intolerance to heat
- excessive perspiration
- rapid heartbeat
- high blood pressure
- increase in appetite
- weight loss
- changes in bowel movements
- irregular or absent menstrual periods
- enlarged thyroid (goiter)

Blood tests and physical examinations help diagnose this condition. Treatment includes anti-thyroid drugs, other medications, called beta-blockers, or radioactive iodine to destroy the thyroid gland. If a goiter is large, surgery may be done. If the thyroid is removed, medication will need to be taken for the rest of the person's life.

5. Describe care guidelines for diabetes

Care of the person with diabetes includes a plan of care associated with every system in the body.

Diabetes must be carefully controlled to prevent complications and serious illness. Follow the care plan closely.

Guidelines
Diabetes

- Observe the skin carefully for sores, blisters, cuts or any other breaks in the skin. Report any of these signs immediately to the nurse (Fig. 23-3). Wounds, skin breaks, and pressure sores must be prevented. A small sore can grow into a large wound, which can require amputation.

- Give frequent skin care. The skin should always be clean and dry.

- Encourage diabetic residents to follow their exercise plans (Fig. 23-4). Exercise will be ordered to help with circulation and maintain a healthy weight. Ambulation, range of motion exercises, or other activity may be ordered. Report any change in the ability to ambulate, muscle weakness, or change in gait.

- Report complaints of pain in the legs immediately to the nurse. This can be a sign of a blood clot.

- Report complaints of numbness and tingling in the arms or legs.

- Perform foot care carefully and as directed. Report any changes in the feet. Never clip or trim any resident's toenails, especially a diabetic's toenails. A nurse or doctor will do this.

- Encourage diabetics to wear proper shoes. Shoes should fit well and not hurt the feet. Shoes made of material that breathes, such as leather or cotton, help prevent moisture build-up. All-cotton socks are best for absorbing sweat. Diabetics should not go barefoot. It is also important for diabetic residents to not wear tight-fitting clothing on the legs and feet.

- As discussed in Chapter 14, carefully following diet instructions is very important to help manage diabetes. Meals must be served at the same time every day. Meals and snacks must be completely eaten in order to keep blood sugar stable. Always report to the nurse if meals and snacks are not being eaten. Report if visitors bring snacks or treats to residents.

Ⓖ The ADA recommends that people with diabetes work with a registered dietitian or a certified diabetes educator (CDE) to help develop individualized meal plans. The Diabetes Food Pyramid may be used to help plan meals. This Pyramid is based on the USDA's old Food Guide Pyramid. The ADA's website has more information.

Ⓖ Keep track of any special tests the resident may have. Tests can affect their diet and insulin dosage. If a resident is fasting for a blood test, for example, food and insulin may need to be withheld until after the test is completed. You may need to notify the nurse immediately when the test has been completed.

Ⓖ Insulin dosage is based upon a variety of factors. Balancing factors like caloric intake, metabolism, exercise levels, the relative condition of the resident and stress levels is important. Report if the resident is not following the care plan exactly.

Ⓖ Perform urine testing and blood glucose tests only as directed and if trained. Not all states allow nursing assistants to perform these tests. Follow facility policy and state regulations on testing.

Ⓖ If any of the following occur, notify the nurse:

- any sign of skin breakdown anywhere on the body, especially on the feet and toes
- visual changes, especially blurred vision
- changes in mobility
- nervousness or anxiety
- dizziness or loss of coordination
- numbness or tingling in the arms and legs
- irritability or confusion
- any changes in appetite or increased thirst

- fruity or sweet-smelling breath
- weight change
- nausea or vomiting
- change in urine output or any signs of urinary tract infection

Fig. 23-3. *Observe the legs and feet carefully when giving care. Poor circulation can increase the risk of infection and the loss of toes, feet, or legs to gangrene.*

Fig. 23-4. *Exercise programs are very important for diabetic residents. They need to increase circulation and maintain a healthy weight.*

Blood Glucose Monitoring

You may assist the nurse with blood glucose monitoring or have special training on how to do this yourself. Monitoring equipment measures the level of glucose in the blood throughout the day. Normal blood glucose is from 70 to 99 mg/dL. Strips are used, along with a blood glucose meter, a special glucose monitoring machine (Fig. 23-5). Make sure that strips have not expired. Always wear gloves when assisting with or performing this procedure. Handle and dispose of sharps and equipment properly.

THE ENDOCRINE SYSTEM

Fig. 23-5. Blood glucose monitoring equipment.

6. Discuss foot care guidelines for diabetes

Quality foot care is vital for people with diabetes. Diabetes weakens the immune system, which reduces resistance to infections. Poor circulation due to the narrowing of the blood vessels also increases the risk of infection. Infections of the feet, when noted in the early stages, can be treated successfully. However, when foot infections are not caught early, amputation of a toe, an entire foot, or a leg may be necessary.

Foot care to prevent infection should be a part of daily care of residents. Keeping the feet clean and dry is a way to help prevent complications. It is important to observe the feet carefully during care.

Guidelines
Safe Diabetic Foot Care

- Inspect and clean resident's feet every day during bathing. Make sure to check between the toes for rashes, cuts, sores, blisters, bruises, or fungus.

- Avoid harsh soaps and hot water when bathing feet. Use only warm water and mild soaps.

- Always dry feet thoroughly, especially between toes. Do not rub the skin; pat it dry.

- Never cut toenails, corns, or calluses for any reason.

- Do not use any object, such as a nail stick, to try to remove dirt from a toenail.

- Use a doctor-recommended cream or lotion on the feet, but avoid the area between the toes. Never use powders.

- Check shoes for rocks or other objects before putting them on residents.

- Remind the resident not to walk around barefoot. Always use clean cotton socks with comfortable shoes or non-skid slippers. Make sure shoes fit properly.

- If any of the following occur, notify the nurse:
  - excessive dryness of the skin of the feet
  - breaks or tears in the skin
  - ingrown nails
  - reddened areas on the feet
  - drainage or bleeding
  - change in color of the skin or nails, especially blackening
  - soft, fragile heels
  - corns, blisters, calluses, or warts
  - blood or drainage on the feet or toes
  - painful, tender, soft, or fragile areas, or burning in the feet

Providing foot care

Equipment: basin, bath mat, soap, lotion, gloves, washcloth, 2 towels, bath thermometer, clean socks

Support the foot and ankle throughout procedure.

1. Identify yourself by name. Identify the resident. Greet the resident by name.

2. Wash your hands.

3. Explain procedure to resident. Speak clearly, slowly, and directly. Maintain face-to-face contact whenever possible. Encourage resident to assist if possible.

4. Provide for the resident's privacy with a curtain, screen, or door.

5. Practice good body mechanics. If the resident is in bed, adjust bed to low level. Lock bed wheels.

6. Fill the basin halfway with warm water. Test water temperature with thermometer or your wrist. Ensure it is safe. Water temperature should be 105° F. Have resident check water temperature. Adjust if necessary.

7. Place basin on the bath mat.

8. Remove resident's socks. Completely submerge resident's feet in water. Soak the feet for five to ten minutes.

9. Put on gloves.

10. Remove one foot from water. Wash entire foot, including between the toes and around nail beds, with soapy washcloth (Fig. 23-6).

Fig. 23-6.

11. Rinse entire foot, including between the toes.

12. Dry entire foot, including between the toes.

13. Repeat steps 10 through 12 for the other foot.

14. Put lotion in hand. Warm lotion by rubbing hands together.

15. Massage lotion into feet (top and bottom), except between the toes, removing excess (if any) with a towel.

16. Assist resident to replace socks.

17. Make resident comfortable.

18. Return bed to low position if raised. Ensure resident's safety. Remove privacy measures.

19. Empty, rinse, and wipe basin. Return to proper storage.

20. Dispose of soiled linen in the proper container.

21. Remove and dispose of gloves properly.

22. Leave call light within resident's reach.

23. Wash your hands.

24. Be courteous and respectful at all times.

25. Report any changes in the resident to the nurse. Document procedure using facility guidelines.

CHAPTER REVIEW

1. Which gland is known as the "master gland" (LO 2)?

2. Where is insulin produced (LO 2)?

3. List four functions of the endocrine system (LO 2).

4. List three normal age-related changes of the endocrine system (LO 3).

5. What are three conditions that make it more likely for a person to have diabetes (LO 4)?

6. List four complications that can result from diabetes (LO 4).

7. What are two ways to delay or prevent pre-diabetes (LO 4)?

8. Which form of diabetes is more common—type 1 or type 2 (LO 4)?

9. List ten symptoms of diabetes (LO 4).

10. List ten symptoms of hypothyroidism (LO 4).

11. List ten symptoms of hyperthyroidism (LO 4).

12. Briefly discuss ten care guidelines for a person with diabetes (LO 5).

13. List seven foot care guidelines for a person with diabetes (LO 6).

14. List ten signs and symptoms to report to the nurse about a resident's feet (LO 6).

24
The Immune and Lymphatic Systems and Cancer

The Amazing Phagocytes

Elie Metchnikoff (1845-1916), a Russian zoologist and microbiologist, discovered that bacteria could be destroyed by certain cells that seemed to consume or "eat" them. He called these cells phagocytes (from Greek meaning "devouring cells") and named the process "phagocytosis." This process is an important part of the immune system's response to harmful bacteria. For this discovery, he won the Nobel Prize in 1908.

"Healing is a matter of time, but it is sometimes also a matter of opportunity."

Hippocrates, 460-377 B.C.

"There are some remedies worse than the disease."

Publilius Syrus, circa 42 B.C.

1. Define important words in this chapter

acquired immune deficiency syndrome (AIDS): disease caused by the human immunodeficiency virus (HIV) in which the body's immune system is weakened and unable to fight infection.

autoimmune disease: a disease in which the body is unable to recognize its own tissue and begins to attack the tissues.

benign: non-cancerous.

biopsy: a removal of a sample of tissue for examination and diagnosis.

cancer: a general term used to describe a disease in which abnormal cells grow in an uncontrolled way.

homophobia: a fear of homosexuality.

human immunodeficiency virus (HIV): a virus that attacks the body's immune system and gradually disables it; eventually causes AIDS.

lymph: a clear yellowish fluid that carries disease-fighting cells called lymphocytes.

malignant: cancerous.

metastasize: to spread from one part of the body to another.

opportunistic infection: an illness caused by organisms due to a person's inability to fight off infection.

tumor: a group of abnormally-growing cells.

2. Explain the structure and function of the immune and lymphatic systems

The Immune System

The immune system protects the body from harmful substances, such as disease-causing bacteria, viruses, and organisms. There are two types of immunity: nonspecific immunity and specific immunity.

Nonspecific Immunity

Nonspecific immunity is present at birth. It protects the body from disease in general. Nonspecific immunity is the first line of defense against invading bacteria or organisms. When foreign materials try to invade the body, it produces a response in which additional white blood cells begin fighting against the disease-causing organisms. Examples of things within the body that help nonspecific immunity are intact (unbroken) skin, saliva, mucous membranes, and tears. The inflammatory response, including redness, swelling, heat and pain is another defense. This removes foreign toxins and other materials and begins tissue repair. Fever also can help fight infection.

Specific Immunity

Specific immunity is a type of immunity that is acquired by the body. Specific immunity is either active or passive. In active immunity, the body manufactures antibodies as a response to an antigen, or foreign substance, in the body. For example, when a person gets chickenpox (varicella-zoster virus), antibodies are created. The body will then "remember" the pathogen each time it is exposed to it in the future. The second time the virus tries to invade the body, the antibodies that had formed during the first illness work to prevent a second infection.

Active immunity is also acquired by a vaccine. Vaccines cause the body to produce antibodies to protect against a particular disease. These antibodies will usually protect the person from getting the disease in the future. Vaccines help people develop immunity to diseases without first having the disease. Vaccines can be made with live organisms or with organisms killed by heat or chemicals.

With passive immunity, a person is given the antibodies needed to defend against the antigen. The antibodies can be passed from mother to baby or via an injection. Passive immunity is temporary because the antibodies have a limited life span.

The Lymphatic System

The lymphatic system is composed of the lymph, lymph vessels, lymph nodes, spleen and the thymus gland. The lymphatic system produces and moves lymph fluid from the body's tissues to the circulatory system. The lymphatic system works to remove excess fluids and waste products from the tissues. It transports fat and vitamins from the gastrointestinal tract to the circulatory system. The lymphatic system also helps the immune system fight infection.

Lymph is a clear yellowish fluid that moves into the lymph system from the tiny capillaries in the circulatory system. Lymph carries disease-fighting cells called lymphocytes. The lymph fluid flows in only one direction.

Lymphatic vessels, or capillaries, are tiny vessels found all over the body. They carry the lymph from the tissues into larger lymphatic vessels. While in the vessels, the lymph travels through and is filtered by the lymph nodes. The larger lymphatic vessels transport lymph into the lymph ducts, from which the lymph drains back into the blood.

The lymph nodes are clumps of lymphatic tissue found in groups along the lymph vessels. These nodes work as filters to cleanse the lymph fluid of microorganisms, such as bacteria, along with other foreign substances. Lymph nodes are strategically located in places where pathogens can be trapped and prevented from harming the body (Fig. 24-1). Tonsils are large clumps of lymphatic tissue at the back of the oral cavity at the entrance to the throat (pharynx). Tonsils work to prevent microorganisms from entering the body, especially through the mouth or nose.

The spleen, an organ, is the biggest cluster of lymph tissue in the human body. One of its main functions is to work as a type of storage shed for blood. The spleen works as a filter to cleanse the blood of old red blood cells and bacteria.

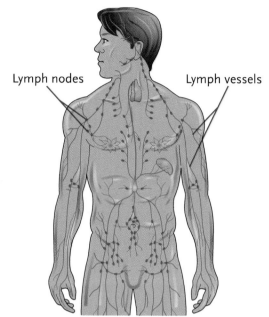

Fig. 24-1. Lymph nodes work as filters and are located throughout the body.

The thymus gland is located in the upper chest, just behind the sternum. Its duty is to make T-cells, or CD4 lymphocytes, which attack and destroy specific types of pathogens. The thymus reaches its greatest size at puberty and shrinks as we become adults. Once its work is completed, the gland turns into fat and other tissue.

The functions of the immune and lymphatic systems are:

- Protect against the invasion of foreign substances and pathogens

- Return extra fluid to the circulatory system

Destination: Homeostasis

A hemorrhage is an excessive, sudden loss of blood, that occurs either externally or internally. When a hemorrhage occurs, the spleen readies for action. The blood that the spleen has held for the body in its reservoir (as much as a full pint), is released into the bloodstream. This release of blood helps the body's blood level and blood pressure return to normal. When bleeding has stopped and the body's blood supply and blood pressure have returned to normal levels, homeostasis is restored.

HOT TIP

Allergies

Allergies occur in people who are hypersensitive to a foreign substance called an allergen. Examples of allergens include pollen, dust, molds, colognes, pets, latex, and certain foods (Fig. 24-2). The immune system responds to the allergen by releasing histamine and other substances that cause the characteristic runny nose and watery eyes. These allergens can trigger a life-threatening response. This is called anaphylaxis, anaphylactic reaction or anaphylactic shock. When this happens, help must be obtained immediately. The bronchi narrow, causing wheezing and difficulty breathing. Loss of consciousness and death may result if not treated promptly.

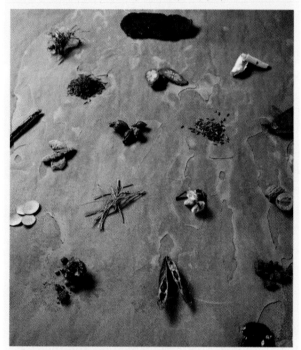

Fig. 24-2. Allergens include pollen, grass, molds, fungi and many other substances.

3. Discuss changes in the immune and lymphatic systems due to aging

Normal age-related changes for the immune and lymphatic systems include the following:

- Immune system weakens, causing increased risk of all types of infections.

- Antibody response slows.

- T-cells decrease in number.

- Response to vaccines decreases.

4. Describe the most common disorder of the immune system

Acquired Immunodeficiency Syndrome (AIDS)

Acquired immune deficiency syndrome (AIDS) is an illness caused by the **human immunodeficiency virus (HIV)**. HIV attacks the body's immune system and damages or destroys its cells. HIV gradually weakens and disables the immune system. AIDS is caused by acquiring the HIV virus through blood or body fluids from an infected person. AIDS is the final stage of HIV infection. It can take years for HIV to develop into AIDS.

High-risk behaviors can spread HIV/AIDS. There are specific behaviors that put people at high risk for HIV/AIDS. The most common methods of transmission of HIV are:

* Unprotected or poorly-protected oral, vaginal or anal sex with an infected person

* Sharing drug needles or syringes

* Transmission from an infected mother to her newborn during pregnancy or birth, or by breastfeeding

In the healthcare setting, infections can be spread through accidental contact with contaminated blood or body fluids, needles or other sharp objects, or contaminated supplies or equipment (Fig. 24-3).

Fig. 24-3. *In health care, contact with contaminated needles or sharps is the most common way for HIV to be transmitted. Handle sharps carefully and dispose of them properly.*

Common Misconceptions About HIV Transmission

The HIV virus cannot survive outside the body for very long. Because of this, the CDC has identified common activities that do not spread HIV:

* hugging another person

* shaking hands

* sitting on a toilet seat

* drinking water from a drinking fountain

* touching a doorknob, telephone, table, or chair

* using drinking glasses or dishes of infected person

* being bitten by mosquitoes

Ways to protect against the spread of HIV/AIDS are:

* Practice Standard Precautions on every person in your care.

* Be careful when handling any type of sharps and dispose of sharps properly.

* Cover any cuts, sores, tears, breaks, or rashes before caring for residents.

* Never share needles or syringes.

* Do not have unprotected sex. Use condoms if you have sex.

* Stay in a monogamous relationship. Monogamous means having only one sexual partner. You and your partner can be tested for bloodborne diseases like AIDS and hepatitis before having sex.

* Practice abstinence. Abstinence means not having sexual contact with anyone.

* Get tested for HIV and re-tested if necessary. Remember that it can take up to six months from the time you are infected for HIV to be detected in the blood.

The beginning stages of HIV show flu-like symptoms along with swollen glands. Symptoms like headache, fever, fatigue and swollen lymph glands can appear, last for a few months, and then disappear. Additional symptoms may appear soon after or they can take many years to develop.

Over time, the HIV virus destroys T-cells, or CD4 lymphocytes, which are a type of white blood cell. Specifically, the virus reduces the number of the T-cells that work to fight infections in the body. This weakens the immune system and makes the person more susceptible to illness. The diagnosis of AIDS is made when the number of T-cells is less than 200 per cubic millimeter of blood. A person will then generally begin to develop other conditions, symptoms, and diseases that are commonly seen with AIDS.

Signs and symptoms of HIV infection and AIDS include the following:

- flu-like symptoms, including fever, cough, and severe or constant fatigue
- headaches
- loss of appetite
- weight loss
- night sweats
- shaking chills
- dry cough
- shortness of breath
- swollen lymph nodes
- sore throat
- cold sores or fever blisters on the lips
- mouth sores
- white patches in the mouth or on the tongue
- cauliflower-like warts on the skin and in the mouth
- bleeding, inflamed gums
- yeast infections
- skin rashes or sores
- bruising that does not go away
- dry skin
- nausea and vomiting
- blurred vision
- memory loss

Other diseases can develop in people who have AIDS. Due to the weakened immune system, opportunistic infections can occur and may be fatal. An **opportunistic infection** is an illness caused by organisms due to a person's inability to fight off infection. Some of these infections do not cause disease in persons with normal immune systems. Lack of treatment for HIV/AIDS can increase the risk of serious complications and death from these diseases.

Other diseases that can develop in people with AIDS are pneumocystis carinii pneumonia (PCP), a lung infection, and cryptococcal meningitis, a nervous system disorder. People with AIDS can also develop certain types of cancers. Cervical cancer and a form of cancer called Kaposi's sarcoma are examples. Kaposi's sarcoma is a form of skin cancer that appears as purple, red, or brown skin lesions (Fig. 24-4). The lesions may be painful.

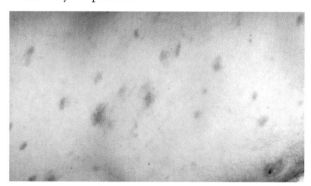

Fig. 24-4. *A purple, red, or brown skin lesion called Kaposi's sarcoma can develop when a person has AIDS.*

In the late stages of AIDS, a form of dementia called AIDS dementia complex (ADC) can develop due to the damage to the central nervous system. Symptoms of ADC include memory loss, limited attention span, irritability, poor coordination, lack of judgment, withdrawal from social situations and depression.

There is no cure for this disease. There is no vaccine to prevent the disease. Without medication, the HIV-infected person's weakened resistance to infections may lead to AIDS and eventually to death. Many people are living longer with HIV by taking combinations of medications every day. HAART, or highly active antiretroviral therapy, has been shown to suppress the HIV virus and has reduced the number of AIDS deaths in the U.S. However, these treatments must generally be taken at specific times throughout the day. They are very expensive and can produce many unpleasant side effects. Gastrointestinal symptoms like nausea, vomiting and diarrhea, as well as fever, and skin rashes are some of the side effects. Certain medications can be effective, but the length of time they will continue to work for each infected person varies.

Autoimmune Diseases

The immune system protects the body from microorganisms and toxic substances. With an **autoimmune disease**, the body is unable to recognize its own tissue. The immune mechanism sees the normal body tissues as foreign and begins to attack the tissues.

Types of organs and tissues that may be affected by this disease are blood cells, the pancreas, the joints, and the skin. Examples of autoimmune diseases are systemic lupus erythematosis (SLE) and rheumatoid arthritis (RA) (Chapter 21).

Autoimmune disorders have no known cause. Some theories suggest that causes are genetic links, specific microorganisms, or medications that trigger these disorders.

Signs and symptoms vary and depend upon the disease and the organ(s) or tissues affected. Fever, fatigue, and dizziness are commonly seen with many disorders.

Specific blood tests help diagnose certain autoimmune disorders. Treatment and outlook will depend upon the disorder. The person may require hormone supplements, medications, blood transfusions, or insulin.

5. Discuss infection control guidelines for a resident with HIV/AIDS

Overall care of a resident with HIV/AIDS involves protection from infections, providing a safe environment, offering emotional support, and managing symptoms. Follow all infection control precautions. It is worth saying again: the most important reason to always follow Standard Precautions is that you cannot tell by looking at

people whether or not they have a bloodborne disease, such as HIV/AIDS. Follow Transmission-Based Precautions if they are ordered in addition to Standard Precautions. See Chapter 6 for more information on Standard and Transmission-Based Precautions.

If you are practicing all infection control precautions correctly, there should be no differences in how you care for a known AIDS resident and how you provide care for other residents. Casual contact cannot spread HIV/AIDS.

Guidelines
Infection Control for HIV/AIDS

Ⓖ Always follow proper infection control procedures and Standard Precautions with all residents.

Ⓖ Per Standard Precautions, wear gloves and other PPE, such as goggles, if you anticipate having contact with blood or other body fluids that might contain blood, like urine and feces (Fig. 24-5). Wear goggles, masks and/or face shields when splashes or spills may occur.

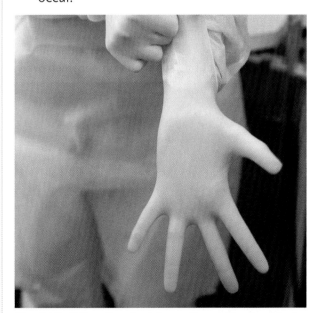

Fig. 24-5. Follow Standard Precautions with all residents in your care. Wear gloves if you may come into contact with blood, body fluids, non-intact skin or mucous membranes.

- Cover all open sores, cuts, abrasions, rashes, or skin breaks or tears with appropriate bandages or dressings before performing care. Notify the nurse if you have cuts, sores, or breaks in the skin before beginning care.

- Wash hands and any other area of the body immediately after contact with blood or other body fluids.

- Handle sharps carefully. Dispose of all sharps properly and safely. Never attempt to re-cap sharps.

- Remind residents and visitors to wash their hands frequently to avoid infection.

- Do not share residents' personal items, such as toothbrushes, hair brushes, razors, etc., with other residents. Put equipment away in its proper place after it has been used.

- Properly disinfect surfaces soiled with blood or body fluids according to facility policy.

RESIDENTS' RIGHTS

HIV Testing and Confidentiality

The right to confidentiality is especially important to people with HIV/AIDS because others may pass judgment on people with this disease. A person with HIV/AIDS cannot be fired from a job because of the disease; however, a healthcare worker with HIV/AIDS may be reassigned to job duties with a lower risk of transmitting the disease and a reduced risk of acquiring certain infections from patients.

HIV testing requires consent. That means no one can force you to be tested for HIV unless you agree. HIV test results are confidential and should not be shared with a person's family, friends, or employer without his or her consent. If you are HIV-positive, consider confiding in your supervisor so your assignments can be adjusted to avoid putting you at high risk for exposure to infections. Everyone has a right to privacy regarding their health status. Do not discuss a resident's status with anyone except during reports and rounds (Chapter 3).

6. Discuss care guidelines for a resident with HIV/AIDS

Helping residents with HIV or AIDS avoid infection and live safely and comfortably is important. Your quality care and attention may go a long way in helping residents with HIV/AIDS.

Guidelines
HIV/AIDS

- Wash your hands often and help residents to wash their hands.

- Disinfect surfaces in the resident's room and bathroom often.

- Protect the resident from people having known contagious diseases, including the common cold virus.

- Change linen whenever it is soiled. Linen should be clean and dry and should lie flat, without wrinkles (Fig. 24-6).

Fig. 24-6. *Hospital corners help keep the flat sheet wrinkle-free, which helps promote comfort and prevent pressure sores.*

- Observe the skin closely for skin breakdown. Keeping skin clean and dry will help prevent skin breakdown. Follow the care plan on the use of soaps and other cleansers.

- Change positions every two hours or as directed. Take great care when moving and positioning residents to reduce bruising.

- Give back rubs for comfort.

- Monitor vital signs often, especially temperature. Fever can occur with infections.

- Residents with HIV/AIDS may have fatigue and severe weakness. Allow enough rest and recognize limitations.

- Ambulate carefully. Provide assistance as needed.

- Allow plenty of time to perform ADLs and help as needed.

- Perform range of motion exercises as ordered (Chapter 25).

- Give quality mouth care frequently. Special mouth rinses can be ordered for mouth sores.

- Use special soft toothbrushes or swabs when cleaning the mouth and performing oral care.

- Because weight loss is a problem for people with HIV/AIDS, special diets may be ordered to assist with maintaining or gaining weight. For example, a high-calorie diet can help increase weight. Special liquid drinks fortified with extra protein can be used. Report to the nurse if a resident does not seem to be eating or enjoying his food.

- Special diets may also be ordered to help prevent complications. For example, a high-fiber diet may aggravate diarrhea, so it will be avoided. Soft or pureed foods may be easier to swallow for residents who have mouth infections. Cool or warm food, rather than hot, may be easier to eat. Eliminating spices and foods high in acids may be ordered. Encourage residents to follow their special diets.

- Give fluids as ordered. Filtered water may be ordered. If so, make sure the resident does not drink regular water or fluids made with regular water, such as iced tea.

- Small meals given throughout the day can help nausea, vomiting and diarrhea. Extra fluids may be ordered to help replace fluid lost. A BRAT diet (bananas, rice, apples, and toast) can also help diarrhea.

- Carefully measure weight and intake and output.

- AIDS residents may be prone to diarrhea. Offer a trip to the bathroom or bedpan as often as needed. A resident with AIDS may benefit from being in the bed nearest the bathroom.

- Encourage residents to be as independent as possible.

- Give emotional support, as well as physical care. A resident with AIDS may have been abandoned by family or friends due to the fear of the disease itself. Some people avoid a person with AIDS due to **homophobia**, or a fear of homosexuality. They may also have lost friends who have died from AIDS. Emotions he or she may be experiencing include anxiety, stress, fear, guilt, sadness, depression, and loneliness. It is important to treat residents with respect and help provide the emotional support they need. Listen if the resident wants to talk.

- Other support systems include family, friends, the person's clergyperson, along with various HIV/AIDS support groups. Special religious or community groups may be of assistance. Depending on your community, many resources and services may be available for people with HIV/AIDS. These include counseling, meal services, access to experimental drugs and other services. Look in the phone book for resources available in your area, or speak to your supervisor if you feel a resident with HIV/AIDS needs more help. Report any comments about suicide immediately to the nurse.

- Notify the nurse if any of the following occur:

  - loss of appetite, nausea, vomiting, or diarrhea

  - weight loss

  - reduced intake of fluids

  - mouth sores or discomfort

  - dysphagia (difficulty swallowing)

  - bleeding from anywhere on the body

  - bruising of the skin

  - pressure sores

  - cracks, breaks, rashes, lumps, or sores anywhere on the skin

  - blood in the stool

  - changes in vital signs, especially fever

  - nervousness, withdrawal, severe mood swings, or depression

  - any behavior that puts themselves or others at risk; suicidal thoughts or comments

Residents' Rights and HIV/AIDS

Spend quality time with residents who have HIV or AIDS. This may mean sitting and listening quietly to their concerns. It can be reading to them if they wish. Encouraging participation in activities of their choice may be helpful. Do not avoid residents who have this disease. HIV/AIDS is not transmitted by breathing the same air as someone who is infected. These residents need the same attentive and thoughtful care you give all of your residents.

Pets and People with HIV/AIDS

Some facilities have one or more cats and/or dogs living on the premises. Due to their weakened immune systems, HIV- or AIDS-infected persons may not be able to be around pets due to the risk of different types of infection. Follow facility policy. Always wash your hands with soap and water after touching a pet, and before touching any resident. Ask visitors to do the same.

For more information about HIV/AIDS and other bloodborne pathogens, see Chapter 6.

7. Describe cancer

Cancer is a general term used to describe a disease in which abnormal cells grow in an uncontrolled way. These cancerous cells do not die like normal cells do. They live longer than normal cells and continue to develop new abnormal cells.

Cancer usually occurs in the form of a tumor that grows on or within the human body. A **tumor** is a group of abnormally-growing cells. Tumors are either **benign** (non-cancerous) or **malignant** (cancerous). Benign tumors grow slowly and do not spread to other parts of the body. Malignant tumors grow rapidly and invade surrounding tissue.

Cancer can act in different ways. It can **metastasize**, or spread, to other areas of the body. Oncology is the branch of medicine that deals with the study of and treatment of cancer.

Risk factors for cancer include the following:

*   Age
*   Race
*   Gender
*   Family history
*   Tobacco use
*   Alcohol use
*   Poor diet/obesity
*   Lack of exercise
*   Chemicals and food additives
*   Radiation
*   Sun exposure (Fig. 24-7)

Fig. 24-7. Prolonged sun exposure puts a person at risk for skin cancer.

There is no known cure for cancer. However, when cancer is caught early, it can be treated effectively and controlled. The American Cancer Society has identified these signs of cancer:

*   fever
*   fatigue
*   unexplained weight loss
*   pain
*   skin changes, such as change in skin color (e.g. jaundice)
*   new mole or a change in the appearance of an existing mole or wart
*   change in bowel/bladder function
*   a sore that does not heal
*   unusual bleeding/discharge

- any thickening in breast, scrotum or other areas
- indigestion, difficulty swallowing
- nagging cough or hoarseness

A diagnosis of cancer is made after various tests, such as a biopsy, have been performed. A **biopsy** is a removal of a sample of tissue for examination and diagnosis (Fig. 24-8). After the diagnosis of cancer is made, the treatment plan is developed. Treatment is based on whether or not the cancer has spread to other parts of the body. The choice of therapy is determined by the person's prognosis, or outlook. Common treatments for cancer, which may be used in combination are as follows:

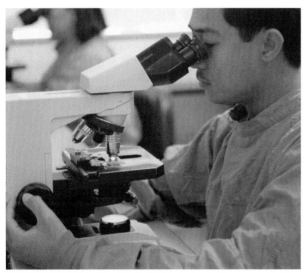

Fig. 24-8. Tissue that is biopsied is checked for malignant cells.

Surgery to remove malignant tumors can be performed for some types of cancer. The goal of the operation(s) is to try to remove as much of the cancer as possible. Surgery is generally performed for cancers of the breast, skin, and colon.

Radiation therapy (radiotherapy) uses high-energy rays to attempt to destroy cancer cells in a specific area (Fig. 24-9). It can also be used to control cancerous growths. Radiation treatments do not cause pain. However, side effects of radiation therapy include skin irritation and burns, which may cause pain. Radiation therapy may also cause an increased risk of infection.

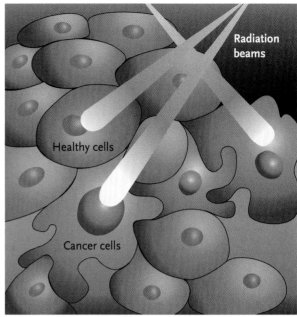

Fig. 24-9. Radiation is targeted at cancer cells, but it also destroys some healthy cells in its path.

Chemotherapy involves chemical agents or medications being administered, usually intravenously, to kill malignant cells and tissues. Chemotherapy is chosen for cancers that have spread. It can also be used to slow growth of a cancer or to prevent the cancer in a certain area from spreading. There are many severe side effects to this treatment, including bone or joint pain, temporary hair loss, nausea and vomiting, diarrhea, fatigue, mouth sores, peripheral neuropathy (Chapter 23), and a higher risk of infections. Chemotherapeutic agents are generally given into a vein through an IV, but some are given by mouth or by injection.

Hormone therapy uses medications to alter the hormones in the body. This can be effective when the tumors rely on specific hormones to survive and grow. Hormone therapy reduces certain hormones in the body. It also changes the ability of the tumors to use the hormones. Side effects include hot flashes, weight gain and fluid retention.

Immunotherapy is another form of cancer treatment. This therapy uses the body's immune system to fight the malignant tumors. One form of immunotherapy is a cancer vaccine. Another is through the administration of antibodies. Immunotherapy works in different ways. One way it works is to interfere with the growth of cancer cells. Side effects depend upon the specific treatment used. They include fever, weakness, and nausea, vomiting and diarrhea. This form of therapy is often combined with chemotherapy or other cancer therapies.

Remission is the reduction in or disappearance of signs and symptoms of cancer. It can be partial or complete.

Palliative care will be provided for someone with advanced cancer. This type of care works to relieve the symptoms and to reduce pain and suffering caused by the disease. See Chapter 27 for more information on palliative care.

8. Discuss care guidelines for a resident with cancer

The resident with cancer will require careful and attentive physical and emotional care.

Guidelines
Cancer

- **Skin care**. Observe the skin carefully to help prevent pressure sores. Follow any special skin care orders exactly (for example: no hot or cold packs, no soap, lotion, or other cosmetics, no garters or tight stockings). Special mattresses or pads used in beds and chairs can help reduce the risk of pressure sores. Keep skin clean and dry. Apply lotion to dry skin if ordered. Do not use lotion on areas having radiation therapy. Do not remove any markings that are used with radiation therapy. If skin problems or infections occur, they can cause odors. Notify the nurse if you observe any signs of infection, such as swelling, warmth, redness, or draining wounds.

- **Self-image**. Hair loss, weakness, changed appearance, and dependency on caregivers can change a person's self-image. Help residents stay clean and well-groomed. Offer wigs, scarves, or hats for hair loss. Assist with application of make-up as requested.

- **Oral care**. Give oral care often and help as needed. Be gentle when brushing teeth; soft brushes or special swabs can help with mouth pain or sores or lip sores. Mild mouth rinses (avoid mouthwashes) can reduce bad taste in the mouth due to medication or vomiting.

- **Pain**. Cancer can cause severe pain. It can affect the ability to sleep, eat, and move about. Medications and other measures are used to treat pain. Be alert for signs of pain and notify the nurse as soon as pain occurs. Provide comfort measures to reduce pain. Give back rubs, and help residents change positions in bed or in a chair. Other measures include playing soft music, reading, or talking quietly with residents.

  Pain medications can cause side effects, including constipation, upset stomach, and fatigue. Notify the nurse if these side effects occur. If a resident has a transdermal patch on the skin to help with pain, report any redness, swelling, or irritation. The nurse is responsible for applying and removing these patches. Notify the nurse if you see more than one patch on the resident's body.

  The resident may be using a PCA pump for pain relief. A PCA pump, or patient-controlled analgesia, allows the person to press a button which releases pain medication (Fig. 24-10). Observe and report redness, swelling, and warmth around the insertion site.

Fig. 24-10. A patient-controlled analgesia (PCA) pump.
(Photo courtesy of McKinley Medical www.mckinleymed.com.)

People with cancer may have a specific type of severe pain, called "breakthrough pain." This type of pain can happen unexpectedly and is often not controlled by regular doses of pain medication. Report signs of pain to the nurse. Guided imagery and relaxation techniques can help with breakthrough pain.

- **Vital signs**. Changes in vital signs can occur with cancer and with cancer therapy. Monitor all vital signs, especially temperature. Fever can occur with some forms of cancer therapy. Report changes in vital signs to the nurse.

- **Mobility**. Residents with cancer may have fatigue and weakness. Allow plenty of time for rest and recognize limitations. Help resident understand why he feels so tired. Gently assist with ambulation if needed. Change position every two hours or as directed. Be careful when moving and positioning residents to reduce bruising.

- **Nutrition**. Good nutrition is important for people with cancer. They need to eat and drink enough to maintain their energy levels. Unintended weight loss can occur with cancer or with cancer treatment. Provide small, frequent meals to reduce nausea and help prevent weight loss. Serve favorite foods and keep nutritious snacks available. Provide food whenever hunger occurs, as allowed. Try cool or cold food if hot foods increase nausea. Cut food into small pieces if necessary. Use plastic utensils if silver utensils cause a bitter taste in the mouth. Weigh residents as ordered, and report weight loss or gain. Encourage fluids as allowed. Fortified liquid supplements may be ordered. Carefully monitor intake and output and report changes.

- **Bladder and bowel changes**. Bladder and bowel habits can be affected in those with cancer. Urine may have blood in it and output may decrease. Urine can become more concentrated and have an odor. Diarrhea can occur, along with blood in the stool. Assist residents to the bathroom or offer the bedpan often. Give catheter care as needed. Carefully measure output. Test stool as ordered for hidden (occult) blood.

- **Mental status and emotional needs**. Some people with cancer want to talk about their diagnosis and treatment; others withdraw and avoid discussing their disease. Be sensitive to this, and follow residents' wishes. Listen and allow them to express their feelings. Spend as much time with residents as possible (Fig. 24-11). Encourage involvement in activities if possible. There are many support groups available for people with cancer. The nurse can ask the social worker to help the resident contact a support group. When talking with residents, do not use clichés such as, "You will be just fine." Provide support during painful episodes and difficult times. Remind residents that there can still be good days and special times ahead. Observe and report signs of depression, including comments about suicide.

Fig. 24-11. *Give residents with cancer as much emotional support as possible.*

- Notify the nurse if the following occur:
  - pain or increased pain
  - changes in vital signs, especially fever
  - signs of any new bumps or lumps or any other changes in the skin
  - rashes, cracks, sores, breaks or reddened areas on the skin
  - odors
  - burns or skin irritation
  - bruising of the skin

- difficulty with ambulation
- fainting
- increased fatigue or weakness
- chest pain or tightness
- shortness of breath
- appetite changes or weight loss
- difficulty chewing or swallowing
- dry, sore mouth and mouth or lip sores
- inflammation or irritation of the mucous membranes in the mouth
- bleeding from gums or anywhere inside the mouth
- nausea or vomiting
- flatus, diarrhea, or constipation
- blood in the stool
- change in output
- any change in the urine or blood in the urine
- urinary tract infection
- change in mental status or confusion
- anxiety, fear or angry feelings
- signs of depression

RESIDENTS' RIGHTS

Cancer

The term "cancer" may frighten you. However, understanding the facts may help lessen your fears. Cancer is not a contagious disease. It cannot be transmitted through touch or hugs or by being close to a person who has it. Do not avoid residents who have cancer. Spend as much time as possible with them. It is the caring and right thing to do.

CHAPTER REVIEW

1. Briefly describe nonspecific immunity and specific immunity (LO 2).
2. Give one example of active immunity and one example of passive immunity (LO 2).
3. What is the function of lymph (LO 2)?
4. List four normal age-related changes of the immune and lymphatic systems (LO 3).
5. How is HIV transmitted (LO 4)?

6. List four risk factors for acquiring HIV (LO 4).
7. List six common activities that do not spread HIV (LO 4).
8. Is there a cure for HIV or AIDS (LO 4)?
9. What is an autoimmune disease (LO 4)?
10. List six infection control guidelines for HIV/AIDS (LO 5).
11. Can a person be forced to be tested for HIV without agreeing to the test (LO 5)?
12. Can an HIV test result be shared with anyone requesting information (LO 5)?
13. List 15 care guidelines for a resident with HIV/AIDS (LO 6).
14. What is the difference between benign and malignant tumors (LO 7)?
15. List nine signs of cancer identified by the ACS (LO 7).
16. Briefly describe five treatments for cancer: surgery, radiation therapy, chemotherapy, hormone therapy, immunotherapy (LO 7).
17. For each of these topics—skin care, self-image, oral care, pain management, vital signs, mobility, nutrition, bladder and bowel changes, mental status and emotional needs—list one way a nursing assistant can help a resident with cancer (LO 8).

25
Rehabilitation and Restorative Care

A View from the Past: Rehabilitation

In 1918 there were so many injured veterans returning from World War I that doctors in the United States developed an idea about how to bring an injured person to the point where he would be able to return to work. Following WWI, the idea of rehabilitation grew. Facilities and programs were created, and when the thousands of victims of the war returned to the U.S. (many without arms or legs), they were able to begin their rehabilitation.

"You cannot run away from a weakness. You must some time fight it out or perish . . ."

Robert Louis Stevenson, 1850-1894

"The best of healers is good cheer."

Pindar, 522-438 B.C.

1. Define important words in this chapter

abduction: moving a body part away from the midline of the body.

active assisted range of motion (AAROM): exercises to put a joint through its full arc of motion that are done by a resident with some help from a staff member.

active range of motion (AROM): exercises to put a joint through its full arc of motion that are done by a resident alone, without help.

adaptive devices: special equipment that helps a person who is ill or disabled perform ADLs; also called assistive devices.

adduction: moving a body part toward the midline of the body.

assistive devices: special equipment that helps a person who is ill or disabled perform ADLs; also called adaptive devices.

dorsiflexion: bending backward.

extension: straightening a body part.

flexion: bending a body part.

foot drop: weakness of muscles in the feet and ankles that interferes with the ability to flex the ankles and walk normally.

hyperextension: extending a joint beyond its normal range of motion.

orthotic devices: devices applied externally to limbs to support, protect, improve function and prevent complications.

passive range of motion (PROM): exercises to put a joint through its full arc of motion that are done by staff, without the resident's help.

physiatrists: doctors who specialize in rehabilitation.

pronation: turning downward.

range of motion (ROM): exercises that put a joint through its full arc of motion.

rehabilitation: care that is managed by professionals to restore a person to the highest possible level of functioning after an illness or injury.

restorative care: care used after rehabilitation to maintain a person's function and increase independence.

rotation: turning the joint.

supination: turning upward.

2. Discuss rehabilitation and restorative care

A disability results from physical, personal, and environmental factors that, when combined, limit a person's ability to function properly. When a person develops a change in his ability to function, rehabilitation may be necessary. **Rehabilitation** is care used to restore a person to his highest level of functioning possible after an accident, illness or injury. Rehabilitation revolves around holistic care, or treating the whole person. All of the person's needs are assessed, including his psychological needs. The type of rehabilitation ordered and how much progress is made depends upon many factors. Some of these factors include the following:

- how soon rehabilitation began

- any pre-existing diseases or injuries that the resident may have

- overall motivation of the resident

- type of facility where the resident is living

- combined efforts of the staff and the resident's family and friends

- attitude of the rehabilitation team

- consistency in following the care plan

For rehabilitation to succeed, all staff members must work together to return the person to his highest level of functioning. The rehabilitation team is made up of highly-skilled and trained professionals, including (Fig. 25-1):

- **physiatrists** (doctors who specialize in rehabilitation) and other doctors

- speech, physical and occupational therapists

- nurses

- social workers

- discharge planners

- nursing assistants

- resident

- resident's family and friends

Fig. 25-1. *A team of specialists, including doctors and physical therapists, helps assist residents with rehabilitation.*

The nursing staff will develop a care plan based on goals for restoring and maintaining the resident's function. Each body system will be considered when creating the care plan. For example, the team will work to prevent contractures, a musculoskeletal condition and a serious complication of immobility.

Goal-setting is done with the participation of all departments. For each task requiring improvement, the team will develop specific steps to meet the goals. The rehabilitation team will carefully follow the goals listed in each resident's care plan. The goals of rehabilitative care include the following:

- Assist the resident in maintaining and/or regaining the ability to perform ADLs

- Promote resident's independence and help resident adapt to the new disability

- Prevent complications of immobility

Nursing assistants are vital members of the rehabilitation team. OBRA states that NAs must be properly trained to work with residents who are in a rehabilitative setting. Not only will they provide quality physical care, they will also help with the resident's emotional needs. Nursing assistants should work to make the environment as safe and secure for the resident as possible.

When the goals of rehabilitation have been met, restorative care may be ordered. **Restorative**

care works to maintain a person's functioning and to increase independence.

During rehabilitation and restorative care, the team must work together to prevent complications. The attitude of staff has a great impact on the success of the program. Follow these guidelines to help give quality care to residents in these programs:

Guidelines
Rehabilitation and Restorative Care

Ⓖ Understand the diagnosis and the disability. Know any limitations the resident may have. Be familiar with the resident's ability to perform ADLs. OBRA requires that residents must receive all of the therapy listed in the care plan each day.

Ⓖ Be patient with the resident and his family and friends. Offer praise frequently, even if the improvement is small. For example, a resident can hold a spoon on Monday. On Tuesday, he is able to lift the spoon. Praise each success.

Ⓖ Maintain a positive attitude at all times. Be empathetic. A happy, optimistic and positive attitude can be contagious (Fig. 25-2). Never become frustrated or angry with the resident or his family or friends. The nursing staff will set the stage for the care.

Ⓖ Spend as much time as possible listening to the resident's thoughts and feelings about the process. Sitting quietly and listening can be very helpful.

Ⓖ Provide plenty of privacy during the process. It helps to avoid distractions and potential embarrassment.

Ⓖ Encourage residents' independence, along with personal choice. They must do as much for themselves as possible. Ask family and friends to encourage residents' independence too. See Learning Objective 3 of this chapter for more on independence.

Ⓖ Encourage as much daily activity as possible. Inactivity causes complications and can cause setbacks in rehabilitation, along with other problems.

Ⓖ Accept that the resident may have setbacks. Each person is different. Focus on the things that the resident can do, and not what they cannot do.

Ⓖ Nursing assistants are often the first staff members who observe a potential problem or complication with the rehabilitative process. Report any of the following signs and symptoms to the nurse:

- lack of motivation
- signs of withdrawal or depression
- any change in ability, positive or negative
- decreased strength
- change in ability to perform range of motion

Fig. 25-2. *Be optimistic and encouraging. Your good attitude has a positive effect on residents.*

HOT TIP

Behavior Management
Residents in rehabilitation may exhibit combative or violent behavior, such as yelling or hitting. When this happens, a behavior management program can be used to try to reduce these behaviors. This is also called behavior modification. General techniques for helping prevent or eliminate difficult behaviors are to praise instances of good behavior and to involve residents in their favorite activities. When combative or inappropriate behavior occurs, try to redirect the resident's attention to something else. If that does not work, quietly remove the resident from the area. See Chapters 4 and 22 for more information on dealing with behavior problems.

The Restorative Environment

A resident's surroundings are very important to the success of rehabilitation. The environment should be set up to encourage a positive outcome. The rehabilitation team should

- Create a secure, quiet, and pleasant rehabilitative environment.
- Encourage residents to make decisions.
- Ensure that residents are bathed, dressed and well-groomed every day.
- Maintain privacy and allow for private visits from family and friends.
- Encourage friendly relationships between residents.
- Spend time with residents as often as possible.
- Encourage participation in appropriate activities.

3. Describe the importance of promoting independence

An injury or illness that results in a loss of function can cause dependence on others for help with daily activities. Residents may never have needed help before with bathing, dressing, eating or other tasks during their entire adult lives. Being required to accept help with ADLs can cause anger, frustration, depression, and embarrassment, as well as a decrease in abilities.

As you have learned, promoting each resident's independence is an important duty of the care team. Encouraging independence has positive effects on self-image, attitude, and abilities. Sometimes it will appear easier for you to do things for residents, rather than allowing them to accomplish tasks independently. However, let residents do as much as they can for themselves, regardless of how long it takes or how poorly they are able to do it. Even if you think you could do a task better or faster, be patient. Encourage each resident to perform as much self-care as possible (Fig. 25-3). Independence helps self-esteem, along with speeding recovery. Self-care also helps the body stay active and prevents complications of immobility.

Fig. 25-3. *Encourage residents to perform self-care no matter how long it takes them to do it.*

Cues

A common approach to promoting independence with rehabilitative care is to try cues. Cues can be verbal or physical. A verbal cue is a short sequence of words that directs the person to complete a specific step. For example, you say, "Take a sip of water." A physical cue is showing the person how to do the activity. For example, you place your hand over the resident's hand around the cup, helping him bring it to his mouth for a drink. Cues may be used with residents during rehabilitation and also for residents with other conditions, such as Alzheimer's disease. See Chapters 14 and 22 for more information on cues.

The Right To Make Choices

Residents should make as many choices as possible. They have the right to choose their food, clothing, doctors, visitors, and how to spend their time. This is not just their legal right; it also helps to encourage independence.

4. Explain the complications of immobility and describe how exercise helps maintain health

Activity is an essential part of a person's life. When a person becomes immobile and inactive, the body does not respond well. Complications that result from a lack of exercise and activity, organized by body system, include the following:

- Integumentary: pressure sores and slow-healing wounds
- Circulatory: blood clots, especially in the legs

- Respiratory: pneumonia
- Musculoskeletal: muscle atrophy and contractures
- Nervous: depression or insomnia
- Endocrine: weight gain
- Urinary: urinary tract infection (UTI)
- Gastrointestinal (GI): constipation

Just as inactivity and immobility have negative effects, regular activity and exercise have many benefits for the body:

- Integumentary: improves the quality and health of the skin
- Circulatory: improves circulation
- Respiratory: reduces the chance of infection, such as pneumonia and improves oxygen level
- Musculoskeletal: increases blood flow to the muscles and improves strength
- Nervous: improves relaxation and sleep
- Endocrine: increases metabolism, helping to maintain healthy weight
- Urinary: improves elimination, helping to decrease infection
- Gastrointestinal (GI): promotes appetite and aids regular elimination

5. Describe canes, walkers, and crutches

Residents may require temporary or permanent walking aids. Canes, walkers and crutches are assistive devices that help a person with ambulation. You first learned about how to assist with ambulation in Chapter 11.

A cane is used to help a person with balance. It is not meant to completely support a person's weight. Residents who use a cane should be able to bear some weight on both legs, even if one leg is weaker. If one leg is weaker, the cane should be held on the stronger side.

Types of canes include the C cane, the functional grip cane, and the quad cane. The C cane is very common and is shaped like a curved

candy cane. It usually has a rubber-tipped bottom to prevent slipping. A functional grip cane is like a C cane, except that it has a straight grip handle, rather than the curved one. This helps the person grip the handle better. A quad cane has four rubber-tipped feet and a rectangular base. Quad canes are able to bear more weight than other canes.

Walkers are walking aids that offer additional support. The walker gives more stability when a person is unsteady or has some weakness. The feet may be rubber-tipped or the walker may have wheels. Walkers are used when a resident can bear some weight on his legs. When using a walker, the walker is moved first, then the weak leg, then the strong leg (Fig. 25-4).

C cane   Quad cane   Walker

Fig. 25-4. Residents who have trouble walking may use canes, walkers, or crutches to help themselves.

Crutches are used when a person can only bear limited weight or cannot bear any weight at all on one leg. Crutches have rubber-tipped feet to prevent sliding. One or two crutches may be used. When a resident uses crutches, stay on his weaker side.

Canes, walkers and crutches are specially fitted to each resident. A physical therapist or a nurse will take measurements for walking aids and will give instructions to residents on how to use this equipment. When helping residents, know how to assist with each device. If you are unsure about anything or have any questions, notify the nurse.

Guidelines

Canes, Walkers and Crutches

- Carefully check cane, walker or crutches for any damage before using these devices. Make sure there are no cracks and that the device is not bent. Make sure any rubber pieces are snugly in place and are in good condition.

- Make sure resident is wearing nonskid shoes, with the laces tied or straps fastened. Clothing should not be so loose or long that it catches in the equipment when moving.

- Watch for and avoid unsafe environmental situations, such as wet floors or clutter in the hallways. Wipe up spills and keep walkways clear.

- Encourage residents to use good posture when walking if possible.

- Do not rush the resident.

- Do not hang purses or clothing on a walker.

- Have the resident use the cane on his stronger side.

- While the resident is ambulating, stay near on the weaker side.

- If the resident has pain while ambulating, move him to a chair or back to the bed, if near, then notify the nurse.

- Return the resident safely back to the bed or chair after activity is completed.

Assisting with ambulation for a resident using a cane, walker or crutches

Equipment: transfer belt, non-skid shoes for resident, cane, walker, or crutches

1. Identify yourself by name. Identify the resident. Greet the resident by name.

2. Wash your hands.

3. Explain procedure to resident. Speak clearly, slowly, and directly. Maintain face-to-face contact whenever possible. Encourage resident to assist if possible.

4. Provide for the resident's privacy with a curtain, screen, or door.

5. Before ambulating, put on and properly fasten non-skid footwear on resident.

6. Adjust bed to a low position so that the resident's feet are flat on the floor. Lock bed wheels.

7. Stand in front of and face resident.

8. Brace resident's lower extremities. Bend your knees. If resident has a weak knee, brace it against your knee.

9. Place transfer belt around resident's waist and grasp the belt, while helping resident to stand.

10. Help as needed with ambulation.

a. **Cane**. Resident places cane about 6 inches, or a comfortable distance, in front of his stronger leg (Fig. 25-5). He brings weaker leg even with cane. He then brings stronger leg forward slightly ahead of cane. Repeat.

Fig. 25-5. *The cane moves in front of the stronger leg first.*

b. **Walker**. Resident picks up or rolls the walker. He places it about 6 inches, or a comfortable distance, in front of him. All four feet or wheels of the walker should be on the ground before resident steps forward to the walker. The walker should not be moved again until the resident has moved both feet forward and is steady (Fig. 25-6). The resident should never put his feet ahead of the walker.

Fig. 25-6. *The walker can be moved after the resident is steady and both feet are forward.*

c. **Crutches.** Resident should be fitted for crutches and taught to use them correctly by a physical therapist or nurse. The resident may use the crutches several different ways. It depends on the weakness. No matter how they are used, weight should be on the resident's hands and arms. Weight should never be on the underarm area (Fig. 25-7).

Fig. 25-7. *When using crutches, weight should be on the hands and arms, not the underarms.*

11. Walk slightly behind and on the weaker side of resident. Hold the transfer belt if one is used.

12. Watch for obstacles in the resident's path. Ask the resident to look ahead, not down at his feet.

13. Encourage resident to rest if he is tired. When a resident is tired, it increases the risk of a fall. Let resident set the pace. Discuss how far he plans to go based on the care plan.

14. After ambulation, remove transfer belt. Help resident to a position of comfort and safety in bed or chair.

15. If in bed, return bed to low position if raised. Ensure resident's safety. Remove privacy measures.

16. Leave call light within resident's reach.

17. Wash your hands.

18. Be courteous and respectful at all times.

19. Report any changes in the resident to the nurse. Document procedure using facility guidelines.

6. Discuss other assistive devices and orthotics

People in rehabilitation may struggle to perform their activities of daily living (ADLs), such as dressing, eating, bathing, oral care, hair care, nail care, toileting, and eating and drinking. The rehabilitation team works to help restore a resident's ability to do ADLs. **Assistive**, or **adaptive**, **devices** can help people who are recovering from an illness or adapting to a physical disability. They also help promote a person's independence. Examples are special combs, plate guards, and prostheses (Chapter 21). There are many types of assistive devices available to assist with ADLs. Examples are shown in Figure 25-8.

Fig. 25-8. *Many assistive devices are available. They help make it easier for residents to adapt to physical changes. (Photos courtesy of North Coast Medical, Inc., www.ncmedical.com, 800-821-9319.)*

Positioning devices are used to help prevent complications from inactivity and immobility. These devices aid in proper body alignment and positioning. They include the following:

- Backrests can be regular pillows or special wedge-shaped foam pillows. They provide support and comfort and maintain proper body alignment.

- Bed cradles or foot cradles are used to keep the bed covers from pushing down on the resident's feet.

- Footboards are padded boards or pillow-like devices placed against the resident's feet to keep them properly aligned. They help prevent foot drop. **Foot drop** is a weakness of muscles in the feet and ankles that interferes with the ability to flex the ankles and walk normally. Footboards are also used to keep linens off the feet (Fig. 25-9).

Fig. 25-9. Footboards help keep the feet properly aligned. (Reprinted with permission of Briggs Corporation, 800-247-2343.)

- Heel protectors are padded protectors wrapped around feet and heels to help prevent rubbing, irritation and pressure sores. They also help keep feet properly aligned, which prevents foot drop (Fig. 25-10).

Fig. 25-10. Padded heel protectors help keep feet properly aligned and prevent pressure sores. (Reprinted with permission of Briggs Corporation, 800-247-2343.)

- Abduction wedges/splints/pads (hip wedges) keep hips in proper position after hip surgery.

- Trochanter rolls are rolled-up bath blankets or towels that prevent the hip and leg from turning outward (Fig. 25-11).

Fig. 25-11. Trochanter rolls prevent the hip and leg from turning outward.

- Handrolls are cloth-covered or rubber grips that keep the hand and/or fingers in a normal and natural position. Handrolls help prevent finger, hand, or wrist contractures (Fig. 25-12).

Fig. 25-12. Handrolls keep the hand and/or fingers in a natural position, helping to prevent contractures. (Reprinted with permission of Briggs Corporation, 800-247-2343.)

- Finger cushions are stuffed devices made of terry cloth or a similar material that keep the fingers separated. They help prevent contractures of the thumb or fingers.

- Elbow protectors are padded protectors wrapped around elbows to help prevent rubbing, irritation and pressure sores.

- **Orthotic devices** are devices applied externally to a limb for support and protection (Fig. 25-13). They keep the joints in the correct position and are used to improve function and prevent complications, such as contractures. Other names for orthotic devices are splints or braces.

REHABILITATION AND RESTORATIVE CARE

Fig. 25-13. *One type of splint. (Photo courtesy of Lenjoy Medical Engineering "Comfy Splints™" www.comfysplints.com, 800-582-5332.)*

7. Discuss range of motion exercises

When a resident is immobile for a period of time, many complications can result, as you learned earlier in the chapter. Range of motion exercises are often ordered to prevent complications from inactivity and immobility. **Range of motion (ROM)** exercises are exercises that put a joint through its full arc of motion. The goal of range of motion exercises is to decrease or prevent contractures and atrophy, increase circulation, and improve strength and movement.

ROM exercises may be ordered at various times during a resident's day. There will also be guidelines for how many times a ROM exercise for a particular joint should be performed each session. The procedure below states that these exercises should be performed at least three times for each joint per session. Follow the care plan and your facility's specific policies, which may require more exercises to be completed.

Three types of range of motion exercises are:

Active range of motion (AROM) exercises put a joint through its full arc of motion that are done by a resident alone, without help.

Active-assisted range of motion (AAROM) exercises put a joint through its full arc of motion and are done by a resident with some help from a staff member.

Passive range of motion (PROM) exercises put a joint through its full arc of motion and are done by staff, without the resident's help. These

are ordered when a resident cannot move on his own.

Range of motion exercises are specific for each body area. Be familiar with the following body movements (Fig. 25-14):

- **Abduction**: moving a body part away from the midline of the body
- **Adduction**: moving a body part toward the midline of the body
- **Extension**: straightening a body part
- **Flexion**: bending a body part
- **Dorsiflexion**: bending backward
- **Pronation**: turning downward
- **Rotation**: turning the joint
- **Supination**: turning upward

Abduction   Adduction   Dorsiflexion   Rotation

Extension   Flexion   Pronation   Supination

Fig. 25-14. *The different range of motion body movements.*

Guidelines
ROM Exercises

- Follow the care plan carefully. A doctor or physical therapist will give the order for ROM exercises to be performed. The head and neck are usually not exercised by NAs without specific instructions from a nurse or doctor.

- Use good body mechanics when performing ROM exercises.

- You will work on both sides of the body, unless instructed otherwise. Begin at the head and work down the body.

- Support the joint, both above and below, while giving ROM exercises.

- Follow instructions for limiting ROM exercises. Do not exercise a joint that is bandaged or has a dressing, cast, or special tubing. Never exercise a joint that has reddened areas, rashes, bruises, sores, or one that is draining fluid.

- Maintain privacy at all times when doing ROM exercises. Expose only the area being exercised at one time.

- Never push the resident to move further than what is comfortable. **Hyperextension**, extending a joint beyond its normal range of motion, can result and can cause injury. Promptly stop and report any complaints of pain or any other problem, such as difficulty breathing, to the nurse.

- Keep the resident's body in good alignment. Use pillows as needed (see Chapter 11).

- Use ROM exercises as an opportunity to provide holistic care to residents. For example, listen to and talk with the resident while performing these exercises. Let the resident voice any problems or concerns he may have. Give praise often.

RESIDENTS' RIGHTS

"No pain, no gain" does not apply to residents.
Range of motion exercises are important to help keep residents' muscles strong and healthy. Make sure you know how to help with these exercises. Doing ROM exercises in an overly-aggressive way may cause pain and injury. Causing unnecessary pain during these exercises is considered abuse. If residents report pain during ROM exercises, stop immediately and inform the nurse.

Assisting with passive range of motion exercises

1. Identify yourself by name. Identify the resident. Greet the resident by name.

2. Wash your hands.

3. Explain procedure to resident. Speak clearly, slowly, and directly. Maintain face-to-face contact whenever possible. Encourage resident to assist if possible.

4. Provide for the resident's privacy with a curtain, screen, or door.

5. Practice good body mechanics. Adjust the bed to a safe level, usually waist high. Lock the bed wheels.

6. Lower the side rail (if bed has one and if it is not already lowered) on side nearest you.

7. Position the resident lying supine—flat on his or her back—on the bed. Position body in good alignment.

8. Repeat each exercise at least 3 times.

9. **Shoulder**. Support resident's arm at elbow and wrist while performing ROM for shoulder. Place one hand under the elbow and the other hand under the wrist. Raise the straightened arm from the side position forward to above the head and return arm to side of the body (flexion/extension) (Fig. 25-15).

Fig. 25-15.

Raise the arm to side position above head and return arm to side of the body (abduction/adduction) (Fig. 25-16).

Fig. 25-16.

10. **Elbow**. Hold the wrist with one hand. Hold the elbow with the other hand. Bend elbow so that the hand touches the shoulder on that same side (flexion). Straighten arm (extension) (Fig. 25-17).

Fig. 25-17.

Exercise forearm by moving it so palm is facing downward (pronation) and then upward (supination) (Fig. 25-18).

Fig. 25-18.

11. **Wrist**. Hold the wrist with one hand. Use the fingers of your other hand to help the joint through the motions. Bend the hand down (flexion). Bend the hand back (extension) (Fig. 25-19).

Fig. 25-19.

Turn the hand in the direction of the thumb (radial flexion). Then turn the hand in the direction of the little finger (ulnar flexion) (Fig. 25-20).

Fig. 25-20.

12. **Thumb**. Move the thumb away from the index finger (abduction). Move the thumb back next to the index finger (adduction) (Fig. 25-21).

Fig. 25-21.

Touch each fingertip with the thumb (opposition) (Fig. 25-22).

Fig. 25-22.

Bend thumb into the palm (flexion) and out to the side (extension) (Fig. 25-23).

Fig. 25-23.

13. **Fingers**. Make the hand into a fist (flexion). Gently straighten out the fist (extension) (Fig. 25-24).

Fig. 25-24.

Spread the fingers and the thumb far apart from each other (abduction). Bring the fingers back next to each other (adduction) (Fig. 25-25).

Fig. 25-25.

14. **Hip**. Support the leg by placing one hand under the knee and one under the ankle. Straighten the leg. Raise it gently upward. Move the leg away from the other leg (abduction). Move the leg toward the other leg (adduction) (Fig. 25-26).

Fig. 25-26.

Gently turn the leg inward (internal rotation). Turn the leg outward (external rotation) (Fig. 25-27).

Fig. 25-27.

15. **Knees**. Support resident's leg under the knee and ankle while performing ROM for knee. Bend the knee to the point of resistance (flexion). Return leg to resident's normal position. (extension) (Fig. 25-28).

Fig. 25-28.

16. **Ankles**. Support the foot and ankle close to the bed while performing ROM for the ankle. Push/pull foot up toward head (dorsiflexion). Push/pull foot down, with the toes pointed down (plantar flexion) (Fig. 25-29).

Fig. 25-29.

Turn inside of the foot inward toward the body (supination). Bend the sole of the foot away from the body (pronation) (Fig. 25-30).

Fig. 25-30.

17. **Toes**. Curl and straighten the toes (flexion and extension) (Fig. 25-31).

Fig. 25-31.

Gently spread the toes apart (abduction) (Fig. 25-32).

Fig. 25-32.

18. While supporting the limbs, move all joints gently, slowly, and smoothly through the range of motion to the point of resistance. Stop exercises if any pain occurs.

19. Return bed to low position if raised. Ensure resident's safety. Return side rails to ordered position. Remove privacy measures.

20. Leave call light within resident's reach.

21. Wash your hands.

22. Be courteous and respectful at all times.

23. Report any changes in the resident to the nurse. Document procedure using facility guidelines.

HOT TIP

No ROM With Osteoporosis

ROM exercises may not be recommended for residents who have osteoporosis or other conditions that cause brittle bones or weak joints. Never perform ROM exercises without a doctor's order. If a resident refuses having these exercises done, notify the nurse.

 CHAPTER REVIEW

1. What factors influence the type of rehabilitation ordered and how much progress is made (LO 2)?

2. List three goals of rehabilitation (LO 2).

3. List seven guidelines for rehabilitation and restorative care (LO 2).

4. How can being dependent on others for help with ADLs affect emotions (LO 3)?

5. List three positive effects that encouraging independence and self-care can have on a resident (LO 3).

6. List one complication for each body system listed that results from a lack of exercise and activity (LO 4).

7. List one benefit for each body system listed that results from regular activity and exercise (LO 4).

8. Briefly describe three types of canes (LO 5).

9. When a resident has one weaker leg, should a cane be held on the resident's weaker or stronger side (LO 5)?

10. After a resident moves a walker, should the weaker or stronger leg follow first (LO 5)?

11. When a resident uses a cane, walker, or crutches, on which side should the nursing assistant stay—the weaker or stronger (LO 5)?

12. List three purposes of assistive, or adaptive, devices (LO 6).

13. What are orthotic devices and what do they do (LO 6)?

14. Look at the adaptive devices in Figure 25-8. Choose one and describe how it might help a resident recovering from or adapting to a physical condition (LO 6).

15. What are the goals of ROM exercises (LO 7)?

16. List and define three types of ROM exercises (LO 7).

17. Define each of the following body movements: abduction, adduction, extension, flexion, dorsiflexion, pronation, rotation, and supination (LO 7).

18. When performing ROM exercises, where on the body should the nursing assistant begin? In which direction should the nursing assistant work (LO 7)?

26
Subacute Care

The Ventilator in Its Infancy

Robert Hooke (1635-1703) developed one of the earliest forms of mechanical ventilators. He attached a bellows to the trachea of a dog and discovered that the dog could be kept alive without any lung or chest motion. This discovery meant that an artificial means of ventilation might someday be used to keep a human being alive, if unable to breathe on his own.

"And in this harsh world draw thy breath in pain . . . "

William Shakespeare, 1564-1616, from *Hamlet*

"Extreme remedies are very appropriate for extreme diseases."

Hippocrates, 460-377 B.C.

1. Define important words in this chapter

artificial airway: any plastic, metal, or rubber device inserted into the respiratory tract for the purpose of maintaining ventilation.

central venous line: a type of intravenous line (IV) that is inserted into a large vein in the body.

chest tubes: hollow drainage tubes that are inserted into the chest to drain air, blood, pus or fluid that has collected inside the pleural space/cavity.

gastrostomy: an opening in the stomach and abdomen.

intubation: the method used to insert an artificial airway; involves passing a plastic tube through the mouth or nose and into the trachea or windpipe.

mechanical ventilator: a machine that breathes for a person.

nasogastric tube: a feeding tube that is inserted through the nose into the stomach.

Percutaneous Endoscopic Gastrostomy (PEG) tube: a tube placed through the skin directly into the stomach to assist with eating.

pulse oximeter: device that measures a person's blood oxygen level and pulse rate.

sedation: the use of medication to calm a person.

severe sepsis: a serious illness caused by an infection, usually bacterial, that requires immediate care.

telemetry: application of a cardiac monitoring device that transmits information about the heart rhythm and heart rate to a central monitoring station for assessment.

total parenteral nutrition (TPN): the intravenous infusion of nutrients in a basic form that is absorbed directly by the cells, bypassing the digestive tract.

tracheostomy: surgically-created opening through the neck into the trachea.

2. Discuss the types of residents who are in a subacute setting

A subacute setting is a special unit or facility that is for people who need more care than most long-term care facilities can provide. Hospitals and nursing homes may offer subacute care. Residents in subacute care settings need a higher level of care than other residents. They will require more direct care and close observation by staff. The cost for subacute care is usually less than care received in a hospital, but more expensive than long-term care.

Recent surgery or chronic illnesses, such as AIDS or cancer, may require subacute care (Fig. 26-1). Other conditions that warrant subacute care are serious burns or dialysis. Dialysis cleanses the body of wastes that the kidneys cannot remove due to chronic renal failure (CRF) (Chapter 16). Residents in subacute units may also be on a **mechanical ventilator**, a machine that breathes for a person.

Fig. 26-1. *Subacute care provides a higher level of care. Subacute care may be necessary for surgery, illness, serious burns, and dialysis.*

3. List care guidelines for pulse oximetry

When residents are on oxygen, require surgery, or have bleeding or breathing problems, a pulse oximeter may be used. A **pulse oximeter** measures a person's blood oxygen level and pulse rate. Blood oxygen is the oxygen level inside the arteries and is also called oxygen saturation. A sensor is clipped on a finger, ear lobe, or toe (Fig. 26-2). The sensor warns of a low blood oxygen level before any observable signs or symptoms develop. It works by moving red and infrared light through the skin. The sensor measures the amount of each type of light absorbed by the hemoglobin in the blood. Blood with oxygen absorbs more of the infrared light, while blood without oxygen absorbs more red light.

Fig. 26-2. *A pulse oximeter.*

Normal blood oxygen levels measure between 95% and 100%. However, normal ranges may differ from person to person. Diseases such as COPD (Chapter 20) can lower a person's blood oxygen levels. Report any increase or decrease in residents' oxygen levels promptly to the nurse.

Guidelines
Pulse Oximeter

- The nurse will set the alarm to identify a resident's low oxygen saturation. If the alarm on the pulse oximeter sounds, report to the nurse immediately.

- Be careful when moving and positioning residents to make sure the oximeter does not come off or move.

- Report dyspnea (difficulty breathing) or shortness of breath.

- Report cyanotic, pale, grayish, or darkening skin or mucous membranes.

- Observe and report any signs of skin breakdown from the device, such as irritation, rash, breaks, cracking, sores, bleeding or drainage. Check the skin around and under the oximeter.

Carefully monitor all vital signs and report changes to the nurse.

4. Describe telemetry and list care guidelines

Telemetry is the application of a cardiac monitoring device that transmits information about the heart's rhythm and rate to a central monitoring station. Monitoring screens are watched constantly by trained staff. A specially-trained team member then assesses the data.

A portable telemetry unit attaches to a resident's chest and is carried in a pack that allows for movement. There are different methods of connecting the device to a person's chest. One type uses sponge-like adhesive pads or patches (also called leads or electrodes) that stick to different parts of the chest. The pad attaches to a wire that is connected to the telemetry battery pack.

Guidelines
Telemetry

- Do not get the unit, wires, pads/patches, or electrodes/leads wet during bathing. Report to the nurse if they become wet.

- If the alarm sounds, notify the nurse. The alarm may sound with movement, a disconnected lead, or a low battery.

- Monitor vital signs carefully as ordered.

- Check pads for loosening. Report if they become loose.

- Check the skin under and around the pads for irritation, rashes, broken skin or cracking. Report these signs to the nurse.

- Remind the resident not to leave the range of the monitoring area during ambulation.

- Notify the nurse if any of the following occur:
  - change in vital signs
  - chest pain or discomfort
  - rapid pulse (tachycardia)
  - sweating
  - shortness of breath
  - dyspnea
  - dizziness

5. Explain artificial airways and list care guidelines

An **artificial airway** is any plastic, metal, or rubber device inserted into the respiratory tract for the purpose of maintaining ventilation. Artificial airways keep the airway open. A clear airway is needed for the lungs to perform air exchange.

An artificial airway is needed when the airway is obstructed from illness, injury, secretions, or aspiration. An artificial airway is inserted during a procedure called **intubation**. It involves a doctor passing a tube through the mouth, nose, or opening in the neck and into the trachea (windpipe). There are different types of artificial airways (Fig. 26-3). One common type is a tracheostomy. A **tracheostomy** is a surgically-created opening through the neck into the trachea. A tracheostomy tube is inserted through this opening, or stoma, into the trachea. It is also called a "trach tube." More information on this type of artificial airway is in the next Learning Objective.

Fig. 26-3. *An endotracheal tube is a type of artificial airway that is inserted through the mouth and then into the trachea. (Photo courtesy of Rusch - A Teleflex Company.)*

Guidelines
Artificial Airways

- Observe resident closely. If tubing falls out, tell the nurse immediately.

- Proper positioning helps reduce the risk of aspiration; orders will depend upon the type of airway, the need for mechanical ventilation, and the level of consciousness. A semi-reclined (semi-Fowler's) or an upright position (Fowler's) may be ordered. Follow orders regarding the positioning of the head and neck; maintain the proper position at all times.

Check vital signs as ordered and report any changes.

Perform oral care as directed at least every two hours.

Watch for biting and tugging on the tube. Report this to the nurse.

Use other methods of communication if the resident cannot speak. Communication boards, writing notes, and drawing pictures can be helpful. Observe for hand or eye signals.

Be supportive and encouraging. Having an artificial airway can be frightening and uncomfortable. It can cause choking and gagging. Be empathetic; try to imagine how you might feel if you had a tube in your nose, mouth, or throat.

Notify the nurse if any of the following occur:

- drainage

- change in vital signs

- wheezing or other unusual breathing sounds or difficulty breathing

- secretions in tubing

- cyanosis, pale, gray or darkening skin or mucous membranes

- nervousness or anxiety

6. Discuss care for a resident with a tracheostomy

A tracheostomy is a common type of artificial airway seen in long-term care (Fig. 26-4). It may be necessary due to an obstruction, tumor, infection, severe injuries, serious allergic reactions, or coma. It may also be used for a person recovering from facial burns or gunshot wounds and to prevent aspiration in an unconscious person. The tracheostomy tube is held in place by a cuff

that attaches to the end of the device in the trachea. The cuff prevents the accidental aspiration of food or fluids.

Fig. 26-4. *A tracheostomy tube is inserted through a surgically-created opening in the neck into the trachea. (Photo courtesy of Rusch - A Teleflex Company.)*

While the tracheostomy is in place, the resident may not be able to speak. Being unable to speak can cause fear and anxiety. Be supportive and responsive. Carefully observe residents who have a tracheostomy. Use other methods of communication if the resident cannot speak, such as notepads, communication boards, or hand signals. Answer call lights promptly.

General tracheostomy care includes keeping the skin around the opening, or stoma, clean, assisting with dressing changes, and helping with the cleansing of the inner part of the device. Suctioning may be needed frequently. Gurgling sounds during breathing may be one sign that suctioning is needed.

Generally, nursing assistants do not perform tracheostomy care or suctioning. However, careful observation and reporting is vital. In addition, follow these guidelines:

Guidelines
Tracheostomies

Answer call lights promptly.

Use alternate methods of communication when needed.

Assist resident into the ordered position. A semi-Fowler's or Fowler's position may be ordered for a conscious resident with a tracheostomy. If the resident is unconscious, a side-lying position (lateral) may be ordered in order to help drain secretions. Gently move and position residents; always get enough help.

- Inspect tape or ties often.
- Report kinks or disconnected tubing.
- Do not get the tracheostomy dressing wet.
- Do not cover the tracheostomy opening.
- Provide good skin care to the site around the tracheostomy. Assist with dressing changes as requested.
- Be careful to prevent aspiration when cleaning the mouth. Use special swabs as needed. Perform oral care at least every two hours.
- Observe for mouth sores, cracks, breaks, or sores on the skin. Apply lubricant to lips as needed.
- Observe skin carefully for paleness, bluish, and darkening skin or mucous membranes.
- Carefully monitor vital signs, if not measured by machine.
- Do not tire resident when performing care.
- Do not move or remove spare tracheostomy tubes or spare bag valve mask (device used to provide ventilation to a person who is not breathing, not breathing adequately, or during power failures to a person on a mechanical ventilator). A special bag valve mask with a removable mask is needed for use with a tracheostomy.
- Notify the nurse if any of the following occur:
    - cyanosis, pale, gray or darkening skin or mucous membranes
    - mouth sores or discomfort
    - cracks, breaks, or sores on the skin
    - gurgling sounds during breathing
    - dyspnea or shortness of breath
    - change in vital signs, especially respiratory rate
    - disconnected tubing
    - loose tape

7. Describe mechanical ventilation and explain care guidelines

A resident in a subacute unit may be on a mechanical ventilator (Fig. 26-5). A ventilator performs the process of breathing for a person who cannot breathe on his own. Many conditions and problems can cause inadequate ventilation, requiring a person to be placed on a mechanical ventilator. Injuries that affect the ability to breathe, such as a spinal cord injury, or diseases such as cancer, are examples.

Fig. 26-5. *A mechanical ventilator. (Photo courtesy of Pulmonetic Systems.)*

Residents on a ventilator will not be able to speak. This is because air will no longer reach the larynx (vocal cords). This can cause intense anxiety. The resident may think that no one will know if he has trouble breathing. Being on a ventilator has been compared to breathing through a straw. Residents will need a lot of support while being connected to the ventilator. Spend as much time as you can with the person. Enter the room often so that the resident can see you. This provides reassurance. Clipboards, pads, and communication boards help with communication.

Residents on a ventilator are often heavily sedated. **Sedation** is the use of medication to calm a person. Sedation helps reduce anxiety and discomfort that can occur with mechanical ventilation. Whether alert or unconscious, continue to speak to the person when providing care. Assume that he is able to understand everything going on around him.

People on ventilators are at a higher risk of getting a type of pneumonia called "ventilator-acquired pneumonia," or VAP. Nursing assistants play a role in preventing this complication. Carefully follow the doctor's orders regarding positioning of the person on a ventilator. For example, the person may need the head of the bed elevated 30 degrees at all times. The resident may need to be turned from side to side at specific times. Frequent mouth care may be ordered. Wash your hands often when working with residents on ventilators. Follow the care plan and the nurse's instructions.

Guidelines
Mechanical Ventilator

- Report to the nurse right away if the alarm sounds.

- Watch for kinks or disconnected tubing; report them immediately.

- Watch for biting on the tube if orally intubated. Report this to the nurse.

- Answer the call light promptly.

- Give frequent oral care as directed. Observe and report mouth sores or discomfort.

- Reposition at least every two hours. Follow instructions carefully when moving and positioning. Keep the resident's head properly elevated in the ordered position, usually semi-Fowler's or Fowler's. Always get enough help when moving a resident. Have the nurse check the resident after repositioning.

- Give regular skin care to prevent pressure sores. Observe for cracks, breaks, or sores in the skin, especially at the intubation site.

- Allow time for rest.

- Be patient during communication. Offer communication aids to assist. Watch for hand or eye signals.

- Provide support during difficult times. Being dependent can cause feelings of despair.

- Do not move or remove spare artificial airway tubes or bag valve masks from the bedside.

- Residents on ventilators will require one-on-one care during a power failure. A bag valve mask and/or a portable oxygen tank will need to be used by the caregiver until the power is restored.

- Notify the nurse if any of the following occur:
  - the alarm sounds
  - a collection of secretions in the tubing
  - mouth sores or discomfort
  - cracks, breaks, or sores anywhere on the skin, especially at the site of intubation
  - change in vital signs
  - nervousness or anxiety
  - depression

Severe Sepsis

Severe sepsis is a life-threatening illness caused by an infection, usually bacterial, that requires immediate care. Symptoms of severe sepsis include early, subtle symptoms such as elevated heart rate, elevated respiratory rate, a slightly-elevated temperature or, in some cases, a low body temperature. Being familiar with residents' normal vital signs will help you better recognize changes. Other symptoms are chills, a general feeling of sickness, weakness, low blood pressure, decreased urine output, headache, skin rash, shortness of breath, and confusion or a change in mental status. If you notice any of these symptoms, report them immediately.

Some of the risks for sepsis are being over the age of 65, chronic disease of the liver or kidneys, diabetes, heart disease, infections, pressure sores, cancer, burns, having a surgical drain, having an indwelling catheter, and recent hospitalization.

Treatment for severe sepsis depends on the type of infection, but includes antibiotics, other medications, IV fluids, oxygen, and careful monitoring of blood glucose. The person may require a ventilator.

8. Describe suctioning and list signs of respiratory distress

Subacute care units include residents who require suctioning by nurses or respiratory therapists. Suctioning is needed when a person has increased secretions that they cannot expel themselves. Suctioning can be performed through the mouth (oropharyngeal), the nasal passages (nasopharyngeal), the trachea and the bronchi (endotracheal). A person with a tracheostomy may also need suctioning.

Suction comes from a wall hook-up or a portable pump. A bottle collects the suctioned material from the airway (Fig. 26-6). Sterile water or sterile saline is normally used to rinse the suction catheter after suctioning. Nurses will change the tubing at least once daily.

Fig. 26-6. *A suctioning pump. Nursing assistants do not perform suctioning. They help by reporting signs of respiratory distress and monitoring vital signs.* (Photo courtesy of Laerdal Medical Corporation.)

A resident who needs frequent suctioning may show signs of respiratory distress. Signs of respiratory distress include gurgling, an elevated respiratory rate, shortness of breath, difficulty breathing (dyspnea), pallor, or cyanosis.

Guidelines
Suctioning

- If you note any signs of respiratory distress, report them immediately. An inability to breathe freely causes great anxiety. It is dangerous to remain in respiratory distress for any length of time.

- Answer call lights promptly.

- Observe skin color carefully for pale, bluish, or darkening skin or mucous membranes.

- Monitor vital signs closely, especially respiratory rate. Report changes.

- Follow Standard Precautions. Wear gloves, gown, mask, or goggles as directed.

- Place resident in position as directed by nurse, normally semi-Fowler's or lateral.

- Place pad or towel under the chin before suctioning; have a wet washcloth ready.

- Give oral and nasal care after suctioning as directed. Apply ordered lubricant to the lips as needed.

- Give support during periods of difficult breathing. Use touch if appropriate.

- Notify the nurse if any of the following occur:

    - change in vital signs, especially respiratory rate

    - gurgling sounds or unusual sounds during breathing

    - change in the color, amount, or quality of secretions coughed up

    - dyspnea or shortness of breath

    - cyanosis, pale, gray or darkening skin or mucous membranes

    - nervousness or anxiety

9. Describe chest tubes and explain related care

Chest tubes are hollow drainage tubes that are inserted into the chest during a sterile procedure. They can be inserted at the bedside or during surgery. Chest tubes are placed between the ribs into the pleural cavity or space to drain air, blood, pus or fluid that has collected inside the cavity. The pleural cavity is the space between the two layers of the pleura, the thin tissue layers covering the lungs. Chest tubes are also inserted to allow a full expansion of the lungs. Some conditions that require chest tube insertion include the following:

- pneumothorax: air or gas in the pleural cavity

- hemothorax: blood in the pleural cavity

- empyema: pus in the pleural cavity

- certain types of surgery

- chest trauma or injuries

A doctor normally inserts chest tubes. The chest tube is connected to a bottle of sterile water. Drainage systems include those using gravity drainage and suction. This system must be sealed so that air cannot enter the pleural cavity. The system must be airtight.

When X-rays show that the air, blood, or fluid has been drained, the tube is removed. Medications may be used to prevent or treat infection.

Guidelines
Chest Tubes

Ⓖ Be aware of the number and location of chest tubes. Tubes may be in the front, back or side of the body.

Ⓖ Check vital signs as directed. Report any changes immediately to the nurse.

Ⓖ Report signs of respiratory distress to the nurse immediately. Report complaints of pain.

Ⓖ Always keep the drainage system below the level of the resident's chest.

Ⓖ Make sure the drainage containers remain upright and level at all times. Inform the nurse right away if containers are not upright.

Ⓖ Make sure tubing is not kinked. Report kinks in tubing to the nurse.

Ⓖ Watch for disconnected tubing. If this happens, report it immediately.

Ⓖ Certain equipment is kept nearby in case the tube is pulled out. This includes special gauze, clamp and bottle(s) of sterile fluid. Do not remove these items from the area.

Ⓖ Observe chest tube drainage for color, amount and consistency of drainage. Report any changes in amount, color, or consistency.

Ⓖ Report if there are clots in the tubing.

Ⓖ Observe the dressings for drainage, saturation or bleeding.

Ⓖ Follow the repositioning schedule. Be very gentle with turning and repositioning. Move the resident and the tubes at the same time to prevent pulling on the tubes so that the tubes do not come out. Always get enough help.

Ⓖ Provide rest periods as needed.

Ⓖ Follow fluid intake orders carefully. Measure intake and output carefully as ordered.

Ⓖ If asked to assist with coughing and deep-breathing exercises, be encouraging and patient. These exercises can cause pain.

Ⓖ Notify the nurse if any of the following occur:

- complaints of pain
- any signs of respiratory distress
- changes in vital signs
- change in oxygen level or alarm sounds on pulse oximetry
- an increase or decrease in bubbling in the drainage system
- disconnected tubing
- kinks in the tubing
- clots in the tubing
- any change in the amount, color, or consistency of chest drainage
- wet or loose dressings
- odor in the chest tube area

10. Describe alternative feeding methods and related care

When a person is unable to consume food normally due to disease or injury, other methods are used. When a person has difficulty swallowing or is unable to swallow, he may be fed through a tube. One tube is called a nasogastric tube (N/G). A **nasogastric tube** is inserted into the nose, down the back of the throat through the esophagus and into the stomach. The tube is secured to the nose with dressing tape and to the gown with tape or a clip. An orogastric tube (O/G) may be used for people who are intubated. It is inserted into the mouth and down the throat, through the esophagus and into the stomach.

Another type of tube that is placed through the skin directly into the abdomen is called a **Percutaneous Endoscopic Gastrostomy (PEG) tube**. The opening in the abdomen and the stomach is called a **gastrostomy** (Fig. 26-7).

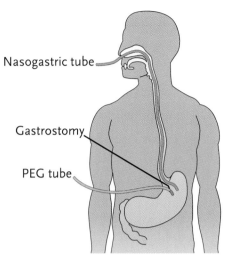

Fig. 26-7. *Nasogastric tubes are inserted through the nose, and PEG tubes are inserted through the skin directly into the stomach.*

Tube feedings are used when residents have swallowing difficulties, but are able to digest food. Other conditions that require tube feedings are coma, cancer, stroke, birth defects, extreme weakness, or refusal to eat.

Nursing assistants do not insert tubes, give the feedings or clean or suction the tubes. However, you may assist the nurse by assembling equipment and supplies and positioning the resident. You may also discard used equipment and clean and store supplies.

Guidelines
Tube Feedings

Ⓖ   Observe carefully for any signs of aspiration during and after a tube feeding (Chapter 14).

Ⓖ   Follow instructions for positioning residents. Generally, they will need to sit upright during feeding and for at least 30 minutes following the feeding to help prevent aspiration.

Ⓖ   Follow fluid orders. The resident may have an order for nothing by mouth (NPO).

Ⓖ   Give frequent nose and mouth care to prevent dryness and irritation. Apply lubricant as ordered.

Ⓖ   Do not pull on or tug tubing. Make sure that tubing is not kinked.

Ⓖ   Observe for tape or clip falling off gown.

Ⓖ   Feeding pumps may be used to administer tube feedings. Pumps help regulate the amount of fluid given. Notify the nurse if an alarm sounds.

Ⓖ   Make conversation or read to residents during tube feedings to help make this time more social.

Ⓖ   Notify the nurse if any of the following occur:

   •   irritation or sores around the nose or mouth

   •   plugged tubing

   •   kinked, cracked, broken, or disconnected tubing

   •   tube comes out of abdomen

   •   dripping or empty bag or container

   •   loose tape

   •   dyspnea or shortness of breath

   •   cyanosis, pale, gray or darkening skin or mucous membranes

   •   nausea, vomiting, or cramping

   •   fluid gathering in the mouth

   •   bleeding or drainage at the gastrostomy site

   •   signs of aspiration such as choking, gagging, or clutching the throat

   •   resident pulling on the tube (increases risk of aspiration)

   •   feeding pump alarm sounds

If a person's digestive system does not function properly, he is unable to eat, or his nutritional needs cannot be met by tube feedings, **total parenteral nutrition (TPN)** may be ordered. With TPN, a resident receives nutrients intravenously, bypassing the digestive tract. The nutrients are in their most basic forms of carbohydrates, proteins and fats and are absorbed directly by the cells.

When this need is expected to continue for a while, a central venous line is often inserted. A **central venous line** is a type of intravenous line (IV) that is placed in one of the larger veins in the body, usually in the upper chest or neck.

SUBACUTE CARE

TPN may be necessary due to surgery, disease, significant weight loss, and coma.

When caring for a resident on TPN, observe and report fever, headache, swelling, redness, bleeding or leaking at the insertion site. Residents on TPN can have fluctuations in their blood sugar. Caregivers will need to watch for signs of hypoglycemia (Chapter 8). Report any change in condition right away. Residents on TPN may find it difficult to be on a restricted diet. Be supportive and positive.

HOT TIP

Gastric Suctioning

Tubes can be inserted into the stomach for reasons other than feeding. Tubes may be used post-operatively for nausea, vomiting, bloating, and to remove materials from the body via suctioning. In addition, poisons can be removed from the stomach with a special wash that is done via a tube.

11. Discuss care guidelines for dialysis

As you learned in Chapter 16, kidney dialysis is a process that cleanses the body of waste that the kidneys cannot remove due to chronic renal failure (CRF). Dialysis can be done via a site in the person's arm (access arm) or a catheter usually inserted into the neck. Central lines in the neck are generally used for temporary dialysis.

When providing care, follow the care plan and the nurse's instructions. Make sure residents avoid putting pressure on the access arm. The resident may be advised to wear loose sleeves. Specific dietary and fluid restrictions may be ordered for a resident on dialysis. Follow instructions for intake and output (I&O) measurement carefully. You may be asked to check vital signs and measure weight daily. Do not take a blood pressure reading on the access arm.

Report to the nurse difficulty breathing, shortness of breath, changes in vital signs, pain, drainage or bleeding from the insertion site, change in I&O, and any swelling of extremities (edema).

 CHAPTER REVIEW

1. What kinds of conditions require subacute care (LO 2)?

2. What does a pulse oximeter measure (LO 3)?

3. List five care guidelines for telemetry (LO 4).

4. What is the purpose of artificial airways (LO 5)?

5. What kinds of alternate methods of communication can be used for residents who have an artificial airway (LO 5)?

6. What does general tracheostomy care involve (LO 6)?

7. List 10 care guidelines for tracheostomies (LO 6).

8. Why is it important to enter the room often when a resident is using a mechanical ventilator (LO 7)?

9. List eight care guidelines for mechanical ventilators (LO 7).

10. List eight symptoms of severe sepsis (LO 7).

11. List five symptoms of respiratory distress (LO 8).

12. What types of materials are drained by chest tubes (LO 9)?

13. What observations should nursing assistants make about chest drainage (LO 9)?

14. Briefly define "nasogastric tube" and "PEG tube" (LO 10).

15. What are generally NOT nursing assistant responsibilities with feeding tubes (LO 10)?

16. How does TPN deliver nutrients (LO 10)?

17. List six signs and symptoms to report about a resident who is on dialysis (LO 11).

27
End-of-Life Care

The Ancient Egyptian Art of Embalming the Dead

Many people in ancient Egypt focused on preparing for the afterlife. Their hope was that the afterlife would be a joyful paradise. The art of embalming dead bodies was common, especially for people of high birth. Embalming consisted of removing and preserving organs, such as the liver and the lungs. They were placed inside jars and then covered. Body cavities were washed out with spices, and then the body was soaked for 70 days with a substance called natron. Natron was made of clay mixed with certain salts. The body was then coated with various gums and wrapped with pieces of fine linen. People who were of lower birth were destined to be buried in the sand without any of these preparations.

"As a well-spent day brings happy sleep, so life well used brings happy death."
Leonardo Da Vinci, 1452-1519

"Men fear death as children fear to go in the dark; and as that natural fear in children is increased with tales, so is the other."
Publilius Syrus, circa 42 B.C.

1. Define important words in this chapter

anticipatory grief: a period of mourning when the dying person or his family is expecting the death.

autopsy: an examination of a body by a pathologist to try to determine the cause of death.

bereavement: the period following a loss in which mourning occurs.

Cheyne-Stokes respirations: alternating slow, irregular respirations followed by rapid, shallow respirations.

complicated grief: grief complicated by disorders or conditions, such as depression and substance abuse.

cremation: the process of burning a dead body until it turns to ash.

grief: a deeply emotional process that is a response to loss.

grief process: the varying emotional responses to grief.

grief therapy: therapy to try to resolve problems due to separation from the deceased.

mourning: the period in which people work to adapt to a loss; influenced by culture, tradition and society.

palliative care: care given to people who have serious, life-threatening diseases; goals are to control symptoms, reduce suffering, prevent side effects and complications, and maintain quality of life.

pathologist: a doctor with advanced training in the examination of organs and tissues.

postmortem care: care of the body after death.

terminal: causing or approaching death.

unresolved grief: grief that continues beyond what is considered a reasonable period of time; can affect the person's ability to function normally.

2. Describe palliative care

Palliative care is care given to people who have serious, life-threatening diseases, such as cancer, AIDS, and congestive heart failure. The goals of palliative care are to control symptoms, reduce suffering, prevent side effects and complications, and maintain the best quality of life possible. Palliative care emphasizes a holistic approach. Both physical and psychosocial needs are considered in palliative care.

It is important to understand that palliative care works to manage symptoms, not to cure the disease. The care plan will include instructions on how to recognize and treat complications early and how to relieve chronic pain and discomfort. This helps to maintain a person's quality of life. Palliative care involves residents' families and friends. Regular care conferences will take place that include the resident, his family and friends, and various staff members who are on the palliative care team. Doctors, nurses, clergy, social workers, dietitians, physical therapists, and nursing assistants are some of the members of the palliative care team. The team will provide access to other specialists. Counseling is made available to residents, families and friends to help them deal with the stress that accompanies a loved one's serious illness.

3. Discuss hospice care

When a serious illness is classified as "**terminal**," or approaching death, hospice care is often the next step. Hospice care is ordered by a doctor when a person has six months or less to live. This type of care is a compassionate way to care for dying people and their families. Hospice care uses a holistic approach, giving physical and emotional care and comfort. The focus is on pain and symptom management, meeting psychosocial needs, and involving family and friends.

Hospice care can be given in a hospital, at a care facility, or in the home (Fig. 27-1). It is available

seven days a week, 24 hours a day. There is always a nurse on call to answer questions, make an additional visit, or solve a problem. Members of the hospice care team include doctors, nurses, social workers, counselors, nursing assistants, therapists, clergy, dietitians and volunteers. Goals of hospice care include the following:

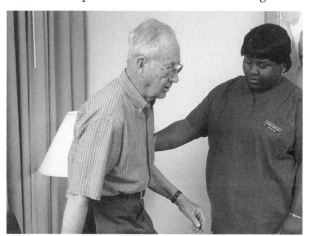

Fig. 27-1. *Hospice care can be given anywhere, even in a person's home. The focus of hospice care is on relieving pain and managing symptoms, rather than on curing an illness.*

- Use a holistic approach to care
- Provide an alternative to traditional hospital care
- Offer medically-directed, team-managed care
- Focus on the resident and family as a unit of care
- Offer compassionate care for a person with a terminal illness
- Focus on soothing and comfort care, rather than curative care
- Emphasize pain and symptom management
- Offer assistance in meeting psychosocial needs for the family
- Help the family obtain financial counseling and legal assistance as needed

Hospice care strives to meet all of the needs of the dying person. Family and friends, as well as the resident, are directly involved in care decisions. The resident is encouraged to participate in family life and decision-making as long as possible.

Hospice care focuses on pain relief by monitoring the administration and effectiveness of medications, which are prescribed by a doctor. Report complaints of pain or signs of pain to the nurse immediately. These observations are related to the doctor and adjustments are made as needed.

Hospice encourages the involvement of the resident's spiritual or religious leader, if the resident has one. Hospice also supports both the family and the dying resident in continuing involvement in social activities. Reading, listening to music, visiting with friends, and learning new skills are encouraged. Residents who are dying need to feel independent for as long as possible. They need to have control over their lives for as long as they are able.

HOT TIP

Hospice cares.

According to the National Hospice and Palliative Care Organization, over 1.2 million people received hospice services in 2005. An estimated 400,000 volunteers provided hospice care in the United States in 2005. Volunteers gave more than 16 million hours of their time to help people who were dying. Hospice volunteers attend a special training program to prepare them for hospice work. Visit www.nhpco.org for more information on hospice care.

4. Discuss the grief process and related terms

Grief is a deeply emotional response to loss. It is an adaptive, or changing, process and is usually healing in some way. Grief includes physical, psychological, emotional, social and spiritual reactions to the loss.

Dr. Elisabeth Kubler-Ross wrote the book *On Death and Dying* in 1969. She developed a theory that dying people experience a common grief process. Her model includes five different emotional stages experienced by a person prior to death. The five stages of grief are denial, anger, bargaining, depression, and acceptance. Not all people go through all of the stages. Some may stay in one stage until death, while others may move back and forth between stages during the process.

Stage 1. Denial: People in the denial stage may refuse to believe they are dying. They may think a mistake has been made and demand that lab work be repeated. They may avoid discussion about their illnesses and simply act like it is not happening. This is the "No, not me" stage.

Stage 2. Anger: Once people start to face the possibility of death, they may become angry. They may be angry because they think they are too young to die or that they have always taken care of themselves. Anger may be directed at staff, visitors, roommates, family, or friends. Anger is a normal reaction. Even though it may be upsetting, do not take anger personally. This is the "Why me?" stage.

Stage 3. Bargaining: Once people have begun to believe that they really are dying, they may start trying to bargain with God or a higher power in hopes of recovery. They may make promises and try to bargain for the ability to attend an important function, such as a wedding. This is the "Yes me, but..." stage.

Stage 4. Depression: As dying people become weaker and their symptoms get worse, they may become deeply sad or depressed. They may cry or become withdrawn (Fig. 27-2). They may be unable to do simple tasks. They need additional physical and emotional support. It is important for you to listen and be understanding.

Fig. 27-2. A dying person may become depressed and withdrawn.

Stage 5. Acceptance: Peace or acceptance may or may not come to a person before he dies. Some people who are dying are eventually able to accept death and prepare for it. They may make arrangements with attorneys, accountants, and/or loved ones for the care of important people or belongings. They may prepare for ceremonies before and/or after death and plan for their last days. At this stage, people who are dying may seem detached.

These stages of dying may not be possible for someone who dies suddenly, unexpectedly, or quickly. You cannot force anyone to move from stage to stage. You can only listen, and be ready to offer any help the person needs.

Terms Associated with Death and Dying

Some terms you may hear that are associated with death and dying include the following:

anticipatory grief: a period of mourning when the dying person or his family is expecting the death.

bereavement: the period following a loss in which mourning occurs.

complicated grief: grief complicated by disorders or conditions, such as depression and substance abuse.

grief process: the varying emotional responses to grief; many models have been developed to explain this process.

grief therapy: therapy to try to resolve problems due to separation from the deceased.

mourning: the period in which people work to adapt to a loss; heavily influenced by culture, tradition and society.

unresolved grief: grief that continues beyond what is considered a reasonable period of time; can affect the person's ability to function normally in daily life.

---

5. Explain the dying person's rights

When a person is dying, there are legal rights that must be respected. Remembering these rights will help you provide proper care, as well as promote the dying person's dignity. Some legal rights to remember when caring for the terminally ill include the following:

The right to have visitors: Residents who are dying have the right to have visitors of their choosing. They can have visits from family, friends, healthcare providers, clergy, members of the community, and others. Visitors must not be prevented from entering the resident's room unless the resident asks them to leave. Normal visiting hours are generally suspended during this difficult time. You may see visitors throughout the night. The only reasons to report a problem with a visitor are if he is upsetting the resident, if he is purposely disruptive to the unit, or if he becomes a threat to other residents, visitors, or staff.

The right to privacy: Dying residents have the right to privacy. Dying individuals may ask one or more people to leave their room. They may ask a spouse to leave during an examination or a procedure. You must honor these requests. If any problem results with a visitor, promptly report this to the nurse.

The right to be free from pain: Dying residents have the right to be free of pain. Pain must be carefully monitored, and medication and pain relief measures must be given to keep the resident as pain-free as possible.

The right to honest and accurate information: Residents who are dying have the right to know the truth about their diagnosis. Information about treatment, possible risks or complications, and side effects must be presented honestly. If residents have questions about their condition, notify the nurse. Avoid answering these difficult questions yourself.

The right to refuse treatment: Dying residents have the right to make choices about their care, including refusing treatment for their illness. Do not judge these decisions, even if you do not agree with them. The choice belongs to the resident and/or his family. See Chapter 2 for more information on Living Wills and Advance Directives.

Other rights of a dying person are listed in Figure 27-3.

I have the right to:

be treated as a living human being until I die.

maintain a sense of hopefulness, however changing its focus may be.

be cared for by those who can maintain a sense of hopefulness, however changing this might be.

express my feelings and emotions about my approaching death in my own way.

participate in decisions concerning my care.

expect continuing medical and nursing attentions even though "cure" goals must be changed to "comfort" goals.

not die alone.

be free from pain.

have my questions answered honestly.

not be deceived.

have help from and for my family in accepting my death.

die in peace and dignity.

retain my individuality and not be judged for my decisions which may be contrary to beliefs of others.

discuss and enlarge my religious and/or spiritual experiences, whatever these may mean to others.

expect that the sanctity of the human body will be respected after death.

be cared for by caring, sensitive, knowledgeable people who will attempt to understand my needs and will be able to gain some satisfaction in helping me face my death.

Fig. 27-3. The Dying Person's Bill of Rights. (This was created at a workshop on "The Terminally Ill Patient and the Helping Person," sponsored by Southwestern Michigan In-service Education Council, and it appeared in the American Journal of Nursing, Vol. 75, January, 1975, p. 99.)

6. Explain how to care for a dying resident

The focus of care for a dying resident is to meet all physical needs, as well as to provide comfort and emotional support. Promoting independence is emphasized in end-of-life care. The dying resident needs to have as much control over his life as possible. When a person's ability to perform his ADLs decreases, staff will meet additional responsibilities as needed. Family and friends may assist with this care.

Guidelines

Dying Resident

- **Skin, Nose and Mouth Care**: Give frequent skin care. Bathe residents often who are perspiring heavily. Change gowns and sheets for comfort. Give incontinence care promptly. Keep resident clean and dry. Turn and reposition resident often to prevent development of pressure sores. Get help with moving the resident as needed due to a decrease in muscle strength and fatigue. Give oral care frequently to rinse secretions and keep mouth moist. Offer ice chips to help keep the mouth moist if ordered. Use light lubricant on the nose and mouth to prevent cracking. A room humidifier can help with dryness in the nose and mouth.

- **Pain Control and Comfort**: Dying residents may be in pain. Pain relief is critical; observe and report signs of pain to the nurse immediately. Residents may be connected to a patient-controlled analgesia (PCA) device (Chapter 24) that they control themselves. They press a button to give themselves a dose of pain medication. Some residents will not be able to communicate that they are in pain. Watch for body language and other signs that they are in pain (Chapter 13). Excessive drowsiness can result from pain medication. Report this to the nurse.

  If body temperature rises, remove heavier blankets if the resident is perspiring. Fever can cause chills; use extra blankets if residents need more warmth.

- **Diminished Senses**: Vision may begin to fail as death nears. Keep the room softly lighted without glare (Fig. 27-4). Verbal communication may become difficult. Try using communication boards, pictures, or hand or eye signals. The sense of hearing is usually the last sense to leave the body. Speak in a normal tone of voice and tell the resident about care that is being performed. Describe what is happening around the resident, but do not expect an answer.

- **Breathing Problems**: Dying residents may have difficulty breathing. They may have alternating slow, irregular respirations followed by rapid, shallow respirations, called

Cheyne-Stokes respirations. They may also have gurgling or rattling sounds as they breathe. This is caused by a build-up of secretions in the throat. Notify the nurse if any of these conditions occur. If coughing becomes severe, notify the nurse. Suctioning may be needed. To ease problems with breathing, elevate the head of the bed and help the resident change positions as ordered. Oxygen therapy and/or a humidifier can be used.

Ⓖ **Food and Fluid Issues**: Feed residents slowly to help prevent choking and aspiration. Small, frequent meals can help. Encourage fluids as desired, as long as residents are not on fluid restrictions. Do not force residents to eat or drink. Residents have the right to refuse food or fluids. Report nausea, vomiting, and diarrhea to the nurse. A clear liquid diet may be ordered. Elevation of the head of the bed can help reduce burping and acid reflux.

Fig. 27-4. Keep a dying resident's room softly lit without glare.

If the resident is constipated, the nurse can provide a stool softener or other medication to help. Bowel obstructions can occur in people who are dying. Report any signs and symptoms of a bowel obstruction to the nurse (see Chapter 15).

HOT TIP

Remember that hearing is the last sense to disappear.

Do not say anything inappropriate around dying residents or their families. The sense of hearing is usually the last sense to leave a person. Be professional. Explain procedures and talk to the resident as you normally would. Never act like the resident is not there or cannot understand you.

7. Discuss factors that influence feelings about death and list ways to meet residents' individual needs

Feelings and attitudes about death differ greatly and are influenced by many factors. These factors include the person's previous experience with death, personality type, religious beliefs, and cultural background (Fig. 27-5).

Cultural groups may have different practices to deal with grieving. For example, some groups grieve openly when a loved one is dying, while others show little or no emotion. Some may want to talk and share stories about the person who is ill (Fig. 27-6). Others will not want to discuss their feelings.

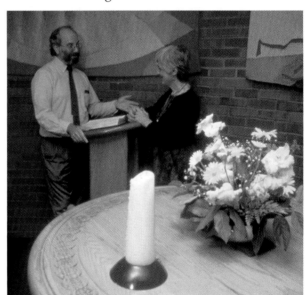

Fig. 27-5. Spiritual beliefs affect a person's feelings about death and dying.

Fig. 27-6. Looking at photos and sharing stories about a person who is dying is one way family and friends may grieve.

After death, cultural and spiritual beliefs play an important part. Some groups share food, play music and talk about the person who has died. Customs may include burying personal items with the body or having specific rules on washing the body after a person has died. Some bury their dead in a coffin, while others prefer to be cremated. **Cremation** is the process of burning a dead body until it turns to ash. Cultural groups may request spiritual or religious leaders, or specific people, be involved in a ceremony after a person has died.

It is important to understand that no matter how residents and their families deal with dying and death, staff members must respect their wishes, preferences and behavior. Honoring cultural traditions whenever possible is important. The care team must always respond in a culturally-sensitive way to different practices and individual beliefs. In addition, follow these guidelines to help meet a dying resident's psychosocial and spiritual needs:

Guidelines

Psychosocial and Spiritual Needs of a Dying Resident

Ⓖ Do not isolate or avoid a dying resident; spend as much time as you can with a resident who is dying.

Ⓖ Listen more; talk less. When dealing with a resident who will die soon, listening is often one of the most important things you can do (Fig. 27-7).

Ⓖ Do not judge anything the resident tells you about his past.

Ⓖ Do not bring your religious beliefs into the conversation. Do not try to change the resident's religious or spiritual beliefs or lack of beliefs.

Ⓖ Notify the nurse immediately if resident requests a visit from a clergy person or any spiritual leader.

Ⓖ Provide privacy for visits from family, friends, or clergy. Let residents and visitors know you will be there if you are needed.

Ⓖ Never share anything private that is said to you by the resident with anyone other than the nurse.

Ⓖ Never share anything about the resident, whether it be conversations, appearance, or anything else about the dying person, with any other person. This includes other staff members, volunteers, your own family and friends, or the media.

Ⓖ If a resident discusses a serious fear of dying with you, tell the nurse immediately. Therapists and other professionals can try to help the resident work through these fears.

Fig. 27-7. Being a good listener can be a great comfort for a resident who is dying.

8. Identify common signs of approaching death

When a person is dying, all body systems are affected. Common signs of approaching death include the following:

- Cyanotic, pale, or darkening skin or mucous membranes

- Cold skin

- Skin that looks bruised (mottling)

- Heavy perspiration

- Fever

- Extreme weakness and exhaustion

- Loss of muscle tone
- Fallen jaw, causing the mouth to stay open
- Decreased sense of touch
- Loss of feeling, beginning in the legs and feet
- Loss of vision
- Pupils dilate and eyes may stare
- Inability to speak
- Extreme drowsiness
- Disorientation or confusion
- Hallucinations
- Low blood pressure
- Increased pulse
- Cheyne-Stokes breathing
- Gurgling and rattling sound when breathing
- Difficulty swallowing
- Decreased appetite and sense of thirst
- Dry mouth
- Nausea, vomiting, and diarrhea
- Incontinence of urine and stool
- Decreased urinary output
- Loss of hearing

9. List changes that may occur in the human body after death

When death occurs, the body will not have a pulse, respiration, or blood pressure. Other physical signs you may see include the following:

- a dropped jaw, which causes the mouth to stay open
- eyelids that are partially open with eyes in a fixed stare
- incontinence of both urine and stool
- fixed and dilated pupils (this means there is no blood flow inside the brain)

Though these things are a normal part of death, they can be unsettling. If you see any of these signs, tell the nurse immediately so that she will confirm the death.

10. Describe ways to help family and friends deal with a resident's death

When a loved one dies, there is a range of emotions that family and friends may experience. These feelings include the following:

- feeling numb or being in shock
- physical reactions or symptoms, such as pain, especially chest pain, nausea, or difficulty breathing (report these to the nurse immediately)
- feelings of guilt, especially if there were any unresolved problems or issues with the relationship
- disbelief or denial of the death
- feelings of relief
- intense sadness and crying
- anxiety or fear
- anger

Family may direct anger at staff members. They may just be reacting to the loss of a loved one. They may blame staff for a problem that they feel was not addressed. Whatever the reason, refer any family complaints to the nurse. Do not try to calm a family member or friend who is upset with staff.

Allowing the family and friends to show their feelings is one of the first steps in the grieving process. Do not ask them to stop crying or to not be upset about their loss. Do not make the family feel embarrassed by their behavior. Treat family and friends with respect and compassion.

Nursing assistants can help families and friends after a loved one dies. Here are some guidelines to follow:

- Be available for the family and friends. Talking is an important part of the grieving process. Listen to them if they want to talk (Fig. 27-8). Let them talk, and only talk if a response is needed. It may not be necessary for you to talk at all.
- Do not be afraid to show your feelings for a resident who has died. Family and friends

may feel better knowing that their loved one was valued by staff.

- Do not say inappropriate comments or use cliches, such as, "This will pass," or "You will get over it." These are painful comments and are not helpful.

- If family or friends make a request to see a spiritual leader or clergyperson, report this to the nurse immediately.

Fig. 27-8. Be available for family and friends if they want to talk. Allow them to express their feelings.

Some facilities have designated staff members available to help families after a resident has died. These people may be social workers, therapists, hospice workers, or spiritual leaders.

11. Describe ways to help staff members cope with a resident's death

Staff members and other residents may be very upset by the death of a beloved resident. Being able to grieve is important. Some facilities offer bereavement therapy to help staff with grieving. This is also called grief counseling. Identifying feelings in a formal setting can help staff work through their loss. Many facilities also allow caregivers and residents to participate in memorial or religious services following a death. Some may be held in the facility.

If you are grieving, it is important not to underestimate your feelings. Do not hesitate to seek out counseling or bereavement therapy to help you work through this difficult time. Do not be ashamed because you feel grief about a resident's death. This grief is a testament to the kind of person you are and the kind of person your resident was. Grieve at your own pace.

Ways that staff can cope with the death of a resident include the following:

- Do not hesitate to express your feelings. Sadness and crying are normal responses to grieving.

- Share important memories about the resident with others.

- Spend quality time with the people you love (Fig. 27-9).

- Do things that make you happy. Be active and exercise regularly. Spend time outside. Take your dog for a walk.

- Talk to a counselor if the need arises.

- Join a special support group for grieving.

- Take care of yourself. Get enough sleep and eat nutritious foods. Do not smoke. Drink only in moderation.

Fig. 27-9. To help cope with your grief, spend time with people you love doing activities you enjoy.

12. Describe postmortem care

Postmortem care is care of the body after death. Be sensitive to the needs of family and friends after death occurs. They may wish to stay with the body for a while. Allow them time to do so. Be aware of any religious and cultural practices that the family wants to observe. Facilities will have different policies on postmortem care.

Ask the nurse for instructions before beginning this type of care. A shroud kit containing a large white piece of material for covering the body may be used. It may include special pads, a chin strap, and ID tags. Follow your facility's policies and procedures. Do only assigned tasks.

An **autopsy** is an examination of a body by a pathologist to try to determine the cause of death. A **pathologist** is a doctor with advanced training in the examination of organs and tissues. If the body is to be autopsied, the person may need to be transferred to another facility.

HOT TIP

Care of the Belongings after Death

Your facility will have a policy for handling residents' personal items after death, such as jewelry, pictures, and other personal belongings. Carefully follow your facility's policy.

Postmortem care

Equipment: two pairs of gloves, drainage pads, shroud kit or sheets, clean gown, toilet tissue, washcloth or wipes, wash basin of warm water, towel, plastic bags for clothing and belongings

1. Identify the resident.

2. Wash your hands.

3. Explain procedure to resident's family and ask them to step outside. Be courteous, respectful, and compassionate at all times.

4. Provide for privacy with a curtain, screen, or door.

5. Practice good body mechanics. Adjust bed to safe working level, usually waist high. Lock bed wheels.

6. Avoid trauma to the resident's body throughout the procedure. Treat the body with the utmost respect.

7. Apply gloves.

8. Turn off any oxygen, suction, or other equipment, if directed by the nurse. Do not remove any tubes or other equipment. A nurse or the funeral home will perform these tasks.

9. Gently close eyes without pressure.

10. Position the body in good alignment, on the back with legs straight. Fold arms across the abdomen.

11. Close the mouth. Place rolled towel under the chin.

12. Gently bathe the body. Be careful to avoid bruising. Replace any dressings only if directed to do so.

13. Comb or brush hair gently without tugging.

14. Place drainage pads where needed. Most often this is under the head and/or under the perineal area and buttocks.

15. Put a clean gown on the body.

16. Cover body to just over the shoulders with sheet. Do not cover face or head.

17. Tidy room so family may visit.

18. Remove all used supplies and linen.

19. Follow your facility's policy for handling or removing personal items. Always have a witness if personal items are removed or given to a family member.

20. Remove gloves and wash hands.

21. Turn lights down and allow family to enter and spend private time with resident. Return bed to low position if raised.

22. Return after family departs and apply clean gloves.

23. Place shroud on resident and follow instructions on completing ID tags.

24. Remove gloves and wash hands.

25. Report and record observations. Document procedure using facility guidelines.

The body will be transported to a morgue or the funeral home. Your responsibilities may include transferring the body on a stretcher to the pickup area. Ask a co-worker to assist you with the transfer. Use the designated elevator and carefully cover with a sheet or shroud during transport. Be careful during the transfer to avoid any bumping or bruising. Behave professionally. Be courteous and respectful at all times.

After the body has been transported, return to the room. Apply gloves. Strip the bed and remove all linen and trash. Open windows to air the room as needed. See Chapter 10 for information on unit cleaning.

HOT TIP

Unexpected Sounds or Movements after Death

After a person dies, the body may make sounds or movements. Breathing sounds, movement of the hands or legs, eyes opening, jaws opening, and bouts of incontinence may occur. It is common for this to happen; try not to be frightened. If you notice anything that concerns you, report promptly to the nurse.

TRIVIA

Two Early Autopsies

Julius Caesar, well-known Roman leader, was killed on March 15th, known as the "Ides of March," in 44 B.C. The first recorded autopsy was done on Julius Caesar by a physician named Antistius. Antistius noted 23 stab wounds, and is thought to have determined that the chest wound was the fatal blow. An early autopsy was performed in 1302 when the nobleman Azzolino died under suspicious circumstances. Bartolomeo da Varignana, a doctor, performed an autopsy to determine the cause of death. He found Azzolino had not died of poisoning, as had been suspected, but from internal bleeding.

CHAPTER REVIEW

1. What are the goals of palliative care (LO 2)?

2. When is hospice care usually ordered by a doctor (LO 3)?

3. List seven goals of hospice care (LO 3).

4. Briefly describe each of the five stages of grief (denial, anger, bargaining, depression, and acceptance) as defined by Elisabeth Kubler-Ross. (LO 4).

5. List five legal rights to remember when caring for the terminally ill (LO 5).

6. For each of the guidelines for caring for a dying person (skin, nose, and mouth care, pain control and comfort, diminished senses, breathing problems, food and fluid issues) list one way that the nursing assistant can help (LO 6).

7. Which sense is usually the last sense to leave the person (LO 6)?

8. List eight ways that nursing assistants can meet a dying resident's psychosocial and spiritual needs (LO 7).

9. List 20 physical signs that a person is approaching death (LO 8).

10. List six physical signs that may occur in the body after death (LO 9).

11. List four ways that nursing assistants can help families and friends after a loved one has died (LO 10).

12. What is bereavement therapy (LO 11)?

13. What are six methods that can help staff members cope with a resident's death (LO 11)?

14. Define "postmortem" (LO 12).

15. What is the goal of an autopsy (LO 12)?

28
Your New Position

The Good Old Days?

Job descriptions of the distant past included things that seem strange and even laughable today. Nurses had to act as wardens to prevent patients from playing cards, stealing from one another, drinking, or fighting. Nurses spent long hours washing and waxing floors. They even had to carry coal and fill lamps with oil. Sometimes they acted as chimney sweeps, too. Nurses were not allowed to openly smoke, drink, or go out socially. In some places, nursing staff were forbidden to meet or see anyone of the opposite sex. So, if you ever find yourself upset about a current challenge, consider the harsh circumstances of the past.

"When men are employed, they are best contented; for on the days they worked they were good-natured and cheerful, and, with the consciousness of having done a good day's work, they spent the evening jollily."

Benjamin Franklin, 1706-1790

"The superior man is the providence of the inferior. He is eyes for the blind, strength for the weak, and a shield for the defenseless. He stands erect by bending above the fallen. He rises by lifting others."

Robert Green Ingersoll, 1833-1899

1. Define important words in this chapter

conflict resolution: the process of resolving conflicts in a positive way so that everyone is satisfied.

constructive criticism: the process of giving opinions about the work of others in a non-aggressive way.

job description: an outline of what will be expected in a job.

résumé: a summary of a person's education and experience.

stress: a mentally or emotionally disruptive or upsetting condition that occurs due to changes in the environment.

stressor: internal or external factors or stimuli that cause stress.

2. Describe how to write a résumé and cover letter

Before you begin a new position as a nursing assistant, you have to look for a job. The first step in any job search is preparing a well-written résumé. A **résumé** is a summary of your education and experience. You will need to include information on these topics when preparing a résumé:

- **Objective**: An objective states your main goals in the field in which you wish to work.

- **Education**: List schools or G.E.D. courses completed, starting from high school and including any college courses.

- **Experience**: Identify the work experience you have had to this point, placing your current job first and moving backwards. A general rule is to list positions you have held for more than six months.

- **Volunteer Work**: Describe all volunteer work, emphasizing any work related to the health-care field.

- **Skills**: List all of your special skills, including things like typing, computer skills, and languages that you speak.
- **References**: State that your references are available upon request.

The following are general rules for writing a résumé:

- Limit your résumé to one page. Use short, precise sentences.
- Do not add borders or color. Use high quality, white paper.
- Use a basic, 12-point, plain font. Boldface your name (you can even make it larger than a 12-point font), and include your address and phone number at the top of the page.
- If using a computer, do not rely on a spell-check program. Use it first, check spelling yourself, then have a friend check the spelling. Read the résumé out loud to make sure you have not made any errors.
- Do not staple anything to your résumé.

An example of a well-written nursing assistant résumé is shown in Figure 28-1. Take time to make your résumé the best it can be.

A cover letter is a letter that will be included with your résumé. A sample cover letter is shown in Figure 28-2. This letter should be brief and serves as your introduction to the interviewer. It should include information on why you are seeking the job and why you are qualified for the position.

After a résumé and cover letter have been created, you will need to identify potential employers. Use the Internet, newspaper, the telephone book, and personal contacts to find employers. Ask your instructor, too; he or she may have some recommendations.

3. Identify information that may be required for filling out a job application

Completing a job application can be stressful. Being prepared will help you present yourself well. To save time and avoid mistakes, take a piece of paper and write down information that you may need for the application. You will take this paper with you, along with a new copy of your résumé, when you go to complete the application. Include the following general information:

- your address and phone number
- your e-mail address if you have one
- your social security number
- salary information from your past and present positions
- names, addresses and telephone numbers of the school or program where you were trained and the date you completed training
- certification numbers and expiration dates from your nursing assistant certification card, CPR card, and first aid cards
- former and present supervisors' and employers' names, titles, addresses and phone numbers
- exact dates of past and current employment and your reasons for leaving each of your former jobs
- complete names, addresses, and phone numbers of personal and professional references
- names of other people you know who work at the facility
- the days and hours you can work (for example, weekdays, nights, or weekends)

Before going to the facility, think about any potential problems in your job application. For example, if you have a time when you did not work at all, an interviewer may ask for the reason for the gap in employment. Imagine being the interviewer and consider the questions you might ask yourself.

When you actually fill out the job application, here are a few steps that can make the process run smoothly:

Sarah Harris
1234 Sandia Court
Albuquerque, NM 87126
505-555-4211

OBJECTIVE:	To secure an entry-level nursing assistant job in a long-term care facility.
EDUCATION:	Hobbs High School, Hobbs, NM, Diploma 2000 Hartman Medical Institute, Albuquerque, NM 2004 Certified Nursing Assistant
EXPERIENCE:	Sunnyvale Nursing Home 2004 - present Albuquerque, NM **Nursing Assistant** • Performed personal care duties and assisted with ADLs. • Worked mostly with residents who have dementia. Happy Home Nursing Center 2002-2004 Austin, Texas **Receptionist** • Managed multi-line phone system. • Made appointments for staff. • Visited residents and read to them. • Made arrangements for resident activities outside of the facility.
SKILLS:	Microsoft Word, Microsoft Excel, Adobe Acrobat, and ACT! database.
VOLUNTEER WORK:	National Diabetes Foundation, Hospice Foundation
REFERENCES:	Available upon request.

Fig. 28-1. *A sample résumé.*

- Fill out the application carefully and neatly (Fig. 28-3). Use a pen to complete it. If you are filling it out at home, use a dictionary to check spelling.

- Never lie on a job application. Tell the truth. Be honest if you have a criminal record. By law the employer is required to do a complete criminal background check. This law is in place to protect residents at facilities. If you do have a record, write a complete explanation in the appropriate section so that they will have your side of the story.

- Do not leave anything blank on the application. You may write N/A (not applicable) if the question does not apply to you. If you do not understand something on the application, ask about it before filling in the space.

November 10, 2007
Sarah Louise Harris
1234 Sandia Court
Albuquerque, NM 87126
505-555-4211

Mr. David Pomazal
Human Resources Manager
Nursing Assistant Finders
PO Box 555
Albuquerque, NM 87102

Dear Mr. Pomazal:

Please consider this letter and the enclosed résumé and application for the nursing assistant position advertised in last Sunday's edition of the *Albuquerque Journal.*

I am an energetic, detail-oriented person who has strong organizational skills, experience, and the ability to work well with people from all walks of life. In addition, I have held positions of responsibility in four community organizations over the last eight years and was chosen the 2005 National Diabetes Foundation Volunteer of the Year.

As you can see from my résumé, I thrive in a busy atmosphere that involves many different tasks, and the opportunity to work with residents. I would appreciate an interview to discuss the possibility of joining your staff. I will call you next week to request an appointment, or you may call me at your convenience at (505) 555-4211.

Thank you for your consideration of my application. I look forward to meeting you soon.

Sincerely,

Sarah Louise Harris
Enclosure

Fig. 28-2. A sample cover letter.

Employment Application

Personal Information		
Name: Rosie Ferguson	Date:	1/15/08

Social Security Number: 555-99-9999

Home Address: 8529 Indian School Rd. NE

City, State, Zip: Albuquerque, NM 87112

Home Phone: 505-291-1274	Business Phone: N/A
US Citizen? Yes	If Not, Give Visa No. & Expiration:

Position Applying For	
Title Nursing Assistant	Salary Desired: $8.50/hr
Referred By: Ms. McClain Instructor, NA Training Center	Date Available: 1/15/08

Education
High School (Name, City, State): Laguna High School Albuquerque, NM
Graduation Date: December 2007
Technical or Undergraduate School: NA Training Center Albuquerque, NM

Dates Attended: July – Dec. 2007	Degree Major:

References
Mr. Robert Castro, Instructor, NA Training Center, 505-291-1284
Ms. Scott, Health Occupations, Laguna HS, 505-555-6255
Kate Crawford, Instructor, NA Training Center, 505-291-1294

Fig. 28-3. *A sample job application.*

4. Discuss proper grooming guidelines for a job interview

In Chapter 1, professional grooming guidelines were identified. Good grooming is equally important when applying for a job. Creating a good first impression can increase your chance of success, so you should look and dress appropriately. Follow these guidelines:

- Bathe and use deodorant.

- Wear clean, nice clothes. Make sure that skirts, dresses, and pants are wrinkle-free and without stains or holes. Dresses and skirts should not be shorter than knee-length. Do not wear jeans or shorts.

- Wash your hands and clean and file your nails. Nails should be medium length or shorter. Do not wear artificial nails.

- Wear simple makeup and jewelry or none at all.

- Wear your hair in a simple style.

- Make sure your shoes are polished. Do not wear sneakers or open-toed sandals.

- Men should shave right before the interview.

- Brush your teeth. Check your teeth right before the interview begins.

- Do not smoke. You will smell like smoke during the interview.

- Do not wear perfume or cologne. Many people dislike or are allergic to scents.

5. List techniques for interviewing successfully

Use these tips to make the best impression at a job interview:

- Practice for the interview with a friend or family member. There are books that have commonly-asked job interview questions. Practice answering these questions.

- Tests may be given during the interview to see how skilled you are for the job. Find out

if there will be a test, and if so, study beforehand to help you feel better prepared.

- Map your way to the interview site. If you are taking the bus, make sure you have bus fare the night before. If you are driving, get gas the day before.

- Arrive ten or fifteen minutes early for the interview.

- Be courteous to other staff members you meet.

- Introduce yourself to the interviewer. Smile and offer to shake hands. Your handshake should be firm and confident (Fig. 28-4).

- Answer questions clearly and completely.

- Do not exaggerate your accomplishments.

- Make eye contact during the interview (Fig. 28-5). Do not look up or down or left or right during the interview. The interviewer may think that you are not telling the truth or are not interested in the conversation. Maintain eye contact to show that you are sincere.

- Do not use slang or curse words.

- Do not eat or chew gum during the interview.

- Be positive and look happy to be there.

- Do not bring children or friends with you.

- Relax. You have worked hard to get this far. You understand the work and what is expected of you. Be confident!

Fig. 28-4. *Smile and shake hands confidently when you arrive at a job interview.*

Fig. 28-5. *Be polite and make eye contact while interviewing.*

During the interview, emphasize what you think you will enjoy about your work as a nursing assistant. Do not speak negatively about a former employer. Ask questions if you are unsure about anything. You may want to write questions down before the interview so that you do not forget.

Take notes during the interview if needed. Most companies will tell you when you can expect to be informed of their decision. After the interview is over, stand up, smile, and shake hands again. Thank the person for taking the time to meet with you.

HOT TIP

It pays to say thank you!
Always write a thank-you letter after every job interview. This shows your continued interest in a job and helps to remind the interviewer who you are. If you haven't heard from a potential employer within the time frame you discussed with the interviewer, call and politely ask if the job has been filled.

6. Describe a standard job description and list steps for following the scope of practice

A **job description** is an outline of what will be expected of you in your job. It can be a long, complex form and you should read it before you sign it. Ask questions if you do not understand anything on the job description.

Nursing assistants have to follow their scope of practice. You learned about this in Chapter 2. A scope of practice lists the tasks that nursing assistants are permitted to perform as allowed by state or federal law. Follow these tips when deciding whether or not to perform a procedure:

- Do not perform a procedure if it is not listed in your job description. Doing things that are beyond your scope of practice could injure a resident, you, or another staff member.

- Do not perform a procedure if you have not been trained to do it.

- Do not perform the procedure if you have forgotten how to do all or part of it. Ask the nurse for a reminder on how to perform the procedure before you do it.

- If you have been trained to perform a procedure that is within your scope of practice, but you believe it may not be appropriate for a certain resident, ask the nurse.

HOT TIP

Organizing Your Days
When you start a new job, you will want to be as organized as possible during your workday. You can purchase an inexpensive nylon or vinyl pocket organizer. These can be found at uniform stores as well as in many uniform catalogs. These are available ready-to-fill or as a complete package, with bandage scissors, penlight, pen, and a small notebook. Some organizers even have room for a stethoscope.

7. Identify guidelines for maintaining certification and explain the state's registry

In order to meet OBRA requirements (Chapter 2), several organizations, including the National Council of State Boards of Nursing, created competency evaluation (testing) programs (CEP). These programs serve as a guide for each state's development of its NA testing program. OBRA requires that nursing assistants complete at least 75 hours of training before being employed. Many states' requirements exceed the minimum 75 hours.

After completing a state's required number of hours of training, NAs may then take the test in that state. A fee may be charged to take this test. Once a nursing assistant has passed both the written and manual skills test, a certificate is issued and mailed to the recipient.

Each state has different requirements for maintaining certification. Know and follow your state's specific requirements. General guidelines on obtaining and keeping nursing assistant certification include the following:

- A nursing assistant has a certain amount of time from the date he or she is employed to take the state test. Your employer will supply you with that information when you are hired. Pay attention to the time frame. If you do not take the test during the time given, you will not be able to work as a nursing assistant until you have passed the tests.

- A nursing assistant usually must take the state test within 24 months of training. If it is not taken during that time period, he or she will have to complete a new training course and state examination.

- A nursing assistant must work for pay during the 24-month certification period. If the nursing assistant does not, a new training program and examination must be completed.

- In most states, a nursing assistant has three chances to pass the state test.

- A nursing assistant must keep his or her certification current if the state requires certification. File a change-of-address with your state agency if you move to make sure you receive your certification renewal. Some states require that you file a change-of-address form within 30 days.

Your employer will require that you show proof of renewal of your certificate each time it expires. Do not allow your certificate to expire. Respond immediately to your state's request to renew your certification. There may be a renewal fee.

In the United States, each state keeps a registry for certified nursing assistants (CNAs). This registry keeps track of every nursing assistant working in that state. Information kept in this registry includes the following:

- a nursing assistant's full name, along with any other names the person may have used

- a nursing assistant's home address and other information, such as date of birth and social security number

- the date that the nursing assistant was placed in the registry and results from the state test

- expiration dates of nursing assistants' certificates

- information about investigations and hearings regarding abuse, neglect, or theft, which becomes a part of a nursing assistant's permanent record

Nursing assistants can ask for a written statement to be added to the file. This includes information explaining events in the nursing assistant's own words. NAs have the right to correct any errors in a registry file.

It is possible for a nursing assistant's certification to be suspended, revoked, or denied. Reasons for this vary. Be familiar with your state's guidelines. A nursing assistant can also voluntarily surrender her certification. If a nursing assistant surrenders her certification or has her certification revoked, she will not be able to practice in that state.

8. Describe continuing education for nursing assistants

The OBRA law requires that nursing assistants must have 12 hours of continuing education each year in order to keep their certification current. Some states require more hours. These classes help keep your knowledge and skills up to date. Your facility is required to provide and document this continuing education, sometimes called in-services.

Some of the subjects covered in continuing education classes include the following:

- Residents' Rights
- Fire safety
- Safety
- CPR
- Infection control
- Confidentiality
- Bloodborne pathogens
- Tuberculosis

Make sure you attend all of the required in-services. Pay attention in class and participate in discussions (Fig. 28-6). Do any required homework or projects. After the in-service is over, keep copies of any certificates and records that show you have successfully completed the class.

Fig. 28-6. *Pay attention and participate during in-service courses.*

HOT TIP

Hepatitis B Vaccine and TB Tests

Employers are required to provide free hepatitis B vaccines to all employees after hire. It is one way to prevent the spread of hepatitis.

At least once per year, employers are required to test all employees for tuberculosis. You will receive a notice when it is time to have a TB skin test. Make sure you promptly take this test and return for follow-up as instructed. For more information on hepatitis and tuberculosis, see Chapters 6 and 20.

9. Describe employee evaluations and discuss criticism

An annual evaluation, sometimes called a performance appraisal or review, is used to evaluate the performance of each employee. Some of the things you will be evaluated on are overall knowledge, conflict resolution, and team effort. Flexibility, friendliness, trustworthiness, and customer service are other qualities considered in an evaluation. A performance review or appraisal may be done after a three-month probationary period and then annually thereafter. As long as you show consistent professionalism, excellent customer service, dependability, and high ethical behavior, you will usually receive a satisfactory evaluation.

Employee evaluations include constructive criticism. **Constructive criticism** is the process of giving opinions about the work of others, which includes helpful suggestions for change. It may involve both positive and negative feedback, but it is done in a non-aggressive way. Constructive criticism should be given in a private setting. It should be work-related; it should not include personal attacks. It is not the same as hostile criticism. Hostile criticism is angry and negative. Constructive criticism is meant to help you improve in your job.

When receiving constructive criticism, be open to suggestions as they will help you grow and be more successful in your work. Try to listen without becoming upset or angry. Consider how you can address or fix the problem; offer ideas during the session (Fig. 28-7). If you are not sure how to avoid a mistake you have made, always ask for suggestions. A person who readily accepts constructive criticism can do well in the workplace.

I'm sorry I've been late several times this month. I know it's inconvenient for you. I am making more of an effort to be on time, and I expect not to be late again.

Fig. 28-7. *Be open to suggestions when receiving constructive criticism.*

It is important for an employee to try each year to improve his or her performance appraisal score. Performance reviews are frequently the basis for salary increases. In addition, a satisfactory review can increase your chances of advancing within the facility. Ask for and keep a copy of every evaluation you receive.

10. Discuss conflict resolution

When you work with a group of people, conflicts can occur. **Conflict resolution** is the process of resolving conflicts in a positive way so that everyone is satisfied with the result. Most people do not like to disagree; however, sometimes it cannot be avoided. Before reacting, think about possible reasons why someone is behaving in an undesirable way. For example, a co-worker may have had a fight with a family member, or an angry resident may be in pain or may be lonely.

When you disagree with a policy at your facility, know that the management makes the best and most informed decisions that they can make. If you have a conflict with your boss or supervisor, understand that this person really wants to help you. However, policy cannot be changed for you at the expense of other staff. In short, conflict resolution works best when you are reasonable with your requests.

Sometimes resolving a conflict means you have to compromise. In order to compromise, think about how important the problem is. What is the worst that could happen if it is not solved your way? Identify the benefits of working with others to solve the issue. Think about whether another person could help resolve the conflict, such as an arbitrator or a mediator.

Conflicts will occur in the workplace. The key to conflict resolution is to think about the issue before reacting. Think about how to best solve the problem. Know when to stand firm, when to walk away, and when it is time to compromise.

HOT TIP

Changing Jobs

If you decide to change jobs, be responsible. Always give your employer at least two weeks written notice that you will be leaving. This helps prevent the facility from being understaffed. It also helps make you a more desirable employee to future employers.

11. Define "stress" and explain ways to manage stress

Many things, both personal and professional, cause stress. **Stress** is a mentally or emotionally disruptive or upsetting condition that occurs due to changes in the environment. Internal factors like worry can also cause stress. Stress causes physical changes in the body. When a person is frightened, anxious, excited, confused, or in danger, stress can occur.

Stress happens because of a stressor. A **stressor** is an internal or external factor or stimulus that causes stress. Anything can be a stressor. Finding out you have a new supervisor can create stress. Being asked to speak in front of fellow employees at a staff meeting can cause stress. A visit from a relative can be stressful.

Stress is linked to many diseases, including hypertension, depression, ulcers, and migraines. It also increases the risk of developing other chronic diseases. Severe stress that does not go away may be linked to premature death.

If stress is unrelieved, burnout can occur. As you learned in Chapter 22, burnout is mental or physical exhaustion due to a prolonged period of stress and frustration.

Signs of burnout include arguing frequently, losing patience, being angry, wanting too much control in situations, and obsessing over small, unimportant things. A person who is experiencing burnout may also be rude, irritated and frustrated. He or she may have trouble focusing on residents and procedures.

It is important to find ways to manage stress. Learning how to recognize stress and its causes is helpful. Avoid things that you know cause stress. People, situations, places, or things can all cause stress.

RESIDENTS' RIGHTS

Leave your stress at home.

When you experience a great deal of stress, it can affect how well you do your job. Not managing stress can cause anger or abusive behavior towards residents, poor relationships with co-workers and residents, and arguments. It is very important to take steps toward managing your stress. Seek help when you need it. Deal with your stress at home, not at work. If you feel that you cannot do this, contact your supervisor. He or she may be able to give you more resources to help manage your stress.

Guidelines

Managing Stress

- Increase your level of exercise (Fig. 28-8).

- Get enough sleep.

- Eat a healthy diet. Eliminate or reduce caffeine in your diet. Caffeine can cause nervousness and irritability, along with increasing anxiety.

- Do not smoke or take illegal drugs. Drink only in moderation.

- Do one task at a time, then move on to the next task. Multi-tasking tends to increase anxiety.

- Develop new hobbies. Riding a bike, dancing, or taking classes can reduce stress. Listening to music can be calming for some people.

- Seek help from others with managing stress (Fig. 28-9). Appropriate people to turn to for help include your supervisor, your doctor, your clergyperson or spiritual leader, your friends, your family, or a local mental health agency. Do not talk to residents or their families about your stress. That is not appropriate.

- Seek counseling if needed. Do not feel embarrassed if you need help. It takes courage to seek help for a problem. Counselors can suggest a variety of methods to reduce stress.

- Set realistic goals. People can set both short-term and long-term goals for themselves and their families.

- Use a personal reward system. When you accomplish something that makes you happy, do something nice for yourself. See a movie, go out to dinner with friends, or visit a loved one.

Fig. 28-8. *Exercising regularly is one healthy way to decrease stress.*

Fig. 28-9. *Support groups can help you deal with different types of stress.*

HOT TIP

Goal-Setting

Setting goals can help manage stress. The key is to make the goals reachable. Do not set only long-term goals. Identify short-term, reachable goals that you can meet in a reasonable time period. The course you are taking right now is an example of a short-term goal, and you are close to meeting this important goal. If you create long-term goals, do not set a time frame of over three to five years. Set only long-term goals that you believe you can meet.

Relaxation Techniques

Abdominal Breathing:

- Stop, sit down, and breathe.
- Rest your hands on your abdomen and close your eyes.
- Breathe slowly and regularly, pushing your hands out with each breath.
- Do this a few times until you feel yourself begin to relax.

Muscle Relaxation:

- Starting with your head and jaw, relax as many muscles as you can.
- Do this one muscle at a time, from top to bottom, until you reach your feet and toes.

12. Describe how to be a valued member of the healthcare community

You have now reached the end of your nursing assistant course. Very soon you will be a practicing nursing assistant. Remember what you have accomplished and know the importance of the work you have chosen to do. You are going to be a valuable member of a care team, a team that literally saves lives every day. It is a noble profession, and one that provides a tremendous service to the community. Be very proud of yourself. As you graduate, make sure you thank your family, friends, instructors and classmates for everything they have done to help you during your course.

As you move forward in your new profession, never stop learning. Learn new things every day. Stay current in your field. Collect reading materials about health care and other topics. Create your own medical library at home.

Value your profession and treat your new position with all of the respect that it deserves. You worked so hard to get where you are—now reward yourself!

CHAPTER REVIEW

1. List six topics you should include when preparing a résumé (LO 2).

2. How long should a résumé be (LO 2)?

3. What are two items that should be included in a cover letter (LO 2)?

4. List six examples of information that you may need in order to complete a job application (LO 3).

5. Why do you think employers are required to do a criminal background check on nursing assistants (LO 3)?

6. List eight grooming guidelines for job interviews (LO 4).

7. List nine guidelines for successful job interviewing (LO 5).

8. List four ways a nursing assistant can make sure she is following her scope of practice before accepting a task (LO 6).

9. How many hours of training does OBRA require a nursing assistant to complete before being employed (LO 7)?

10. Within how many months of training is a nursing assistant usually required to take the state test (LO 7)?

11. List the information about nursing assistants that is kept in the state registry (LO 7).

12. How many hours of continuing education for nursing assistants is required by the federal government each year (LO 8)?

13. List four areas on which a nursing assistant may be evaluated in an annual employee performance appraisal (LO 9).

14. What is constructive criticism (LO 9)?

15. Before reacting to a conflict, what should a nursing assistant do (LO 10)?

16. What is stress (LO 11)?

17. List three signs of burnout (LO 11).

18. List ten ways to manage stress (LO 11).

Abbreviations

ABCD	airway, breathing, circulation, defibrillation
abd	abdomen
ABR	absolute bedrest
ac, a.c.	before meals
AD	Alzheimer's disease
ad lib	as desired
adm.	admission
ADLs	activities of daily living
AIDS	acquired immune deficiency syndrome
AMA	against medical advice, American Medical Association
amb	ambulate, ambulatory
as tol	as tolerated
ax.	axillary (armpit)
BID, b.i.d.	two times a day
BM	bowel movement
BP, B/P	blood pressure
BPM	beats per minute
BR	bedrest
BRP	bathroom privileges
BSC	bedside commode
c̄	with
cath.	catheter
CBR	complete bedrest
C. diff	*clostridium difficile*
CHF	congestive heart failure

ck ✔	check
cl liq	clear liquid
c/o	complains of, in care of
CNA	certified nursing assistant
COPD	chronic obstructive pulmonary disease
CPR	cardiopulmonary resuscitation
CS	Central Supply
CVA	cerebrovascular accident, stroke
CVP	central venous pressure
CXR	chest X-ray
DAT	diet as tolerated
DM	diabetes mellitus
DNR	do not resuscitate
DON	director of nursing
Dr., DR	doctor
drsg	dressing
Dx/dx	diagnosis
EMS	emergency medical services
exam	examination
FF	force fluids
ft	foot
F/U, f/u	follow-up
geri chair	geriatric chair
h, hr, hr.	hour
H$_2$0	water
HBV	hepatitis B virus
HIPAA	Health Insurance Portability and Accountability Act

HIV	human immunodeficiency virus
HOB	head of bed
HS/hs	hour of sleep
ht	height
HTN	hypertension
hyper	above normal, too fast, rapid
hypo	low, less than normal
inc	incontinent
I&O	intake and output
IV, I.V.	intravenous (within a vein)
isol	isolation
L, lt	left
lab	laboratory
lb.	pound
lg	large
LPN	licensed practical nurse
LTC	long-term care
LVN	licensed vocational nurse
M.D.	medical doctor
MDS	minimum data set
meds	medications
MI	myocardial infarction
min	minute
mm HG	millimeters of mercury
mL	milliliter
mod	moderate
MRSA	methicillin-resistant *staphylococcus aureus*

MSDS	material safety data sheet
NA	nursing assistant
N/C	no complaints, no call
NG, ng	nasogastric
NKA	no known allergies
NPO	nothing by mouth
NVD	nausea, vomiting and diarrhea
OBRA	Omnibus Budget Reconciliation Act
OOB	out of bed
OSHA	Occupational Safety and Health Administration
oz.	ounce
p̄	after
pc, p.c.	after meals
per os	by mouth
peri care	perineal care
PHI	Protected Health Information
PO	by mouth
PPE	personal protective equipment
p.r.n., prn	when necessary
q̄	every
qh, qhr	every hour
qhs	every night at bedtime
q2h	every two hours
q3h	every three hours
q4h	every four hours
q.i.d., qid	four times a day
R, rt.	right

R	respirations, rectal
rehab	rehabilitation
res.	resident
resp.	respiration
RF	restrict fluids
RN	Registered Nurse
R/O	rule out
ROM	range of motion
RR	respiratory rate
s̄	without
SOB	shortness of breath
SP	Standard Precautions
spec.	specimen
ss	one-half
S&S, S/S	signs and symptoms
stat, STAT	immediately
std. prec.	Standard Precautions
T., temp	temperature
TB	tuberculosis
t.i.d., tid	three times a day
TLC	tender loving care
TPR	temperature, pulse and respiration
U/A, u/a	urinalysis
UTI	urinary tract infection
VRE	vancomycin-resistant *enterococcus*
VS, vs	vital signs
w/c, W/C	wheelchair
wt.	weight

Symbols

©	copyright
&	and
☣	biohazard
△	change, heat
°	degree
♀	female
♂	male
%	percent
☢	radiation

Appendix

In life, it is important to continue to improve oneself and to strive to learn something new each day. This section includes a brief review of many basic skills; you may or may not already be familiar with this material. Feel free to refer to it any time you need a refresher on writing, studying, note-taking, and many other topics.

Grammar, Punctuation and Capitalization

It is important to speak well and to use grammar correctly. Grammar is the correct use of the rules of a language. Here are some basic grammatical terms and their definitions:

- A noun is a person, place, or thing. Examples: car, home, lipstick, school.

- An adjective is a word that describes a noun. Examples: *blonde* hair, *gray* sweater.

- A pronoun is a word that takes the place of a noun. Examples: I, he, him, she, them, we.

- A verb is a word that expresses an action or the condition of a person. Examples: jumps, drives, lifts.

- An adverb is a word that describes a verb, adjective, or adverb. Examples: He smiled *happily*. She skated *quickly*.

- A conjunction is a connecting word. Examples: and, but, neither, nor, or.

- A sentence is a group of words with a subject and verb that expresses a complete thought. Example: The fireman rescued the cat from the tree.

Punctuation is the use of marks in writing to separate words and ideas. Here are some common punctuation marks and their definitions:

- A period (.) is the punctuation mark placed at the end of sentences and other statements thought to be complete. Examples: Hello. Welcome to the nursing assistant training class.

  Periods are also placed after many abbreviations. For example, "Dr." is an abbreviation for the word "Doctor."

- A comma (,) separates thoughts or items in a list, such as a list of adjectives. Example: The hospital sat on top of a tall, grassy hill.

- A semicolon (;) connects two sentences with closely related ideas. Example: John has great patience; we appreciate him.

- A colon (:) introduces a list or indicates that an addition is coming. Examples: Kelley picked up these items: a comb, a razor, and soap. There was only one thing they needed to make their family complete: a pet.

- An apostrophe (') shows possession (ownership). It also shows where letters are missing in contractions. Examples: Susan took Sarah's toy. Elizabeth wasn't trained to do that task (contraction of "was not").

- Quotation marks ("") show you are quoting what someone has said or written. Example: The resident said, "I am having pain in my shoulder."

Capitalization is the writing of a word with its first letter as an upper case letter and the remaining letters in lowercase letters. You should capitalize the following:

- The first word of a sentence, question, or quote. Example: The gate is open.

- Proper names and titles. Example: "Hello, Mr. Dickens. How are you and Margaret today?"

- Names of peoples. Example: Asian

- Names of religious groups and of sacred texts. Examples: Protestants, Catholics, the Bible, the Koran

- Names of countries, states, cities, or areas. Examples: Italy, Massachusetts, Dallas, the Pacific Northwest

- Names of streets or roads. Example: Thatcher Road
- Names of buildings, organizations, colleges, schools. Examples: Yale University, the United Nations, Roosevelt High School, the White House
- Holidays, historical and special events, and holy days. Examples: Labor Day, Passover, the Civil War
- Days of the week and months of the year. Examples: Tuesday, May
- Trade names. Examples: Arby's, Target, Nike

Reading Skills

Reading well is an important part of being a nursing assistant. In the healthcare field, you must be able to read assignments, care plans, menus, activity schedules, and many other documents. Improving your reading skills can help in these situations, and reading well will also help with doing homework and studying for exams.

Choose a place to read in your home where you can concentrate. If one is not available, try a library. When you read your textbook, follow these guidelines:

- Know yourself. Choose the site where you can read best.
- Use glasses or contact lenses if you need them.
- Have enough light to read.
- Sit comfortably so that you do not hurt your back or neck. Use supportive pillows if needed.
- Take notes if you need to.
- Practice saying words you do not know. Do not be embarrassed to ask for help pronouncing a word.
- Refer to a dictionary when you need help.

When reading textbooks, make sure to separate and organize important information. First, look at the objectives for the chapter or unit; this will help you understand its primary goals. Complete each chapter section or learning objective before moving on to the next one. After all notes are taken and the sections for that chapter are finished, complete the chapter review. If you can successfully answer the questions asked in the review, move on to the next chapter.

Note-Taking

People take notes all the time. You may take notes while in class or while reading this textbook. There are many ways to take notes. Here are three methods that can make this process easier:

1. **Outline Method**: Write down the subject. Then put all sentences about that subject under it in outline form (see the box below). Use a highlighting marker to highlight the subjects and words or points you need to remember.

Taking Notes—Outline Method

I. Positioning of Residents
    a.   Purpose
    b.   Preparation

2. Types of Positions
    a.   Supine
    b.   Lateral
    c.   Dorsal recumbent
    d.   Knee-chest
    e.   Prone
    f.   Sims'
    g.   Fowler's/Semi-fowler's
    h.   Lithotomy

3. Positions Requiring Doctor's Order
    a.   Trendelenburg
    b.   Reverse trendelenburg

2. **Index Card Method**: Write down all of your notes neatly on large index cards. Use one card for each topic. To keep cards together, use rubber bands or punch a hole in the corner and use rings (one ring for every chapter).

3. **Rewrite Method**: Rewrite your notes neatly in a spiral notebook to keep them together. Rewriting them may help you remember more material.

Studying Effectively

It is not enough to simply sit down and start studying; having the proper tools will help. The following tips may help you study more effectively:

- Keep a large pad of paper to write down questions or notes.

- Use pens and highlighters. After making notes, highlight all important words and main subjects in your notes.

- Tape your thoughts and ideas about each chapter. This may help you to remember them. Some people replay their thoughts while resting.

- Take regular breaks, such as every 30 minutes or once per hour. Get a drink of water, take a walk, etc.

- Keep a regular dictionary and a medical dictionary close by. Write new words down in a notepad or on index cards. Look up any terms you do not know and write down their meanings. Review these words each time you study.

Taking Exams

Sometimes so much effort is put into mental preparation for a test that people forget to prepare their bodies as well. Physical condition affects mental abilities.

Before taking a test, get plenty of rest and watch what you eat and drink. On the day of the exam, eat a good breakfast. It is hard to think if you are hungry. Eat things such as whole grain breads, cereals, and proteins. Avoid simple sugars like candy, doughnuts, and soda.

Being in good physical shape allows more blood to get to your brain. A person who gets regular physical exercise will have a body that uses oxygen more effectively than someone who is completely out of shape. Even exercising for a few days in a row before a test can make a noticeable difference in your thinking powers.

Decrease your stress level before an exam. Fill up the car with gas or get correct bus fare the day before. Make lunch the night before. In short, try to avoid stress on the day of an exam. Stress may affect your grade.

When taking the exam, listen carefully to any instructions given. Be sure to read the directions. When taking a multiple-choice test, first eliminate answers you know are wrong. Since your first choice is usually correct, do not change your answers unless you are sure of the correction.

Do not spend too much time on any one question. If you do not understand it, move on and go back if time allows. Remember to leave that question blank on your answer sheet. Be careful to answer the next question in the proper space.

When you are done with a test, go over the entire answer sheet. Check to make sure you have circled an answer for each question. Make sure you have placed an answer for each question on the answer sheet in the correct space.

Basic Math Skills

Some people have been out of school for a while and begin to overuse calculators. They start to rely on them too much. Nursing assistants need math skills when doing certain tasks, such as recording how much a resident eats and drinks. A basic math review is listed below.

Addition

```
    3,457              11,999
+     398          +    7,657
    3,855              19,656
```

Subtraction

```
   27,785             179,746
−   9,358          −   37,437
   18,427             142,309
```

Multiplication

```
    3,754                 92
x     129          x      37
   33,786                644
   75,080          +   2,760
+ 375,400              3,404
  484,266
```

Division

```
          49                   33
  26 ) 1,274           16 )   528
     − 1,040                 − 480
        234                    48
      − 234                  − 48
          0                     0
```

Converting Decimals, Fractions, and Percentages

Decimals, fractions, and percentages are all related. A decimal is a fraction whose denominator is a power of 10. A percentage is a way of expressing a fraction as a whole number, by using 100 as the denominator. To express one-half (½) as a decimal, we would say 0.50. To express one-half (½) as a percentage, we would say 50% or 50/100.

Here are some examples:

Example: ½=0.5=50%

To get the decimal 0.5 from ½, divide the denominator (2) into the numerator (1).

To change 0.5 into a percent, move the decimal sign two places to the right and add the percent sign.

0.5 = 50%

Example: ¼ = 0.25 = 25%

To change 0.25 into a percent, move the decimal sign two places to the right and add the percent sign.

0.25 = 25%

Example: ¾ = .75 = 75%

To change 0.75 into a percent, move the decimal sign two places to the right and add the percent sign.

0.75 = 75%

Other Useful Information

Multiplication Table

1	2	3	4	5	6	7	8	9	10	11	12
2	4	6	8	10	12	14	16	18	20	22	24
3	6	9	12	15	18	21	24	27	30	33	36
4	8	12	16	20	24	28	32	36	40	44	48
5	10	15	20	25	30	35	40	45	50	55	60
6	12	18	24	30	36	42	48	54	60	66	72
7	14	21	28	35	42	49	56	63	70	77	84
8	16	24	32	40	48	56	64	72	80	88	96
9	18	27	36	45	54	63	72	81	90	99	108
10	20	30	40	50	60	70	80	90	100	110	120
11	22	33	44	55	66	77	88	99	110	121	132
12	24	36	48	60	72	84	96	108	120	132	144

Conversions: Volume

1 milliliter (mL) = 1 cubic centimeter (cc)

1 ounce (oz.) = 30 mL (cc)

¼ cup = 2 oz. = 60 mL (cc)

½ cup =4 oz. = 120 mL (cc)

1 cup = 8 oz. = 240 mL (cc)

1 Liter = 1000 mL (cc)

Conversions: Weight

2 pints = 1 quart (qt.) = 960 mL (cc)

2 quarts = ½ gallon (gal.) = 1920 cc = 2 liters (L)

4 quarts = 1 gallon (gal.)

2.2 pounds (lbs.) = 1 Kilogram (kg)

1 gram (g) = 1000 milligrams (mg)

Conversions: Length

1 inch (in) = 2.54 centimeters (cm)
(or round off to 2.5)

12 inches = 1 foot

3 feet = 1 yard

10 millimeters (mm) = 1 centimeter (cm)

100 centimeters (cm) = 1 meter

24-hour urine specimen: a urine specimen consisting of all urine voided in a 24-hour period.

abdominal girth: a measurement of the circumference around the abdomen at the umbilicus (navel).

abdominal thrusts: the method of attempting to remove an object from the airway of someone who is choking.

abduction: moving a body part away from the midline of the body.

absorption: the digestive process in which digestive juices and enzymes break down food into materials the body can use.

abuse: purposely causing physical, mental, or emotional pain or injury to someone.

accountable: answerable for one's actions.

acquired immune deficiency syndrome (AIDS): disease caused by the human immunodeficiency virus (HIV) in which the body's immune system is weakened and unable to fight infection.

active assisted range of motion (AAROM): exercises to put a joint through its full arc of motion that are done by a resident with some help from a staff member.

active listening: a way of communicating that involves giving a person your full attention while he is speaking and encouraging him to give information and clarify ideas; includes nonverbal communication.

active neglect: purposely harming a person physically, mentally, or emotionally by failing to provide needed care.

active range of motion (AROM): exercises to put a joint through its full arc of motion that are done by a resident alone, without help.

activities of daily living (ADLs): personal daily care tasks, including bathing, dressing, mouth care, hair care, toileting, and eating and drinking.

acute care: 24-hour skilled care for temporary illnesses or injuries; generally given in hospitals and ambulatory surgical centers.

adaptive devices: special equipment that helps a person who is ill or disabled perform ADLs; also called assistive devices.

additive: a substance added to another substance, changing its effect.

adduction: moving a body part toward the midline of the body.

admission: the initial entry of a resident into a facility or a unit.

admission pack: personal care items supplied upon a resident's admission.

adult daycare: care given to adults at a facility during daytime work hours.

advance directives: written documents or oral statements that allow people to decide what kind of medical care they wish to have if they are unable to make those decisions themselves.

ageism: stereotyping of, prejudice toward, and/or discrimination against the elderly.

age-related macular degeneration (AMD): a condition in which the macula degenerates, gradually causing central vision loss.

agitated: the state of being excited, restless, or troubled.

agnostic: a person who claims that he does not know or cannot know if God exists.

airway: the natural passageway for air to enter into the lungs.

alveoli: tiny, grape-like sacs in the lungs where the exchange of oxygen and carbon dioxide occurs.

Alzheimer's disease (AD): a progressive, degenerative, and irreversible disease that is a form of dementia; there is no cure.

ambulation: walking.

amputation: the surgical removal of an extremity.

anal incontinence: an inability to control the muscles of the bowels, which leads to an involuntary passage of stool or gas; also called fecal incontinence.

anatomy: the study of body structure.

anemia: a condition in which the red blood cells or the hemoglobin in red blood cells is very low.

angina pectoris: chest pain.

anticipatory grief: a period of mourning when the dying person or his family is expecting the death.

anti-embolic stockings: special stockings used to help prevent swelling and blood clots and aid circulation; also called elastic stockings.

antimicrobial: able to destroy or resist pathogens.

anxiety: uneasiness or fear, often about a situation or condition.

apathy: a lack of interest.

apical pulse: the pulse on the left side of the chest, just below the nipple.

apnea: the absence of breathing; may be temporary.

artery: vessel that carries blood away from the heart.

arthritis: a general term that refers to inflammation of the joints.

artificial airway: any plastic, metal, or rubber device inserted into the respiratory tract for the purpose of maintaining ventilation.

aspiration: the inhalation of food or drink into the lungs; can cause pneumonia or death.

assault: threatening to harm a person or leading a person to feel threatened that he or she will be touched without his or her permission.

assisted living: a setting for people who require some help with daily care, but who need less care than a long-term care facility offers.

assistive devices: special equipment that helps a person who is ill or disabled perform ADLs; also called adaptive devices.

asthma: a chronic and episodic inflammatory disease that makes it difficult to breathe and causes coughing and wheezing.

atheist: a person who claims that there is no God.

atria: the upper two chambers of the heart.

atrophy: the wasting away, decreasing in size, and weakening of muscles from lack of use.

autoclave: machine creating steam or a type of gas that kills all microorganisms.

autoimmune disease: a disease in which the body is unable to recognize its own tissue and begins to attack the tissues.

autopsy: an examination of a body by a pathologist to try to determine the cause of death.

axilla: underarm or armpit area.

barrier: block or obstacle; object(s) worn by healthcare providers to prevent the transmission of infectious diseases.

baseline: initial value that can be compared to future measurements.

battery: the actual touching of another person without the person's permission.

bedridden: confined to bed.

benign: non-cancerous.

benign prostatic hypertrophy: a disorder in which the prostate becomes enlarged, causing problems with urination and/or emptying the bladder.

bereavement: the period following a loss in which mourning occurs.

biohazard container: hard, leakproof containers into which sharp objects and items contaminated with infectious material are placed.

biology: the study of all life forms.

biopsy: a removal of a sample of tissue for examination and diagnosis.

biorhythms: natural rhythms or cycles related to bodily functions.

bipolar disorder: a type of depression that causes a person to have mood swings, changes in energy levels and the ability to function; also called manic depression.

bloodborne pathogens: microorganisms found in human blood that can cause infection and disease in humans.

Bloodborne Pathogen Standard: federal law requiring that healthcare facilities protect employees from bloodborne health hazards.

body alignment: body positioning that promotes proper body functioning; posture.

body fluids: tears, saliva, sputum (mucus coughed up), urine, feces, semen, vaginal secretions, and pus or other wound drainage.

body language: all of the conscious or unconscious messages your body sends as you communicate, such as facial expressions, shrugging your shoulders, and wringing your hands.

body mechanics: the way the parts of the body work together when you move.

body systems: groups of organs that perform specific functions in the human body.

bones: rigid connective tissue that make up the skeleton, lend support to body structures, allow the body to move, and protect the organs.

bony prominences: areas of the body where the bone lies close to the skin.

bowel elimination: the physical process of releasing or emptying the colon or large intestine of stool or feces.

BPM: the abbreviation for "beats per minute."

brachial pulse: the pulse inside the elbow; used to measure blood pressure.

bradycardia: a slow heart rate; under 60 beats per minute.

brain: the part of the nervous system housed in the skull that is responsible for motor activity, memory, thought, speech, and intelligence, along with regulation of vital functions, such as heart rate, blood pressure, and breathing.

bridge: a type of dental appliance that replaces missing or pulled teeth.

bronchi: branches of the passages of the respiratory system that lead from the trachea into the lungs.

bronchiectasis: a condition in which the bronchi become permanently dilated (wider) and damaged.

bronchitis: an irritation and inflammation of the lining of the bronchi.

Buddhism: a religion that follows the teachings of Buddha.

burnout: mental or physical exhaustion due to a prolonged period of stress and frustration.

bursae: tiny sacs of fluid that are located near joints and help reduce friction.

bursitis: a condition in which the bursae become inflamed and painful.

calculi: kidney stones.

cancer: a general term used to describe a disease in which abnormal cells grow in an uncontrolled way.

capillaries: tiny blood vessels in which the exchange of gases, nutrients, and waste products occurs between blood and cells.

cardiac arrest: the medical term for the stopping of the heartbeat.

cardiomyopathy: a condition in which the heart muscle is diseased and no longer pumps effectively.

care conference: a meeting to share and gather information about residents in order to develop a care plan.

care plan: a written plan for each resident created by the nurse; outlines the steps taken by the staff to help the resident reach his or her goals.

care team: the group of people with different kinds of education and experience who provide resident care.

carrier: person who carries a pathogen without signs or symptoms of an illness or disease and who can spread the disease.

cartilage: the protective substance that covers the ends of bones and makes up the discs that are found between vertebrae.

cataract: a condition in which the lens of the eye becomes cloudy, causing vision loss.

catastrophic reaction: reacting to something in an unreasonable, exaggerated way.

catheter: tube inserted through the skin or into a body opening; used to add or drain fluid.

C. difficile (C. diff, clostridium difficile): a bacterial illness that can cause diarrhea and colitis; spread by spores in feces that are difficult to kill.

cells: the basic structural unit of all organisms.

Celsius: the centigrade temperature scale in which the boiling point of water is 100 degrees and the freezing point of water is 0 degrees.

Centers for Disease Control and Prevention (CDC): federal government agency responsible for improving the overall health and safety of the people of the United States.

central nervous system: part of the nervous system made up of the brain and spinal cord.

central venous line: a type of intravenous line (IV) that is inserted into a large vein in the body.

cerebrovascular accident (CVA): a condition caused when the blood supply to the brain is cut off suddenly by a clot or a ruptured blood vessel; also called a stroke.

chain of command: the order of authority within a facility.

charge nurse (nurse-in-charge): a nurse responsible for a team of healthcare workers.

chart: written legal record of all care received within a facility.

charting: the act of noting care and observations; documenting.

chemical restraint: medications used to control a person's behavior.

chest percussion: clapping the chest to help lungs drain with the force of gravity.

chest tubes: hollow drainage tubes that are inserted into the chest to drain air, blood, pus or fluid that has collected inside the pleural space/cavity.

Cheyne-Stokes respirations: alternating slow, irregular respirations followed by rapid, shallow respirations.

chlamydia: a sexually-transmitted disease caused by bacteria.

Christianity: a religion that follows the teachings of Jesus Christ.

chronic: the term for an illness or condition that is long-term or long-lasting.

chronic obstructive pulmonary disease (COPD): a chronic, progressive, and incurable lung disease that causes difficulty breathing.

chronic renal failure (CRF): progressive condition in which the kidneys cannot filter certain waste products; also called chronic kidney failure.

chyme: semi-liquid substance made as a result of the chemical breakdown of food in the stomach.

circadian rhythm: the 24-hour day-night cycle.

cite: to find a problem through a survey.

civil law: private law; law between individuals.

clean: a condition in which an object has not been contaminated with pathogens.

clean-catch specimen: a urine specimen that does not include the first and last urine that is voided; also called mid-stream.

clean technique: process of removing pathogens; also called medical asepsis.

closed bed: bed completely made with the bedspread and blankets in place.

closed wound: wound in which the skin's surface is not broken.

code: when a group of specially-trained staff is called to provide advanced life support to a resident.

code status: whether a resident has a signed advance directive or not.

code team: group of people chosen for a particular shift that respond to resident emergencies.

cognition: the ability to think clearly and logically.

colon: the large intestine.

colostomy: surgically-created opening into the large intestine to allow feces to be expelled; causes stool to be semi-solid.

coma: state of unconsciousness in which a person is unable to respond to any change in the environment, including pain.

combative: violent or hostile.

combustion: the process of burning.

communicable disease: disease transmitted when a pathogen is spread from one person to another.

complicated grief: grief complicated by disorders or conditions, such as depression and substance abuse.

concussion: a head injury that occurs from a banging movement of the brain against the skull.

condom catheter: a catheter that has an attachment on the end that fits onto the penis; also called an external or Texas catheter.

conflict resolution: the process of resolving conflicts in a positive way so that everyone is satisfied.

confusion: the inability to think clearly and logically.

congestive heart failure (CHF): a condition in which the heart muscle is damaged and does not pump effectively; blood backs up into the heart instead of circulating; can occur on one or both sides of the heart.

conscientious: guided by a sense of right and wrong; principled.

conscious: the state of being mentally alert and having awareness of surroundings, sensations, and thoughts.

constipation: the difficult and often painful elimination of a hard, dry stool.

constructive criticism: the process of giving opinions about the work of others in a non-aggressive way.

contagious disease: a communicable disease that is spread easily from person to person.

contaminated: soiled, unclean; having disease-causing organisms or infectious material on it.

continuity of care: coordination of care for a resident over time, during which the care team is always exchanging information about the resident and working toward shared goals.

contracture: the permanent and often painful shortening of a muscle, usually due to a lack of activity.

coronary artery disease (CAD): a condition in which blood vessels in the coronary arteries narrow, lowering blood supply to the heart and depriving it of oxygen and nutrients.

courteous: polite, kind, considerate.

CPR (cardiopulmonary resuscitation): medical procedures used when a person's heart or lungs have stopped working.

cremation: the process of burning a dead body until it turns to ash.

criminal law: public law; related to committing a crime against the community.

critical thinking: the process of reasoning and analyzing in order to solve problems; for the nursing assistant, critical thinking means making good observations and promptly reporting all potential problems.

Crohn's disease: a disease that causes the wall of the intestines (large or small) to become inflamed (red, sore and swollen).

cross-infection: acquiring an infection from someone else; also called cross-contamination.

cultural diversity: the variety of people living and working together in the world.

culture: a set of learned beliefs, values, traditions, and behaviors shared by a social, ethnic, or age group.

cyanosis: blue or pale skin and/or mucous membranes due to decreased oxygen in the blood.

dandruff: excessive shedding of dead skin cells from the scalp.

dangling: position with the resident sitting up with the feet over the side of the bed to regain balance, equalize blood flow in the body, and return blood flow to the head; helps prevent dizziness and lightheadedness that can cause fainting.

defecation: the process of eliminating feces from the rectum through the anus.

defense mechanisms: unconscious behaviors used to release tension and/or help a person cope with stress.

dehydration: a condition that occurs when a person does not have enough fluid in the body.

delegation: transferring authority to a person for a specific task.

delirium: a sudden state of severe confusion due to a change in the body; also called acute confusional state or acute brain syndrome.

delusion: a belief in something that is not true, or is out of touch with reality.

dementia: a serious, progressive loss of mental abilities such as thinking, remembering, reasoning, and communicating.

dentures: artificial teeth.

depressant: a substance that causes calmness and drowsiness.

depression: an illness that causes social withdrawal, lack of energy, and loss of interest in activities, as well as other symptoms.

dermis: the inner layer of the two main layers of tissue that make up the skin.

developmental disability: a chronic condition that restricts physical and/or mental abilities.

diabetes: a condition in which the pancreas does not produce insulin or does not produce enough insulin; causes problems with circulation and can damage vital organs.

diabetic ketoacidosis: a life-threatening complication of diabetes that can result from undiagnosed diabetes, not enough insulin, eating too much, not getting enough exercise, and stress; also known as ketoacidosis or hyperglycemia.

diagnosis: the identification of a disease by its signs and symptoms and from the results of different tests.

dialysis: a process that cleanses the body of wastes that the kidneys cannot remove due to kidney failure.

diarrhea: frequent elimination of liquid or semi-liquid feces.

diastole: phase when the heart muscle relaxes.

diastolic: second measurement of blood pressure; phase when the heart relaxes.

diet cards: cards that list residents' names and information about special diets, allergies, likes and dislikes, and any other dietary instructions.

digestion: the process of breaking down food so that it can be absorbed into the cells.

dilate: to widen.

direct contact: way to transmit pathogens through touching the infected person or his or her secretions.

direct spread: method of transmission of disease from one person to another.

dirty: a condition in which an object has been contaminated with pathogens.

discharge: a doctor's order that releases a resident to leave a facility to go home or to another facility.

disinfection: a measure used to decrease the spread of pathogens and disease by destroying pathogens.

disorientation: confusion about person, place, or time; may be permanent or temporary.

disposable: designed to be thrown away after one use.

disruptive behavior: any behavior that disturbs others.

diuretics: medications that reduce fluid volume in the body.

diverticulitis: inflammation of sacs that develop in the wall of the large intestine due to diverticulosis.

diverticulosis: a disorder in which sac-like pouchings develop in weakened areas of the wall of the large intestine (colon).

DNR (do-not-resuscitate): an order that tells medical professionals not to perform CPR.

domestic violence: abuse by spouses, intimate partners, or family members; can be physical, sexual, or emotional.

dorsal recumbent: position with the person flat on her back with knees flexed and slightly separated; feet are flat on bed.

dorsiflexion: bending backward.

douche: a rinsing of the vagina in order to cleanse the vaginal tract or to introduce medication into the vagina; also called a vaginal irrigation.

drainage: flow of fluids from a wound or cavity.

draw sheet: an extra sheet placed on top of the bottom sheet; used for moving residents.

duodenum: the first part of the small intestine where the common bile duct enters the small intestine.

Durable Power of Attorney for Health Care: a signed, dated, and witnessed paper that appoints someone to make the medical decisions for a person in the event he becomes unable to do so.

dysphagia: difficulty in swallowing.

dyspnea: difficulty breathing.

eczema: a temporary or a chronic skin disorder that results in redness, itching, burning, swelling, cracking, weeping, and lesions; also called dermatitis.

edema: swelling in body tissues caused by excess fluid.

edentulous: lacking teeth; toothless.

electrolytes: chemical substances that are essential to maintaining fluid balance and homeostasis in the body.

elimination: the process of expelling wastes.

elopement: the act of wandering away from the facility in which a resident with Alzheimer's disease lives.

emesis: the medical term for vomit or vomitus.

empathetic: identifying with and understanding another's feelings.

emphysema: a chronic, incurable lung disease in which the alveoli in lungs become filled with trapped air; usually results from smoking and chronic bronchitis.

end-stage renal disease (ESRD): condition in which kidneys have failed and dialysis or transplantation is required.

enema: a specific amount of water, with or without an additive, introduced into the colon to eliminate stool.

epidermis: the outer layer of the two main layers of tissue that make up the skin.

epilepsy: a general term used to describe a pattern of repeated seizures.

epistaxis: the medical term for a nosebleed.

ergonomics: the science of designing equipment and setting up areas to make them safer and to suit the worker's abilities.

ethics: the knowledge of what is right and wrong; standards of conduct.

etiquette: the code of proper behavior and courtesy in a certain setting.

eupnea: normal respirations.

expiration: the process of exhaling air out of the lungs.

exposure control plan: plan that identifies the step-by-step method of what to do if exposed to infectious material; also includes specific work practices that must be followed.

exposure incident: situation that occurs when a person is exposed to infectious blood or material.

expressive aphasia: inability to express needs to others through speech or written words.

extension: straightening a body part.

Fahrenheit: a temperature scale where the boiling point of water is 212 degrees and the freezing point of water is 32 degrees.

fainting: loss of consciousness; also called syncope.

false imprisonment: unlawfully restraining or confining someone against his or her will.

farsightedness: the ability to see distant objects more clearly than objects that are near; also called hyperopia.

fasting: a period of time during which food is given up voluntarily.

fecal impaction: a mass of dry, hard stool that remains packed in the rectum and cannot be expelled.

feces: solid body waste excreted through the anus from the large intestine; also called stool.

financial abuse: stealing, taking advantage of, or improperly using the money, property, or other assets of another.

first aid: care given by the first people to respond to an emergency.

first impression: a way of classifying or categorizing people at the first meeting.

flammable: easily ignited and capable of burning quickly.

flatulence: air in the intestine that is passed through the rectum; also called gas or flatus.

flexion: bending a body part.

fluid balance: taking in and eliminating equal amounts of fluid.

fluid overload: a condition in which the body cannot eliminate the fluid consumed.

fomite: an object that is contaminated with a pathogen and can now spread the pathogen to another person.

foot drop: weakness of muscles in the feet and ankles that interferes with the ability to flex the ankles and walk normally.

force fluids: a medical order for a person to drink more fluids.

Fowler's: position with the person lying on his or her back with the head of bed elevated about 45 to 60 degrees.

fracture: a broken bone.

fracture pan: a bedpan that is flatter than a regular bedpan; used for small or thin people or those who cannot lift their buttocks onto a standard bedpan.

full weight-bearing (FWB): able to support full body weight on both legs.

functional nursing: method of care assigning specific tasks to each team member.

gait belt: a belt made of canvas or other heavy material used to help residents walk; also called a transfer belt.

gangrene: death of tissue caused by infection or lack of blood flow.

gastroesophageal reflux disease (GERD): a chronic condition in which the liquid contents of the stomach back up into the esophagus.

gastrointestinal tract: a continuous tube from the opening of the mouth all the way to the anus, where solid wastes are eliminated from the body.

gastrostomy: an opening in the stomach and abdomen.

generalized anxiety disorder (GAD): an anxiety disorder characterized by chronic anxiety, excessive worrying, and tension, even when there is no cause for these feelings.

genital herpes: a sexually-transmitted disease caused by a virus; cannot be cured.

genital HPV infection: a sexually-transmitted disease caused by human papillomavirus (HPV).

gingivitis: an inflammation of the gums.

gland: an organ that produces and secretes hormones.

glaucoma: a condition in which the pressure in the eye increases, damaging the optic nerve and causing blindness.

glucose: natural sugar.

gonads: the male and female sexual reproductive glands.

gonorrhea: a sexually-transmitted disease caused by bacteria.

graduate: a measuring container.

grief: a deeply emotional process that is a response to loss.

grief process: the varying emotional responses to grief.

grief therapy: therapy to try to resolve problems due to separation from the deceased.

grooming: practices to care for oneself, such as caring for fingernails and hair.

halitosis: bad-smelling breath.

hallucinations: seeing or hearing things that are not really there.

hand hygiene: handwashing with either plain or antiseptic soap and water and using alcohol-based hand rubs.

health: state of physical, mental, and social well-being.

healthcare-associated infection (HAI): an infection associated with various healthcare settings, such as long-term care facilities, hospitals, ambulatory settings and home care.

hearing aid: a battery-operated device that amplifies sound.

heart: four-chambered pump that is responsible for the flow of blood in the body.

heart attack: a condition in which all or part of the blood flow to the heart is blocked and muscle cells die; also called a myocardial infarction.

heartburn: a condition that results from a weakening of the sphincter muscle which joins the esophagus and the stomach; also known as acid reflux.

hemianopsia: loss of vision on one-half of the visual field due to CVA, tumor or trauma.

hemiparesis: weakness on one side of the body.

hemiplegia: paralysis of one side of the body.

hemoptysis: the coughing up of blood from the respiratory tract.

hemorrhoids: enlarged veins in the rectum that can cause itching, burning, pain, and bleeding.

hepatitis: inflammation of the liver caused by infection.

Hinduism: a religion that believes in the unity of everything and that all are a part of God.

HIPAA (Health Insurance Portability and Accountability Act): law passed to protect the privacy of health information and to facilitate the transferring of protected health information (PHI) for payment and research needs.

hoarding: collecting and putting things away in a guarded way.

holistic: care that involves the whole person; this includes his or her physical, social, emotional, and spiritual needs.

home health care: care that takes place in a person's home.

homeostasis: the condition in which all of the body's systems are balanced and are working at their best.

homophobia: a fear of homosexuality.

hormones: chemical substances created by the body that control numerous body functions.

hospice care: care for people who have six months or less to live.

human immunodeficiency virus (HIV): a virus that attacks the body's immune system and gradually disables it; eventually causes AIDS.

hygiene: methods of keeping the body clean.

hyperextension: extending a joint beyond its normal range of motion.

hyperglycemia: a life-threatening complication of diabetes that can result from undiagnosed diabetes, not enough insulin, eating too much, not getting enough exercise, and stress; also known as diabetic ketoacidosis (DKA) or ketoacidosis.

hypertension: a condition in which blood pressure consistently measures 140/90 or higher; also known as high blood pressure.

hyperthyroidism: a condition in which the thyroid gland produces too much thyroid hormone, which causes body processes to speed up and metabolism to increase.

hypoglycemia: a life-threatening complication of diabetes that can result from either too much insulin or too little food; also known as insulin reaction and insulin shock.

hypotension: low blood pressure.

hypothermia: a condition in which body temperature drops below the level required for normal functioning; severe sub-normal body temperature.

hypothyroidism: a condition in which the body lacks thyroid hormone, which causes body processes to slow down.

hypoxia: a condition in which the body does not receive enough oxygen.

ileostomy: surgically-created opening into the end of the small intestine, the ileum, to allow feces to be expelled; causes stool to be liquid.

immunity: resistance to infection by a specific pathogen.

impairment: a loss of function or ability; can be a partial or complete loss.

impotence: the inability to have or maintain a penile erection.

incident: an accident, problem, or unexpected event during the course of care.

incident report: a written report documenting the incident and the response to the incident.

incontinence: the inability to control the bladder or bowels, which leads to an involuntary loss of urine or feces.

incubation period: the period of time between the time the pathogen enters a body and the time it causes an infection.

indirect contact: a way to transmit pathogens from touching something contaminated by the infected person.

indirect spread: method of transmission of disease from an object, insect, or animal to a person.

indwelling catheter: a catheter that stays inside the bladder for a period of time; urine drains into a bag.

infection: the state resulting from pathogens invading and growing within the human body.

infection control: set of methods used to control and prevent the spread of disease.

infectious disease: any disease caused by growth of a pathogen.

ingestion: the process of taking food or fluids into the body.

input: the fluid a person consumes; also called intake.

insomnia: the inability to fall asleep or remain asleep.

inspiration: the process of inhaling air into the lungs.

insulin reaction: a life-threatening complication of diabetes that can result from either too much insulin or too little food; also known as hypoglycemia or insulin shock.

intake: the fluid a person consumes; also called input.

integument: natural protective covering.

inter-generational care: mixing children and the elderly in the same care setting.

intervention: a way to change an action or development.

intubation: the method used to insert an artificial airway; involves passing a plastic tube through the mouth or nose and into the trachea or windpipe.

invasion of privacy: a violation of the right to be left alone and the right to control personal information.

involuntary seclusion: confinement or separation from others in a physical space; done without consent or against one's will.

irreversible: term used to refer to a disease or condition that cannot be cured.

irritable bowel syndrome (IBS): a chronic condition of the gastrointestinal tract that is worsened by stress.

ischemia: a lack of blood supply to an area.

Islam: a religion that follows the prophet Muhammad and the Five Pillars of Islam.

isolate: to keep something separate, or by itself.

job description: an outline of what will be expected in a job.

Joint Commission: a not-for-profit organization that evaluates and accredits different types of healthcare facilities.

joints: the points where two bones meet; provide movement and flexibility.

Judaism: a religion that follows the teachings of God as given to Moses in laws and commandments.

ketones: chemical substances that the body produces when it does not have enough insulin in the blood.

kilogram: 1000 grams; 1 kilogram = 2.2 pounds.

knee-chest: position with the person lying on his abdomen with knees pulled up towards the abdomen and with legs separated; arms are pulled up and flexed; the head is turned to one side.

lactose intolerance: the inability to digest lactose, a type of sugar in milk and other dairy products.

lateral: position with person on his or her side.

laws: rules set by the government to help protect the public.

length of stay: the number of days a person stays in a healthcare facility.

lesion: an area of abnormal tissue or an injury or wound.

liability: a legal term that means a person can be held legally responsible for harming someone else.

licensed practical nurse (LPN) or licensed vocational nurse (LVN): licensed nurse who has completed one to two years of education; LPN/LVN passes medications, gives treatments, and may supervise daily care of residents.

ligaments: strong bands of fibrous connective tissue that connect bones and support the joints and joint movement.

lithotomy: position with the person on her back with her hips at the edge of the exam table; legs are flexed and feet are in padded stirrups.

Living Will: a document that states the medical care a person wants, or does not want, in case he or she becomes unable to make those decisions.

localized infection: infection limited to a specific part of the body; has local symptoms.

logrolling: moving a person as a unit, without disturbing the alignment of the body.

long-term care: 24-hour care, provided usually in nursing homes, for people with ongoing conditions.

lungs: main organs of respiration responsible for the exchange of oxygen and carbon dioxide.

lymph: a clear yellowish fluid that carries disease-fighting cells called lymphocytes.

malabsorption: a condition in which the body cannot absorb or digest a particular nutrient properly.

malignant: cancerous.

malnutrition: poor nutrition due to insufficient food intake or an improper diet.

malpractice: a negligent or improper act by a doctor or other medical professional that results in damage or injury to a person.

mandated reporters: people who are legally required to report suspected or observed abuse or neglect due to their regular contact with vulnerable populations, such as the elderly in nursing homes.

masturbation: to touch or rub sexual organs in order to give oneself or another person sexual pleasure.

Material Safety Data Sheet (MSDS): sheets that provide information on the safe use, hazards, and emergency steps to take when using chemicals.

mechanical lift: special equipment used to lift and move or lift and weigh a person.

mechanical ventilator: a machine that breathes for a person.

medical asepsis: process of removing pathogens; also called clean technique.

melanin: the pigment that gives skin its color.

melanocyte: cell in the skin that produces and contains the pigment called melanin.

menopause: the point at which a woman's menstrual periods stop permanently and she can no longer conceive.

menstruation: the shedding of the lining of the uterus that occurs approximately every 28 days; also known as the menstrual cycle or period.

mental health: refers to the normal function of emotional and intellectual abilities.

mental illness: a disease that disrupts a person's ability to function at a normal level in the family, home, or community.

metabolism: the process of utilizing all nutrients that enter the body to provide energy, growth, and maintenance.

metastasize: to spread from one part of the body to another.

metric: system of weights and measures based upon the meter.

microbe: a tiny living thing visible only by microscope; also called a microorganism.

microorganism (MO): a tiny living thing not visible to the eye without a microscope; also called a microbe.

micturition: the process of emptying the bladder of urine; also called urination or voiding.

Minimum Data Set (MDS): a detailed form with guidelines for assessing residents in nursing homes; also details what to do if resident problems are identified.

misappropriation: the act of taking what belongs to someone else and using it illegally for one's own gain.

mores: the accepted traditional customs of a particular social group.

mourning: the period in which people work to adapt to a loss; influenced by culture, tradition and society.

MRSA (methicillin-resistant *Staphylococcus aureus*) infection: an infection caused by bacteria that are resistant to many antibiotics; can develop when people do not take all of the medication prescribed to them.

MSDs: acronym that stands for work-related musculoskeletal disorders.

mucous membranes: the membranes that line body cavities that open to the outside of the body, such as the linings of the mouth, nose, eyes, rectum, and genitals.

multidrug-resistant organisms (MDROs): microorganisms, mostly bacteria, that are resistant to one or more antimicrobial agents.

multidrug-resistant TB (MDR-TB): disease that occurs when the full course of medication is not taken for tuberculosis (TB).

multiple sclerosis (MS): a progressive disease in which the protective covering for the nerves, spinal cord, and white matter of the brain breaks down over time; without this covering, nerves cannot send messages to and from the brain in a normal way.

muscles: groups of tissues that contract and relax, allowing motion, supporting the body, protecting organs, and creating heat.

muscular dystrophy: an inherited, progressive disease that causes a gradual wasting of muscle, weakness and deformity.

myocardial infarction (MI): a condition in which all or part of the blood flow to the heart is blocked and muscle cells die; also called a heart attack.

myocardial ischemia: a condition in which the heart muscle does not receive enough blood and lacks oxygen; can cause angina pectoris.

nasogastric tube: a feeding tube that is inserted through the nose into the stomach.

NATCEP (Nurse Aide Training and Competency Evaluation Program): part of OBRA that sets minimum requirements for nursing assistants for training and testing.

nearsightedness: the ability to see objects that are near more clearly than distant objects; also called myopia.

necrosis: the death of living cells or tissues caused by lack of nourishment to tissues.

need: something necessary or required.

negligence: actions, or a failure to act or give care, that results in injury to a person.

neuron: the basic nerve cell of the nervous system.

nitroglycerin: medication that relaxes the walls of the coronary arteries.

non-communicable disease: a disease not capable of being spread from one person to another.

non-intact skin: skin that is broken by abrasions, cuts, rashes, acne, pimples, lesions, surgical incisions or boils.

nonverbal communication: communication without words, such as gestures and facial expressions.

non-weight-bearing (NWB): unable to support any weight on one or both legs.

normal flora: the microorganisms that normally live in and on the body and do not cause harm in a healthy person.

nosocomial infection: an infection acquired in a hospital.

nurse practitioner (CNP): a registered nurse with advanced education who is able to see patients and write prescriptions.

nursing assistant: an important member of the care team who performs assigned nursing tasks and gives personal care.

nursing process: an organized method used by nurses to determine residents' needs, plan the appropriate care to meet those needs, and evaluate how well the plan of care is working; five steps are assessment, diagnosis, planning, implementation, and evaluation.

nutrient: substance in food that enables the body to use energy for metabolism.

nutrition: the taking in and using of food by the body to maintain health.

objective information: factual information collected using the senses of sight, hearing, smell, and touch; also called signs.

OBRA (Omnibus Budget Reconciliation Act): law originally passed in 1987; includes minimum standards for nursing assistant training, staffing requirements, resident assessment instructions, and information on rights for residents.

obsessive-compulsive disorder (OCD): a disorder characterized by repetitive behavior used to cope with anxiety.

obstructed airway: a condition in which a person has something blocking the tube through which air enters the lungs.

occlusion: a complete obstruction of a blood vessel.

occult: hidden.

Occupational Safety and Health Administration (OSHA): a federal government agency that makes rules to protect workers from hazards on the job.

occupied bed: a bed made while the resident is in the bed.

ombudsman: person assigned by law as the legal advocate for residents.

open bed: bed made with linen folded down to the foot of the bed.

open wound: wound in which the skin's surface is not intact.

opportunistic infection: an illness caused by organisms due to a person's inability to fight off infection.

organ: a structural unit in the human body that performs a specific function.

orthopnea: shortness of breath when lying down that is relieved by sitting up.

orthostatic hypotension: a sudden drop in blood pressure that occurs when a person stands up; also called postural hypotension.

orthotic devices: devices applied externally to limbs to support, protect, improve function and prevent complications.

osteoarthritis: a type of arthritis that usually affects weight-bearing joints, especially the hips and knees; also called degenerative joint disease (DJD).

osteoporosis: a condition in which the bones become brittle and weak; may be due to age, lack of hormones, not enough calcium in bones, or lack of exercise.

ostomy: surgical creation of an opening from an area inside the body to the outside.

outpatient care: care usually given for less than 24 hours to people who have had treatments or surgery.

output: fluid that is eliminated each day through urine, feces, and vomitus, as well as perspiration; also includes suction material and wound drainage.

ovum: female sex cell or egg.

oxygen therapy: the administration of oxygen to increase the supply of oxygen to the lungs.

pacing: walking back and forth in the same area.

palliative care: care given to people who have serious, life-threatening diseases; goals are to control symptoms, reduce suffering, prevent side effects and complications, and maintain quality of life.

panic disorder: an anxiety disorder that causes repeated episodes of intense fear for no known reason.

paranoid schizophrenia: a form of mental illness characterized by hallucinations and delusions.

paraplegia: a loss of function of lower body and legs.

parasomnias: sleep disorders.

Parkinson's disease: a progressive disease that causes a portion of the brain to degenerate; causes rigid muscles, shuffling gait, pill-rolling, mask-like face, and tremors.

partial bath: bath that includes washing the face, underarms, and hands, and performing perineal care.

partial weight-bearing (PWB): able to support some body weight on one or both legs.

PASS: acronym for use of a fire extinguisher; stands for Pull-Aim-Squeeze-Sweep.

passive neglect: unintentionally harming a person physically, mentally, or emotionally by failing to provide needed care.

passive range of motion (PROM): exercises to put a joint through its full arc of motion that are done by staff, without the resident's help.

pathogen: the microorganisms that cause disease.

pathologist: a doctor with advanced training in the examination of organs and tissues.

pathophysiology: the study of the disorders that occur in the body.

pediculosis: an infestation of lice.

Percutaneous Endoscopic Gastrostomy (PEG) tube: a tube placed through the skin directly into the stomach to assist with eating.

perineal care: care of the genitals and anal area.

peripheral nervous system: part of the nervous system made up of the nerves that extend throughout the body and connect to the spinal cord.

peripheral vascular disease (PVD): a condition in which the legs, feet, arms or hands do not have enough blood circulation.

peristalsis: muscular contractions that push food through the gastrointestinal tract.

perseveration: the repetition of words, phrases, questions, or actions.

pet therapy: the practice of bringing pets into a facility or home to provide stimulation and companionship.

phantom limb pain: pain in a limb (or extremity) that has been amputated.

phantom sensation: itching or tingling feeling from a body part that has been amputated.

phlebitis: inflammation of the veins in the lower extremities.

physiatrists: doctors who specialize in rehabilitation.

physical abuse: intentional or unintentional treatment that causes harm or injury to a person's body.

physiology: the study of how body parts function.

pillaging: taking things that belong to someone else; not considered stealing.

plaque: a substance that forms in a brief period of time if oral care is not done regularly.

pneumonia: acute inflammation in the lung tissue caused by a bacterial, viral, or fungal infection and/or chemical irritants.

policy: a course of action to be followed.

portable commode: a chair with a toilet seat and a removable container underneath.

positioning: helping people into positions that will be comfortable and healthy for them.

postmortem care: care of the body after death.

post-traumatic stress disorder (PTSD): anxiety-related disorder caused by a traumatic experience.

postural support: device that maintains good posture or body alignment; also considered a restraint.

pound: measurement of weight equal to 16 ounces.

PPE (personal protective equipment): a barrier between a person and disease; includes gloves, gowns, masks, goggles, and face shields.

pre-diabetes: a condition in which a person's blood glucose levels are above normal but not high enough for a diagnosis of type 2 diabetes.

prefix: a word part added to the beginning of a root to create a new meaning.

prehypertension: a condition in which a person has a systolic measurement of 120–139 mm Hg and a diastolic measurement of 80–89 mm Hg; indicator that the person does not have high blood pressure now but is likely to have it in the future.

pressure points: areas of the body that bear much of its weight.

pressure sore: a serious wound resulting from skin breakdown; also known as decubitus ulcer or bed sore.

primary nursing: method of care in which the registered nurse gives much of the daily care to residents.

prioritize: to place things in order of importance.

procedure: a method, or way, of doing something.

professionalism: the act of behaving properly for a certain job.

progressive: something that continually gets worse or deteriorates.

pronation: turning downward.

prone: position with person lying on his or her stomach.

prosthesis: a specially-fitted artificial body part that replaces a missing limb or extremity.

Protected Health Information (PHI): information that can be used to identify a person and relates to the patient's past, present, or future physical or mental condition, including any health care that patient has had, or payment for that health care.

protective device: another word for a physical restraint or postural support.

psoriasis: a chronic skin condition caused by skin cells growing too quickly which results in red, white or silver patches, itching and discomfort.

psychological abuse: harming a person by threatening, scaring, insulting, humiliating, or treating him or her as a child; also includes verbal abuse.

psychosocial needs: needs which involve social interaction, emotions, intellect, and spirituality.

puberty: the period when a person develops secondary sex characteristics.

pulmonary edema: a condition in which there is an accumulation of fluid in the lungs; usually due to heart failure.

pulse oximeter: device that measures a person's blood oxygen level and pulse rate.

puree: to chop, blend, or grind food into a thick paste of baby food consistency.

quadriplegia: loss of function of legs, trunk, and arms.

RACE: acronym for steps taken during a fire; stands for Remove-Activate-Contain-Extinguish.

radial pulse: the pulse on the inside of the wrist, where the radial artery runs just beneath the skin.

range of motion (ROM): exercises that put a joint through its full arc of motion.

reality orientation: type of therapy that uses calendars, clocks, signs, and lists to help people with Alzheimer's disease remember who and where they are.

receptive aphasia: inability to understand what others are communicating through speech or written words.

registered nurse (RN): a licensed nurse who has completed two to four years of education; RNs assess residents, monitor progress, provide skilled nursing care, give treatments, and supervise the care given by nursing assistants and other members of the care team.

rehabilitation: care that is managed by professionals to restore a person to the highest possible level of functioning after an illness or injury.

reinfection: being infected a second time with an infection the person already had.

religion: a set of beliefs and practices followed by a group of people.

reminiscence therapy: type of therapy that encourages people with Alzheimer's disease to remember and talk about the past.

remotivation therapy: type of therapy that promotes self-esteem, self-awareness, and socialization in groups for people with Alzheimer's disease.

resident: a person living in a long-term care facility.

resident-focused care: method of care in which the resident is the primary focus; team members are cross-trained in skills, allowing residents to see many of the same people performing their care.

Residents' Council: a group of residents who meet regularly to discuss issues related to the nursing home.

Residents' Rights: rights identified by OBRA for residents in long-term care facilities; purpose is to inform residents and others of their rights within these facilities and to provide an ethical code of conduct for healthcare workers.

resistance: the body's ability to prevent infection and disease.

respiration: the process of inhaling air into the lungs (inspiration) and exhaling air out of the lungs (expiration).

respiratory arrest: the medical term for the stopping of breathing.

restorative care: care used after rehabilitation to maintain a person's function and increase independence.

restraint: a physical or chemical way to restrict voluntary movement or behavior.

restraint alternatives: measures used instead of physical or chemical restraints.

restraint-free care: an environment in which restraints are not kept or used for any reason.

restrict fluids: a medical order that limits the amount of fluids a person takes in.

résumé: a summary of a person's education and experience.

rheumatoid arthritis: a type of arthritis in which joints become red, swollen, and very painful; movement is restricted and deformities of the hands are common.

ringworm: a fungal infection that causes red scaly patches to appear in a ring shape, generally on the upper body, or the hands and feet.

root: the main part of a word that gives it meaning.

rotation: turning the joint.

rounds: physical movement of staff from room to room to discuss each resident and the plans of care.

routine urine specimen: a urine specimen that can be collected any time a person voids.

rummaging: going through items that belong to other people.

sandwich generation: people responsible for the care of both their children and aging relatives.

sanitation: ways communities maintain clean, hygienic conditions that help prevent disease, such as the disposal of sewage and solid waste.

scabies: a contagious skin infection caused by mites burrowing into the skin that results in pimple-like irritations, rashes, intense itching, and sores.

scalds: burns caused by very hot liquids.

schizophrenia: a form of chronic mental illness that may have acute episodes; affects a person's ability to think, communicate, make decisions, and understand reality.

scope of practice: the tasks that nursing assistants are permitted to perform as allowed by state or federal law.

sedation: the use of medication to calm a person.

sentinel event: an unexpected occurrence involving death or serious physical or psychological injury.

sequential compression device (SCD): special stockings used to improve circulation and prevent blood clots; may be applied during or after surgery.

severe sepsis: a serious illness caused by an infection, usually bacterial, that requires immediate care.

sexual abuse: forcing a person to perform or participate in sexual acts against his or her will.

sexual harassment: any unwelcome sexual advance or behavior that creates an intimidating, hostile or offensive working environment.

sexually-transmitted diseases (STDs): diseases passed through sexual contact; also called venereal diseases.

sexually-transmitted infections (STIs): infections caused by sexual contact; infected person may not show signs or symptoms of disease.

shearing: rubbing or friction resulting from the skin moving one way and the bone underneath it remaining fixed or moving in the opposite direction.

shingles: a viral infection caused by the same virus that causes chickenpox; causes pain, itching, rashes, and possibly fever and chills.

shock: a condition in which there is decreased blood flow to organs and tissues.

Sims': position with person lying on his or her left side with one leg drawn up.

sitz bath: a warm soak of the perineal area to cleanse perineal wounds and reduce inflammation and pain.

skilled care: medically necessary care given by a skilled nurse or therapist.

sleep: natural period of rest for the mind and body during which energy is restored.

slip knot: a special quick-release knot used to tie restraints.

social anxiety disorder: a disorder in which a person has excessive anxiety about social situations; also called social phobia.

special diet: a diet for people who have certain illnesses or conditions; also called therapeutic or modified diet.

specific gravity: a test performed to measure the density of urine.

specimen: a sample, such as of tissue, blood, urine, stool, or sputum, used for analysis and diagnosis.

sperm: male sex cells.

sphincter: a ring-like muscle that opens and closes an opening in the body.

sphygmomanometer: a device that measures blood pressure.

spinal cord: the part of the nervous system inside the vertebral canal that conducts messages between the brain and the body and controls spinal reflexes.

spirituality: of or relating to the concerns of the spirit, the sacred, or the soul.

sputum: mucus coughed up from the lungs.

stable angina: chest pain that occurs when a person is active or under severe stress.

Standard Precautions: a method of infection control in which all blood, body fluids, non-intact skin (like abrasions, pimples, or open sores), and mucous membranes (lining of mouth, nose, eyes, rectum, or genitals) are treated as if they were infected with a disease.

stereotype: a biased generalization about a group that is usually based on opinions and distorted ideas.

sterilization: a measure used to decrease the spread of pathogens and disease by destroying all microorganisms, including pathogens.

stethoscope: an instrument used to hear sounds in the human body, such as the heartbeat or pulse, breathing sounds, or bowel sounds.

stimulant: a drug that increases or quickens actions of the body.

stoma: an artificial opening in the body.

straight catheter: a catheter that does not stay inside the person; it is removed immediately after urine is drained or sampled.

stress: a mentally or emotionally disruptive or upsetting condition that occurs due to changes in the environment.

stressor: internal or external factors or stimuli that cause stress.

subacute care: care given in a nursing home or a hospital; used for people who need a higher level of care and observation than some long-term care facilities can give.

subjective information: information collected from residents, their family members and friends; information may or may not be true but is what the person reported; also called symptoms.

substance abuse: the use of legal or illegal substances in a way that is harmful to oneself or others.

suffix: a word part added to the end of a root or a prefix to create a new meaning.

suffocation: death from a lack of air or oxygen.

sundowning: a condition in which a person gets restless and agitated in the late afternoon, evening, or night.

supination: turning upward.

supine: position with person lying flat on his or her back.

suppository: a medication given rectally to cause a bowel movement.

surgical asepsis: method that makes an area or an object completely free of microorganisms; also called sterile technique.

surgical bed: bed made so that a person can easily move onto it from a stretcher.

syncope: loss of consciousness; also called fainting.

synthetic: artificial or man-made.

syphilis: a sexually-transmitted disease caused by bacteria.

systemic infection: an infection that occurs when pathogens enter the bloodstream and move throughout the body; causes general symptoms, such as chills and fever.

systole: phase where the heart is at work, contracting and pushing blood out of the left ventricle.

systolic: first measurement of blood pressure; phase when the heart is at work, contracting and pushing blood out of the left ventricle.

tachycardia: a fast heartbeat, over 100 beats per minute.

tachypnea: rapid respirations.

tartar: hard deposits on the teeth that are filled with bacteria and may cause gum disease and loose teeth if they are not removed.

team leader: a nurse in charge of a group of residents for one shift of duty.

team nursing: method of care in which a nurse acts as a leader of a group of people giving care.

telemetry: application of a cardiac monitoring device that transmits information about the heart rhythm and heart rate to a central monitoring station for assessment.

tendons: tough fibrous bands that connect muscle to bone.

terminal: causing or approaching death.

thermometer: a device used for measuring the degree of heat or cold.

tissues: a group of cells that performs similar tasks.

total hip replacement (THR): a surgery that replaces the head of the femur (long bone of the leg) where it joins the hip.

total knee replacement (TKR): a surgery that replaces a damaged or painful knee with artificial parts.

total parenteral nutrition (TPN): the intravenous infusion of nutrients in a basic form that is absorbed directly by the cells, bypassing the digestive tract.

trachea: an air passage that goes from the throat (pharynx) to the bronchi; also called the windpipe.

tracheostomy: surgically-created opening through the neck into the trachea.

transfer: an order that moves a resident from one unit to another within the same facility.

transfer belt: a belt made of canvas or other heavy material used to assist residents who are weak, unsteady, or uncoordinated; also called a gait belt.

transmission: transfer of a disease.

trichomoniasis: a sexually-transmitted disease caused by protozoa (single-celled animals).

trigger: a situation that leads to agitation.

trustworthy: deserving the trust of others.

tuberculosis: a contagious lung disease caused by a bacterium that is transmitted through the air; causes coughing, difficulty breathing, fever, and fatigue.

tumor: a group of abnormally-growing cells.

ulcerative colitis: a chronic inflammatory disease of the large intestine.

unoccupied bed: a bed made while no resident is in the bed.

unresolved grief: grief that continues beyond what is considered a reasonable period of time; can affect the person's ability to function normally.

unstable angina (USA): chest pain that occurs while a person is at rest and not exerting himself.

ureterostomy: a type of urostomy in which a surgical creation of an opening from the ureter through the abdomen is made for urine to be eliminated.

urinary incontinence: the inability to control the bladder, which leads to an involuntary loss of urine.

urinary tract infection (UTI): a disorder that causes inflammation of the bladder; also called cystitis.

urostomy: the general term used for any surgical procedure that diverts the passage of urine by re-directing the ureters.

vaccine: a substance prepared from weakened or killed microbes that is used to give immunity to disease.

vaginal irrigation: a rinsing of the vagina in order to cleanse the vaginal tract or to introduce medication into the vagina; also called a douche.

validating: giving value to or approving.

validation therapy: a type of therapy that lets people with Alzheimer's disease believe they are living in the past or in imaginary circumstances.

vegans: vegetarians who do not eat any animal products, including milk, cheese, other dairy items, or eggs; vegans may also not use or wear any animal products, including wool, silk, and leather.

vegetarians: people who do not eat meat, fish, or poultry for religious, moral, or health reasons; they may or may not eat eggs and dairy products.

vein: vessel that carries blood to the heart.

ventricles: the lower two chambers of the heart.

verbal abuse: oral or written words, pictures, or gestures that threaten or embarrass a person.

verbal communication: communication involving the use of spoken or written words or sounds.

violent: word to describe actions that include attacking, hitting, or threatening someone.

vital signs: measurements that monitor the function of the vital organs of the body.

voiding: the process of emptying the bladder of urine; also called urination or micturition.

VRE (vancomycin-resistant *enterococcus*): a mutant strain of the bacterium *enterococcus*; it is a resistance caused by a person not taking all of a powerful antibiotic Vancomycin.

wandering: walking around a facility without any known goal or purpose.

wart: contagious rough, hard bump caused by a virus.

wellness: successfully balancing things that happen in everyday life; includes five different types: physical, social, emotional, intellectual, and spiritual.

withdrawal: the physical and mental symptoms caused by ceasing to use a particular addictive substance.

workplace violence: the abuse of staff by other staff members, residents, or visitors; includes both physical and verbal abuse.

Index